Cardiovascular Disorders: A Clinical Handbook

Cardiovascular Disorders: A Clinical Handbook

Edited by Adrian Nolan

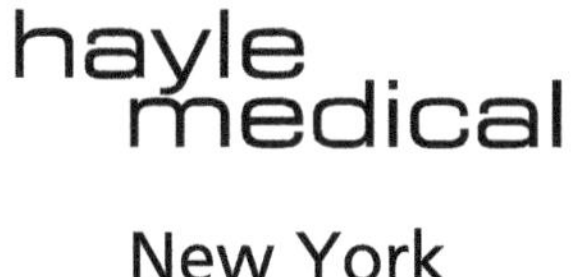

New York

Hayle Medical,
750 Third Avenue, 9th Floor,
New York, NY 10017, USA

Visit us on the World Wide Web at:
www.haylemedical.com

ISBN: 978-1-63241-555-4

Cataloging-in-Publication Data

Cardiovascular disorders : a clinical handbook / edited by Adrian Nolan.
p. cm.
Includes bibliographical references and index.
ISBN 978-1-63241-555-4
1. Cardiovascular system--Diseases. 2. Cardiovascular system--Diseases--Treatment.
3. Cardiology. I. Nolan, Adrian.
RC667 .C37 2019
616.1--dc23

Table of Contents

Preface

Cardiovascular disorders (CVDs) are diseases of the heart or the blood vessels, such as coronary artery diseases (CADs) which include myocardial infarction and angina. Conditions such as heart failure, stroke, cardiomyopathy, rheumatic heart disease, venous thrombosis, etc. are also cardiovascular diseases. The mechanism involved in the manifestation of each CVD is different for each disease. A variety of factors can contribute to the incidence of CVDs, such as poor diet, lack of exercise, lifestyle choices and excessive alcohol consumption, among others. Most of these conditions are preventable. However, cardiovascular diseases remain the dominant cause of death in the world today. This book discusses the fundamentals as well as modern approaches in the study of cardiovascular disorders. It aims to shed light on some of the unexplored aspects of CVDs and the recent researches in this domain. It is a complete source of knowledge on the present status of this important set of diseases.

This book unites the global concepts and researches in an organized manner for a comprehensive understanding of the subject. It is a ripe text for all researchers, students, scientists or anyone else who is interested in acquiring a better knowledge of this dynamic field.

I extend my sincere thanks to the contributors for such eloquent research chapters. Finally, I thank my family for being a source of support and help.

Editor

1

Predictors of high-cost hospitalization in the treatment of acute coronary syndrome in Asia: findings from EPICOR Asia

Stephen Jan[1*], Stephen W-L. Lee[2], Jitendra P. S. Sawhney[3], Tiong K. Ong[4], Chee Tang Chin[5], Hyo-Soo Kim[6], Rungroj Krittayaphong[7], Vo T. Nhan[8], Stuart J. Pocock[9], Ana M. Vega[10], Nobuya Hayashi[11] and Yong Huo[12]

Abstract

Background: The EPICOR Asia (long-tErm follow-uP of antithrombotic management patterns In acute CORonary syndrome patients in Asia) study (NCT01361386) was an observational study of patients hospitalized for acute coronary syndromes (ACS) enrolled in 218 hospitals in eight countries/regions in Asia. This study examined costs, length of stay and the predictors of high costs during an ACS hospitalization.

Methods and results: Data for patients hospitalized for an ACS ($n = 12,922$) were collected on demographics, medical history, event characteristics, socioeconomic and insurance status at discharge. Patients were followed up at 6 weeks' post-hospitalization for an ACS event to assess associated treatment costs from a health sector perspective. Primary outcome was the incurring of costs in the highest quintile by country and index event diagnosis, and identification of associated predictors. Cost data were available for 10,819 patients. Mean length of stay was 10.1 days. The highest-cost countries were China, Singapore, and South Korea. Significant predictors of high-cost care were age, male sex, income, country, prior disease history, hospitalization in 3 months before index event, no dependency before index event, having an invasive procedure, hospital type and length of stay.

Conclusions: Substantial variability exists in healthcare costs for hospitalized ACS patients across Asia. Of concern is the observation that the highest costs were reported in China, given the rapidly increasing numbers of procedures in recent years.

Keywords: Acute coronary syndrome, Asia, Health insurance, Costs, Hospitalization

Background

Ischemic heart disease is associated with a substantial healthcare burden worldwide, in terms of both deaths and disability-adjusted life years [1], while the costs of treating acute coronary syndromes (ACS) also represent a major burden for healthcare systems globally [2–6]. With the increasing prevalence of lifestyle-related chronic-disease risk factors, increasing healthcare costs, technological innovation, and growing consumer and patient expectations regarding access to twenty-first century healthcare, it is expected this burden will likely continue to increase [5]. This will have implications for the future financial sustainability of healthcare systems globally. These pressures are particularly pronounced in low- and middle-income countries in Asia where large-scale policies are underway or in planning; notably, in India and China to achieve universal coverage through the expansion of financial coverage for treatments to previously under-served populations. Such reforms, while critical in promoting social protection and equity of access to healthcare, come with significant resource requirements and will inevitably magnify future health sector financing challenges.

In addressing issues of cost and financial sustainability, understanding of the factors that drive variation in resource

* Correspondence: sjan@georgeinstitute.org
[1]The George Institute for Global Health, Sydney Medical School, University of Sydney, King George V Building, 83–117 Missenden Rd, Camperdown, NSW 2050, Australia
Full list of author information is available at the end of the article

use is important, particularly those factors that contribute to higher treatment costs. Notably, only very few studies have examined the factors associated with variation in treatment costs for ACS. Evidence from the US, comparing inpatient resource use for ACS in patients who died in hospital with that for a surviving ACS cohort, indicated that inpatient mortality for ACS is associated with a 47% greater duration of hospital stay along with an incremental cost of around US$43,000 [7]. Similarly, in a study conducted in Italy, which followed up patients for 12 months' post-hospitalization for ACS, patients who died of a cardiovascular event had an average cost of around €16,000 compared with an average cost of around €11,000 for the entire ACS cohort [8]. In China, a small study in a single hospital in Shandong found that increased age was associated with increased treatment costs and poorer clinical outcomes [9]. In a study in the US of over 12,000 patients with ACS, which compared those with and without diabetes, the presence of diabetes was reported to incur significant additional hospitalization costs of $32,577 versus no diabetes $29,150 [10]. Although evidence from such studies helps to clarify how resource use varies for patients with differing clinical presentations, the implications for policy are limited insofar as they reinforce the well-acknowledged relationship between more severe and complex illness and higher healthcare costs.

Investigation into the broader socioeconomic and regional health systems factors that influence costs is generally limited. Notably, however, a study in India using national administrative and household survey data reported that costs of hospitalization for cardiovascular disease were significantly higher in private health centers, in patients of high-fertility status, and in those of high socioeconomic status [11]. Studies of this kind, which examine broader healthcare systems and socioeconomic drivers of healthcare costs, provide potential policy lessons by addressing disparities in costs that reflect possible inefficiencies in healthcare systems, and are thus amenable to policy intervention.

In this study we assessed hospitalization costs associated with treating ACS patients across eight countries/regions in Asia: China, Hong Kong, India, Malaysia, Singapore, South Korea, Thailand, and Vietnam. The aim was to highlight variations in care costs across different healthcare settings and by different categories of ACS (ST-elevation myocardial infarction [STEMI], non-STEMI [NSTEMI] and unstable angina [UA]), and to determine the clinical, socioeconomic, and healthcare system factors that predict whether patients incur a level of treatment cost equivalent to the highest quintile by country and type of ACS.

Methods

The EPICOR Asia (long-tErm follow-uP of antithrombotic management patterns In acute CORonary syndrome patients in Asia) study (NCT01361386; registration, May 26, 2011), was a prospective, multinational, observational, cohort study of patients hospitalized for ACS enrolled in 218 hospitals in eight countries/regions in Asia [12]. These countries represent a combination of high- (Singapore, Hong Kong, Republic of Korea), upper-middle (China, India, Malaysia), and lower-middle (India, Vietnam) income settings. EPICOR Asia recruited consecutive patients hospitalized for ACS within 48 h of symptom onset and who were discharged with a final diagnosis of STEMI, NSTEMI, or UA, with 2-yearfollow-up. Data collection occurred between 2011 and 2014.

The study was conducted in compliance with the principles of the Declaration of Helsinki, International Conference on Harmonization Good Clinical Practice guidelines and applicable legislation on non-interventional studies in participating countries and regions. The protocol, including the informed consent form, was approved in writing by the applicable ethics committee of the participating centers in accordance with local regulations in each country. The ethics committee also approved any other non-interventional study documents in accordance with local regulations. A list of participating centers is provided in Additional file 1: Table S1. Patients provided written informed consent at discharge and completed a contact order form agreeing to be contacted for regular follow-up interviews post-discharge.

Data were collected from 12,922 patients on demographics, medical history, event characteristics, and socioeconomic and insurance status at discharge. Patients were followed up at 6 weeks following hospitalization for the index event in regard to treatment course. Costs associated with hospitalization were estimated from a health sector perspective based on health system payments for individual items at each specific hospital. Such payments reflect the outlay required of payers and are therefore of primary relevance from a policy standpoint. Costs were converted into US dollars at the prevailing exchange rates (see footnote to Table 2). These have not been converted into international dollars although prevailing purchasing power parities (PPPs) are presented to enable the reader to make such a conversion. In spite of potentially skewed distributions, mean costs were reported in accordance with economic theory which deems that the arithmetic mean (unlike the median) best informs resource allocation given a budgetary constraint [13–17].

The primary outcome was whether a patient incurred costs in the highest quintile for their specific country and index event diagnosis. This type of binary outcome, standardized against country and condition-specific norms, facilitated the pooling of data from multiple countries with differences in living standards and cost structures.

We assessed the association between the outcomes variable and several demographic, socioeconomic, health and clinical systems variables through univariate analyses. These variables included age, sex, smoking status, income (defined by country-specific quintiles based on country-specific income distributions, with quintile 1 representing the lowest income group, and quintile 5 the highest), country, place of residence (rural versus metropolitan), insurance status, cardiovascular disease history, hospitalization in the 3 months prior to the index event, dependence before the index event, index event medical management (invasive, non-invasive or unknown), type of hospital (regional/community/rural, non-university general hospital, university general hospital, other type of hospital/clinic), number of beds within the facility, and length of stay. A multivariable logistic regression model was constructed using stepwise selection, forcing in a variable of interest – health insurance status. A conditional binary regression model [18] to conduct a matched analysis was not used because the objective in this study was not to estimate a treatment effect.

Analyses were undertaken using SAS® v8.2 or later (SAS Institute, Cary, USA).

Results

Cost data were available for 10,819 participants; data from Malaysia ($n = 42$ patients) were excluded as costs were incorrectly recorded. Overall, 71% of participants were from China and 21% from India. Hong Kong, South Korea, Thailand, and Vietnam comprised between 1.2–2.3% of participants, with Singapore representing the fewest participants (0.6%).

Participant mean age was 60 years, 77% were males and 33% were current smokers compared with 20% former smokers, and 40% who had never smoked. Most participants were concentrated in the second (42%) and third (25%) income quintiles. Quintile 1 comprised less than 1% of participants, quintile 4 had 2% and quintile 5 had 24% (Table 1).

The majority (65%) of participants were resident in metropolitan areas compared with 35% in rural areas; 83% of participants had health insurance; 28% had some cardiovascular disease history; 7% had been hospitalized in the 3 months before the index event; 13% had some degree of dependence before the index event; and 83% underwent an invasive procedure during hospitalization. In terms of hospital type, 5% were admitted to a regional/community/rural hospital, 23% to a non-university general hospital, 56% to a university general hospital, and 17% to a 'other' type of hospital or clinic. The mean number of beds was 1312, and mean length of stay was 10.1 days, with little difference between STEMI (10.3 days), NSTEMI (10.2 days) and UA (9.8 days) (Table 1).

When compared in US dollars, the highest-cost countries were China (STEMI mean cost = $7790; NSTEMI = $7450; UA = $6585), Singapore ($6978; $4910; $3394), the Republic of Korea ($4300; $4621; $3552), and Thailand ($4427; $3321; $2008); across the three index-event types, UA generally represented the lowest-cost category except in India where it was the highest, albeit modestly (Fig. 1). In Hong Kong, all emergency admissions for ACS are subsidised by the Government and although the real cost incurred is not clear, health system payments to the patient are generally low. In terms of invasive interventional procedures, the highest costs were associated with (in descending order) coronary artery bypass graft, percutaneous coronary intervention (PCI) with one drug-eluting stent, PCI with one bare metal stent, and angiography; the costs for these procedures being highest in China, Hong Kong, Singapore, and Thailand (Table 2; also, conversion of these costs based on purchasing power parities (PPP) into international dollars is provided in Additional file 1: Table S2). Univariate analyses indicated that high-cost utilization was significantly associated with income, hospitalization in the 3 months prior to the index event, degree of dependence before the index event, index-event medical management, length of stay, sex, type of hospital and disease history (Table 3).

In controlling for all these variables at once, a multivariate analysis indicates the significant predictors of high-cost care were age (odds ratio [OR] = 1.10 per 10-year increment), being male (OR = 1.17), income (quintile 2 versus 5: OR = 0.76), prior disease history (OR = 1.25), hospitalization in the 3 months prior to index event (OR = 1.48), no dependency prior to index event (OR = 1.96), having an invasive procedure (OR = 5.48), hospital type (community versus university general: OR = 1.74), country (Hong Kong versus China: OR = 1.92; India versus China: OR = 2.54; Thailand versus China: OR = 1.52) and length of stay (OR = 1.06 per day) (Table 4).

Discussion

This study in more than 10,000 participants represents one of the largest prospective cost analyses of ACS and one of only few such analyses to provide cross-country comparisons. We found substantial variations across countries/regions and index diagnosis in healthcare costs incurred by patients during hospitalization for treatment of an ACS event. This is perhaps to be expected given the milieu of high, upper-middle and lower-middle income countries included in EPICOR Asia. What seems surprising is that the cost of treating ACS appeared relatively high in China across all three index-event types, exceeding those recorded for high-income countries/regions such as Singapore, the Republic of Korea, and Hong Kong. Interestingly, in contrast to Hong Kong and Singapore, costs in China were generally similar across all three index-event types. This suggests stratification of patients may not

Table 1 Baseline characteristics by final diagnosis of index event – all patients with cost data

	STEMI (*n* = 5478)	NSTEMI (*n* = 2030)	UA (*n* = 3311)	Total (*n* = 10,819)
Age, mean (SD)	58.5 (11.7)	61.9 (11.95)	61.4 (10.44)	60.0 (11.48)
Male, n (%)	4532 (82.7)	1520 (74.9)	2247 (67.9)	8299 (76.7)
Smoker, n (%)				
Current	2197 (40.1)	649 (32.0)	742 (22.4)	3588 (33.2)
Former	964 (17.6)	398 (19.6)	775 (23.4)	2137 (19.8)
Never	1896 (34.6)	855 (42.1)	1602 (48.4)	4353 (40.2)
Unknown	421 (7.7)	128 (6.3)	192 (5.8)	741 (6.8)
Income, n (%)				
Quintile 1	14 (0.3)	21 (1.0)	18 (0.5)	53 (0.5)
Quintile 2	2352 (42.9)	849 (41.8)	1342 (40.5)	4543 (42.0)
Quintile 3	1253 (22.9)	471 (23.2)	965 (29.1)	2689 (24.9)
Quintile 4	70 (1.3)	61 (3.0)	31 (0.9)	162 (1.5)
Quintile 5	1271 (23.2)	463 (22.8)	805 (24.3)	2539 (23.5)
Country, n (%)				
China	3716 (67.8)	1234 (60.8)	2754 (83.2)	7704 (71.2)
Hong Kong	75 (1.4)	45 (2.2)	5 (0.2)	125 (1.2)
India	1341 (24.5)	527 (26.0)	415 (12.5)	2283 (21.1)
Singapore	25 (0.5)	36 (1.8)	4 (0.1)	65 (0.6)
South Korea	101 (1.8)	70 (3.4)	76 (2.3)	247 (2.3)
Thailand	124 (2.3)	81 (4.0)	30 (0.9)	235 (2.2)
Vietnam	96 (1.8)	37 (1.8)	27 (0.8)	160 (1.5)
Place of residence, n (%)				
Rural	2088 (38.1)	624 (30.7)	1067 (32.2)	3779 (34.9)
Metropolitan	3390 (61.9)	1406 (69.3)	2244 (67.8)	7040 (65.1)
Insurance status, n (%)				
Yes	4396 (80.2)	1620 (79.8)	2950 (89.1)	8966 (82.9)
No	1082 (19.8)	410 (20.2)	361 (10.9)	1853 (17.1)
Disease history, n (%)	1008 (18.4)	630 (31.0)	1437 (43.4)	3075 (28.4)
Myocardial infarction	354 (6.5)	247 (12.2)	421 (12.7)	1022 (9.4)
Prior PCI	201 (3.7)	173 (8.5)	455 (13.7)	829 (7.7)
Prior CABG	43 (0.8)	39 (1.9)	70 (2.1)	152 (1.4)
CAG diagnostic for CAD	233 (4.3)	216 (10.6)	606 (18.3)	1055 (9.8)
Chronic angina	484 (8.8)	299 (14.7)	1018 (30.7)	1801 (16.6)
Heart failure	63 (1.2)	71 (3.5)	135 (4.1)	269 (2.5)
Atrial fibrillation	47 (0.9)	45 (2.2)	62 (1.9)	154 (1.4)
TIA/stroke	212 (3.9)	101 (5.0)	166 (5.0)	479 (4.4)
Peripheral vascular disease	24 (0.4)	24 (1.2)	41 (1.2)	89 (0.8)
Chronic renal failure	59 (1.1)	70 (3.4)	38 (1.1)	166 (1.5)
Hospitalization in 3 months prior to index event, n (%)	206 (3.8)	126 (6.2)	458 (13.8)	790 (7.3)
Dependence degree (need of help for daily activities) prior to index event, n (%)				
Some dependence	715 (13.1)	318 (15.7)	367 (11.1)	1400 (12.9)
No dependence	4601 (84.0)	1659 (81.7)	2826 (85.4)	9086 (84.0)
Unknown	162 (3.0)	53 (2.6)	118 (3.6)	333 (3.1)

Table 1 Baseline characteristics by final diagnosis of index event – all patients with cost data *(Continued)*

	STEMI (*n* = 5478)	NSTEMI (*n* = 2030)	UA (*n* = 3311)	Total (*n* = 10,819)
Index event medical management, n (%)				
Invasive	4713 (86.0)	1598 (78.7)	2612 (78.9)	8923 (82.5)
Non-invasive	724 (13.2)	422 (20.8)	617 (18.6)	1763 (16.3)
Unknown	41 (0.7)	10 (0.5)	82 (2.5)	133 (1.2)
Type of hospital, n (%)				
Regional/community/rural hospital	296 (5.4)	111 (5.5)	76 (2.3)	483 (4.5)
Non-university general hospital	1269 (23.2)	368 (18.1)	792 (23.9)	2429 (22.5)
University general hospital	2931 (53.5)	1074 (52.9)	2092 (63.2)	6097 (56.4)
Other type of hospital/clinic	982 (17.9)	477 (23.5)	351 (10.6)	1810 (16.7)
Number of beds, mean (95% CI)	1307.1 (1280.0, 1334.2)	1223.1 (1181.9, 1264.3)	1374.5 (1338.6, 1410.5)	1311.9 (1292.7, 1331.2)
Length of stay, mean (95% CI)	10.3 (10.2, 10.5)	10.2 (9.9, 10.6)	9.8 (9.6, 10.0)	10.1 (10.0, 10.3)

CABG Coronary artery bypass graft, *CAD* Coronary artery disease, *CAG* Coronary angiogram, *CI* Confidence interval, *NSTEMI* Non-ST-elevation myocardial infarction, *PCI* Percutaneous coronary intervention, *STEMI* ST-elevation myocardial infarction, *TIA* Transient ischemic attack, *UA* Unstable angina

have been optimal, with patients at high- and lower-risk variably receiving high-level interventional therapy, and of variable cost. This may be compounded by inaccurate recording as to whether percutaneous transluminal coronary angioplasty was provided with or without stenting. Further detailed study is required to establish the multifarious factors underlying the apparent high costs of treatment in China and alleviate any concerns to decision makers given the increasing burden of ACS and growing proliferation of treatment. For example, between 2007 and 2011, there was a virtual doubling in the number of PCI procedures performed from 180,000 to 330,000 [19].

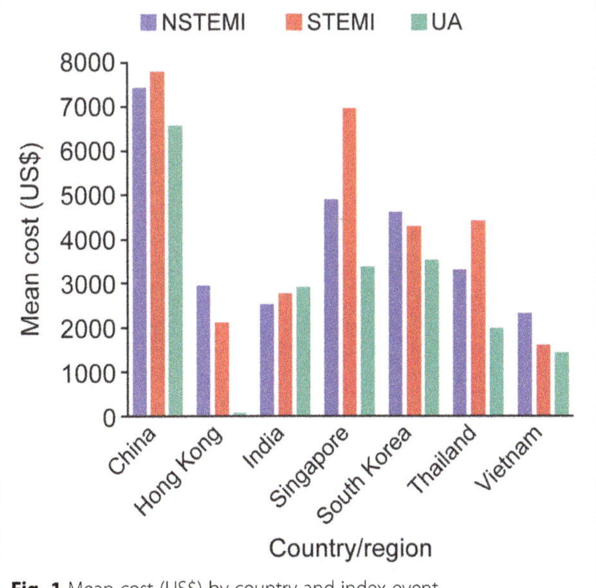

Fig. 1 Mean cost (US$) by country and index event. *NSTEMI* non-ST-elevation myocardial infarction, *STEMI* ST-elevation myocardial infarction, *UA* unstable angina

The finding that age is a positive predictor of high cost is consistent with potentially greater complexity and severity of illness, some of which may not have been captured and thus controlled for in the model. This is perhaps further evidenced by the positive association between hospitalization in the 3 months prior to the index event and high costs. Similar findings for male sex are consistent with a study in Italy where costs incurred by men were significantly greater than that for women, irrespective of index-event type [8]. Reports that women who present with ACS may be evaluated less intensively than men, may go some way towards explaining this [20].

The findings reported here also provide evidence of a potential income effect in that patients on relatively high income appear more likely to be categorized as highest cost. Odds ratios relative to income quintile 5 of 0.45 for quintile 1; 0.76 for quintile 2; 0.97 for quintile 3; 0.80 for quintile 4 (although only statistically significant in relation to quintile 2), ostensibly indicate a pattern in which the odds of incurring high costs increase with income. Such a finding, again, accords with expectations that wealthier patients will seek and have access to higher-cost treatments.

The findings that longer length of stay and having an invasive procedure (versus non-invasive medical management) were both positively associated with odds of incurring high costs is consistent with expectations and reflects, perhaps obviously, resource needs associated with longer treatment duration and need for an invasive procedure. Less intuitive is the finding that those patients who required no help with daily activities prior to hospitalization for their index condition ("no dependence") had significantly higher odds of being in the highest-cost category. Here, it is possible that patients with dependency at

Table 2 Mean (95% confidence interval [CI]) individual center-specific cost ($) per procedure by country[a]

	Country/Region							
	China ($n = 7704$)	Hong Kong ($n = 125$)	India ($n = 2283$)	Singapore ($n = 65$)	South Korea ($n = 247$)	Thailand ($n = 235$)	Vietnam ($n = 160$)	All ($n = 10{,}819$)
ECG	4.2 (3.9, 4.4)	43.7 (38.1, 49.3)	3.2 (2.8, 3.6)	35.0 (NA)	7.6 (5.5, 9.7)	8.8 (6.6, 11.0)	1.2 (0.7, 1.7)	5.9 (4.9, 6.8)
Cardiac markers	32.9 (30.2, 35.5)	51.5 (41.8, 61.1)	26.7 (23.0, 30.4)	84.0 (NA)	30.3 (22.6, 38.0)	15.5 (11.9, 19.0)	7.8 (0.9, 14.6)	35.8 (22.5, 49.1)
Echocardiography	53.9 (42.5, 65.3)	261.6 (226.9, 296.3)	25.2 (22.1, 28.3)	443.0 (NA)	184.9 (167.5, 202.3)	72.4 (65.7, 79.0)	9.3 (5.7, 12.9)	69.5 (59.3, 79.6)
Angiography	666.4 (613.1, 719.6)	1536.0 (816.9, 2255.1)	343.8 (203.6, 484.0)	4674.0 (NA)	667.0 (376.0, 958.0)	645.2 (539.3, 751.1)	284.2 (209.8, 358.6)	621.4 (549.6, 693.3)
PCI with 1 drug eluting stent	3072.8 (2820.6, 3325.1)	4359.2 (2615.1, 6103.3)	3696.7 (2251.7, 5141.8)	17,590.0 (NA)	1980.9 (1464.5, 2497.4)	4261.4 (3456.8, 5066.1)	3233.3 (2729.3, 2737.4)	3308.1 (2918.5, 3697.7)
PCI with 1 bare metal stent	2174.9 (1924.9, 2425.0)	1942.4 (617.2, 3715.6)	2192.2 (1858.5, 2525.9)	7995.0 (NA)	1752.4 (1291.4, 2213.4)	3247.6 (2609.0, 3886.1)	1900.0 (1542.6, 2257.4)	2251.1 (2067.0, 2435.3)
CABG	8864.1 (8173.1, 9555.1)	7561.0 (4368.2, 10,753.8)	3265.1 (2918.4, 3611.7)	29,520.0 (NA)	4458.6 (2879.3, 6038.0)	7240.7 (4485.7, 9995.7)	4160.0 (2980.1, 5339.9)	6906.7 (6284.3, 7529.0)
Stay in CCU per day	164.5 (119.7, 209.2)	1482.0 (1233.7, 1730.3)	90.7 (72.5, 108.8)	861.0 (NA)	123.2 (73.4, 173.0)	109.7 (59.3, 160.0)	35.3 (4.4, 72.3)	231.3 (102.1, 360.5)

CABG Coronary artery bypass graft, *CCU* Critical care unit, *ECG* Electrocardiogram, *NA* Not available, *PCI* Percutaneous coronary intervention
[a]Exchange rate conversion based on (March 2013): 1 USD = 6.2943 CNY; 7.7681 HKD; 53.060 INR; 3.1690 SGD; 1158.1 KRW; 31.545 THB; 21,030 VND

Table 3 Model-based point estimates for high-cost healthcare expenditure[a] using logistic models – univariate analysis (excluding Malaysia)

Factor	Odds ratio	95% CI	*P* value
Age, per 10-year increment	1.04	0.99, 1.08	0.0925
Sex, male versus female	1.18	1.06, 1.33	0.0038
Income (versus quintile 5)			< 0.0001
Quintile 1	0.45	0.19, 1.06	
Quintile 2	0.76	0.67, 0.85	
Quintile 3	0.97	0.85, 1.11	
Quintile 4	0.80	0.53, 1.20	
Health insurance, yes versus no	1.02	0.90, 1.16	0.7074
Residence, rural versus non-rural	1.02	0.92, 1.12	0.7516
Smoker (versus never)			0.2418
Current	0.92	0.83, 1.03	
Former	1.02	0.89, 1.15	
Disease history, yes versus no	1.15	1.04, 1.28	0.0068
Hospitalization in the 3 months prior to index event, yes versus no	1.37	1.16, 1.62	0.0002
Dependence degree before index event, none versus some	1.74	1.48, 2.05	< 0.0001
Index event medical management, invasive versus non-invasive	4.62	3.78, 5.64	< 0.0001
Type of hospital (versus UGH)			0.0030
Regional/community/rural hospital	0.92	0.72, 1.17	
Non-UGH	1.13	1.01, 1.27	
Other type of hospital/clinic	1.24	1.09, 1.40	
Number of beds	1.00	1.00, 1.00	0.5995
Length of stay	1.04	1.03, 1.05	< 0.0001
Country (versus China)			0.8569
Hong Kong	1.00	0.64, 1.56	
India	1.09	0.97, 1.23	
Singapore	0.91	0.48, 1.70	
South Korea	1.00	0.72, 1.36	
Thailand	1.00	0.72, 1.38	
Vietnam	0.96	0.65, 1.43	

UGH University general hospital, CI Confidence interval
[a]high cost defined as the top quintile within a country

baseline would have the ongoing support of a "carer" to rely on. The potential lack of such support for patients without dependency at baseline may have led to greater costs due to a greater need for in-hospital rehabilitation and extensive discharge planning.

Another ostensibly unexpected observation was that the odds of incurring high-cost treatment, relative to those encountered in patients admitted to a university general hospital, were higher for those patients admitted to all "other" categories of hospital, e.g. regional/community/rural hospitals, non-university general hospitals and other type of clinics. Here, it is possible that the multivariable analysis used in this study effectively controlled for factors implicated in higher costs seen in teaching (university) hospitals, such as size of facility, treatment mode, disease history and length of stay. Our findings suggest, therefore, that the independent effect of university status of a hospital was to lower costs, very likely associated with efficiency and an established degree of expertise in such centers.

The lack of significant association between insurance status and high-cost care may allay potential concerns about the inflationary effects of national programs to expand insurance coverage, e.g. due for instance to incentives created by a third-party payer for providers to overcharge/over-service (provider moral hazard) and patients to overuse (patient moral hazard) [21]. Although this study focuses only on ACS patients, the findings of

Table 4 Model-based point estimates for high-cost healthcare expenditure[a] using logistic models – multivariate analysis (excluding Malaysia)

Factor	Odds ratio	95% CI	*P* value
Age, per 10-year increment	1.10	1.05, 1.16	< 0.0001
Sex, male versus female	1.17	1.02, 1.33	0.0224
Income (versus quintile 5)			< 0.0001
Quintile 1	0.43	0.15, 1.19	
Quintile 2	0.76	0.67, 0.86	
Quintile 3	0.96	0.83, 1.11	
Quintile 4	0.74	0.45, 1.23	
Health insurance, yes versus no	1.11	0.89, 1.38	0.3686
Disease history, yes versus no	1.25	1.11, 1.41	0.0002
Hospitalization in the 3 months prior to index event, yes versus no	1.48	1.23, 1.77	< 0.0001
Dependence degree before index event, none versus some	1.96	1.60, 2.40	< 0.0001
Index event medical management, invasive versus non-invasive	5.48	4.34, 6.92	< 0.0001
Type of hospital (versus UGH)			0.0016
Regional/community/rural hospital	1.74	1.25, 2.41	
Non-UGH	1.13	0.99, 1.29	
Other type of hospital/clinic	0.97	0.79, 1.19	
Length of stay	1.06	1.04, 1.06	< 0.0001
Country (versus China)			< 0.0001
Hong Kong	1.92	1.04, 3.53	
India	2.54	1.98, 3.25	
Singapore	1.58	0.77, 3.24	
South Korea	1.21	0.76, 1.95	
Thailand	1.52	1.05, 2.20	
Vietnam	0.90	0.57, 1.42	

UGH University general hospital
[a]Defined as the top quintile within a country

this study found no evidence of an inflationary impact associated insurance coverage. Further country-specific research is needed to determine whether the roll out of social insurance programs will increase costs to any significant degree.

There were several limitations in the present study. First, inclusion only of patients alive and followed up at 6 weeks might suggest a possible survivor bias to the findings. As mentioned, earlier studies have reported in-hospital mortality to be associated with higher costs, suggesting our estimates of average costs may have been underestimated. In addition, the costs examined in this study reflect only health system cost whereas a broader societal perspective would have considered costs to households and the community associated with indirect loss of income and reduced productivity. Also, the costs included in this analysis were confined to hospitalization for the index condition and excluded costs of potential re-hospitalizations for ACS; in the US, such costs have been estimated at over 30% [22], suggesting there are significant costs associated with ACS outside of the scope of this analysis. Furthermore, the costs of sub-acute follow-up care were not included. These may vary across countries due to differences in treatment norms, funding models and other health system characteristics. Despite these potential limitations in capturing the high costs to health systems associated with ACS, the study highlights the major policy challenges associated with a high burden of illness in Asia. Some countries in this analysis were represented by a relatively small number of participants, thus precluding detailed country-specific analyses. Thus, the way in which the primary outcome for this study was specified (i.e. occurrence of cost in the highest quintile specific to each country and index condition) served as a standardized outcome that facilitated the pooling of data across all countries. An alternative approach would have been to adjust for differences in purchasing power by converting into international dollars; however, the problem with such a strategy is that costs reported in international dollars lack meaning for local policy makers since they do not reflect actual budgetary implications (nevertheless the conversions are provided in Additional file 1: Table S2 for reference). The inclusion of hospital length of stay as an explanatory variable and the likelihood of it being highly correlated with cost is a potential weakness in the modelling [23], as we may not be able to identify factors that affect the cost through the hospital length of stay. However, it is an important variable of interest and its inclusion is justified as it allows us to estimate the direct effect of other factors included in the model. Finally, without accounting for clustering in the analysis, variance and confidence intervals could be slightly underestimated. However, in international studies of this kind, it is conventional that such adjustments are not made.

Conclusion

The present analysis highlights the drivers of high-cost treatment for ACS in Asia. It represents an advance in this area by examining factors beyond the clinical drivers of costs. The study further identifies health-system factors including hospital type, and health insurance and socioeconomic status, providing evidence to policy makers of the financial implications of current and future reforms; notably programs in Asia to expand health insurance coverage to underserved populations. The value of prevention programs in avoiding hospitalizations for ACS is also considered to highlight population groups (e.g. men, high-income groups, and uninsured) in whom effective prevention may yield the greatest financial savings.

Abbreviations

ACS: Acute coronary syndromes; CABG: Coronary artery bypass graft; CAD: Coronary artery disease; CAG: Coronary angiogram; CCU: Critical care unit; CI: Confidence interval; ECG: Electrocardiogram; NA: Not available; NSTEMI: Non-ST-elevation myocardial infarction; OR: Odds ratio; PCI: Percutaneous coronary intervention; STEMI: ST-elevation myocardial infarction; TIA: Transient ischemic attack; UA: Unstable angina; UGH: University general hospital

Acknowledgements

The authors would like to thank the patients, their families and all investigators involved in this study. Medical writing and editorial support, including assisting authors with incorporation of comments, fact checking, referencing, figure preparation, formatting, proofreading, and submission was provided by Carl V Felton PhD, Prime Global (Knutsford, Cheshire, UK), supported by AstraZeneca according to Good Publication Practice guidelines (Link). The Sponsor was involved in the study design, collection, analysis and interpretation of data, as well as data checking of information provided in the manuscript. However, ultimate responsibility for opinions, conclusions, and data interpretation lies with the authors.

Funding

The EPICOR Asia study and editorial support were supported by AstraZeneca.

Authors' contributions

All authors, SJ, SW-LL, JPPS, TKO; CTC; H-SK, RK, VTN, SJP, AMV, NH, and YH made substantial contributions to the analysis and interpretation of the data, and to the preparation, review and final approval of this manuscript. SJ led the analysis of the data and was the major contributor in writing the manuscript: SW-LL, JPPS, TKO; CTC; H-SK, RK, VTN, SJP, AMV, and YH all provided critical review and intellectual comment; and NH undertook statistical analysis and provided critical review. All authors read and approved the final manuscript.

Competing interests

JPSS has been a consultant or advisory board member for AstraZeneca, Lupin, and Intas. TKO has acted as a consultant or advisory board member for Sanofi-Aventis, Abbott Vascular, Boston Scientific, Boehringer Ingelheim, Novartis, and AstraZeneca. CTC has received research support from Eli Lilly, honoraria from Medtronic, and has been a consultant or advisory board member for AstraZeneca. RK has been a consultant or advisory board member for AstraZeneca and Boehringer Ingelheim. VTN has received research grants from AstraZeneca, Servier, Sanofi, and Boston Scientific, and has been a consultant or advisory board member for AstraZeneca, Pfizer, Sanofi, Boehringer Ingelheim, Servier, MSD, Abbott, Bayer, Novartis, Merck Serono, Biosensor, Biotronic, Boston Scientific, Terumo, and Medtronic. SJP receives research funds from AstraZeneca. AMV and NH are employees of AstraZeneca. All other authors declare that they have no competing interests.

Author details

[1]The George Institute for Global Health, Sydney Medical School, University of Sydney, King George V Building, 83–117 Missenden Rd, Camperdown, NSW 2050, Australia. [2]Queen Mary Hospital, Hong Kong, SAR, China. [3]Sir Ganga Ram Hospital, New Delhi, India. [4]Sarawak General Hospital, Kuching, Malaysia. [5]National Heart Centre Singapore, Singapore, Singapore. [6]Seoul National University Hospital, Seoul, South Korea. [7]Siriraj Hospital, Bangkok, Thailand. [8]Cho Ray Hospital, Ho Chi Minh City, Vietnam. [9]London School of Hygiene and Tropical Medicine, London, UK. [10]Observational Research Centre, Global Medical Affairs, AstraZeneca, Madrid, Spain. [11]AstraZeneca, Osaka, Japan. [12]Peking University First Hospital, Beijing, China.

References

1. Vedanthan R, Seligman B, Fuster V. Global perspective on acute coronary syndrome: a burden on the young and poor. Circ Res. 2014;114:1959–75.
2. Roggeri DP, Roggeri A, Rossi E, Cinconze E, De Rosa M, Maggioni AP, et al. Direct healthcare costs and resource consumption after acute coronary syndrome: a real-life analysis of an Italian subpopulation. Eur J Prev Cardiol. 2014;21:1090–6.
3. Wieser S, Ruthemann I, De Boni S, Eichler K, Pletscher M, Radovanovic D, et al. Cost of acute coronary syndrome in Switzerland in 2008. Swiss Med Wkly. 2012;142:w13655.
4. Kim J, Lee E, Lee T, Sohn A. Economic burden of acute coronary syndrome in South Korea: a national survey. BMC Cardiovasc Disord. 2013;13:55.
5. Xi B, Liu F, Hao Y, Dong H, Mi J. The growing burden of cardiovascular diseases in China. Int J Cardiol. 2014;174:736–7.
6. Wang S, Petzold M, Cao J, Zhang Y, Wang W. Direct medical costs of hospitalizations for cardiovascular diseases in Shanghai, China: trends and projections. Medicine. 2015;94:e837.
7. Page RL II, Ghushchyan V, Van Den Bos J, Gray TJ, Hoetzer GL, Bhandary D, et al. The cost of inpatient death associated with acute coronary syndrome. Vasc Health Risk Manag. 2016;12:13–21.
8. Roggeri A, Gnavi R, Dalmasso M, Rusciani R, Giammaria M, Anselmino M, et al. Resource consumption and healthcare costs of acute coronary syndrome: a retrospective observational administrative database analysis. Crit Pathw Cardiol. 2013;12:204–9.

9. Fan GQ, Fu KL, Jin CW, Wang XZ, Han L, Wang H, et al. A medical costs study of older patients with acute myocardial infarction and metabolic syndrome in hospital. Clin Interv Aging. 2015;10:329–37.
10. Zhao Z, Zhu B, Anderson J, Fu H, LeNarz L. Resource utilization and healthcare costs for acute coronary syndrome patients with and without diabetes mellitus. J Med Econ. 2010;13:748–59.
11. Srivastava A, Mohanty SK. Age and sex pattern of cardiovascular mortality, hospitalisation and associated cost in India. PLoS One. 2013;8:e62134.
12. Huo Y, Lee SW, Sawhney JP, Kim HS, Krittayaphong R, Nhan VT, et al. Rationale, design, and baseline characteristics of the EPICOR Asia study (long-tErm follow-uP of antithrombotic management patterns in acute CORonary syndrome patients in Asia). Clin Cardiol. 2015;38:511–9.
13. Mani K, Lundkvist J, Holmberg L, Wanhainen A. Challenges in analysis and interpretation of cost data in vascular surgery. J Vasc Surg. 2010;51:148–54.
14. Thompson SG, Barber JA. How should cost data in pragmatic randomised trials be analysed? BMJ. 2000;320:1197–200.
15. Ramsey S, Willke R, Briggs A, Brown R, Buxton M, Chawla A, et al. Good research practices for cost-effectiveness analysis alongside clinical trials: the ISPOR RCT-CEA task force report. Value Health. 2005;8:521–33.
16. Hurley J. Chapter 2: An overview of normative economics of the health care sector. In: Culyer A, Newhouse J, editors. Handbook of health economics: volume 1A. 1st ed. Amsterdam: Elsevier Science BV; 2000.
17. Glick H, Doshi J, Sonnad S, Polsky D. Economic evaluation in clinical trials. Oxford: Oxford University Press; 2007.
18. Breslow NE, Day NE, Halvorsen KT, Prentice RL, Sabai C. Estimation of multiple relative risk functions in matched case-control studies. Am J Epidemiol. 1978;108:299–307.
19. Li H, Ge J. Cardiovascular diseases in China: current status and future perspectives. IJC Heart & Vasculature. 2015;6:25–31.
20. Elsaesser A, Hamm CW. Acute coronary syndrome: the risk of being female. Circulation. 2004;109:565–7.
21. Cutler DM, Zeckhauser RJ. The anatomy of health insurance. In: Handbook of health economics: volume 1A. First edn. Edited by Culyer AJ and Newhouse JP: Elsevier, Oxford; 2000: 563–643.
22. Berenson K, Ogbonnaya A, Casciano R, Makenbaeva D, Mozaffari E, Lamerato L, et al. Economic consequences of ACS-related rehospitalizations in the US. Curr Med Res Opin. 2010;26:329–36.
23. Polverejan E, Gardiner JC, Bradley CJ, Holmes-Rovner M, Rovner D. Estimating mean hospital cost as a function of length of stay and patient characteristics. Health Econ. 2003;12:935–47.

2

Safety and efficacy of ultrathin strut biodegradable polymer sirolimus-eluting stent versus durable polymer drug-eluting stents

Ping Zhu, Xin Zhou, Chenliang Zhang, Huakang Li, Zhihui Zhang* and Zhiyuan Song*

Abstract

Background: The Orsiro biodegradable polymer sirolimus-eluting stent (O-SES) is a new-generation biodegradable polymer drug-eluting stent with the thinnest strut thickness to date developed to improve the percutaneous treatment of patients with coronary artery disease. We perform a meta-analysis of randomized clinical trials (RCTs) comparing the efficacy and safety of an ultra-thin, Orsiro biodegradable polymer sirolimus-eluting stent (O-SES) compared with durable polymer drug-eluting stents (DP-DESs).

Methods: Medline, Embase, and CENTRAL databases were searched for randomized controlled trials comparing the safety and efficacy of O-SES versus DP-DES. Paired reviewers independently screened citations, assessed risk of bias of included studies, and extracted data. We used the Mantel-Haenszel method to calculate risk ratio (RR) by means of a random-effects model.

Results: Six RCTs with a total of 6949 patients were selected. All included trials were rated as low risk of bias. The O-SES significantly reduced the risk of myocardial infarction (RR 0.78, 95% confidence interval [CI] 0.62–0.98; $I^2 = 0\%$; 10 fewer per 1000 [from 1 fewer to 18 fewer]; high quality) compared with the DP-DES. There was no significant difference between O-SES and DP-DES in the prevention of stent thrombosis (RR: 0.75; 95% CI: 0.52–1.08), cardiac death (RR: 0.93; 95% CI: 0.63–1.36), target lesion revascularization (RR 1.10, 95% CI 0.86–1.42) and target vessel revascularization (RR 0.97, 95% CI 0.78–1.21).

Conclusion: Among patients undergoing percutaneous coronary intervention, O-SES resulted in significantly lower rates of myocardial infarction than DP-DES and had a trend toward reduction in stent thrombosis.

Keywords: Meta-analysis, Biodegradable polymer, Durable polymer, Percutaneous coronary intervention

Background

The implantation of a drug-eluting stent (DES) that prevent restenosis by the release of antiproliferative agents from polymers is considered the standard approach for percutaneous coronary intervention [1]. After DES implantation, however, the lifelong presence of a durable polymer (DP) might induce chronic inflammation, cell proliferation, delay arterial healing, long-term endothelial dysfunction, and occasionally cause cardiovascular events such as myocardial infarction (MI) and stent thrombosis (ST) [2, 3]. Raising awareness of this risk motivated the improvements of stents with biodegradable polymer (BP) allowing elimination of the polymer by degradation. Despite these iterations, the potential benefits for BP-DES remain largely unproven. BP-DES has shown superior profiles over bare-metal stents and first-generation DP-DES [4–6] but shares a similar efficacy and safety profile compared with second-generation DP-DES [7, 8].

The Orsiro biodegradable polymer sirolimus-eluting stent (O-SES; Biotronik, Bülach, Switzerland) is a novel DES consisting of an ultrathin strut cobalt chromium design with a bioresorbable, poly-Llactic acid polymer coating that releases sirolimus [9]. Furthermore, O-SES

* Correspondence: xyzpj@126.com; zysong2010@126.com
Department of Cardiology, Southwest Hospital, Third Military Medical University (Army Medical University), Chongqing, China

has the thinnest strut thickness to date (60 μm), and thus provides good flexibility and deliverability. Preclinical study has reported that thin struts reduced both intimal proliferation and thrombus formation [10]. Evidence in the bare-metal stent era suggested reduced arterial injury and angiographic restenosis with low stent strut thickness [11]. The reduced strut thickness of 40% has been reported to improve outcomes compared with early generation drug-eluting stents [12]. Thus, the use of thin struts might reduce the risk of potentially fatal complications, such as ST and MI [10].

Recently, the safety and efficacy of O-SES compared with contemporary DP-DES has been assessed in randomized controlled trials (RCTs) [13–18]. However, the results of these trials were controversial. Early, modest-sized studies in this field failed individually to prove that O-SES was super to DP-DES [13–15, 17, 18]. In late 2017, a new trial has endorsed the safety and effectiveness of O-SES compared with DP-everolimus-eluting stents (EES) [16]. Therefore, we conducted a meta-analysis to compare the efficacy and safety of O-SES to DP-DES.

Methods

The registered study protocol is available on PROSPERO (CRD42017081107). The findings of the meta-analysis was reported according to the Preferred Reporting Items for Systematic Reviews and Meta-Analyses (PRISMA) [19].

Eligibility criteria

Inclusion criteria

1) Population: adult participants (≥18 years) with percutaneous coronary intervention.
2) Intervention: percutaneous coronary intervention with O-SES.
3) Comparison intervention: percutaneous coronary intervention with DP-SES.
4) Outcome: Primary outcome was MI, as defined by the individual trials. Secondary outcomes were definite or probable ST, cardiac death, target vessel revascularization (TVR), and target lesion revascularization (TLR).
5) Study design: RCT.

Exclusion criteria

We excluded duplicate reports and post hoc analyses.

Search strategy

Medline, EMBASE, and the Cochrane Library at the CENTRAL Register of Controlled Trials were searched with the assistance of a professional librarian. The last electronic search was performed on October 20, 2017. We also reviewed the reference lists of the original trials, prior meta-analysis, and review articles. There were no restrictions on language. For the search strategy, we used, in various relevant combinations, MeSH terms and keywords pertinent to the intervention of interest: "biodegradable polymer", "Orsiro", "drug-eluting stent", "sirolimus", "durable polymer", "controlled trials" and "randomized controlled trial." (Table 3 in Appendix 1).

Study selection

Two investigators performed the study selection independently. They screened titles and abstracts for initial study inclusion. They screened the full text of potentially relevant trials. Disagreements were resolved by consensus with a senior author. Follow-up of all outcomes was at 12 months.

Data collection process

Two investigators independently extracted data from the included RCTs using a standardized electronic form. Disagreements between the two investigators were resolved by consensus with a third investigator. Authors of studies were contacted when suitable data were not available.

Assessment of risk of bias and quality of evidence

Two investigators assessed the risk of bias of the trials by using the risk of bias tool of The Cochrane Collaboration [20]. Disagreements were discussed with a third author. Trials with more than two high-risk components were considered as a moderate risk of bias, and trials with more than four high-risk components as having a high risk of bias.

We used the GRADE approach to rate the quality of evidence and generate absolute estimates of effect for the outcomes [21]. We used detailed GRADE guidance to assess the overall risk of bias, indirectness, inconsistency, imprecision and publication bias and summarized results in an evidence profile.

Outcomes

The safety outcomes of the analysis included MI, definite or probable ST, and cardiac death, and the efficacy outcomes included TVR and TLR. The primary outcome was MI, which was defined by the individual trials.

Data synthesis

Computations were performed with RevMan- v 5.3.3 (a freeware available from The Cochrane Collaboration). Analyses for all outcomes were done on an intention-to-treat basis. The meta-analysis was done using random effect models regardless of the level of heterogeneity. The risk ratios (RR) along with 95% confidence intervals (CI) was calculated for dichotomous data. We assessed heterogeneity with the Chi^2 test (threshold $p = 0.10$) and the I^2 tests, I^2 values lower than 25%, 25–50%, and higher than 75% represented low, moderate, and high heterogeneity, respectively [22]. A 2-tailed P value of < 0.05 was set for statistical significance.

We conducted trial sequential analysis (TSA) for primary outcome (MI) using TSA software (version 0.9.5.9; Copenhagen Trial Unit, Copenhagen, Denmark) [23]. We used the O'Brien-Fleming approach to compute the trial sequential monitoring boundaries. An optimal information size was set to a two-sided alpha of 0·05, beta 0·80, relative risk reduction of 20%.

If a pooled analysis included 10 or more studies, we planned to use a funnel plot to explore the possibility of published bias.

We performed a subgroup analysis according to the different types of DP-DES (Everolimus versus Zotarolimus).

We planned sensitivity analyses:1. by performing meta-analysis using both fixed-effect models; 2. using alternative imputation methods; 3 using odds ratios instead of risk ratios;

Results

Study selection and characteristics

The search strategy yielded 331 manuscript abstracts (Fig. 1). Excluding 316 non-pertinent titles or abstracts, 15 studies were assessed according to the selection criteria. Six trials [13–18] were included in the meta-analysis.

Study characteristics

The baseline characteristics of included trials have been summarized in Table 1 and Tables 4 and 5 in Appendices 2 and 3. All trials published from 2015 to 2017. A total of 3120 patients receiving DP-SES compared with 3829 patients treated with O-SES. The types of DP-DES included zotarolimus-eluting stents (ZES, 2 trials) and everolimus-eluting stents (EES, 4 trials). All trials reported outcomes at 12-months follow-up, whereas one [15] of them even reported outcomes at 24-months follow-up. To decrease heterogeneity, we included only outcomes at 12-months follow-up in the meta-analysis.

Risk of bias and quality of evidence

All six trials were at low risk of bias (Fig. 2). The greatest risk of bias came from blinding. The nature of the trial

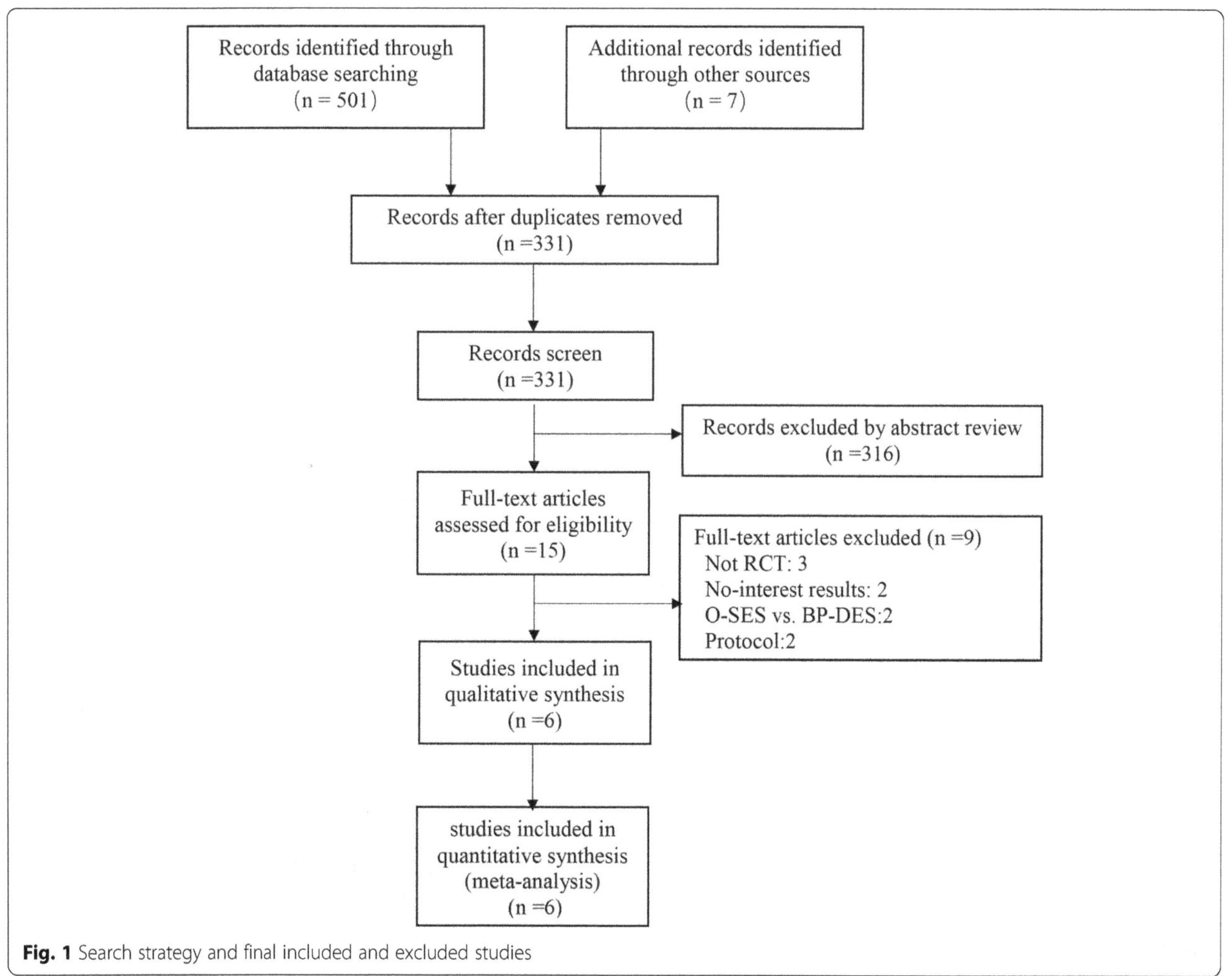

Fig. 1 Search strategy and final included and excluded studies

Table 1 Characteristics of patients in eligible studies

Trial	Year	No. of Patients		Follow-up (months)	DAPT (Months)	O-DES Characteristics			DP-DES Characteristics		
		O-SES	DP-DES			Stent	Thickness	Drug	Stent	Thickness	Drug
BIO-RESORT	2016	1169	1173	12	6	Orsiro	60	Sirolimus	Resolute Integrity	91	zotarolimus
BIOFLOW II	2015	298	154	12	> 6	Orsiro	60	Sirolimus	Xience Prime	81	Everolimus
BIOFLOW V	2017	884	450	12	> 6	Orsiro	60	Sirolimus	Xience Prime	81	Everolimus
BIOSCIENCE	2016	1063	1056	12	12	Orsiro	60	Sirolimus	Xience Prime	81	Everolimus
ORIENT	2017	250	122	12	> 12	Orsiro	60	Sirolimus	Resolute Integrity	91	zotarolimus
PRISON IV	2017	165	165	12	> 12	Orsiro	60	Sirolimus	Xience Prime	81	Everolimus

interventions precluded blinding of their physicians; whereas five of trials stated that blinding of outcome assessment was used and the other one was unclear. GRADE summary findings for all outcomes is showed in Table 2. We did not use funnel plots to assess the existence of possible publication bias because there were only six trials included in our meta-analysis.

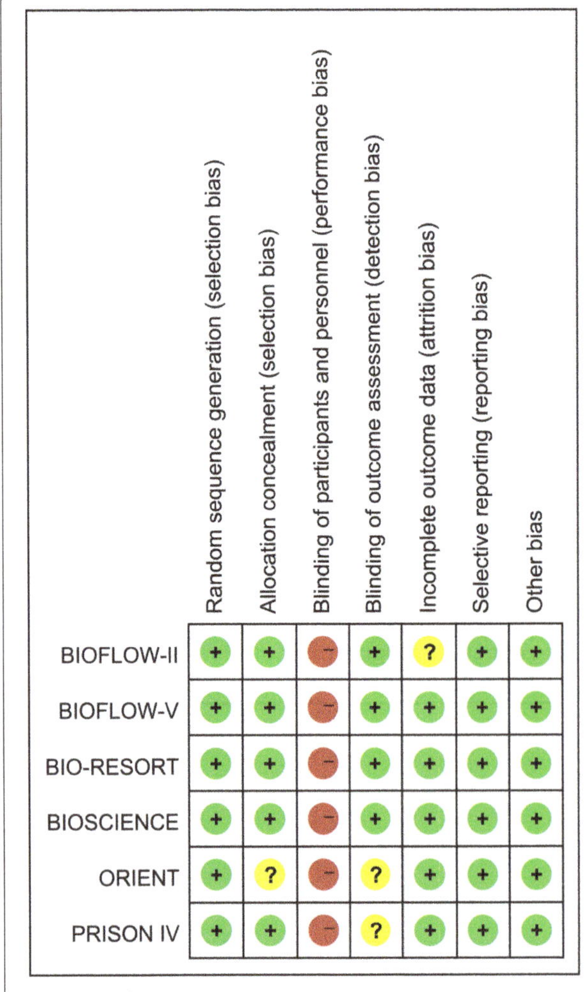

Fig. 2 Risk of bias summary

Safety endpoints: MI, ST, and cardiac mortality

The associations between O-SES versus DP-DES and safety outcomes are shown in Fig. 3. All six trials reported safety outcomes. MI occurred in 142 of 3777(3.8%) participants randomized to the O-SES group and 147 of 3095(4.8%) participants randomized to the medical therapy group. The risk ratio (RR) for MI also confer an advantage of O-SES over DP-DES (RR 0.78, 95% CI 0.62–0.98; I^2 = 0%; 10 fewer per 1000 [from 1 fewer to 18 fewer]; high quality). Sensitivity analyses using an alternative statistical method (Inverse Variance; RR 0.78, 95% CI 0.62–0.97; I^2 = 0%), effect measure (Odds Ratio 0.77, 95% CI 0.60–0.97; I^2 = 0%), and analysis model showed similar results of MI (Fixed; RR 0.78, 95% CI 0.62–0.98; I^2 = 0%). TSA confirmed that the required information size was not met (Fig. 5 in Appendix 4).

The meta-analysis showed no significant difference between O-SES and DP-SES on ST (RR: 0.75; 95% CI: 0.52–1.08; I^2 = 0%) or cardiac mortality (RR: 0.93; 95% CI: 0.63–1.36; I^2 = 0%).

Efficacy outcomes: TVR and TLR

All the included studies presented outcomes of TVR and TLR, showing that there was no statistically significant difference between O-SES and DP-DES regarding TVR (RR 0.97, 95% CI 0.78–1.21) and TLR (RR 1.10, 95% CI 0.86–1.42). (Fig. 4).

Subgroup analysis

We performed a subgroup analysis based on various DES types (everolimus and zotarolimus). Like the overall analysis, this subgroup analysis showed that O-SES has certain benefit in reducing risk of MI compared to DP-EES (RR 0.75, 95% CI 0.58–0.96; I^2 = 0%, Fig. 6 in Appendix 5) but this benefit did not show in cardiac mortality, ST, TVR, or TLR. There is no significant difference between O-SES and DP-ZES in the risks of MI, cardiac mortality, TVR, or TLR.

Table 2 GRADE evidence profile of outcomes, O-SES versus DP-DES

Outcome	No. of patients (Studies)		Study results (95% CI) and measurements	Absolute effect estimates (per 1000)			Quality	Importance
	O-SES	DP-DES		O-SES	DP-DES	Absolute Risk (95% CI)		
Myocardial infarction	142/3777 (3.8%)	147/3095 (4.7%)	RR 0.78 (0.62 to 0.98)	37	47	10 fewer (from 1 fewer to 18 fewer)	⊕⊕⊕⊕ High	Critical
Stent thrombosis	50/3767 (1.3%)	63/3095 (2%)	RR 0.75 (0.52 to 1.08)	15	20	5 fewer (from 10 fewer to 2 more)	⊕⊕⊕⊖ Moderate[a]	Important
Cardiac death	50/3777 (1.3%)	50/3095 (1.6%)	RR 0.93 (0.63 to 1.36)	15	16	1 fewer (from 6 fewer to 6 more)	⊕⊕⊕⊖ Moderate[a]	Important
Target vessel revascularization	166/3778 (4.4%)	141/3092 (4.6%)	RR 0.97 (0.78 to 1.21)	45	46	1 fewer (from 10 fewer to 10 more)	⊕⊕⊕⊕ High	Important
Target lesion revascularization	129/3777 (3.4%)	101/3094 (3.3%)	RR 1.1 (0.86 to 1.42)	36	33	3 more (from 5 fewer to 14 more)	⊕⊕⊕⊕ High	Important

CI Confidence interval, *RR* Risk ratio, *O-SES* Orsiro biodegradable polymer sirolimus-eluting stent, *DP-DES* Durable polymer drug-eluting stents;
High quality: Further research is very unlikely to change our confidence in the estimate of effect. Moderate quality: Further research is likely to have an important impact on our confidence in the estimate of effect and may change the estimate. Low quality: Further research is very likely to have an important impact on our confidence in the estimate of effect and is likely to change the estimate. Very low quality: We are very uncertain about the estimate
[a]Serious imprecision

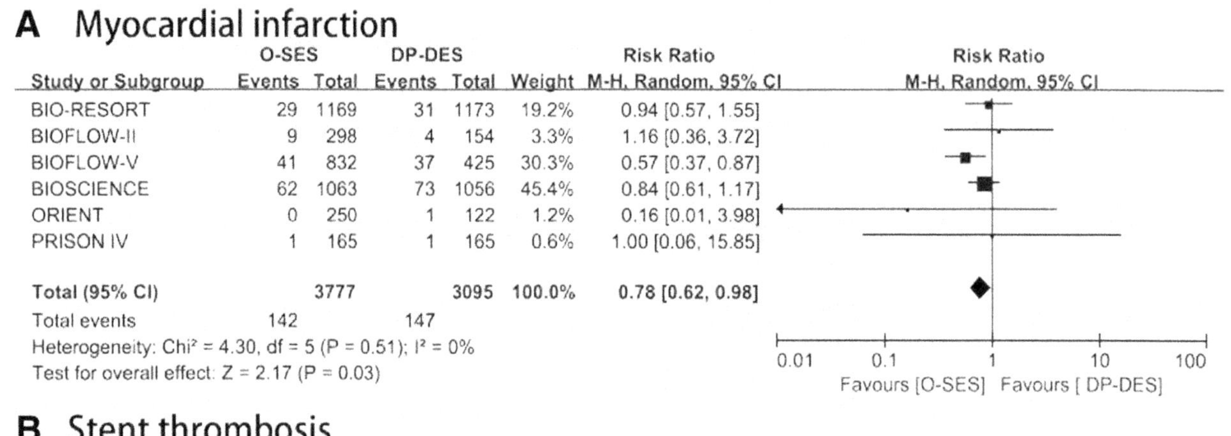

A Myocardial infarction
O-SES DP-DES Risk Ratio Risk Ratio
Study or Subgroup Events Total Events Total Weight M-H, Random, 95% CI M-H, Random, 95% CI
BIO-RESORT 29 1169 31 1173 19.2% 0.94 [0.57, 1.55]
BIOFLOW-II 9 298 4 154 3.3% 1.16 [0.36, 3.72]
BIOFLOW-V 41 832 37 425 30.3% 0.57 [0.37, 0.87]
BIOSCIENCE 62 1063 73 1056 45.4% 0.84 [0.61, 1.17]
ORIENT 0 250 1 122 1.2% 0.16 [0.01, 3.98]
PRISON IV 1 165 1 165 0.6% 1.00 [0.06, 15.85]
Total (95% CI) 3777 3095 100.0% 0.78 [0.62, 0.98]
Total events 142 147
Heterogeneity: Chi² = 4.30, df = 5 (P = 0.51); I² = 0%
Test for overall effect: Z = 2.17 (P = 0.03)
0.01 0.1 1 10 100
Favours [O-SES] Favours [DP-DES]

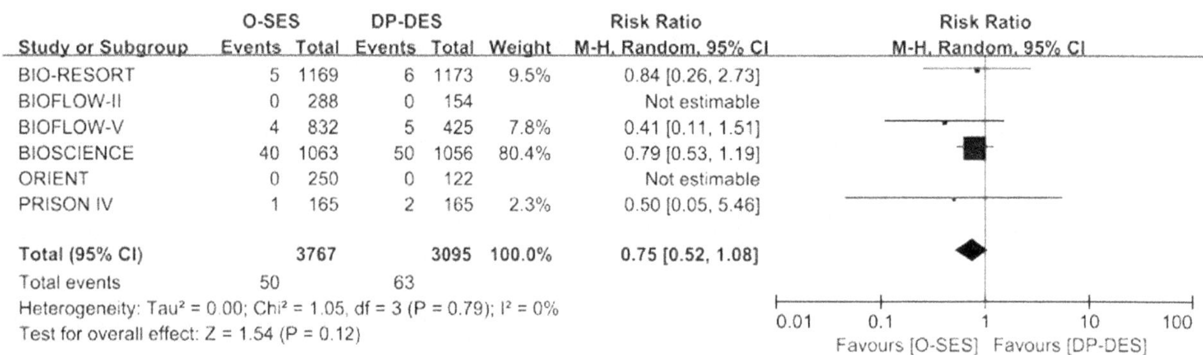

B Stent thrombosis
O-SES DP-DES Risk Ratio Risk Ratio
Study or Subgroup Events Total Events Total Weight M-H, Random, 95% CI M-H, Random, 95% CI
BIO-RESORT 5 1169 6 1173 9.5% 0.84 [0.26, 2.73]
BIOFLOW-II 0 288 0 154 Not estimable
BIOFLOW-V 4 832 5 425 7.8% 0.41 [0.11, 1.51]
BIOSCIENCE 40 1063 50 1056 80.4% 0.79 [0.53, 1.19]
ORIENT 0 250 0 122 Not estimable
PRISON IV 1 165 2 165 2.3% 0.50 [0.05, 5.46]
Total (95% CI) 3767 3095 100.0% 0.75 [0.52, 1.08]
Total events 50 63
Heterogeneity: Tau² = 0.00; Chi² = 1.05, df = 3 (P = 0.79); I² = 0%
Test for overall effect: Z = 1.54 (P = 0.12)
0.01 0.1 1 10 100
Favours [O-SES] Favours [DP-DES]

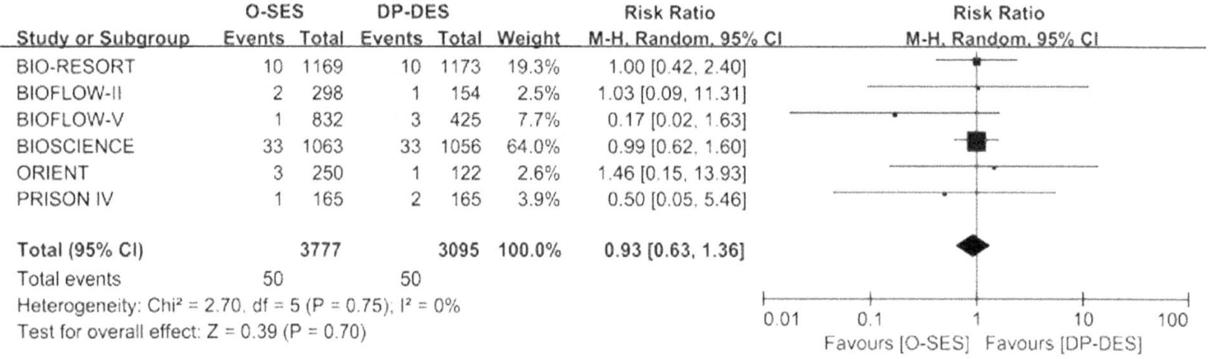

C Cardiac death
O-SES DP-DES Risk Ratio Risk Ratio
Study or Subgroup Events Total Events Total Weight M-H, Random, 95% CI M-H, Random, 95% CI
BIO-RESORT 10 1169 10 1173 19.3% 1.00 [0.42, 2.40]
BIOFLOW-II 2 298 1 154 2.5% 1.03 [0.09, 11.31]
BIOFLOW-V 1 832 3 425 7.7% 0.17 [0.02, 1.63]
BIOSCIENCE 33 1063 33 1056 64.0% 0.99 [0.62, 1.60]
ORIENT 3 250 1 122 2.6% 1.46 [0.15, 13.93]
PRISON IV 1 165 2 165 3.9% 0.50 [0.05, 5.46]
Total (95% CI) 3777 3095 100.0% 0.93 [0.63, 1.36]
Total events 50 50
Heterogeneity: Chi² = 2.70, df = 5 (P = 0.75); I² = 0%
Test for overall effect: Z = 0.39 (P = 0.70)
0.01 0.1 1 10 100
Favours [O-SES] Favours [DP-DES]

Fig. 3 Forest plot assessing safety outcomes. A: myocardial infarction, B: definite or probable stent thrombosis, C: cardiac death. CI = confidence interval; M-H = Mantel-Haenszel; SE = standard error

Discussion

In this meta-analysis of 6 RCTs, we found that MI was significantly lower in patients with O-SES than in patients with DP-DES. There was no evidence of a difference between groups concerning cardiac mortality, ST, TLR, and TVR.

Possibly our most important finding was the significant risk reduction for MI in patients with O-SES compared with DP-DES. Contrary to our meta-analysis, however, recent meta-analyses showed that BP-DES were similar regarding cardiovascular outcomes including MI compared to second-generation DP-DES [8, 24]. Similarly, a meta-analysis comparing BP-SES with DP-DES found there was no significant difference in the risk of MI [25]. The different results regarding MI between our meta-analysis and previous meta-analyses may be explained by the different eligibility criteria. Our meta-analysis included trials comparing O-SES with DP-DES rather than BP-DES (or BP-SES) with DP-DES. O-SES has the thinnest strut thickness to date. It is probable that the thinner stent struts of the O-SES (60 μm) compared with DP-DES (81–91 μm) lead to the lower risk of MI. The effect of stent strut thickness has been well established. In fact, compared to the thicker struts, thinner struts have been

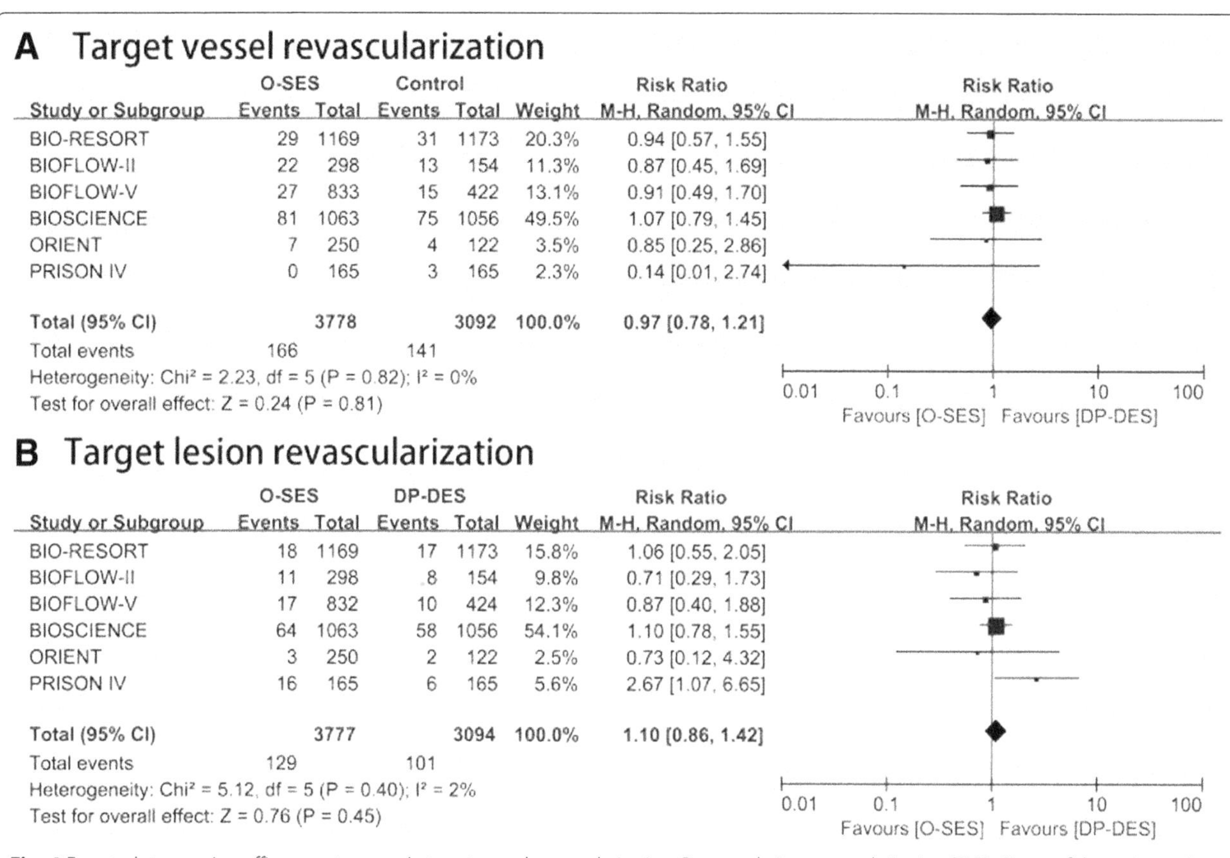

A Target vessel revascularization
O-SES Control
Risk Ratio
Risk Ratio
Study or Subgroup Events Total Events Total Weight M-H, Random, 95% CI
M-H, Random, 95% CI
BIO-RESORT 29 1169 31 1173 20.3% 0.94 [0.57, 1.55]
BIOFLOW-II 22 298 13 154 11.3% 0.87 [0.45, 1.69]
BIOFLOW-V 27 833 15 422 13.1% 0.91 [0.49, 1.70]
BIOSCIENCE 81 1063 75 1056 49.5% 1.07 [0.79, 1.45]
ORIENT 7 250 4 122 3.5% 0.85 [0.25, 2.86]
PRISON IV 0 165 3 165 2.3% 0.14 [0.01, 2.74]
Total (95% CI) 3778 3092 100.0% 0.97 [0.78, 1.21]
Total events 166 141
Heterogeneity: Chi² = 2.23, df = 5 (P = 0.82); I² = 0%
Test for overall effect: Z = 0.24 (P = 0.81)
0.01 0.1 1 10 100
Favours [O-SES] Favours [DP-DES]
B Target lesion revascularization
O-SES DP-DES
Risk Ratio
Risk Ratio
Study or Subgroup Events Total Events Total Weight M-H, Random, 95% CI
M-H, Random, 95% CI
BIO-RESORT 18 1169 17 1173 15.8% 1.06 [0.55, 2.05]
BIOFLOW-II 11 298 8 154 9.8% 0.71 [0.29, 1.73]
BIOFLOW-V 17 832 10 424 12.3% 0.87 [0.40, 1.88]
BIOSCIENCE 64 1063 58 1056 54.1% 1.10 [0.78, 1.55]
ORIENT 3 250 2 122 2.5% 0.73 [0.12, 4.32]
PRISON IV 16 165 6 165 5.6% 2.67 [1.07, 6.65]
Total (95% CI) 3777 3094 100.0% 1.10 [0.86, 1.42]
Total events 129 101
Heterogeneity: Chi² = 5.12, df = 5 (P = 0.40); I² = 2%
Test for overall effect: Z = 0.76 (P = 0.45)
0.01 0.1 1 10 100
Favours [O-SES] Favours [DP-DES]

Fig. 4 Forest plot assessing efficacy outcomes. A: target vessel revascularization, B: target lesion revascularization (TLR). CI = confidence interval; M-H = Mantel-Haenszel; SE = standard error

shown to reduce vessel injury, inflammation, neointimal proliferation, and thrombus formation [10, 11, 26, 27]. Reduction in strut thickness from stainless steel (132–140 μm) to chromium alloys (81–91 μm) contributed to a decreased risk of MI by about 40–80% [28–31].

Our meta-analysis has reported results suggestive of a protective effect of O-SES on ST compared with DP-DSE but failed to show the statistical significance of this association. One explanation for this fail was the small number of events during the follow-up. New generation DES have the most favourable safety and efficacy outcomes to date, adverse events have become less frequent in the past decade. Thus, to find a significant difference in management strategy, additional RCTs needs to follow patients for a long duration or enrol substantial numbers.

Our study did not show a significant decrease of TVR or TLR in O-SES compared with DP-DES. Indeed, two prior network meta-analyses have demonstrated a reduced risk of TVR and TLR of BP-DES compared to DP-DES [4, 32]. But, BP-SES were not included in the two network meta-analyses. A meta-analysis comparing BP-SES with DP-DES found similar efficacy profiles between those groups [25].

Strengths and limitations

Strengths of our meta-analysis included duplicate assessment of risk of bias, eligibility, and data abstraction. The meta-analysis included a rigorous assessment of the quality of evidence. We have evaluated relative and absolute risks, which are crucial for making decisions between O-SES and DP-DES.

First, different DP-DES platforms were used for comparison in the RCTs included in our meta-analysis. However, authors attempted to overcome these differences by performing a subgroup analysis based on DP-DES. We found O-SES significantly decreased MI compared to DP-EES but not to DP-ZES.

Second, a small number (6 RCTs, 6949 patients) and short follow-up duration (12 months) of included trials might afford insufficient ability to detect differences in rare events. For example, our results might suggest a reduced ST in O-SES but failed to show the statistical significance of this association. Thus, longer duration of follow-up and larger populations are required for further research.

Third, the limited number of included RCTs lead to insufficiently detect the presence of publication bias. However, publication bias is unlikely as most included RCTs had negative results.

Fourth, previous meta-analysis suggested a possible increased midterm risk for ST and MI with BP-DES [33]. However, we did not report mid- and long-term outcomes in this topic, because follow-up data of longer than 1 year is limited. Thus, the mid- and long-term safety and efficacy of O-SES vs. DP-DES is not clealy established.

Fifth, although the statistical heterogeneity was very low in most outcomes ($I^2 = 0$), there may be substantially clinical heterogeneity, which was driven by differences in methodological and clinical features between trials. For example, the duration and the type of dual antiplatelet therapy may have an influence on outcomes; however, we cannot perform a subgroup analyses on dual antiplatelet therapy because of lack of data from included trials. Sixth, TSA found that the required information size was not met. Thus, this review mirrors the lack of quantity of the included trials. The results of ongoing and future well designed, large randomized clinical trials are needed.

Conclusions

Compared with DP-DES, O-SES showed a significantly reduced risk of MI and a trend toward reduction in ST.

Appendix 1

Table 3 Search strategy on PubMed

#1	"Percutaneous Coronary Intervention"[Mesh]
#2	"Coronary Disease"[Mesh]
#3	"PCI"
#4	"CAD"
#5	(#1) OR (#2) OR (#3) OR (#4)
#6	"biodegradable"[tiab]
#7	"degradable"[tiab]
#8	"bioabsorbable"[tiab]
#9	"absorbable"[tiab]
#10	"absorptive"[tiab]
#11	" orsiro"[tiab]
#12	"O-SES"[tiab]
#13	"dissolvable"[tiab]
#14	(#6) OR (#7) OR (#8) OR (#9) OR (#10) OR (#11) OR (#12) OR (#13)
#15	"Polymers"[Mesh] OR "Polymer"[tiab] OR "coating"[tiab]
#16	(#14) AND (#15)
#17	"BioMatrix" OR "NOBORI" OR "Axxess" OR "Supralimus" OR "Infinnium" OR "BioMime" OR "Orsiro" OR "DESyne" OR "SYNERGY" OR "MiStent" OR "Excel" OR "Firehawk" OR "NOYA" OR "Inspiron" OR "Tivoli" OR "BuMA" OR "Svelte" OR "Custom" OR "NEVO" OR "Elixir" OR "JACTAX" OR "CORACTO"
#18	(#16)) OR (#17)
#19	"randomized controlled trial"[pt] OR "controlled clinical trial"[pt] OR "randomized"[tiab] OR "randomly"[tiab] OR "trial"[tiab] OR " clinical trials as topic"[sh]
#20	# (5) AND # (18) AND # (19)

Appendix 2

Table 4 Characteristics of patients in eligible studies

	Age	Male sex (%)	Hypertension (%)	Diabetes mellitus (%)	Smoker (%)	Previous MI (%)	ACS (%)	Stable angina (%)
BIO-RESORT	64 ± 11	72	46	18	30	19	70	30
BIOFLOW II	63 ± 10	77	78	28	27	27	NR	NR
BIOFLOW V	65 ± 10	74	80	35	23	27	51	48
BIOSCIENCE	66 ± 12	77	68	23	29	20	53	31
ORIENT	65 ± 11	72	65	26	27	NR	45	55
PRISON IV	63 ± 10	78	56	20	33	30	17	70

Appendix 3

Table 5 Primary and second outcomes of the Included Trials

	Primary outcome	Second outcomes
BIO-RESORT	target vessel failure at 12 months	target lesion failure, death, myocardial infarction, coronary revascularization, major adverse cardiac events, patient-oriented composite endpoint, definite or probable stent thrombosis
BIOFLOW II	in-stent late lumen loss at 9 months	in-segment late lumen loss and in-stent and in-segment minimal luminal diameter, percent diameter stenosis, and binary restenosis. Cardiac death, procedure-related deaths, myocardial infarction, target-lesion revascularization.
BIOFLOW V	target lesion failure at 12 months	major adverse cardiac events (all-cause death, myocardial infarction or ischemia-driven target lesion revascularization), target vessel failure, the individual components of the composite endpoints at 30 days and 12 months, and definite or probable stent thrombosis according to academic research consortium (arc) criteria.
BIOSCIENCE	target-lesion failure at 12 months	all-cause death, cardiac death, myocardial infarction, target vessel mi, coronary revascularization, major adverse cardiac events, patient-oriented composite endpoint, stent thrombosis, target lesion revascularization, target vessel revascularization, repeat revascularization, target vessel failure, cerebrovascular event
ORIENT	in-stent late lumen loss at 9 months,	in-segment late lumen loss, percentage diameter stenosis, and binary restenosis at 9 months; all-cause death, cardiac death, myocardial infarction, repeat revascularization, ischemic stroke, hemorrhagic stroke, bleeding, stent thrombosis, target lesion failure, target vessel failure
PRISON IV	in-segment late lumen loss at 9 months	in-stent late lumen loss, in-stent and in-segment percentage of diameter stenosis, binary restenosis, and re-occlusions at 9 months; clinically indicated target lesion, revascularization or target vessel revascularization, myocardial infarction, death (cardiac and noncardiac), stent thrombosis, target vessel failure, and major adverse cardiac events.

Appendix 4

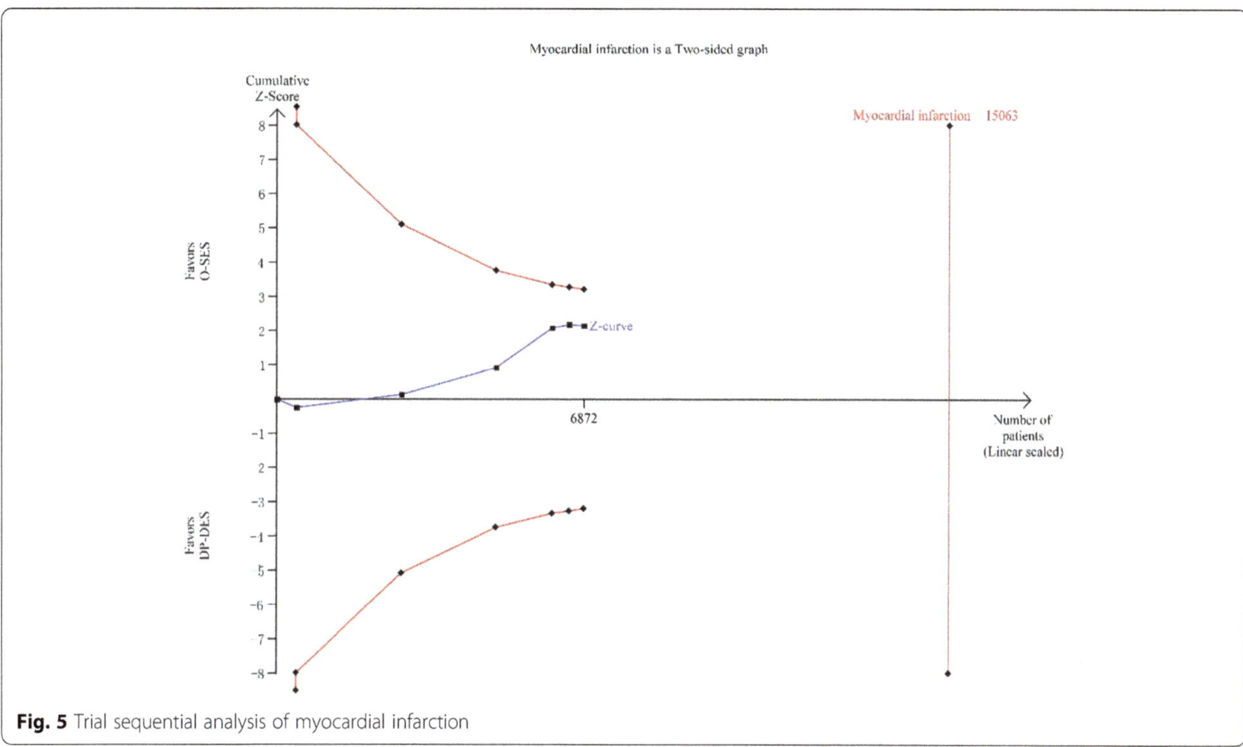

Fig. 5 Trial sequential analysis of myocardial infarction

Appendix 5

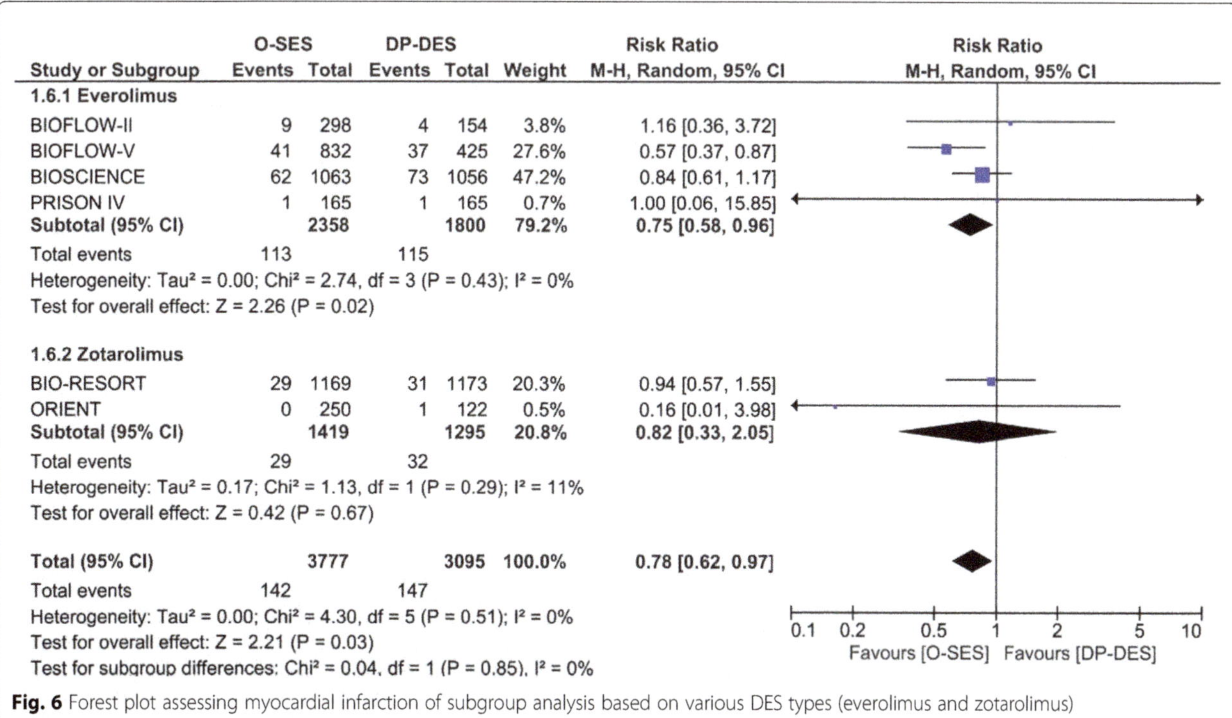

Fig. 6 Forest plot assessing myocardial infarction of subgroup analysis based on various DES types (everolimus and zotarolimus)

Abbreviations

BP: Biodegradable polymer; CI: Confidence intervals; DES: Drug-eluting stent; DP: Durable polymer; EES: Everolimus-eluting stents; MI: Myocardial infarction; O-SES: Orsiro biodegradable polymer sirolimus-eluting stent; RCTs: Randomized controlled trials; RR: Risk ratios; ST: Stent thrombosis; TLR: Target lesion revascularization; TVR: Target vessel revascularization; ZES: Zotarolimus-eluting stents

Funding

This work is supported by Southwest Hospital Project: SWH2016JSTSZD-09.

Authors' contributions

PZ and ZS had the idea for the review, and PZ and XZ managed the literature search and data extraction. PZ, XZ, CZ, HL, ZZ and ZS developed the analysis plan. PZ and XZ conducted the analysis and developed the figures. HL, PZ, and ZS wrote the original draft of the manuscript. PZ, XZ, and ZS determined the study approach, interpreted the results, and critically reviewed the manuscript. All authors read and approved the final manuscript.

Competing interests

The authors declare that they have no competing interests.

References

1. Byrne RA, Stone GW, Ormiston J, Kastrati A. Coronary balloon angioplasty, stents, and scaffolds. Lancet. 2017;390(10096):781–92.
2. Joner M, Finn AV, Farb A, Mont EK, Kolodgie FD, Ladich E, Kutys R, Skorija K, Gold HK, Virmani R. Pathology of drug-eluting stents in humans: delayed healing and late thrombotic risk. J Am Coll Cardiol. 2006;48(1):193–202.
3. Finn AV, Nakazawa G, Joner M, Kolodgie FD, Mont EK, Gold HK, Virmani R. Vascular responses to drug eluting stents: importance of delayed healing. Arterioscler Thromb Vasc Biol. 2007;27(7):1500–10.
4. Navarese EP, Tandjung K, Claessen B, Andreotti F, Kowalewski M, Kandzari DE, Kereiakes DJ, Waksman R, Mauri L, Meredith IT, et al. Safety and efficacy outcomes of first and second generation durable polymer drug eluting stents and biodegradable polymer biolimus eluting stents in clinical practice: comprehensive network meta-analysis. BMJ. 2013;347:f6530.
5. Kang SH, Park KW, Kang DY, Lim WH, Park KT, Han JK, Kang HJ, Koo BK, Oh BH, Park YB, et al. Biodegradable-polymer drug-eluting stents vs. bare metal stents vs. durable-polymer drug-eluting stents: a systematic review and Bayesian approach network meta-analysis. Eur Heart J. 2014;35(17):1147–58.
6. Palmerini T, Benedetto U, Biondi-Zoccai G, Della Riva D, Bacchi-Reggiani L, Smits PC, Vlachojannis GJ, Jensen LO, Christiansen EH, Berencsi K, et al. Long-term safety of drug-eluting and bare-metal stents: evidence from a comprehensive network meta-analysis. J Am Coll Cardiol. 2015;65(23): 2496–507.
7. Stefanini GG, Holmes DR Jr. Drug-eluting coronary-artery stents. N Engl J Med. 2013;368(3):254–65.
8. El-Hayek G, Bangalore S, Casso Dominguez A, Devireddy C, Jaber W, Kumar G, Mavromatis K, Tamis-Holland J, Samady H. Meta-analysis of randomized clinical trials comparing biodegradable polymer drug-eluting stent to second-generation durable polymer drug-eluting stents. JACC Cardiovasc Interv. 2017;10(5):462–73.
9. Stefanini GG, Taniwaki M, Windecker S. Coronary stents: novel developments. Heart. 2014;100(13):1051–61.
10. Kolandaivelu K, Swaminathan R, Gibson WJ, Kolachalama VB, Nguyen-Ehrenreich KL, Giddings VL, Coleman L, Wong GK, Edelman ER. Stent thrombogenicity early in high-risk interventional settings is driven by stent design and deployment and protected by polymer-drug coatings. Circulation. 2011;123(13):1400–9.
11. Kastrati A, Mehilli J, Dirschinger J, Dotzer F, Schuhlen H, Neumann FJ, Fleckenstein M, Pfafferott C, Seyfarth M, Schomig A. Intracoronary stenting and angiographic results: strut thickness effect on restenosis outcome (ISAR-STEREO) trial. Circulation. 2001;103(23):2816–21.
12. Windecker S, Stortecky S, Stefanini GG, da Costa BR, Rutjes AW, Di Nisio M, Silletta MG, Maione A, Alfonso F, Clemmensen PM, et al. Revascularisation versus medical treatment in patients with stable coronary artery disease: network meta-analysis. BMJ. 2014;348:g3859.
13. Windecker S, Haude M, Neumann FJ, Stangl K, Witzenbichler B, Slagboom T, Sabate M, Goicolea J, Barragan P, Cook S, et al. Comparison of a novel biodegradable polymer sirolimus-eluting stent with a durable polymer everolimus-eluting stent: results of the randomized BIOFLOW-II trial. Circ Cardiovasc Interv. 2015;8(2):e001441.
14. von Birgelen C, Kok MM, van der Heijden LC, Danse PW, Schotborgh CE, Scholte M, Gin R, Somi S, van Houwelingen KG, Stoel MG, et al. Very thin strut biodegradable polymer everolimus-eluting and sirolimus-eluting stents versus durable polymer zotarolimus-eluting stents in allcomers with coronary artery disease (BIO-RESORT): a three-arm, randomised, non-inferiority trial. Lancet. 2016;388(10060):2607–17.
15. Zbinden R, Piccolo R, Heg D, Roffi M, Kurz DJ, Muller O, Vuilliomenet A, Cook S, Weilenmann D, Kaiser C, et al. Ultrathin strut biodegradable polymer Sirolimus-eluting stent versus durable-polymer Everolimus-eluting stent for percutaneous coronary revascularization: 2-year results of the BIOSCIENCE trial. J Am Heart Assoc. 2016;5(3):e003255.
16. Kandzari DE, Mauri L, Koolen JJ, Massaro JM, Doros G, Garcia-Garcia HM, Bennett J, Roguin A, Gharib EG, Cutlip DE, et al. Ultrathin, bioresorbable polymer sirolimus-eluting stents versus thin, durable polymer everolimus-eluting stents in patients undergoing coronary revascularisation (BIOFLOW V): a randomised trial. Lancet. 2017;390(10105):1843–52.
17. Kang SH, Chung WY, Lee JM, Park JJ, Yoon CH, Suh JW, Cho YS, Doh JH, Cho JM, Bae JW, et al. Angiographic outcomes of Orsiro biodegradable polymer sirolimus-eluting stents and resolute integrity durable polymer zotarolimus-eluting stents: results of the ORIENT trial. EuroIntervention. 2017;12(13):1623–31.
18. Teeuwen K, van der Schaaf RJ, Adriaenssens T, Koolen JJ, Smits PC, Henriques JP, Vermeersch PH, Joe T, Gin RM, Scholzel BE, Kelder JC, et al. Randomized multicenter trial investigating angiographic outcomes of hybrid Sirolimus-eluting stents with biodegradable polymer compared with Everolimus-eluting stents with durable polymer in chronic Total occlusions: the PRISON IV trial. JACC Cardiovasc Interv. 2017;10(2):133–43.
19. Liberati A, Altman DG, Tetzlaff J, Mulrow C, Gotzsche PC, Ioannidis JP, Clarke M, Devereaux PJ, Kleijnen J, Moher D. The PRISMA statement for reporting systematic reviews and meta-analyses of studies that evaluate healthcare interventions: explanation and elaboration. BMJ. 2009;339:b2700.
20. Shinichi A. Cochrane handbook for systematic reviews of interventions. Online Kensaku. 2014;35(3):154–5.
21. Guyatt GH, Oxman AD, Vist GE, Kunz R, Falck-Ytter Y, Alonso-Coello P, Schunemann HJ. GRADE: an emerging consensus on rating quality of evidence and strength of recommendations. BMJ. 2008;336(7650):924–6.
22. Higgins JP, Thompson SG. Quantifying heterogeneity in a meta-analysis. Stat Med. 2002;21(11):1539–58.
23. Brok J, Thorlund K, Gluud C, Wetterslev J. Trial sequential analysis reveals insufficient information size and potentially false positive results in many meta-analyses. J Clin Epidemiol. 2008;61(8):763–9.
24. Pandya B, Gaddam S, Raza M, Asti D, Nalluri N, Vazzana T, Kandov R, Lafferty J. Biodegradable polymer stents vs second generation drug eluting stents: a meta-analysis and systematic review of randomized controlled trials. World J Cardiol. 2016;8(2):240–6.
25. Yang Y, Lei J, Huang W, Lei H. Efficacy and safety of biodegradable polymer sirolimus-eluting stents versus durable polymer drug-eluting stents: a meta-analysis of randomized trials. Int J Cardiol. 2016;222:486–93.
26. Soucy NV, Feygin JM, Tunstall R, Casey MA, Pennington DE, Huibregtse BA, Barry JJ. Strut tissue coverage and endothelial cell coverage: a comparison between bare metal stent platforms and platinum chromium stents with and without everolimus-eluting coating. EuroIntervention. 2010;6(5):630–7.

27. Pache J, Kastrati A, Mehilli J, Schuhlen H, Dotzer F, Hausleiter J, Fleckenstein M, Neumann FJ, Sattelberger U, Schmitt C, et al. Intracoronary stenting and angiographic results: strut thickness effect on restenosis outcome (ISAR-STEREO-2) trial. J Am Coll Cardiol. 2003;41(8):1283–8.
28. Kandzari DE, Leon MB, Popma JJ, Fitzgerald PJ, O'Shaughnessy C, Ball MW, Turco M, Applegate RJ, Gurbel PA, Midei MG, et al. Comparison of zotarolimus-eluting and sirolimus-eluting stents in patients with native coronary artery disease: a randomized controlled trial. J Am Coll Cardiol. 2006;48(12):2440–7.
29. Stone GW, Midei M, Newman W, Sanz M, Hermiller JB, Williams J, Farhat N, Mahaffey KW, Cutlip DE, Fitzgerald PJ, et al. Comparison of an everolimus-eluting stent and a paclitaxel-eluting stent in patients with coronary artery disease: a randomized trial. Jama. 2008;299(16):1903–13.
30. Leon MB, Mauri L, Popma JJ, Cutlip DE, Nikolsky E, O'Shaughnessy C, Overlie PA, McLaurin BT, Solomon SL, Douglas JS Jr, et al. A randomized comparison of the Endeavor zotarolimus-eluting stent versus the TAXUS paclitaxel-eluting stent in de novo native coronary lesions 12-month outcomes from the ENDEAVOR IV trial. J Am Coll Cardiol. 2010;55(6):543–54.
31. Stone GW, Rizvi A, Newman W, Mastali K, Wang JC, Caputo R, Doostzadeh J, Cao S, Simonton CA, Sudhir K, et al. Everolimus-eluting versus paclitaxel-eluting stents in coronary artery disease. N Engl J Med. 2010;362(18):1663–74.
32. Bangalore S, Toklu B, Amoroso N, Fusaro M, Kumar S, Hannan EL, Faxon DP, Feit F. Bare metal stents, durable polymer drug eluting stents, and biodegradable polymer drug eluting stents for coronary artery disease: mixed treatment comparison meta-analysis. *BMJ*. 2013;347:f6625.
33. Cassese S, Byrne RA, Ndrepepa G, Kufner S, Wiebe J, Repp J, Schunkert H, Fusaro M, Kimura T, Kastrati A. Everolimus-eluting bioresorbable vascular scaffolds versus everolimus-eluting metallic stents: a meta-analysis of randomised controlled trials. *Lancet*. 2016;387(10018):537–44.

3

Association between periodontitis and peripheral artery disease

Shuo Yang[†], Li Sheng Zhao[†], Chuan Cai, Quan Shi, Ning Wen[*] and Juan Xu[*]

Abstract

Background: Inflammation is a common feature of both peripheral arterial disease (PAD) and periodontitis. Some studies have evaluated the association between PAD and periodontitis. However, there is still no specialized meta-analysis that has quantitatively assessed the strength of the association. Thus, we conducted this meta-analysis to critically assess the strength of the association between PAD and periodontitis.

Methods: PubMed, Embase, and the Cochrane Library were searched for observational studies of the association between periodontitis and PAD in February 2018. Risk ratios (RRs) and their 95% confidence intervals (CIs) from included studies were pooled to evaluate the strength of the association between periodontitis and PAD. Weighted mean differences (WMDs) and their 95% CIs were pooled to compare the difference in periodontal-related parameters between PAD and non-PAD patients.

Results: Seven studies including a total of 4307 participants were included in the meta-analysis. The pooled analysis showed that there was a significant difference in the risk of periodontitis between PAD patients and non-PAD participants (RR = 1.70, 95% CI = 1.25–2.29, $P = 0.01$). There was also a significant difference in number of missing teeth between PAD patients and non-PAD participants (WMD = 3.75, 95% CI = 1.31–6.19, $P = 0.003$). No significant difference was found in clinical attachment loss between PAD patients and non-PAD participants (WMD = – 0.05, 95% CI = – 0.03–0.19, $P = 0.686$).

Conclusion: In conclusion, the results of this meta-analysis revealed a significant relationship between periodontitis and PAD. Moreover, our study indicated that PAD patients had more missing teeth than control subjects did. Further high-quality and well-designed studies with specific inclusion and exclusion criteria are required to strengthen the conclusions of this study.

Keywords: Periodontitis, Peripheral arterial disease, Inflammation, Risk factor, Meta-analysis

Background

Periodontitis, a chronic inflammatory disease, is primarily characterized by the destruction of tooth-supporting tissues [1, 2]. Without treatment, periodontitis typically causes a loss of connective tissue attachment, erosion of the alveolar bone and, ultimately, tooth loss [3]. In the US, nearly half of the population aged > 30 years have periodontal problems, and nearly 10% of them have severe periodontitis [4]. The findings from current studies indicate that periodontitis is associated with a wide range of systemic diseases, including pulmonary disease, diabetes mellitus, myocardial infarction, rheumatoid arthritis, and systemic lupus erythematosus [5–8]. The World Health Organization (WHO) has stated that oral health, including periodontal health, is an essential part of general health [9].

Higher levels of serum IL-6, C-reactive protein (CRP), TNF-α and IL-1β have been reported among periodontitis patients in several studies [10, 11]. Additionally, the serum IL-6 and CRP levels have a positive association with the extent of periodontitis [12]. These results suggest that as a chronic inflammatory condition, periodontitis may contribute to increased serum inflammatory markers.

Peripheral artery disease (PAD), which is usually associated with atherosclerosis, results in a significant

* Correspondence: wenningchn@163.com; newxj@hotmail.com
[†]Shuo Yang and Li Sheng Zhao contributed equally to this work.
Department of Stomatology, Chinese People's Liberation Army General Hospital, 28 Fuxing Road, Beijing 100853, China

reduction of the lumen of peripheral arteries, and its most common symptom is intermittent claudication [13]. Studies have shown that PAD is associated with elevated morbidity and mortality with cardiovascular disease (CVD) [14, 15]. The presence of PAD leads to a three- to six-fold increase in the risk of CVD mortality [16]. PAD shares the same underlying pathology as CVD and cerebrovascular diseases [17, 18]. Systemic hyperinflammation plays an important role in the onset of these diseases. It has been reported that elevated circulating levels of IL-6, TNF-α and CRP are associated with the progression of CVD, PAD and cerebrovascular disease [19–21].

The relationship between periodontitis and CVD has been investigated in many studies, and there is strong evidence that periodontitis is associated with CVD [22–24], as PAD and CVD are both chronic infammatory conditions, and they share similar infammatory factors with periodontitis. We hypothesized that there may also exist an association between PAD and periodontitis. Mendez et al. [25] was the first to report that subjects with clinically significant periodontitis at baseline had a 2.27-fold possibility of developing PAD (OR = 2.27, 95% CI = 1.32–3.9). In a case–control study conducted by Soto-Barreras et al. [26], periodontitis, defined as a clinical attachment loss (CAL) ≥4 mm in at least 30% of the six measured sites, was strongly associated with PAD risk (OR = 8.18, 95% CI = 1.21–35.23). Similar findings have proliferated in recent years [27, 28]. However, no specialized meta-analysis has quantitatively assessed the strength of the association between PAD and periodontitis. Thus, we conducted this meta-analysis to evaluate the possible association between PAD and periodontitis. The results of our study will expand the current knowledge of the etiology of PAD and will provide clinicians with better evidence-based recommendations and management strategies.

Methods

We conducted this meta-analysis in accordance with the Preferred Reporting Items for Systematic Reviews and Meta-Analyses statement (PRISMA) [29]. The checklist of the PRISMA guidelines has been put into the supplemental material (Additional file 1). This study was conducted according to the Population, Intervention, Control and Outcome (PICO) format, in order to answer the following focused PICO question:

> Are people (P) with periodontitis (I) more likely to get PAD (O)?
> Population: humans with or without PAD
> Intervention: participants with periodontitis
> Comparison: non-PAD participants with periodontitis
> Outcome: PAD

Literature-search strategy

We performed a literature search in February 2018, and the search language was restricted to English. PubMed, Embase, and the Cochrane Library were searched using the following key words: "periodontitis," "periodontal disease," "peripheral vascular disease," and "peripheral arterial disease." In addition, we identified additional studies by checking the reference lists of the related studies. The search strategy (Additional file 2) has been put into the supplemental material.

Inclusion and exclusion criteria

We included studies that (1) reported the relationship between periodontitis and risk of PAD; (2) defined PAD by ankle brachial pressure index (ABI) or angiographic findings or clinical symptoms [30]; (3) defined periodontitis using at least one of several clinical definitions according to the International Workshop for the Classification of Periodontal Disease [31] or by self-report using questionnaires or clinical diagnosis by a periodontist; (4) were observational, including those with a cross-sectional, case-control, or cohort design; and (5) had data that could be extracted.

The exclusion criteria were (1) animal model or in vitro studies; (2) reviews, case reports or comments; (3) non-English-language studies; and (4) studies without available data.

Study selection methods

To select studies, we first excluded duplicated studies from the literature search. Then, we screened the titles and abstracts and excluded obviously irrelevant studies. After assessing the full texts of potentially eligible studies, we only included studies that met the inclusion criteria. The entire process was conducted by 2 reviewers, and any disagreements were resolved by discussion with a third reviewer.

Data extraction and quality assessment

Two authors (SY and LSZ) independently assessed the characteristics of included studies. The following information was extracted from each included study: first author's name and year of publication; country of study; study design; characteristics of the study participants, including number of patients and controls, age range, and sex; study population; definition of PAD and periodontitis; and adjusted or matched factors.

The Newcastle-Ottawa Scale (NOS) [32] was used by two authors (CC and QS) to complete the quality assessment of all eligible studies. The NOS ratings (Additional file 3) has been put into the supplemental material. In this assessment tool, study selection, comparability, and outcome were used to appraise the methodological quality of the included studies, with a maximum of

9 points for each study. NOS scores of 1–3, 4–6, and 7–9 indicated low, moderate, and high study quality, respectively.

Statistical analysis

Statistical analyses were performed using the Stata 12.0 software (Stata Corporation, College Station, TX, USA). The risk ratios (RRs) and 95% confidence intervals (CIs) from the included studies were pooled to evaluate the strength of the association between periodontitis and PAD. As the parameters used for evaluating periodontal status were continuous variables, weighted mean differences and their 95% CIs were pooled to compare the difference in periodontal status between PAD and non-PAD patients.

The I^2 statistic was used to assess the degree of heterogeneity among studies. The values 25, 50, and 75% corresponded to low, moderate, and high heterogeneity, respectively. A fixed effects model was applied if $I^2 < 50\%$, and a random effects model was used if $I^2 > 50\%$.

Results

Literature selection

The detailed literature selection process is shown in Fig. 1. Based on the search strategy, 273 potentially relevant studies were selected from the electronic database. Of these studies, 140 were excluded after removing duplicates. After screening titles and abstracts, 119 irrelevant studies were excluded because they failed to meet the eligibility criteria. Twelve studies were subsequently assessed by full text review, and 5 studies were removed for various reasons. Ultimately, 7 studies were included in our meta-analysis [25–28, 30, 33, 34].

Study characteristics

The characteristics of the included studies are shown in Tables 1 and 2. A total of 4307 participants were included in the meta-analysis, for a total of 493 participants with PAD and 3814 participants without PAD. The publication dates of the included studies ranged from 1998 to 2017. Of the seven included studies, four [26, 27, 30, 33] were case-control studies, two [28, 34] were cross-sectional studies, and one [25] was a prospective cohort study. Three studies [27, 28, 30] were conducted in Asian countries, two studies [25, 26] were conducted in American countries, and two [33, 34] were conducted in European countries. One study [25] enrolled male participants only, and one [33] enrolled female participants only.

The quality of the included studies was assessed using the NOS; the results are shown in Table 2. Four case-control studies [26, 27, 30, 33] and one cohort study [25] scored more than 6 points and were considered to be of high quality. Two cross-sectional studies [28, 34] scored 6 points and were considered to be of moderate quality.

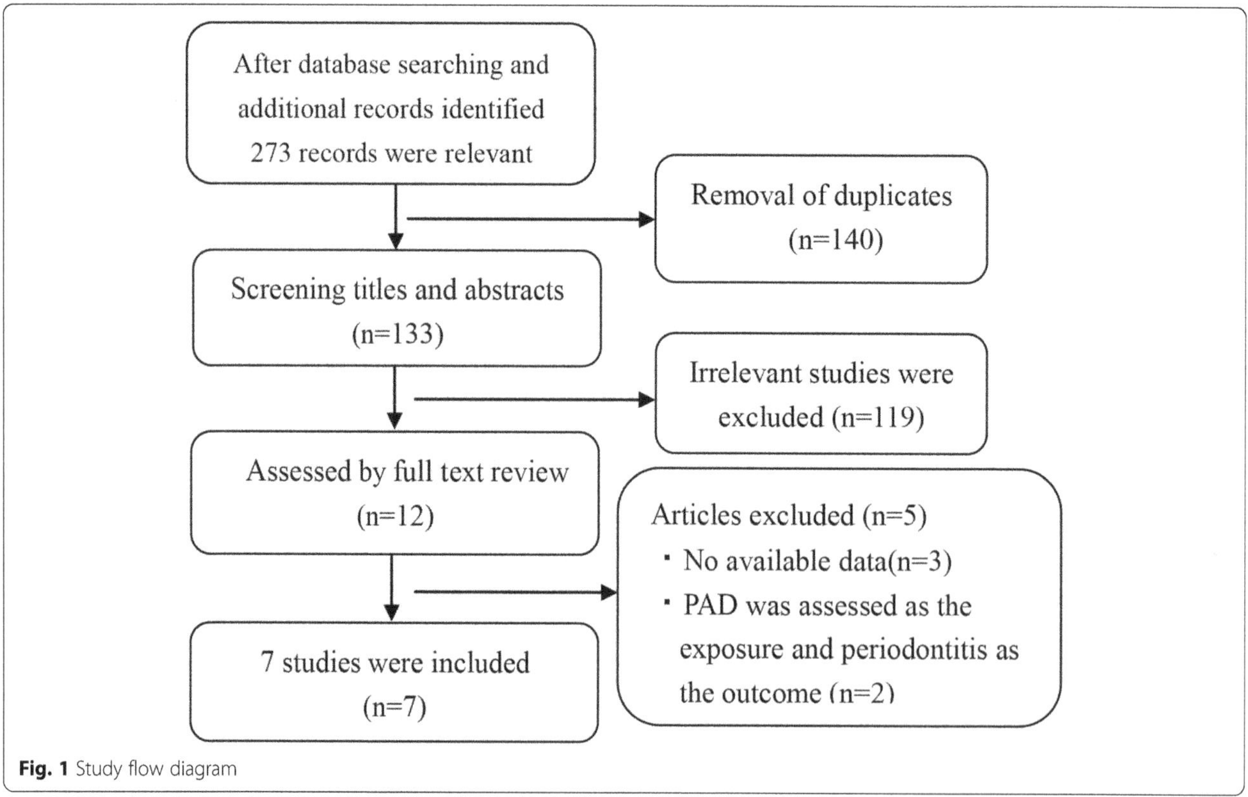

Fig. 1 Study flow diagram

Table 1 Characteristics of included studies

Study (Author, Year)	Country	Study population	Study Design	PAD[a] patients		Control	
				Number (M/F)[b]	Age (SD[c] or Range)	Number (M/F)	Age (SD or Range)
Aoyama et al. 2017 [22]	Japan	hospital-based	cross-sectional	34 (23/11)	65.6 ± 11.8	956 (693/263)	64.4 ± 13.0
Çalapkorur et al. 2017 [34]	Turkey	hospital-based	cross-sectional	40 (32/8)	60.45 ± 9.94	20 (18/2)	57.40 ± 11.16
Ahn et al. 2016 [27]	South Korea	population-based	case-control	72 (28/44)	NR[d]	1271 (473/798)	NR
Soto-Barreras et al. 2013 [26]	Mexico	hospital-based	case-control	30 (8/22)	61.86 ± 8.49	30 (9:21)	63.23 ± 9.06
Chen et al. 2008 [30]	Japan	hospital-based	case-control	25 (21/4)	67.6 ± 10	32 (28/4)	63.1 ± 10
Bloemenkamp et al. 2002 [33]	Netherlands	population-based	case-control	212 (0/212)	48.2 ± 7.0	475 (0/475)	45.5 ± 8.1
Mendez et al. 1998 [25]	USA	population-based	cohort	80 (80/0)	44.2 (29–62)	1030 (1030/0)	42.7 (23–80)

[a]PAD, peripheral arterial disease
[b]M/F, male/female
[c]SD, standard deviation
[d]NR, not report

Table 2 Characteristics of included studies

Study (Author, Year)	Defnition of PAD	Defnition of periodontitis	Adjusted or matched factors	NOS score
Aoyama et al. 2017 [22]	PAD was diagnosed based on clinical symptoms, ABI, and angiographic fndings	NR	age, sex, smoking, hypertension, dyslipidemia and HbA1c levels	6
Çalapkorur et al. 2017 [34]	Patients with ABI values of ≤0.90 were diagnosed as having PAD	Periodontitis was defined as the presence of at least five teeth with one or more sites with a PD of ≥5 mm, a CAL of ≥2 mm, the presence of BOP and 30% radiographic bone loss	age, gender, diabetes, hypertension and BMI	6
Ahn et al. 2016 [27]	PAD was evaluated by using ABI lower than 1.0	The radiographic alveolar bone loss 4 mm at two or more interproximal sites, not on the same tooth	age, sex, education level, tooth loss, smoking, drinking, central obesity	7
Soto-Barreras et al. 2013 [26]	Patients with ABI values of ≤0.90 were diagnosed as having PAD	The diagnosis of periodontitis was determined when the attachment loss was ≥4 mm in ≥30% of measured sites.	age, sex, BMI,smoking, and diabetes mellitus	8
Chen et al. 2008 [30]	PAD was diagnosed based on clinical symptoms, ABI, and angiographic fndings	Participants who presented with at least one probing site with PD 4 mm or CAL 4 mm in each quadrant were defined as periodontitis patients	Smoking, age, gender, and diabetes	7
Bloemenkamp et al. 2002 [33]	PAD was angiographically confirmed when a stenotic lesion causing more than 50% reduction of the lumen was present in at least one major peripheral artery	NR	Smoking, age, gender, and diabetes	7
Mendez et al. 1998 [25]	PAD was defined as one or more of the following: (1) intermittent claudication; (2) extracranial erebrovascular disease; (3) atherosclerosis (including aortic, renal, and mesenteric disease); and (4) arterial embolism and thrombosis.	Periodontitis was considered present if the mean whole mouth alveolar bone loss was>20%.	age, BMI, family history of heart disease, and smoking exposure	8

ABI ankle brachial pressure index, *PAD* peripheral arterial disease, *PD* probing depth, *CAL* clinical attachment loss, *BOP* bleeding on probing, *BMI* body mass index, *NR* not report

Meta-analysis

PAD and periodontitis prevalence

Six studies [25–27, 30, 33, 34] that had available data to calculate the RRs and 95% CIs were included in the meta-analysis to evaluate the strength of the association between PAD and periodontitis. The pooled analysis indicated a significant difference in the risk of periodontitis between PAD patients and non-PAD participants (RR = 1.70, 95% CI = 1.25–2.29, $P = 0.01$, Fig. 2). However, considering the high heterogeneity ($I^2 = 78.3\%$) of the included studies, a random effects model was used.

Missing teeth

Three studies [26–28] compared the number of missing teeth in PAD patients and non-PAD participants. The meta-analysis showed that PAD patients lost more teeth than non-PAD participants did, and the difference was statistically significant (WMD = 3.75, 95% CI = 1.31–6.19, $P = 0.003$, Fig. 3). Considering the high heterogeneity ($I^2 = 56.9\%$) of the included studies, a random effects models was used.

Clinical attachment loss (CAL)

Two studies [28, 34] reported CAL results in PAD patients and non-PAD participants. The pooled analysis showed that there was no significant difference in clinical attachment loss between PAD patients and non-PAD participants (WMD = – 0.05, 95% CI = – 0.03–0.19, $P = 0.686$, Fig. 4). Considering the low heterogeneity ($I^2 = 0.0\%$) of the included studies, a fixed effects model was used.

Discussion

In this meta-analysis, we found a statistically significant increased risk of periodontitis in PAD patients compared to non-PAD participants, suggesting that there was a significant association between PAD and periodontitis. Moreover, we found that PAD patients had more missing teeth than non-PAD participants did. However, there was no statistical difference in CAL between PAD patients and controls.

Our finding that periodontitis was associated with PAD is in agreement with other studies focused on this relationship. Ahn et al. [27] reported that periodontitis was a risk factor for PAD; their study showed that patients with periodontitis had a 2.03-fold increase in the risk of PAD (95% CI = 1.05–3.93). Çalapkorur et al. [34] showed that periodontitis raised the odds ratio for developing PAD to 5.84 (95% CI = 1.56–21.91). Chen et al. [30] conducted a case-control study and found that periodontitis was associated with a relative risk of 5.45 (95% CI = 1.57–18.89) for developing PAD.

In this meta-analysis, we also compared periodontal parameters, such as the CAL and number of missing teeth, to reflect the periodontal status of PAD patients and non-PAD participants. CAL is well known as a gold-standard measurement for periodontitis in both clinical research and clinical work [35]. However, this meta-analysis failed to find a difference in CAL between PAD patients and non-PAD participants. This null finding may have been caused by the heterogeneity of the study groups and the limited number of related studies. Hence, further well-designed studies are needed to evaluate this relationship.

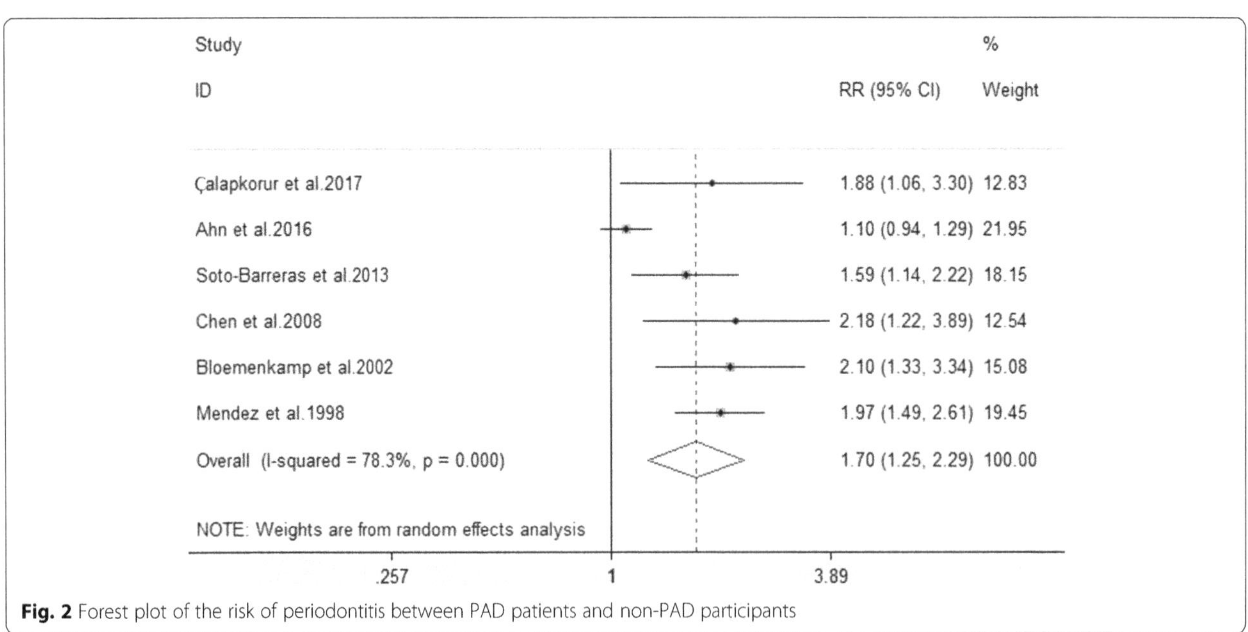

Fig. 2 Forest plot of the risk of periodontitis between PAD patients and non-PAD participants

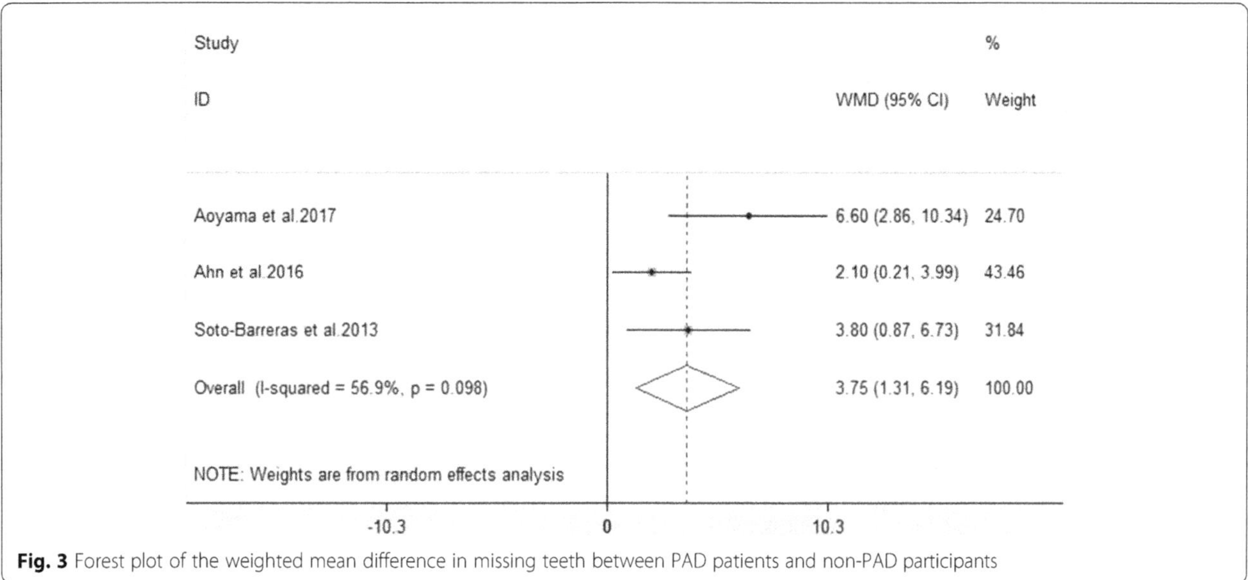

Fig. 3 Forest plot of the weighted mean difference in missing teeth between PAD patients and non-PAD participants

Missing teeth can reflect an irreversible condition in the end-stage of periodontitis [36]. Our meta-analysis indicated that PAD patients typically have more missing teeth than non-PAD participants do. It is well known that the most important cause of missing teeth is periodontitis. This result, in turn, may illustrate the close relationship between periodontitis and PAD.

The mechanism by which periodontitis causes PAD is not yet fully understood. However, elevated levels of inflammatory mediators such as IL-6, IL-1β and TNF-α in systemic circulation within PAD patients suggests that chronic infection in the body that may play an important role [11, 30, 37]. Periodontitis is a chronic inflammatory disease, and it is believed that periodontitis has the ability to induce local and host immune responses and to cause both transient bacteremia and the release of inflammatory mediators such as ILs and TNF-α. These mediators can subsequently damage endothelial tissues and eventually lead to PAD [11, 38].

However, we observed high heterogeneity among the studies included in the meta-analysis. The observed heterogeneity may have been due to several factors. First, diagnostic criteria and methods of evaluating periodontitis were different among the included studies, and in some studies, the methods were not reported. These different criteria and evaluation methods for periodontitis lead to variation in the outcome measures and thus cause heterogeneity.

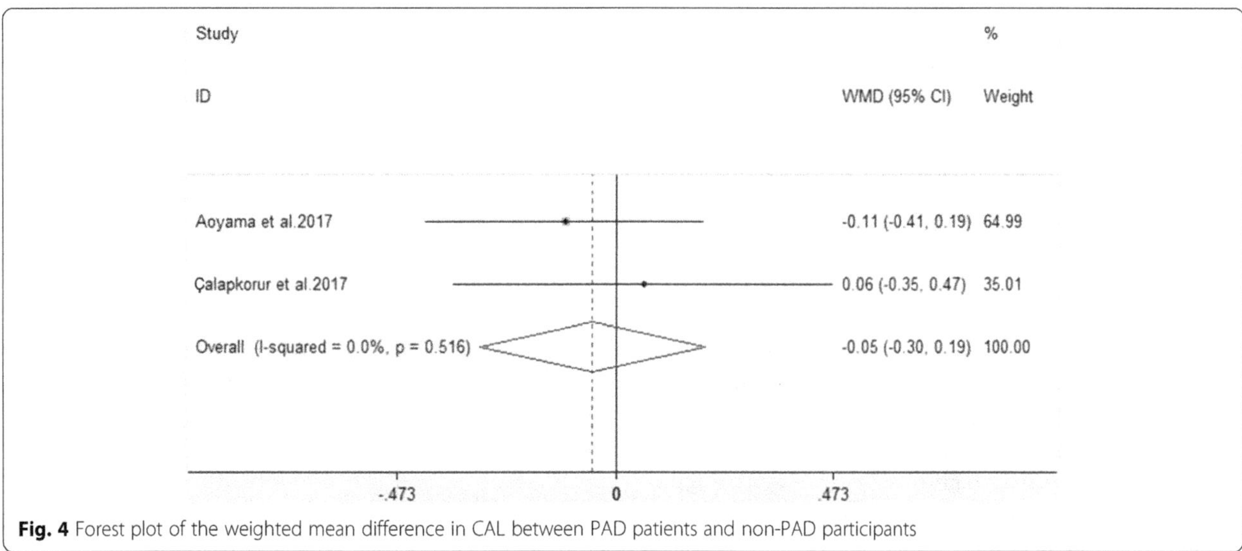

Fig. 4 Forest plot of the weighted mean difference in CAL between PAD patients and non-PAD participants

Second, different types of observational studies and study populations were included in this study. We included cross-sectional, case-control, and cohort studies in this meta-analysis, and the hospital-based or population-based subjects were recruited in different studies. Third, different adjustments for confounding factors may play a role in heterogeneity. Some factors can affect both PAD and periodontitis independently, such as diabetes, tobacco and age. Moreover, unmeasured confounders may exist and could lead to heterogeneity. Fourth, the limited patient numbers in some studies may have contributed to the inconsistent results and resulted in high heterogeneity.

To our knowledge, this is the first meta-analysis to estimate the association between periodontitis and PAD. Our results showed a significant relationship between periodontitis and PAD. Additionally, our study indicated that PAD patients had more missing teeth than control subjects did. Furthermore, a study conducted by Blum et al. [39] found that treating periodontitis effectively improved the function of the vascular endothelium and may play a protective role in vascular injury and prevent PAD. From the perspective of public health, periodontitis is a disease that can be prevented and treated; thus, the effective implementation of prevention programs and treatment measures could not only improve oral health but may also reduce the risk of PAD. It should be noted that the current evidence only reveals a potential association of periodontitis and PAD. The specific mechanisms by which the two diseases are associated remain unknown, and further experimental studies to investigate pathologic mechanisms underlying periodontitis and PAD are needed.

The current meta-analysis has some limitations. First, high heterogeneity among the included studies was detected during analysis. Second, sensitivity analysis, meta-regression, and publication bias analyses were not performed due to the limited number of included studies. Third, the included studies were published in English; thus, relevant studies published in other languages may have been overlooked, causing selection bias.

Conclusions

In conclusion, the results of this meta-analysis revealed a significant relationship between periodontitis and PAD. Moreover, our study demonstrated that PAD patients had more missing teeth than control subjects did. However, the results should be viewed with caution because of the high heterogeneity and limited number of included studies. Further high-quality and well-designed studies with specific inclusion and exclusion criteria are required to strengthen the conclusions of this study.

Abbreviations

ABI: Ankle brachial pressure index; CAL: Clinical attachment loss; CIs: Confidence intervals; CRP: C-reactive protein; CVD: Cardiovascular disease; NOS: Newcastle-Ottawa Scale; PAD: Peripheral arterial disease; PRISMA: Preferred Reporting Items for Systematic Reviews and Meta-Analyses statement; RRs: Risk ratios; WHO: World health organization; WMDs: Weighted mean differences

Acknowledgements

Not applicable.

Funding

This study was supported by grant from the National Natural Science Foundation of China (No.51472270).

Authors' contributions

SY and LSZ carried out the literature research and drafted the manuscript. LSZ, CC and QS completed the data extraction and performed the statistical analysis. NW and JX are the corresponding author, and they designed this meta-analysis and helped to draft the manuscript. All authors read and approved the final manuscript.

Competing interests

The authors declare that they have no competing interests.

References

1. Lundmark A, Davanian H, Bage T, Johannsen G, Koro C, Lundeberg J, et al. Transcriptome analysis reveals mucin 4 to be highly associated with periodontitis and identifies pleckstrin as a link to systemic diseases. Sci Rep. 2015;5:18475.
2. Williams RC. Periodontal disease. N Engl J Med. 1990;322(6):373–82.
3. Pihlstrom BL, Michalowicz BS, Johnson NW. Periodontal diseases. Lancet (London, England). 2005;366(9499):1809–20.
4. Eke PI, Zhang X, Lu H, Wei L, Thornton-Evans G, Greenlund KJ, et al. Predicting periodontitis at state and local levels in the United States. J Dent Res. 2016;95(5):515–22.
5. Rutter-Locher Z, Smith TO, Giles I, Sofat N. Association between systemic lupus erythematosus and periodontitis: a systematic review and meta-analysis. Front Immunol. 2017;8:1295.
6. Hobbins S, Chapple IL, Sapey E, Stockley RA. Is periodontitis a comorbidity of COPD or can associations be explained by shared risk factors/behaviors? IntJ Chron Obstruct Pulmon Dis. 2017;12:1339–49.
7. Shi Q, Zhang B, Huo N, Cai C, Liu H, Xu J. Association between myocardial infarction and periodontitis: a meta-analysis of case-control studies. Front Physiol. 2016;7:519.

8. Cardoso EM, Reis C, Manzanares-Cespedes MC. Chronic periodontitis, inflammatory cytokines, and interrelationship with other chronic diseases. Postgrad Med. 2018;130(1):98–104.
9. Petersen PE, Kwan S. The 7th WHO global conference on health promotion: towards integration of oral health (Nairobi, Kenya, 2009). Community Dent Health. 2010;27(Suppl 1):1–9.
10. Ebersole JL, Machen RL, Steffen MJ, Willmann DE. Systemic acute-phase reactants, C-reactive protein and haptoglobin, in adult periodontitis. Clin Exp Immunol. 1997;107(2):347–52.
11. Gorska R, Gregorek H, Kowalski J, Laskus-Perendyk A, Syczewska M, Madalinski K. Relationship between clinical parameters and cytokine profiles in inflamed gingival tissue and serum samples from patients with chronic periodontitis. J Clin Periodontol. 2003;30(12):1046–52.
12. Loos BG, Craandijk J, Hoek FJ, Wertheim-van Dillen PM, van der Velden U. Elevation of systemic markers related to cardiovascular diseases in the peripheral blood of periodontitis patients. J Periodontol. 2000;71(10):1528–34.
13. Ouma GO, Jonas RA, Usman MH, Mohler ER 3rd. Targets and delivery methods for therapeutic angiogenesis in peripheral artery disease. Vasc Med (London, England). 2012;17(3):174–92.
14. Howell MA, Colgan MP, Seeger RW, Ramsey DE, Sumner DS. Relationship of severity of lower limb peripheral vascular disease to mortality and morbidity: a six-year follow-up study. J Vasc Surg. 1989;9(5):691–6. discussion 696-697
15. McKenna M, Wolfson S, Kuller L. The ratio of ankle and arm arterial pressure as an independent predictor of mortality. Atherosclerosis. 1991; 87(2–3):119–28.
16. Hirsch AT, Criqui MH, Treat-Jacobson D, Regensteiner JG, Creager MA, Olin JW, et al. Peripheral arterial disease detection, awareness, and treatment in primary care. JAMA. 2001;286(11):1317–24.
17. Blaizot A, Vergnes JN, Nuwwareh S, Amar J, Sixou M. Periodontal diseases and cardiovascular events: meta-analysis of observational studies. Int Dent J. 2009;59(4):197–209.
18. Sfyroeras GS, Roussas N, Saleptsis VG, Argyriou C, Giannoukas AD. Association between periodontal disease and stroke. J Vasc Surg. 2012; 55(4):1178–84.
19. Botti C, Maione C, Dogliotti G, Russo P, Signoriello G, Molinari AM, et al. Circulating cytokines present in the serum of peripheral arterial disease patients induce endothelial dysfunction. J Biol Regul Homeost Agents. 2012; 26(1):67–79.
20. Moreno VP, Subira D, Meseguer E, Llamas P. IL-6 as a biomarker of ischemic cerebrovascular disease. Biomark Med. 2008;2(2):125–36.
21. Kofler S, Nickel T, Weis M. Role of cytokines in cardiovascular diseases: a focus on endothelial responses to inflammation. Clini Sci (London). 2005; 108(3):205–13.
22. Aoyama N, Suzuki JI, Kobayashi N, Hanatani T, Ashigaki N, Yoshida A, et al. Associations among tooth loss, systemic inflammation and antibody titers to periodontal pathogens in Japanese patients with cardiovascular disease. J Periodontal Res. 2018;53(1):117-22.
23. Li C, Lv Z, Shi Z, Zhu Y, Wu Y, Li L, et al. Periodontal therapy for the management of cardiovascular disease in patients with chronic periodontitis. Cochrane Database Syst Rev. 2017;11:Cd009197.
24. Almeida A, Fagundes NCF, Maia LC, Lima RR. Is there an association between periodontitis and atherosclerosis in adults? A systematic review. Curr Vasc Pharmacol. 2017. https://doi.org/10.2174/ 1570161115666170830141852. Epub ahead of print.
25. Mendez MV, Scott T, LaMorte W, Vokonas P, Menzoian JO, Garcia R. An association between periodontal disease and peripheral vascular disease. Am J Surg. 1998;176(2):153–7.
26. Soto-Barreras U, Olvera-Rubio JO, Loyola-Rodriguez JP, Reyes-Macias JF, Martinez-Martinez RE, Patino-Marin N, et al. Peripheral arterial disease associated with caries and periodontal disease. J Periodontol. 2013; 84(4):486–94.
27. Ahn YB, Shin MS, Han DH, Sukhbaatar M, Kim MS, Shin HS, et al. Periodontitis is associated with the risk of subclinical atherosclerosis and peripheral arterial disease in Korean adults. Atherosclerosis. 2016;251:311–8.
28. Aoyama N, Suzuki JI, Kobayashi N, Hanatani T, Ashigaki N, Yoshida A, et al. Periodontitis deteriorates peripheral arterial disease in Japanese population via enhanced systemic inflammation. Heart Vessel. 2017;32(11):1314–9.
29. Liberati A, Altman DG, Tetzlaff J, Mulrow C, Gotzsche PC, Ioannidis JP, et al. The PRISMA statement for reporting systematic reviews and meta-analyses of studies that evaluate healthcare interventions: explanation and elaboration. BMJ (Clinical research ed). 2009;339:b2700.
30. Chen YW, Umeda M, Nagasawa T, Takeuchi Y, Huang Y, Inoue Y, et al. Periodontitis may increase the risk of peripheral arterial disease. Eur J Vasc Endovasc Surg. 2008;35(2):153–8.
31. Armitage GC. Development of a classification system for periodontal diseases and conditions. Northwest Dent. 2000;79(6):31–5.
32. Wells GA, Shea B, O'Connell D, Peterson J, Welch V, Losos M, Tugwell P. The Newcastle-Ottawa Scale (NOS) for assessing the quality of nonrandomised studies in meta-a nalyses. In: Clinical epidemiology The Ottawa Hospital. 2018. http://www.ohri.ca/programs/clinical_epidemiology/oxford.ASp. Accessed 3 Mar 2018.
33. Bloemenkamp DG, van den Bosch MA, Mali WP, Tanis BC, Rosendaal FR, Kemmeren JM, et al. Novel risk factors for peripheral arterial disease in young women. Am J Med. 2002;113(6):462–7.
34. Calapkorur MU, Alkan BA, Tasdemir Z, Akcali Y, Saatci E. Association of peripheral arterial disease with periodontal disease: analysis of inflammatory cytokines and an acute phase protein in gingival crevicular fluid and serum. J Periodontal Res. 2017;52(3):532–9.
35. Savage A, Eaton KA, Moles DR, Needleman I. A systematic review of definitions of periodontitis and methods that have been used to identify this disease. J Clin Periodontol. 2009;36(6):458–67.
36. Hyde S, Dupuis V, Mariri BP, Dartevelle S. Prevention of tooth loss and dental pain for reducing the global burden of oral diseases. Int Dent J. 2017;67(Suppl 2):19–25.
37. Dye BA, Choudhary K, Shea S, Papapanou PN. Serum antibodies to periodontal pathogens and markers of systemic inflammation. J Clin Periodontol. 2005;32(12):1189–99.
38. Jimenez M, Krall EA, Garcia RI, Vokonas PS, Dietrich T. Periodontitis and incidence of cerebrovascular disease in men. Ann Neurol. 2009;66(4):505–12.
39. Blum A, Kryuger K, Mashiach Eizenberg M, Tatour S, Vigder F, Laster Z, et al. Periodontal care may improve endothelial function. Eur J Intern Med. 2007; 18(4):295–8.

4

Non-adherence to antihypertensive pharmacotherapy in Buea, Cameroon: a cross-sectional community-based study

Nkengla Menka Adidja[1,2†], Valirie Ndip Agbor[3,4†], Jeannine A. Aminde[1,5], Calypse A. Ngwasiri[6,7], Kathleen Blackett Ngu[4] and Leopold Ndemnge Aminde[8*]

Abstract

Background: Hypertension is a challenging public health problem with a huge burden in the developing countries. Non-adherence to antihypertensive treatment is a big obstacle in blood pressure (BP) control and favours disease progression to complications. Our objectives were to determine the rate of non-adherence to antihypertensive pharmacotherapy, investigate factors associated with non-adherence, and to assess the association between non-adherence and BP control in the Buea Health District (BHD), Cameroon.

Methods: A community-based cross-sectional study using stratified cluster sampling was conducted in the BHD from November 2013 – March 2014. Eligible consenting adult participants had their BP measured and classified using the Joint National Committee VII criteria. The Morisky medication adherence scale was used to assess adherence to BP lowering medication. Multivariable logistic regression models were used to predict non-adherence.

Results: One hundred and eighty-three participants were recruited with mean age of 55.9 years. Overall, 67.7% (95% CI: 59.8–73.6%) of participants were non-adherent to their medications. After adjusting for age, sex and other covariates, forgetfulness (aOR = 7.9, 95%CI: 3.0–20.8), multiple daily doses (aOR = 2.5, 95%CI: 1.2–5.6), financial constraints (aOR = 2.8, 95%CI: 1.1–6.9) and adverse drug effects (aOR = 7.6, 95%CI: 1.7–33.0) independently predicted non-adherence to anti-hypertensive medication. BP was controlled in only 21.3% of participants and was better in those who were adherent to medication (47.5% versus 8.2%, $p < 0.01$).

Conclusion: At least two of every three hypertensive patients in the Buea Health District are non-adherent to treatment. Forgetfulness, multiple daily doses of medication, financial constraints and medication adverse effects are the major predictors of non-adherence in hypertensive patients. These factors should be targeted to improve adherence and BP control, which will contribute to stem hypertension-related morbidity and mortality.

Keywords: Hypertension, Medication adherence, Non-adherence, Morisky scale, Cameroon

Background

Hypertension is an important public health challenge worldwide. In 2010, the global prevalence of hypertension was estimated at 1.39 billion representing 31.1% in the adult population [1]. This implies one in three adults suffer from hypertension. Low- and middle-income countries are more affected than high income countries [2]. Compared with Caucasians, Africans with hypertension have lower hypertension control rates and higher prevalence of hypertension-related complications [3]. The prevalence of hypertension in Africa was estimated at 30.8% in 2014 [4]. Studies done in specific populations in Cameroon have equally revealed prevalence rates as high as 37.8% [5] and 57.3% in an elderly population [6]. In fact, it is projected that by 2025, 31.9% of Cameroonians (approximately 5.6 million people) will be living with hypertension [7].

Adherence to a medication regimen is generally defined as the extent to which patients take medications as

* Correspondence: amindeln@gmail.com
†Nkengla Menka Adidja and Valirie Ndip Agbor contributed equally to this work.
[8]Faculty of Medicine, School of Public Health, The University of Queensland, Brisbane, Australia
Full list of author information is available at the end of the article

prescribed by their health care providers [8]. Non-adherence is the main obstacle for controlling hypertension in the community, and a significant barrier to effective hypertension management [9–11]. Good adherence is therefore crucial to improve hypertension controls rates and prevent complications such as cerebrovascular accidents, coronary artery disease, aneurysms and heart failure [12, 13].

Several studies conducted globally on this topic have produced a wide range of results. The non-adherence rate in a global study conducted was 45% and a significant number of the hypertensive patients with co-morbidities were non-adherent to treatment [14]. The non-adherence rate from community-based studies in Bangladesh and Vietnam were as high as 85 and 49.8% respectively [15, 16]. About 66.7% of participants in a study conducted in both Nigeria and Ghana were non-adherent to treatment [17]. Similar studies conducted in Cameroon have reported low adherence rates of 43.9% [18] and 12.9% [19]. Several factors have been associated with non-adherence including but not limited to forgetfulness, lack of motivation due to the incurable nature of the disease, absence of symptoms, use of herbal preparation, physical disability, presence of complications, low level of education, poor knowledge of the disease and ignorace on the need for longterm treatment [17–20].

Hypertension accounts for a significant disease burden in Cameroon and control rates for blood pressure (BP) are poor. Adherence to medication is a key patient-factor in enhancing BP control, and community-based studies that have explored medication adherence in hypertensive populations in Cameroon are scant. We conducted this study to bridge the knowledge gap on the prevalence and factors associated with non-adherence to antihypertensive medication in Cameroon.

Methods

Study design and setting

This was a cross-sectional analytic study conducted from 12 November 2013 to 11 March 2014, a period of four months in the Buea Health District (BHD).

Buea is located at the eastern slope of the base of Mount Cameroon and is the capital of the South West Region. The BHD shares boundaries with Mount Cameroon to the west and north, Mutengene to the south, and Ekona to the east. Its population is estimated at 86,272 [21], and is made up of seven health areas including Buea road, Muea, Molyko, Bova, Buea Town, Bokwaongo and Tole.

Sample size, sampling and eligibility

Using the following formula: $n = \frac{p(1-p)z^2}{d^2}$

We estimated a minimum acceptable sample size (n) of 174 participants for this study. The standard normal variate for significance (z) was 1.96 and margin of error (d) set at 5%, and the prevalence (p) of adherence rate was considered to be 13% according to a community-based study conducted by Ekram et al. [22].

Participants were recruited using a two-staged cluster randomised sampling technique. The preliminary stage involved random selection through balloting to select four out of the seven aforementioned health areas. The Tole, Muea, Bokwaongo and Bova health areas were selected. With the permission of the local leaders, the objective of our study was channeled to the community through the local radio stations, focal person for communication, churches and meeting houses. This was followed by an exhaustive invitation of consenting eligible participants in every household. For every household, we inquired about the hypertension status of all adults who were 21 years and older. Participants who attested to have been diagnosed with hypertension and placed on treatment were required to state the name(s) and physically present the drug(s) they were taking for hypertension. This information was then confirmed with the participants' hospital records. Only one participant was required per household. In case there was more than one person in a household who were eligible for this study, balloting was done to select the final participant to be included.

Inclusion criteria

Consenting participants at least twenty-one years old living with hypertension who were on hypertensive medication(s) for at least one month were recruited for this study.

Exclusion criteria

We excluded pregnant women, individuals who declared being hypertensive but had no proof that they were on or had been prescribed drugs, those who had smoked, or consumed alcohol or other cardiostimulants 30 min prior to data collection, and individuals who could not express themselves in either English or French.

Data items and study procedure

Using a predesigned questionnaire, data was collected in two steps. First, through a one-on-one interview, data on socio-demographic characteristics (age, gender, marital status, religion, educational status, occupational status), clinical parameters (BP, duration of treatment, number of tablets and number of doses per day), level of adherence using the Morisky 8-item validated questionnaire [23], and factors potentially associated with non-adherence (like forgetfulness, absence of symptoms, use of herbal medicine, smell and taste of drugs, lack of funds to purchase drugs, busy schedule, and adverse drug effects) were collected. Second, the BP was measured respecting standardized protocol. For every participant, two BP readings were recorded at least 10 min apart using an automatic machine (Medical Rossmax-Automatic Upper Arm Blood Pressure Monitor, Model AK150f, manufactured by Rossmax International Ltd., Botzstrasse 6,D-07743 Jena, Germany) approximated to the nearest 1 mmHg. The average of both readings was then computed and used for analysis.

Definition of operational variables

A controlled BP was defined as a systolic BP and diastolic BP below 140 mmHg and 90 mmHg, respectively.

Adherence to antihypertensive pharmacotherapy was defined as a Morisky score of ≤2 while non-adherence was defined as a Morisky score above 2.

Occupational status was categorised as low (require no expert training or no technical expertise like farming), medium (a technical expertise is required but no expert training e.g. carpentry, commercial bike riding and commercial taxi, etc.) and high (for professionals and require advanced training e.g. health personnel, teachers, accountants etc.).

Ethical considerations

Ethical approval was granted by the Faculty of Health Sciences, Institutional Review Board (IRB) of the University of Buea (reference number: 2013/0106/UB/FHS/IRB) prior to conducting this study. In addition, administrative authorization was obtained from the South West Regional Delegation of Public Health before data collection.

Data analysis

Data was entered in a Microsoft Excel 2007 spreadsheet and imported to the Statistical Package for Social Sciences (SPSS) version 20 software for analysis. Categorical variables were presented as frequencies and percentages. On the other hand, quantitative variables were reported as mean or median with their corresponding standard deviation (SD) or interquartile ranges (IQR), respectively. The chi squared or Fisher's exact test and the student t-test were used for group comparisons for categorical and continuous variables, respectively. To determine predictors of non-adherence to antihypertensive medication, while adjusting for age, sex and other confounders, a multivariate logistic regression model using forward selection was built using variables with p-values below 0.25 on univariate analysis. The level of statistical significance was set at a p-value of 0.05.

Results

General characteristics

Table 1 portrays the socio-demographic and clinical characteristics of our study population. Out of 183 participants, 118 (64.5%) were females and the mean age was 55.9 ± 12.3 years. The ages of the participants ranged from 21 to 90 years. One hundred and twenty-six (68.9%) of the participants were married. One hundred and sixty-three (89.1%) were Christians. Majority ($n = 139$, 79.9%) of the participants had only up to primary school level of education. Ninety-five (51.9%) were employed.

Prevalence of non-adherence to antihypertensive pharmacotherapy

Out of 183 participants, 122 were non-adherent to their blood pressure lowering medication according to the Morisky medication adherence tool, giving a non-adherence prevalence of 66.7% (95%CI: 59.8–73.6%).

Factors associated with non-adherence to antihypertensive pharmacotherapy

The following candidate variables were used in univariate analysis to test their association with non-adherence: multiple daily doses, multiple antihypertensive drugs, use of herbs, cost of treatment, absence of symptoms, forgetfulness, adverse drug effects, busy schedule. We found that forgetfulness (adjusted odds ratio (aOR) = 7.9; 95% confidence interval (CI): 3–20.8, $p < 0.001$), lack of finances (aOR = 2.8; CI: 1.1–6.9, $p = 0.024$), multiple daily doses (aOR =2.5; 1.2–5.6, p = 0.02) and drug side effects (aOR = 7.0 CI: 1.7–33.6, $p = 0.007$) were independent predictors of non-adherence after controlling for potential confounders in multivariate analysis. Our model, shown in Table 2, explained about 32.7% of the variability in the outcome variable (non-adherence). When adjusted for age, gender, number of antihypertensive medications and duration on medications, participants who were adherent to medication were more likely to have good BP control (OR = 13.82; 95% CI = 5.46–34.95; $p < 0.001$), Table 3.

Discussion

In this community-based study assessing adherence to antihypertensive medication among adults in the BHD, we found that two-thirds of our study participants were non-adherent to antihypertensive pharmacotherapy and this was mainly driven by forgetfulness to take medications, lack of funds to buy medications, antihypertensive regimens requiring multiple daily dosing and drug side effects. In addition, non-adherence was associated with poor blood pressure control.

Two-thirds (66.7%) of our study population were non-adherent to treatment. This prevalence was similar to studies carried out in Ghana and Nigeria and Nigeria

Table 1 Characteristics of the study population

Variables	Category	Frequency ($n = 183$)	Proportion (%)
Age (years)	20–39	15	8.2
	40–59	89	48.6
	≥ 60	79	43.2
Gender	Male	65	35.5
	Female	118	64.5
Marital status	Single	17	9.3
	Married	126	68.9
	Divorced	3	1.6
	Widow/widower	37	20.2
Religion	Christian	163	89.1
	Muslim	15	8.2
	None	5	2.7
Educational status	None	72	39.3
	Primary	67	36.6
	Secondary	31	16.9
	Tertiary	13	7.1
Employment status	Employed	95	51.9
	Unemployed	88	48.1
SBP (in mmHg) Mean (SD)			162.72 (26.1)
DBP (in mmHg) Mean (SD)			98.3 (17.7)
Daily dose frequency Median (IQR)			2(1–3)
Number of antihypertensive drugs Median (IQR)			1 (1–2)
Duration of treatment in years Median (IQR)			3 (2–4)

SBP Systolic blood pressure, *DBP* Diastolic blood pressure, *SD* Standard deviation, *IQR* Interquartile range

[17, 20], but higher than the values reported from studies in Czech Republic (31.5%), United Kingdom (41.6%) [24] and Canada (23%) [25]. These difference in the prevalence of non-adherence rates is probably due to better access to health care, availability of basic drugs for cardiovascular disorders in contrast to our setting where less than 60% of cardiovascular drugs are available [26], better standards of living with majority being insured and low illiteracy rates in these high income countries. In addition, we noted a higher non-adherence rate than the 13% prevalence rate obtained from a community-based study in Rajshashi in Bangladesh [22]. This discrepancy could be attributed to a difference in the methods used to assess non-adherence in both studies. In our study, the Morisky questionnaire was used to evaluate non-adherence while in the study done in Bangladesh, a participant was considered non-adherent if he/she missed his/her medication(s) on any day of the month. Furthermore, the high non-adherence rate in our study could be attributed to the fact that most of our study participants were just between 2 and 4 years of antihypertensive pharmacotherapy. Indeed, the adherence rate has been shown to increase with the duration on antihypertensive pharmacotherapy [27, 28].

After multivariable regression analysis, forgetfulness was significantly associated with non-adherence to antihypertensive pharmacotherapy. This is similar to the finding in Ghana where patients reported forgetfulness as the main reason for non-adherence [29]. The use of alarm clocks and/or education of other household members about when the drug(s) should be taken could improve adherence. Lack of finances was equally a predictor of medication non-adherence amongst our study population. Lack of finances appears to be a major predictor of non-adherence in sub-Saharan Africa [30–32] and other developing countries [33]. Unlike highly active antiretroviral drugs used in the management of the human immunodeficiency virus that are free, it is not the case with antihypertensive medications. These (hypertensive) patients need to buy their drugs out of their pockets. The absence of universal healthcare schemes and high unemployment rates in Africa [34] are chiefly

Table 2 Predictors of medication non-adherence among hypertensive patients in univariate and multivariate logistic regression

Variables	Non-adherent		OR	95% CI	*p*-value	AOR	95% CI	*p*-value
	Yes (*N* = 122)	No (*N* = 61)						
Age (in years) Mean (SD)	57.0 (12.3)	53.8 (12.2)	1.02	1.0–1.04	0.108	1.02	0.98–1.06	0.264
Gender								
Male	48 (39.3)	17 (26.2)	1.7	0.9–3.3	0.128	1.1	0.4–2.6	0.814
Female	74 (60.7)	44 (72.1)	Ref					
Marital status								
Single	11 (9.0)	6 (9.8)	Ref			–		
Married	86 (70.5)	40 (65.6)	0.9	0.3–3.0	0.857			
Divorced	2 (1.6)	1 (1.6)	0.8	0.4–1.6	0.489			
Widow/Widower	23 (18.9)	14 (23.0)	0.9	0.1–9.9	0.877			
Level of education								
None	47 (38.5)	25 (41.0)	Ref			–		
Primary	44 (36.1)	23 (37.7)	1.0	0.5–2.0	0.961			
Secondary	21 (17.2)	10 (16.4)	1.1	0.5–2.7	0.809			
Tertiary	10 (8.2)	3 (4.9)	1.8	0.4–7.0	0.415			
Employment status								
Unemployed	63 (51.6)	25 (41.0)	1.5	0.8–2.9	0.175	1.4	0.3–1.6	0.477
Employed	59 (48.4)	36 (59.0)	Ref					
Occupational status								
Low	38 (64.4)	23 (63.9)	0.8	0.3–2.5	0.735	–		
Medium	9 (15.3)	7 (19.4)	0.6	0.2–2.6	0.534			
High	12 (20.3)	6 (16.7)	Ref					
Daily dose frequency								
Mean (SD)	1.7 (0.6)	1.4 (0.6)	2.6	1.4–4.6	**0.001***	2.5	1.2–5.6	**0.021***
Number of antihypertensive								
Mean (SD)	1.7 (0.8)	1.3 (0.6)	2.5	1.4–4.3	**0.001***	1.3	0.6–2.9	0.477
Duration of treatment (in years)								
Mean (SD)	3.1 (1.3)	2.8 (1.4)	0.2	0.9–1.5	0.215	0.9	0.7–1.3	0.590
Forgetfulness								
Yes	86 (72.3)	13 (21.7)	10.0	5.1–20.2	**< 0.001***	7.9	3.0–20.8	**< 0.001***
No	33 (27.7)	47 (78.3)	Ref			Ref		
Lack of funds								
Yes	67 (56.3)	18 (29.5)	3.3	1.7–5.0	**0.001***	2.8	1.1–6.9	**0.024***
No	52 (43.7)	43 (70.5)	Ref			Ref		
Busy schedule								
Yes	44 (37.0)	8 (13.3)	3.3	1.7–10.1	**0.002***	2.0	0.6–6.5	0.247
No	75 (63.0)	52 (86.7)	Ref			Ref		
Experiencing side effects								
Yes	40 (33.6)	3 (4.8)	10.2	2.5–25.1	**< 0.001***	7.6	1.7–33.0	**0.007***
No	79 (66.4)	58 (95.1)	Ref			Ref		
Belief in the efficacy of the drug								
Yes	102 (85.7)	57 (95.0)	0.3	0.1–1.1	0.075	4.9	0.9–26.9	0.066
No	17 (14.3)	3 (5.0)	Ref			Ref		
Herbs								

Table 2 Predictors of medication non-adherence among hypertensive patients in univariate and multivariate logistic regression *(Continued)*

Variables	Non-adherent		OR	95% CI	*p*-value	AOR	95% CI	*p*-value
	Yes ($N = 122$)	No ($N = 61$)						
Yes	25 (21.0)	13 (22.0)	1.1	0.5–2.3	0.875	–		
No	94 (79.0)	46 (78.0)	Ref					
Taste and smell of the drug								
Yes	1 (1.7)	3 (2.5)	0.7	0.1–6.5	0.717	–		
No	59 (98.3)	116 (97.5)						

SD Standard deviation, *OR* Odds ratio, *AOR* Adjusted Odd's ratio, *CI* Confidence interval
*significant *p*-value; $N = 183$; df = 1, $p < 0.001$, $R^2 = 0.453$

responsible for the inability of hypertensive patients to afford their medications in a timely manner, and consequently achieve a good hypertensive control. Instituting a universal health insurance scheme is likely to improve access to, and utilization of healthcare facilities as well as drug availability.

People who experienced side effects of the drugs were more likely to be non-adherent than their counterparts. This corroborates with the findings of Okoro and Ngong in Nigeria whereby, feeling worse (side effects of antihypertensive drugs) and feeling better were independent predictors of non-adherence [35]. This finding is supported by those of other sub-Saharan countries [36] and elsewhere [37]. Health care providers need to devote time in educating patients about this chronic disorder and its management. Affected individuals should be enlightened on the need to report to the hospital in case of any inconveniences posed by the drug rather than personally stopping the drugs without medical advice. Patients should also be given regular appointments for proper follow up and those who miss their appointments should be contacted or strategies put in place to ensure retention in care and limit loss to follow-up.

Evidence on the association between multiple factors including age and gender, and non-adherence to antihypertensive medication is controversial and warrants careful interpretation [11, 28]. Caro [38] and Gupta [24] found that females were more likely to be non-adherent to antihypertensive pharmacotherapy, contrary to the report of other authors in which males were more adherent to treatment than females [39–41]. On the other hand, some authors have reported no association between gender and adherence rate [42–44]. In a recent global meta-analysis on non-adherence to antihypertensive pharmacotherapy assessed using the MMAS-8 tool, Abegaz et al. reported that males were 1.3 times more likely to be non-adherent after a gender subgroup analysis, however their findings were not statistically significant [45]. Generally, younger age has been associated with greater odds of non-adherence in a number of studies [24, 42, 44], whereas in line with our findings, others have revealed no significant association [46]. These discrepancies with age as a predictor of non-adherence to antihypertensive pharmacotherapy could be attributed, in part, to the dichotomization of age, which results in loss of statistical power and precision [39, 47]. Furthermore, failure to explore this association using a multivariable logistic regression analysis to account for potential confounders [39, 42], differences in the technic or tool used to assess medication adherence [48] or the difference in sample sizes across studies are other alternate explanations.

Non-adherence was associated with poor blood pressure control. This finding accords with several results obtained in other countries in sub-Saharan Africa [17] and elsewhere [46, 49, 50]. The importance of adhering to medication cannot be overemphasized in the fight to prevent hypertension-related morbidity and mortality, as adequate

Table 3 Association between non-adherence to medication and blood pressure control[a]

Covariate	Blood pressure control status		OR (95% CI)	*P*-value
	Controlled ($N = 40$)	Uncontrolled ($N = 143$)		
Age in years, Mean (SD)	53.8 (14.0)	56.5 (11.8)	0.99 (0.96–1.04)	0.975
Gender (Male), N (%)	10 (25.0)	55 (38.5)	1.57 (0.63–3.90)	
Duration on treatment in years, Mean (SD)	2.75 (1.4)	3.06 (1.3)	0.86 (0.63–1.18)	0.353
Number of antihypertensive, mean (SD)	1.55 (0.7)	1.56 (0.6)	1.93 (0.98–3.77)	0.056
Adherence (Yes)	30 (75.0)	31 (78.3)	13.82 (5.46–34.95)	< 0.001**

OR Odd's ratio, *SD* Standard deviation, *CI* Confidence interval
[a]Model adjusted for age, gender, number of antihypertensive drugs and duration of treatment; **Significant *p*-value; $R^2 = 0.328$

treatment and control of BP has been highlighted among the strategies to reduce burden of CVD by 25% by the year 2025 [51]. However, this finding disagrees with that from other sub-Saharan countries [27] which could be attributed to a difference in study setting (community- versus hospital-based) and frequency of BP measurements (single versus multiple BP measures). For example, Mekonnen et al. 2017 [27] measured the BP just once. The average of multiple BP readings is critical to reduce type 1 error.

Strengths and limitations

Our study had a number of limitations. First, our cross-sectional design precluded assessment of temporality; rather we could only obtain associations. Second, only a single questionnaire was used to assess adherence in this study. The use of a second scale to measure medication adherence, such as the Medication Adherence Rating Scale would potentially have improved on the reliability of our findings. Third, pathologies such as chronic kidney disease, which can influence blood pressure control and indirectly adherence rates, were not excluded. Fourth, all seven health areas of this district could not be sampled due to financial restrictions, which limited a more complete picture on antihypertensive medication non-adherence in this health district. However, the authors believe that with a random selection of four out of the seven health areas gave each health area a fairly equal probability to be included. Fifth, participants on antihypertensive pharmacotherapy for just a year were recruited in this study. This could be a source of bias. Indeed, shorter treatment durations have been associated with higher non-adherence rates. In addition, predictors of medication non-adherence such as a poor patient-provider relationship was not captured in this study [11]. The Morisky medication adherence scale (MMAS) is largely based on self-report, making it liable to recall bias. Additionally, this can potentially lead to misclassification with individuals providing inaccurate responses. Despite these shortcomings, the MMAS has been widely validated in patients with hypertension [23] and other chronic diseases [52] with fairly good performance (sensitivity of 93% and specificity of 53%) in the clinic setting. It is thus the most widely accepted self-report tool for assessing medication adherence, especially to detect medication non-adherence with good blood pressure control data [23].

Conclusions

Two-thirds of our study population were non-adherent to antihypertensive pharmacotherapy. Forgetfulness, multiple daily doses, lack of finances, and side effects of drugs were associated with non-adherence. Non-adherence to medication was associated with uncontrolled blood pressure. The use of reminders like alarms, prescription of generic drugs, less complex regimens and intensive patient/carer education are of paramount importance in tackling these factors. Lessons from interventions promoting retention in care and medication adherence among persons living with HIV could be applied for hypertensive populations. In addition, institution of a universal insurance scheme is likely to improve patient accessibility to healthcare facilities and the availability of antihypertensive drugs.

Abbreviations

BHD: Buea Health District; BP: Blood pressure; CVD: Cardiovascular disease; HIV: Human immunodeficiency virus; LMIC: Low-income and middle-income countries; MMAS: Morisky medication adherence scale; OR: odds ratio

Acknowledgements

Our sincere gratitude goes to all the participants who sacrificed their time in order to take part in this study.

Authors' contributions

Study design and conception: NMA and LNA; data collection: NMA; data analysis and interpretation: VNA, JAA and LNA; manuscript drafting: NMA, VNA, LNA; critical revision of the manuscript: VNA, JAA, CAN, KNB, LNA. All authors read and approved the final manuscript.

Competing interests

The authors declare that they have no competing interests.

Author details

[1]Faculty of Health Sciences, University of Buea, Buea, Cameroon. [2]Djeleng Sub-divisional Hospital, Bafoussam, Cameroon. [3]Ibal Sub-divisional Hospital, Oku, Cameroon. [4]Faculty of Medicine & Biomedical Sciences, University of Yaoundé 1, Yaoundé, Cameroon. [5]Etoug-Ebe Baptist Hospital, Yaoundé, Cameroon. [6]Bamendjou District Hospital, Bamendjou, Cameroon. [7]Clinical Research Education, Networking & Consultancy (CRENC), Douala, Cameroon. [8]Faculty of Medicine, School of Public Health, The University of Queensland, Brisbane, Australia.

References

1. Bloch MJ. Worldwide prevalence of hypertension exceeds 1.3 billion. J Am Soc Hypertens. 2016;10:753–4.
2. Mills KT, Bundy JD, Kelly TN, Reed JE, Kearney PM, Reynolds K, et al. Global disparities of hypertension prevalence and control: a systematic analysis of population-based studies from 90 countries. Circulation. 2016;134:441–50.
3. Akintunde AA, Akintunde TS. Antihypertensive medications adherence among Nigerian hypertensive subjects in a specialist clinic compared to a general outpatient clinic. Ann Med Health Sci Res. 2015;5:173–8.

4. Adeloye D. An estimate of the incidence and prevalence of stroke in Africa: a systematic review and meta-analysis. PLoS One. 2014;9:e100724.
5. Lemogoum D, Van de Borne P, Lele CEB, Damasceno A, Ngatchou W, Amta P, et al. Prevalence, awareness, treatment, and control of hypertension among rural and urban dwellers of the far north region of Cameroon. J Hypertens. 2018;36:159–68.
6. Tianyi FL, Agbor VN, Njamnshi AK. Prevalence, awareness, treatment, and control of hypertension in Cameroonians aged 50 years and older: A community-based study. Health Sci Rep. 2018;1:e44.
7. Jingi A, Dzudie A, Noubiap JJ, Menanga AP, Aminde L, Fesuh B, et al. [PS 03–24] Hypertension prevalence, awareness and control in Cameroon: a systematic review with projections for 2025 and 2035. J Hypertens. 2016;34:e132.
8. Osterberg L, Blaschke T. Adherence to medication. N Engl J Med. 2005;353: 487–97.
9. van Veen WA. Treatment adherence in hypertension: problems and research. J R Coll Gen Pract Occas Pap. 1980;(12):22–5.
10. Burnier M, Wuerzner G, Struijker-Boudier H, Urquhart J. Measuring, analyzing, and managing drug adherence in resistant hypertension. Hypertension. 2013;62:218–25.
11. van der Laan DM, Elders PJM, Boons CCLM, Beckeringh JJ, Nijpels G, Hugtenburg JG. Factors associated with antihypertensive medication non-adherence: a systematic review. J Hum Hypertens. 2017;31:687–94.
12. Agbor VN, Essouma M, Ntusi NAB, Nyaga UF, Bigna JJ, Noubiap JJ. Heart failure in sub-Saharan Africa: a contemporaneous systematic review and meta-analysis. Int J Cardiol. 2018;257:207–15.
13. Nyaga U, Bigna JJR, Agbor VN, Essouma M, NAB N, Noubiap JJ. Data on the epidemiology of heart failure in Sub-Saharan Africa. Int J Cardiol. 2018; https://doi.org/10.1016/j.dib.2018.01.100.
14. Tadesse M, Eyob A, Akshay S, Asim A. Nonadherence to antihypertensive drugs. A systematic review and meta-analysis. Medicine. 2017;96:e5647.
15. Hussanin SM, Boonshuyar C, Ekram A. Non-adherence to antihypertensive treatment in essential hypertensive patients in Rajshahi, Bangladesh. Anwer Khan Modern Med Coll J. 2011;2:9–14.
16. Nguyen T-P-L, Schuiling-Veninga CCM, Nguyen TBY, Vu T-H, Wright EP, Postma MJ. Adherence to hypertension medication: quantitative and qualitative investigations in a rural northern Vietnamese community. PLoS One. 2017;12:e0171203.
17. Boima V, Ademola AD, Odusola AO, Agyekum F, Nwafor CE, Cole H, et al. Factors Associated with Medication Nonadherence among Hypertensives in Ghana and Nigeria. Int J Hypertens [Internet]. 2015; Available from: https://www.hindawi.com/journals/ijhy/2015/205716/. [cited 29 May 2018]
18. Akoko BM, Fon PN, Ngu RC, Ngu KB. Knowledge of hypertension and compliance with therapy among hypertensive patients in the Bamenda Health District of Cameroon: a cross-sectional study. Cardiol Ther. 2017;6:53–67.
19. Mbouemboue O, Tamanji M, Gambara R, Lokgue Y, Ngoufack J. Determinants of therapeutic nonadherence to antihypertensive treatment: a hospital-based study on outpatients in northern Cameroon. 2015.
20. Busari O, Olanrewaju T, Desalu O, Opadijo O, Kayode J, Agboola S, et al. Impact of PatientsAND#8217; Knowledge, Attitude and Practices on Hypertension on Compliance with Antihypertensive Drugs in a Resource-poor Setting. 2010.
21. Agbornkwai N. An assessment of the knowledge, attitutes and practice of preventive measures against HIV/AIDS among students of the University of Buea. Buea: University of Buea; 2012.
22. Ekram AS, Hussain SM, Boonshuyar C. Preliminary report on non-adherence to antihypertensive treatment in essential hypertensive patients: a community based survey. 2009.
23. Morisky DE, Ang A, Krousel-Wood M, Ward HJ. Predictive validity of a medication adherence measure in an outpatient setting. J Clin Hypertens (Greenwich). 2008;10:348–54.
24. Gupta P, Patel P, Štrauch B, Lai FY, Akbarov A, Marešová V, et al. Risk factors for nonadherence to antihypertensive TreatmentNovelty and significance. Hypertension. 2017;69:1113–20.
25. Natarajan N, Putnam W, Van Aarsen K, Beverley Lawson K, Burge F. Adherence to antihypertensive medications among family practice patients with diabetes mellitus and hypertension. Can Fam Physician. 2013;59:e93–100.
26. Jingi AM, Noubiap JJN, Onana AE, Nansseu JRN, Wang B, Kingue S, et al. Access to diagnostic tests and essential medicines for cardiovascular diseases and diabetes care: cost, Availability and Affordability in the West Region of Cameroon. PLOS ONE. 2014;9:e111812.
27. Mekonnen HS, Gebrie MH, Eyasu KH, Gelagay AA. Drug adherence for antihypertensive medications and its determinants among adult hypertensive patients attending in chronic clinics of referral hospitals in Northwest Ethiopia. BMC Pharmacol Toxicol. 2017;18:27.
28. Fitz-Simon N, Bennett K, Feely J. A review of studies of adherence with antihypertensive drugs using prescription databases. Ther Clin Risk Manag. 2005;1:93–106.
29. Jambedu HA. Adherence to anti-hypertensive medication regimens among patients attending the G.P.H.A. Hospital in Takoradi - Ghana. [Internet]. Thesis. 2006; Available from: http://ir.knust.edu.gh/xmlui/handle/123456789/677. [cited 31 May 2018]
30. Wariva E, January J, Maradzika J. Medication adherence among elderly patients with high blood pressure in Gweru, Zimbabwe. J Public Health Africa. 2014;5(1):304.
31. Ohene KB, Matowe L, Plange-Rhule J. Unaffordable drug prices: the major cause of non-compliance with hypertension medication in Ghana. J Pharm Pharm Sci. 2004;7:350–2.
32. Amira CO, Okubadejo NU. Factors influencing non-compliance with anti-hypertensive drug therapy in Nigerians. Niger Postgrad Med J. 2007;14:325–9.
33. Al-Ramahi R. Adherence to medications and associated factors: a cross-sectional study among Palestinian hypertensive patients. J Epidemiol Glob Health. 2015;5:125–32.
34. Dokainish H, Teo K, Zhu J, Roy A, AlHabib KF, ElSayed A, et al. Heart failure in Africa, Asia, the Middle East and South America: the INTER-CHF study. Int J Cardiol. 2016;204:133–41.
35. Okoro R, Ngong K. Assessment of patient's antihypertensive medication adherence level in non-comorbid hypertension in a tertiary hospital in Nigeria. 2012.
36. Chelkeba L, Dessie S. Antihypertension medication adherence and associated factors at Dessie hospital, north East Ethiopia, Ethiopia. International journal of research in medical. Sciences. 2017;1:191–7.
37. Jokisalo E, Kumpusalo E, Enlund H, Halonen P, Takala J. Factors related to non-compliance with antihypertensive drug therapy. J Hum Hypertens. 2002;16:577–83.
38. Caro JJ, Speckman JL, Salas M, Raggio G, Jackson JD. Effect of initial drug choice on persistence with antihypertensive therapy: the importance of actual practice data. Can Med Assoc J. 1999;160:41–6.
39. Khayyat SM, Khayyat SMS, Alhazmi RSH, Mohamed MMA, Hadi MA. Predictors of medication adherence and blood pressure control among Saudi hypertensive patients attending primary care clinics: a cross-sectional study. PLoS One. 2017;12:e0171255.
40. Benson S, Vance-Bryan K, Raddatz J. Time to patient discontinuation of antihypertensive drugs in different classes. Am J Health Syst Pharm. 2000;57:51–4.
41. Wogen J, Krelick CA, Livornese RC, Yokoyama K, Frech F. Patient adherence with amlodipine, Lisinopril, or valsartan therapy in a usual-care setting. J Manag Care Pharm. 2003;9:424–9.
42. Al Ghobain M, Alhashemi H, Aljama A, Bin Salih S, Assiri Z, Alsomali A, et al. Nonadherence to antihypertensive medications and associated factors in general medicine clinics. Patient Prefer Adherence. 2016;10:1415–9.
43. Tong X, Chu EK, Fang J, Wall HK, Ayala C. Nonadherence to antihypertensive medication among hypertensive adults in the United States—HealthStyles, 2010. J Clin Hypertens. 2016;18:892–900.
44. Degli Esposti E, Sturani A, Di Martino M, Falasca P, Novi MV, Baio G, et al. Long-term persistence with antihypertensive drugs in new patients. J Hum Hypertens. 2002;16:439–44.
45. Abegaz TM, Shehab A, Gebreyohannes EA, Bhagavathula AS, Elnour AA. Nonadherence to antihypertensive drugs: A systematic review and meta-analysis Medicine (Baltimore). 2017;96(4):e5641.
46. Hedna K, Hakkarainen KM, Gyllensten H, Jönsson AK, Sundell KA, Petzold M, et al. Adherence to antihypertensive therapy and elevated blood pressure: should we consider the use of multiple medications? PLoS One. 2015;10:e0137451.
47. Department of biostatistics, Vanderbilt University. Problems Caused by Categorizing Continuous Variables [Internet]. Available from: http://biostat.mc.vanderbilt.edu/wiki/Main/CatContinuous. [cited 4 June 2018]
48. Agbor VN, Takah NF, Aminde LN. Prevalence and factors associated with medication adherence among patients with hypertension in sub-Saharan Africa: protocol for a systematic review and meta-analysis. BMJ Open. 2018; 8:e020715.
49. Bramley TJ, Gerbino PP, Nightengale BS, Frech-Tamas F. Relationship of blood pressure control to adherence with antihypertensive monotherapy in 13 managed care organizations. J Manag Care Pharm. 2006;12:239–45.

5

Managing patients with prediabetes and type 2 diabetes after coronary events: individual tailoring needed

John Munkhaugen[1,10*], Jøran Hjelmesæth[2,3], Jan Erik Otterstad[4], Ragnhild Helseth[5,6], Stina Therese Sollid[7], Erik Gjertsen[7], Lars Gullestad[8,6], Joep Perk[9], Torbjørn Moum[10], Einar Husebye[7] and Toril Dammen[10]

Abstract

Background: Understanding the determinants associated with prediabetes and type 2 diabetes in coronary patients may help to individualize treatment and modelling interventions. We sought to identify sociodemographic, medical and psychosocial factors associated with normal blood glucose (HbA1c < 5.7%), prediabetes (HbA1c 5.7–6.4%), and type 2 diabetes.

Methods: A cross-sectional explorative study applied regression analyses to investigate the factors associated with glycaemic status and control (HbA_{1c} level) in 1083 patients with myocardial infarction and/or a coronary revascularization procedure. Data were collected from hospital records at the index event and from a self-report questionnaire and clinical examination with blood samples at 2–36 months follow-up.

Results: In all, 23% had type 2 diabetes, 44% had prediabetes, and 33% had normal blood glucose at follow-up. In adjusted analyses, type 2 diabetes was associated with larger waist circumference (Odds Ratio 1.03 per 1.0 cm, $p = 0.001$), hypertension (Odds Ratio 2.7, $p < 0.001$), lower high-density lipoprotein cholesterol (Odds Ratio 0.3 per1.0 mmol/L, $p = 0.002$) and insomnia (Odds Ratio 2.0, $p = 0.002$). In adjusted analyses, prediabetes was associated with smoking (Odds Ratio 3.3, $p = 0.001$), hypertension (Odds Ratio 1.5, $p = 0.03$), and non-participation in cardiac rehabilitation (Odds Ratio 1.7, $p = 0.003$). In patients with type 2 diabetes, a higher HbA_{1c} level was associated with ethnic minority background (standardized beta [β] 0.19, $p = 0.005$) and low drug adherence (β 0.17, $p = 0.01$). In patients with prediabetes or normal blood glucose, a higher HbA_{1c} was associated with larger waist circumference (β 0.13, $p < 0.001$), smoking (β 0.18, $p < 0.001$), hypertension (β 0.08, $p = 0.04$), older age (β 0.16, $p < 0.001$), and non-participation in cardiac rehabilitation (β 0.11, $p = 0.005$).

Conclusions: Along with obesity and hypertension, insomnia and low drug adherence were the major modifiable factors associated with type 2 diabetes, whereas smoking and non-participation in cardiac rehabilitation were the factors associated with prediabetes. Further research on the effect of individual tailoring, addressing the reported significant predictors of failure, is needed to improve glycaemic control.

Keywords: Secondary prevention, Coronary heart disease, Type 2 diabetes, Prediabetes, HbA_{1c}, Risk factor control, Glycaemic control, Psychosocial factors

* Correspondence: johmun@vestreviken.no
[1]Department of Medicine, Drammen Hospital, Vestre Viken Health Trust, Dronninggata 41, 3004 Drammen, Norway
[10]Department of Behavioural Sciences in Medicine and Faculty of Medicine, University of Oslo, Oslo, Norway
Full list of author information is available at the end of the article

Background

The prevalence of type 2 diabetes (T2D) is rapidly increasing with the obesity epidemic [1]. Diabetes is associated with doubled long-term mortality risk after coronary heart disease (CHD) events [2] and increases the risk of both macro- (i.e. cardiovascular events) and micro- (i.e. retino-, nephro- and neuropathy) vascular complications linearly with increasing blood levels of glycated haemoglobin (HbA_{1c}) [3, 4]. Intensive glycaemic control by multidrug treatment regimen, as performed in randomized controlled trials, reduces the risk of micro- and macro-vascular complications in T2D patients [5], but no improvement in cardiovascular or all-cause mortality has been demonstrated.

Attempts to delay the onset of T2D and prevent or delay microvascular and macrovascular complications drew attention to prediabetes, an intermediate form of dysglycaemia between normal blood glucose and overt diabetes [6]. In the most recent US guidelines, prediabetes is defined as HbA_{1c} between 5.7 and 6.4% (39–47 mmol/mol) [7]. Prediabetes may progress to T2D in up to 50% of cases within 5 years [8]. Also, patients with prediabetes are at increased risk of subsequent cardiovascular events after myocardial infarction [9]. Healthy lifestyle changes and treatment with antidiabetic drugs, as previously shown in clinical trials, may prevent or reduce the risk of T2D and its complications by 40–70% [10], emphasising the need for early disease detection and optimal management.

A complex array of demographic, psychosocial and behavioural factors influences T2D management [11–13], in addition to the causal risk factors increasing age, family history of diabetes, and obesity [7]. It remains to be studied carefully how these factors are associated with prediabetes and T2D, in particular within the CHD patient cohorts. The determinants of these diabetic manifestations may help to identify patients at risk, and to develop individualized interventions that may prevent prediabetes to progress to T2D and the subsequent cardiovascular events in both groups.

The NORwegian CORonary (NOR-COR) Prevention Study identifies sociodemographic, medical, and psychosocial factors associated with unfavourable risk factor control after CHD events in a cohort representing daily clinical practice (phase I). Moreover, the project aims to apply the factors of importance for risk factor control in developing tailored interventions (phase II) [14]. The present cross-sectional exploratory analysis sought to identify factors associated with glycaemic status and control among CHD patients. We hypothesise that potentially modifiable factors of importance for glycaemic status and control may be identified for those with prediabetes and T2D.

Methods

Design and population

The design, methods, and baseline patient characteristics of the NOR-COR Study have been described elsewhere [14]. In brief, 1789 consecutive patients undergoing a first or recurrent coronary event or treatment (i.e. acute myocardial infarction, coronary artery bypass graft operation, or percutaneous coronary intervention) were identified from the hospital medical records over the 3 years (2011–14) prior to study inclusion. All coronary angiograms and revascularization procedures were performed by experienced invasive cardiologists and thoracic surgeons at Oslo University Hospital. Reasons for exclusion of 423 patients were cognitive impairment ($n = 28$), psychosis ($n = 18$), drug abuse ($n = 10$), short life expectancy due to end-stage organ failure, malignant disease ($n = 136$), death following discharge from index hospitalization to invitation for the follow-up visit ($n = 160$), not being able to understand Norwegian ($n = 44$), or other reasons ($n = 27$). Of the remaining 1366 eligible patients, 1127 (83%) gave their informed consent to participate in a clinical visit and complete a comprehensive questionnaire [14]. Data on glycaemic status at follow-up were missing in 26 patients, while 18 patients with type 1 diabetes were excluded due to the different pathophysiology. Thus, a total of 1083 (96.1%) patients were included in the present study.

The study was conducted at two Norwegian hospitals (Drammen and Vestfold Hospital Trust) with a total catchment area of 380,000 inhabitants, corresponding to approximately 7% of the Norwegian population. The catchment areas have a blend of city and rural district population representative of Norwegian geography, economy, age distribution, morbidity, and mortality [15]. The level of education in this coronary population is in line with national data on cardiovascular disease patients [15].

Outcome assessment

The primary outcome variables were glycaemic status (T2D, prediabetes or normal blood glucose) and glycaemic control (HbA_{1c}) at follow-up. The diagnosis of T2D was defined as either i) treatment with antidiabetic drugs or a T2D diagnosis recovered from hospital records at the time of the index event or ii) the presence of $HbA_{1c} \geq 6.5\%$ (≥48 mmol/mol) at the follow-up visit. Normal blood glucose was defined by $HbA_{1c} < 5.7\%$ (< 39 mmol/mol), and prediabetes by HbA_{1c} between 5.7 and 6.4% (39–47 mmol/mol) at follow-up, without T2D diagnosis at the index event [7]. HbA_{1c} was categorized based on a single blood test. Non-fasting venous whole blood sampled in an EDTA-tube was analysed on a clinical chemistry analyzer (Tosoh G8, Tosoh Medics Inc., San Francisco, CA, US) at Drammen Hospital to avoid inter-laboratory bias [14].

Covariates (sociodemographic, medical, and psychosocial factors)

Demographic and medical factors registered from hospital medical records at the time of the index event:

- Demographic factors (age, sex, ethnic minority background defined as 1st and 2nd generation patients born in Asia, Africa or South America). Coronary history and treatment, cardiovascular medication, antidepressant medication, and somatic comorbidity summarized according to the Charlson comorbidity index.
- Participation in cardiac rehabilitation programs was confirmed by the hospital medical records and separate lists from the cardiac rehabilitation departments. In Drammen, cardiac rehabilitation includes a multidisciplinary one-day 'heart school' and exercise training twice per week for 6 weeks with start-up 2–6 weeks following the index event. Vestfold provides a comprehensive, multi-disciplinary program with individual and group approaches, motivational interviewing, education and exercise described previously [14]. Start-up is 2–3 weeks after the index event, followed by visits twice per week for 5 weeks, with exercise duration up to 6 months.

At follow-up 2–36 months after the index event, the following study factors were provided from:

- *Blood samples:* Total cholesterol, low density lipoprotein (LDL) cholesterol, high density lipoprotein (HDL) cholesterol, HbA_{1c}, and C-reactive Protein (CRP).
- *Clinical examination*: systolic and diastolic blood pressure measured with standardized procedures using a validated digital sphygmomanometer (Welch Allyn WA Connex ProBP 3400). Weight (nearest 0.5 kg), height (nearest 0.5 cm), waist circumference (nearest 0.5 cm).
- The self-report questionnaires [14, 16]:
  - Socio-demographic factors: marital status and education (low education was defined by completion of primary and secondary school only).
  - Medical factors: smoking, physical activity, current treatment with cardiovascular drugs, drug related side-effects and adherence (Poor drug adherence was defined by a score of > 2 on the Morisky 8-item medication adherence questionnaire).
  - Psychosocial factors: quality of life (Short-Form 12), anxiety and depression (Hospital Anxiety and Depression Scale (HADS), Type D personality (DS-14), insomnia (Bergen Insomnia Scale), illness perception (Brief illness perception questionnaire), and perceived risk perception.

The sociodemographic variables, somatic comorbidity including coronary history and treatment are descriptive factors, while the remaining medical and psychosocial factors are regarded as potentially modifiable [14]. The NOR-COR Study explores a comprehensive set of study factors in relation to the following six well-established modifiable risk factors of CHD: smoking, body mass index ≥30 kg/m^2, low or no physical activity (i.e. < 30 min moderate activity 2–3 times/week and never or < 1 time/week, respectively) [17], blood pressure ≥ 140/90 [80 in T2D] mmHg, LDL-cholesterol ≥1.8 mmol/L, and unfavourable glycaemic control (i.e.T2D and prediabetes). In the present study, addressing the risk factors T2D and prediabetes as primary independent variables, the remaining five risk factors are included as co-variates as indicated.

Statistical analyses

The descriptive associations between covariates and glycaemic status are presented as frequencies (%) and mean ± standard deviation (SD), as appropriate. The χ^2 test was used to compare proportions, and independent samples t-test to compare mean differences between groups. To identify the sub-set of predictors, in which all variables were statistically significant when multivariately controlled, a backwards stepwise elimination procedure was used to fit a multivariable logistic model, starting with the set of all socio-demographic, medical, and psychosocial factors with a p-value < 0.10 in bivariate analyses. Odds ratios (OR) and 95% confidence intervals (CI) for unfavourable glycaemic status by study factors were calculated. A similar backwards-stepwise elimination procedure was used to explore the linear association between HbA_{1c} and study factors in patients with T2D and prediabetes or neither, respectively. Beta (β) coefficients (standard error) for unfavourable glycaemic control by study factors were calculated. P-values < 0.05 were considered significant. Statistical interactions between study factors in ordinary least squares regressions, using HbA1c as dependent variable, were tested by entering two-way interaction terms in the equation, one at a time. Somatic co-morbidity and number of coronary events prior to the index event were not included in the regression models, as they could be direct effects rather than putative causes of T2D and unfavorable glycemic control. Statistical analyses were performed using SPSS version 21.

Results

Baseline sociodemographic, medical, and psychosocial factors differed by glycaemic status are shown in Table 1 and Table 2. ST-elevation myocardial infarction, non-ST-elevation myocardial infarction and stable/unstable angina were the index coronary events in 30% (n = 324), 50% (n = 542) and 20% (n = 217) of the patients, respectively. At the index hospitalization 16 % (n = 175) had a diagnosis of T2D recorded in the hospital records, whereas information about prediabetes was not available. The prevalence of T2D was 22% (n = 243) at follow-up

2–36 (median 16) months after the coronary event compatible with a further 6% ($n = 68$) having new-onset T2D, defined by $HbA_{1c} \geq 6.5\%$ (≥46 mmol/mol). Prediabetes (HbA1c 5.7–6.4% [39–47 mmol/mol]) was present in 44% ($n = 484$) at follow-up. Mean age at follow-up in patients with T2D and prediabetes was 62.3 (SD 9.1) years and 63.3 (SD 8.9) years, respectively, while 19% ($n = 69$) and 22% ($n = 108$) were women. Mean HbA_{1c} was 7.4% (57 mmol/mol) (SD 1.3) in subjects with T2D, and 55% ($n = 134$) did not reach the recommended treatment target of $HbA_{1c} < 7.0\%$ (< 53 mmol/mol), while 35% ($n = 85$) had $HbA_{1c} > 8\%$ (> 64 mmol/mol). Antidiabetic medication was prescribed to 70% ($n = 122$) of those with T2D at the index hospitalization, of whom 9% ($n = 15$) used combination therapy with insulin.

Compared to patients with prediabetes, those with T2D were more frequently of ethnic minority background, had more somatic comorbidities, lower coronary risk factor control, and higher levels of CRP. They also had a higher cardiac rehabilitation participation rate, and reported insomnia more frequently. Compared to patients with normal glucose levels, those with prediabetes were significantly older, less educated, had more somatic co-morbidity, lower cardiac rehabilitation participation rate, higher prevalence of daily smoking, and more unfavourable blood pressure control.

A multi-adjusted logistic regression analysis showed the independent determinants of T2D compared to prediabetes, as well as of prediabetes compared to normal blood glucose (Table 3). Larger waist circumference, unfavourable blood pressure control, lower HDL cholesterol, insomnia, and perceived restriction in future activities due to the coronary disease were statistically significant study factors associated with T2D. The quality of life mental component was inversely related to T2D. Older age, non-participation in cardiac rehabilitation, current smoking, and unfavourable blood pressure control were statistically significantly associated with prediabetes.

A multi-adjusted linear regression analysis showed the independent determinants of HbA_{1c} in patients with T2D and in patients with either prediabetes or normal blood glucose level (Table 4). Ethnic minority background and low drug adherence were statistically significant study factors associated with higher HbA_{1c} levels in patients with T2D. Older age, higher waist circumference, current smoking, non-participation in cardiac rehabilitation and unfavourable blood pressure control were factors associated with higher HbA_{1c} in patients with prediabetes or normal blood glucose. The positive gradient between HbA1c and age was significantly stronger among those with prediabetes or normal blood glucose compared to those with T2D (F 32.4, $p < 0.001$). A corresponding stronger association between HbA1c and non-participation in cardiac rehabilitation (F 18.2, $p < 0.001$) and unfavourable blood pressure control (F 7.6, $p = 0.006$) was found. The positive association between HbA1c and ethnic minority background (F 17.2, $p < 0.001$) and low drug adherence (F 29.2, $p < 0.001$) was significantly stronger among those with T2D compared to those with prediabetes or optimal blood sugar.

Discussion

In this cohort representing routine clinical practice, 2 of 3 patients had either prediabetes or T2D 2–36 months after hospitalization for a coronary event. The novelty of the present study is the detailed analysis of sociodemographic, medical and psychosocial factors providing new knowledge that potentially may improve risk factor control in the CHD population with disturbed glucose metabolism. The stratification of CHD patients into T2D, prediabetes and normal glucose control has been reported only once previously, in a US population without cardiovascular disease [18], and thus contributes to the originality of the present findings. Differences in the strength of associations of the potentially modifiable factors across the levels of glycemic status are demonstrated in the present study. For example, non-participation in cardiac rehabilitation emerges as a particular challenge in patients with prediabetes, while insomnia seems to be of particular importance for patients with T2D. The small sub-group of patients with ethnic minority background deserves particular attention due to their high risk of T2D and poor glycaemic control, as previously reported [19]. Patients with prediabetes at a cardiac event emerge as a particularly relevant subgroup to address more carefully in future secondary prevention of CHD.

The coronary index events in the present study are a ST-elevation myocardial infarction [20], and angina/non-ST-elevation myocardial infarction diagnoses [21]. Differences in pathophysiology, presentation and acute and long-term management of prediabetes and T2D could potentially influence our study results [20, 21]. Even though the relative number of patients with prediabetes and T2D varied by the coronary index diagnosis, the type of index event was not associated with glycemic status or control in adjusted analyses. An elegant randomised controlled study by Marfella R et al. demonstrated that optimal peri-procedural glycemic control up-regulated endothelial progenitor cell level and differentiation during acute ST-elevation myocardial infarction, with the results supporting the notion that tight glycemic control may improve myocardial salvage [22]. In our study, however, glycaemic status was assessed 2–36 months after the coronary event, and whether these mechanisms may explain any potential beneficial effect of tight glycemic control several months after the acute event is unknown.

Table 1 Sociodemographic and medical factors in coronary patients with normal blood glucose, prediabetes and type 2 diabetes

	Normal blood glucose	Prediabetes	Type 2 diabetes	*P*-Value	
	(*n* = 356, 32.4%)	(*n* = 484, 44.1%)	(*n* = 243, 22.4%)	Normal blood glucose vs. prediabetes	Type 2 diabetes vs. prediabetes
Socio-demographic factors					
Age in years at index event, mean (SD)	59.4 (9.9)	63.3 (8.9)	62.3 (9.1)	***	N.S.
Number of months from index event to follow-up, mean (SD)	16.2 (10.3)	17.0 (10.5)	18.3 (10.5)	N.S.	N.S.
Female sex, n (%)	69 (19.4)	108 (22.3)	49 (20.2)	N.S.	N.S.
Ethnic minority, n (%)[a]	5 (1.4)	10 (2.1)	18 (7.4)	N.S.	***
Living alone, n (%)	57 (16.0)	84 (17.4)	50 (21.7)	N.S.	N.S.
Low education, n (%)[b]	221 (62.1)	346 (71.5)	181 (76.1)	**	N.S.
Medical factors					
Coronary index diagnosis, n (%)					
Non-ST elevation myocardial infarction	170 (47.8)	247 (51.0)	123 (40.1)	N.S.	*
ST-elevation myocardial infarction	111 (31.1)	148 (30.6)	58 (23.9)	N.S.	N.S.
Stable or unstable angina	75 (21.1)	89 (18.4)	62 (25.5)	N.S.	N.S.
> 1 coronary event prior to the index event, n (%)	91 (25.6)	119 (24.6)	113 (46.5)	N.S.	***
Participation in cardiac rehabilitation, n (%)	183 (51.4)	206 (42.6)	139 (57.2)	*	***
Charlson co-morbidity score, mean (SD)	3.6 (1.4)	4.1 (1.3)	4.8 (1.5)	***	***
Chronic kidney disease (eGFR < 60), n (%)	30 (8.4)	58 (12.0)	45 (20.3)	N.S.	*
Antidepressant medication at the time of the index event, n (%)	16 (4.5)	16 (3.3)	21 (8.6)	N.S.	**
Coronary risk factors and medication at interview					
Low density lipoprotein cholesterol mmol/L, mean (SD)	2.15 (0.73)	2.09 (0.80)	2.07 (0.84)	N.S.	N.S.
Low density lipoprotein cholesterol ≥1.8 mmol/L, n (%)	222 (62.4)	273 (56.4)	122 (51.0)	N.S.	N.S.
High density lipoprotein cholesterol mmol/L, mean (SD)	1.19 (0.34)	1.16 (0.32)	1.02 (0.30)	N.S.	***
Current smoking, n (%)	49 (13.8)	115 (23.8)	53 (22.7)	***	N.S.
C-reactive protein in mg/L, mean (SD)	2.06 (2.13)	2.37 (2.73)	3.22 (2.89)	N.S.	***
C-reactive protein ≥2 mg/L, n (%)	123 (35.5)	172 (36.6)	131 (56.5)	N.S.	***
Physical activity < 30 min of moderate activity 2–3 times a week, n (%)	158 (44.5)	227 (48.4)	129 (54.2)	N.S.	N.S.
Physical activity < 1 time a week, n (%)	53 (14.9)	73 (15.1)	59 (24.9)	N.S.	**
Blood pressure ≥ 140/90 (80 in diabetes) mmHg, n (%)	118 (33.1)	198 (44.0)	129 (60.6)	***	***
Waist circumference, mean (SD)	100.1 (11.1)	101.3 (12.1)	108.5 (12.6)	N.S.	***
Waist circumference ≥ 102/88 cm in men/ women, n (%)	168 (51.5)	258 (57.5)	164 (76.6)	N.S.	***
Body Mass Index ≥30 kg/m^2, n (%)	84 (23.6)	133 (27.5)	116 (54.2)	N.S.	***
Fruit and vegetables < 2 units/day, n (%)	132 (37.6)	187 (38.6)	92 (39.7)	N.S.	N.S.
Fish meals < 3 times/week, n (%)	171 (48.0)	213 (44.0)	118 (48.6)	N.S.	N.S.
Medication at interview, n (%)					
Statin, n (%)	332 (93.3)	451 (93.2)	224 (92.2)	N.S.	N.S.
High-intensity statin therapy, n (%)	168 (47.2)	247 (51.0)	104 (55.9)	N.S.	N.S.
Aspirin, n (%)	351 (98.6)	467 (96.5)	235 (96.7)	N.S.	N.S.
Beta-blockers, n (%)	248 (69.7)	349 (72.1)	188 (77.4)	N.S.	N.S.

Table 1 Sociodemographic and medical factors in coronary patients with normal blood glucose, prediabetes and type 2 diabetes *(Continued)*

	Normal blood glucose	Prediabetes	Type 2 diabetes	*P*-Value	
	(*n* = 356, 32.4%)	(*n* = 484, 44.1%)	(*n* = 243, 22.4%)	Normal blood glucose vs. prediabetes	Type 2 diabetes vs. prediabetes
ACE-inhibitors or ARB, n (%)	166 (46.6)	232 (47.9)	143 (58.8)	N.S.	**
Low Morisky Score[c], n (%)	38 (10.7)	40 (8.3)	22 (9.6)	N.S.	N.S.

SD standard deviation, *NS* not significant, *eGFR* estimated glomerular filtration rate, *ACE* angiotensin converting enzyme, *ARB* angiotensin receptor blocker. *$p < 0.05$, **$p < 0.01$, ***$p < 0.001$

[a]Ethnic minority was defined as 1st and 2nd generation patients born in Asia, Africa and South America

[b]Low education was defined as completion of primary and secondary school only

[c]Scores: > 2 on the Morisky 8-item medication adherence questionnaire, indicating low adherence

Table 2 Psychosocial factors, quality of life, illness and risk factor perception in coronary patients with normal blood glucose, prediabetes and type 2 diabetes

Study factors	Normal blood glucose	Prediabetes	Type 2 diabetes	*P*-Value	
	(*n* = 356, 32.4%)	(*n* = 484,44.1)	(*n* = 243, 22.4%)	Prediabetes vs. normal blood glucose	Type 2 diabetes vs. prediabetes
Psychosocial factors and quality of life					
Hospital Anxiety and Depression Score-Anxiety ≥8, n (%)	66 (19.2)	99 (21.5)	53 (22.9)	NS	NS
Hospital Anxiety and Depression Score-Depression ≥8, n (%)	49 (14.0)	62 (13.3)	40 (17.2)	NS	NS
Type D personality disorder, n (%)	62 (17.4)	82 (16.9)	44 (18.7)	NS	NS
Worry score (Penn State Worry Questionnaire), mean (SD)	37.8 (12.4)	38.0 (13.0)	38.9 (12.5)	NS	NS
Insomnia, n (%)[a]	157 (44.1)	186 (38.4)	124 (54.1)	NS	***
Quality of life (SF-12), physical component summary, mean (SD)	39.0 (4.7)	38.3 (4.6)	37.9 (5.1)	*	NS
Quality of life (SF-12), mental component summary, mean (SD)	45.9 (6.1)	46.5 (6.4)	45.0 (6.8)	NS	**
Illness and risk factor perception (1–10 Likert scale), mean (SD)					
What do you feel is the likelihood of having a new heart attack over the next 12 months?	2.5 (2.3)	2.7 (2.4)	3.1 (2.6)	NS	NS
How much do you feel you can help reduce your risk of having another heart attack?	6.4 (2.7)	6.6 (2.8)	6.1 (2.8)	NS	*
How much do you think you will have to restrict your activities in the long-term due to your heart condition?	3.0 (2.7)	3.3 (2.7)	4.1 (2.9)	NS	***
Brief Illness Perception (1–10 Likert scale), mean (SD)					
How much does your illness affect your life? (consequences)	3.6 (2.8)	3.6 (2.8)	4.3 (2.9)	NS	**
How long do you think your illness will continue? (timeline)	7.7 (3.3)	7.6 (3.3)	7.9 (3.0)	NS	NS
How much control do you feel you have over your illness? (personal control)	5.9 (2.8)	5.9 (2.9)	5.9 (2.7)	NS	NS
How much do you think your treatment can help you? (treatment control)	7.3 (2.3)	7.4 (2.4)	7.2 (2.4)	NS	NS
How much do you experience symptoms from your illness? (identity)	3.0 (2.5)	3.0 (2.7)	4.0 (2.9)	NS	***
How concerned are you about your illness? (concern)	3.5 (2.8)	3.6 (3.0)	4.0 (3.1)	NS	NS
How well do you feel you understand your illness? (understanding)	6.9 (2.6)	7.0 (2.6)	6.7 (2.5)	NS	NS
How much does your illness affect you emotionally? (emotional response)	3.4 (3.0)	3.4 (3.0)	4.0 (3.0)	NS	*

SD standard deviation, *NS*; not significant, *SF* short form*$p < 0.05$, **$p < 0.01$, ***$p < 0.001$

[a]Insomnia (Bergen insomnia scale): a 7 -item self-report inventory designed to assess primary insomnia

Table 3 Multivariable[a] odds ratios (confidence intervals and *p*-values) for prediabetes and type 2 diabetes by study factors

Study factors	Prediabetes (1) vs. normal blood glucose (0)		Type 2 diabetes (1) vs. prediabetes (0)	
	Odds ratio (95% CI)		Odds ratio (95% CI)	
Age at index event per 1.0 year	1.05 (1.03–1.07)	< 0.001		NS
Waist circumference per 1.0 cm		NS	1.03 (1.01–1.05)	0.001
Non-participation in cardiac rehabilitation	1.69 (1.19–2.40)	0.003		NS
Current smoking	3.29 (2.00–5.42)	0.001		NS
Blood pressure ≥ 140/90 (80 in diabetes) mmHg	1.48 (1.04–2.11)	0.030	2.67 (1.74–4.11)	0.001
Quality of life (SF-12), mental component per 1.0 points		NS	0.97 (0.94–0.99)	0.042
Insomnia[b]		NS	1.98 (1.30–3.05)	0.002
How much do you think you will have to restrict your activity in the long term due to your heart condition? per 1.0 points[c]		NS	1.14 (1.06–1.23)	0.001

SD standard deviation, *NS*: not significant, *CI* confidence interval
[a]Multi-adjusted models using backward step-wise elimination in binary logistic regression analyses adjusted for study and starting with risk factors showing $p < 0.1$ in bivariate association
[b]Insomnia (Bergen insomnia scale): a 7 -item self-report inventory designed to assess primary insomnia
[c]Measured by the Perceived risk perception Questionnaire (1–10 Likert scale)

Although long-term mortality after coronary events has declined in line with improved acute treatment and better risk factor management, patients with T2D are at particular risk for recurrent cardiovascular events [23]. Similarly, a meta-analysis has also demonstrated that compared to subjects with normal glycaemic status, those with prediabetes experienced a 20% increased risk for cardiovascular disease [9]. The mechanisms behind the poor prognosis in patients with T2D and prediabetes are not completely understood, but a higher prevalence of complications in combination with lack of appropriate secondary preventive treatment contribute [24]. It was therefore not unexpected that patients with T2D had most somatic comorbidty and poorest overall risk factor control, followed by subjects with prediabetes. Subjects with normal blood glucose had least comorbidity and best coronary risk profile. Interestingly, T2D patients were characterized by central obesity, unfavourable blood pressure, and low levels of HDL cholesterol, which constitute important components of the metabolic syndrome [25].

The T2D patients in our study were characterized by subclinical inflammation. The association between high-sensitivity CRP and T2D, however, was no longer significant when adjusting for somatic comorbidity and other cardiovascular risk factors in our study. Inflammation, particularly in diabetes, plays a pivotal role in the series of events that result in plaque disruption and thus influence the incidence and severity of cardiovascular events in T2D patients [26]. The involvement of the gene regulating transcription factor sirtuin 6 in the inflammatory

Table 4 HbA1c regressed on study factors by multi-adjusted[a] linear regression analysis

	Prediabetes or normal blood glucose ($n = 840$)			Type 2 diabetes ($n = 243$)		
Study factors	b (standard error)	Standardized β		b (standard error)	Standardized β	
Age at index event per year	0.006 (0.001)	0.157	$p < 0.001$			
Ethnic minority background			NS	1.06 (0.370)	0.193	$p = 0.005$
Non-participation in cardiac rehabilitation	0.074 (0.027)	0.106	$p = 0.005$			NS
Waist circumference per 1.0 cm	0.003 (0.001)	0.131	$p < 0.001$			NS
Current smoking	0.157 (0.033)	0.177	$p < 0.001$			NS
Blood pressure ≥ 140/90 (80 in diabetes) mmHg	0.056 (0.027)	0.079	$p = 0.037$			NS
Low self-report drug adherence[b]			NS	0.668 (0.265)	0.168	$p = 0.012$

NS not significant
Unstandardized (b) and standardized (β) regression coefficients. [a]Adjusted for all variables with $p \leq 0.10$ retained in backward elimination linear regression analysis
[b]Scores: > 2 on the Morisky 8-item medication adherence questionnaire indicating low adherence

diabetic atherosclerotic lesions was recently established. Incretin-based therapies (i.e. GLP-1 receptor agonists, and dipeptidyl peptidase-4 inhibitors) resulted in a greater sirtuin 6 expression and less inflammation and oxidative stress in carotid plaques of diabetic versus non-diabetic patients, indicating a more stable plaque phenotype [27]. The prevalence and predictors of culprit coronary plaque rupture identified by optical coherence tomography in patients undergoing coronary angiography was recently described in a meta-analysis by Iannaccone et al. which showed high rates of plaque rupture in patients with acute coronary syndrome [28]. Hypertension was the only clinical predictor for ST-elevation myocardial infarction, whereas increasing age, diabetes and hyperlipidemia were clinical predictors in non- ST-elevation myocardial infarction and unstable angina [28]. Another interesting endocrinological aspect of inflammation is the association with subclinical hypothyroidism independent of the traditional risk factors, as demonstrated by Marfella et al. [29]. Their study showed a potential interplay between subclinical hypothyroidism and inflammatory activity in atherosclerotic plaque progression towards instability, and that synthetic levothyroxine replacement therapy might contribute to plaque stabilization and thus improved prognosis by inhibiting the immunity-dependent plaque rupture in patients with subclinical hypothyroidism [29].

Low self-reported drug adherence was significantly associated with higher HbA_{1c} level in T2D, but not in prediabetic patients. Among patients with T2D having HbA_{1c} > 8.0% (64 mmol/mol), 30% did not use antidiabetic drugs, while only 9% used combination therapy with antidiabetic drugs and insulin. Intensified antidiabetic treatment and strategies to improve drug adherence therefore appear to be the major factors needed to improve glycaemic control in T2D patients. The newer hypoglycemic drugs, in particular incretins, are recommended for T2D patients with established CHD [6], and their potential beneficial pleiotropic effects on atherosclerotic plaque functionality and thus clinical outcome was recently documented in patients with a non-obstructive coronary artery stenosis non-ST-elevation myocardial infarction event [30].

In a long-term follow-up of patients with T2D and microalbuminuria without CHD participating in the Steno-2 trial, Gæde et al. showed that intensive target-driven intervention with multiple drug combinations and behaviour modification had sustained beneficial effects on the incidence of cardiovascular events and mortality compared to conventional multifactorial treatment [31]. The intensive drug regimen included higher dosages of statins and ACE-inhibitors than that of conventional treatment, resulting in lower LDL cholesterol and systolic blood pressure. These findings emphasize the importance of adequate prescription of and adherence to secondary preventive drug therapy in T2D patients.

The risk factors obesity, smoking and unfavorable blood pressure control were also significantly associated with increasing HbA_{1c} level in the group of patients with prediabetes or normal blood glucose, but not in those with T2D. The pharmacological treatment of T2D, aiming at HbA_{1c} control, may partly account for these differences at group level. The present finding thus emphasizes the particular need to address glycemic control through appropriate lifestyle changes and drug treatement, even in CHD patients without T2D [10].

Participation in multidisciplinary cardiac rehabilitation programme is strongly recommended and has proven beneficial for several cardiovascular risk factors in CHD patients with and without diabetes [32]. Participation in a comprehensive cardiac rehabilitation program was associated with improved risk profile as well as drug adherence in a recent publication derived from our data set [33]. In the present study, the participation rate in cardiac rehabilitation was lowest in patients with prediabetes, and was significantly related to increasing HbA_{1c} level. Even though patients with T2D had the highest participation rate in cardiac rehabilitation, more than 40% did not participate. Efforts to increase the participation rate in effective preventive cardiac rehabilitation programs are of particular importance for both patients with prediabetes and T2D, as non-participation appears to contribute to poor risk factor control.

No differences in psychosocial factors (i.e. anxiety, depression, worry, type D personality illness perception) were found in patients with prediabetes or with T2D in the present study, apart from the higher prevalence of insomnia among T2D compared with prediabetic patients. Psychosocial factors like diabetes distress, depression, and anxiety are prevalent in general populations with diabetes [34], and associated with increased risk of developing T2D in subjects with prediabetes [35]. The present selection of CHD patients may in part account for differences when compared with studies of diabetic populations. Furthermore, the level of psychosocial distress may decrease with increasing time since CHD events [36] and the association between psychosocial factors and glycaemic status may potentially be different if these factors had been assessed at the time of the index event. According to a recent study [12], depression and other psychosocial factors were not associated with the HbA_{1c} level in patients with T2D. Diabetes distress has recently been suggested to be more important for glycaemic control in patients with diabetes than clinical depression or depressive symptoms [13, 37].

The prevalence of insomnia accords to previous reports from the general population [38] and T2D patients [39]. A significant relationship between sleep problems and increased HbA_{1c} has been found in most, but not all, studies [40]. Patients with T2D and sleep problems have been considered a high-risk group for disease progression and might have resistance to standard treatment for T2D [40]. The pathways linking insomnia and glycaemic control remain unknown and are not determined in our study applying a cross-sectional design. The high prevalence of insomnia in T2D in the present study favours the previous recommendation that screening for sleep disturbance should be part of the management of T2D [41]. Sleep disorders are in general likely to be under-recognized and under-reported in the health care system [38]. Effective interventions to improve insomnia (pharmacotherapy and cognitive behaviour therapy) are available [40]. Interestingly, few studies have addressed the relationship between sleep and prediabetes. We did not find a significant association between insomnia and prediabetes, as reported by two previous studies excluding patients with CVD [42, 43]. Selection bias and differences in assessment methods may explain the differences. Separate insomnia symptoms (e.g. sleep onset, maintenance, early awakening, feeling adequately rested) were not explored separately in the present study. Which insomnia/sleep symptoms may have the strongest associations with prediabetes and T2D should be explored in future studies.

Immigrants from Asia and Africa living in Europe have a higher prevalence of T2D and are diagnosed earlier in life compared to native Europeans [44, 45]. In line with this, our coronary population had a three times higher prevalence of first and second generation ethnic minorities among patients with T2D compared to those with normoglycemia or prediabetes. Similar to several earlier studies [19], our study also found ethnic minorities with T2D to have inferior glycaemic control. Ethnic disparities in sociodemographic, cultural, and psychosocial factors may contribute to the observed ethnic inequalities in diabetes management [46]. In this respect, the high frequency of clinically significant symptoms of anxiety (29%), depression (24%), and insomnia (75%) observed in the subgroup with ethnic minority background, is a potentially important observation in the present study. Although these results must be interpreted with care due to the small numbers, the findings call for further studies to explore the role of psychosocial factors in ethnic minorities. Furthermore, these findings may encourage clinicians to recognize psychosocial distress as a potential barrier to secondary prevention in cardiovascular disease and in the management of T2D.

The proportion of patients with known T2D at the time of the index event (16%) was lower than reported in the latest EuroAspire survey (33%) [47], with comparable inclusion criteria including age distribution, and prevalence of obesity. Patient inclusion from largely academic centres [47] with potentially more focus on coronary prevention as well as more systematically screening for T2D than in everyday clinical practice, may, in part, account for the difference. At follow-up, an additional 6% of our patients fulfilled the diagnostic criteria for T2D, whereas the prevalence of undetected T2D in EuroAspire was 19%. Differences in prevalence rates may be explained by differences in measurements, as the latter study also screened the patients by an oral glucose tolerance test [47]. Systematic screening with both HbA_{1c} and oral glucose tolerance test has recently been proven to identify more individuals with T2D than each of them alone [48]. Thus, more patients with T2D would potentially have been diagnosed in the present study if screened by both tests. This highlights the need for better integration of systematic screening strategies for T2D after hospitalization for coronary events.

Study limitations and strengths

Most study factors in the present study were measured at one point in time and are thus prone to measurement and recall bias. However, a reproducibility study of the NOR-COR questionnaire demonstrated highly acceptable test-retest values for all key items and instruments [16]. The sample size does not allow sub-group analyses (e.g. age and gender) in the subgroup with T2D. The validity of using a single HbA1c measurement for the diagnosis of diabetes is suboptimal, as WHO guidelines advocate at least one additional HbA1c or plasma glucose test result with a value in the diabetic range in order to confirm the diagnosis; either fasting, from a random (casual) sample, or from the oral glucose tolerance test (OGTT) [49]. For the index hospitalization, however, diabetic status was based upon treatment with antidiabetic drugs or a T2D diagnosis recovered from hospital records at the time of the index event. Since diabetes diagnostics were not performed routinely at the time of the index event, the proportion of patients receiving their first T2D diagnosis during the index hospitalization remains unknown. Due to this limitation of the diagnostic test, some asymptomatic patients with diabetes may have been missed at follow-up. Our diagnostic criteria are, however, in accordance with the most recent US guidelines [7] and those of the WHO [49]. Furthermore, reporting bias of the T2D diagnosis in the hospital medical records might have occurred. Accordingly, some of the patients classified as new-onset T2D based HbA_{1c} at follow-up may have also had known T2D at the time of the index event. Our study design did not incorporate echocardiographic measurements in order to detect possible deterioration in left ventricular function in patients with ST-elevation myocardial infarction who had conventional glycaemic control. Although this study provides a comprehensive evaluation of determinants associated with prediabetes and T2D, additional confounders should be considered, including family history of diabetes, the duration of T2D and details on T2D management in general practice. Moreover, information about the different oral antidiabetic drugs prescribed at the time of the index coronary event and the reasons for admission to or non-participation with cardiac rehabilitation were not available. We did not assess sleep duration and objective measures of sleep and did not control for use of hypnotics, sedative, use of caffeine and obstructive sleep apnoea syndrome. The retrospective design with follow up times of 2–36 months after the index coronary event gives some indication of how HbA_{1c} and the study factors vary by time. A prospective design with repeated measurements is required to explore the influence of time properly. The representative cohort from routine clinical practice, the high participation rate (i.e. 83%) and the comprehensive data set are important strengths of the study.

Conclusion

Prediabetes and T2D are prevalent conditions both prior and subsequent to coronary events. Along with obesity and hypertension, insomnia and low drug adherence were the major modifiable factors associated with T2D, whereas smoking and non-participation in cardiac rehabilitation were the factors associated with prediabetes. Further research on the effect of individual tailoring, addressing the reported significant predictors of failure, is needed to improve glycaemic control.

Abbreviations

CHD: Coronary heart disease; CRP: C-reactive protein; HbA_{1c}: Glycated haemoglobin; HDL-C: High-density lipoprotein-cholesterol; LDL-C: low-density lipoprotein-cholesterol; T2D: Type 2 diabetes

Acknowledgements

The NOR-COR project originates from the Department of Medicine, Drammen Hospital Trust, with the study carried out at both Drammen and Vestfold Hospitals. The project developed through collaboration with research communities at the University of Oslo. The authors thank the study patients for participating and the study personnel for their invaluable contribution. The authors also thank Matthew McGee at the Center for Morbid Obesity at Vestfold Hospital for proofreading the manuscript.

Funding

The study was funded by grants from the Department of Medicine, Drammen Hospital Trust (grant number 1703001 project 9603003) and the Department for Cardiology, Vestfold Hospital Trust (grant number 703110 project 19440). Munkhaugen receives funding from the National Association for Public Health ("Nasjonalforeningen for Folkehelsen").

Authors' contributions

TD, JEO, JP, LG, EG, EH and JM contributed to the design of the study. JM, TM and RH contributed to the analysis, while all authors (TD, JEO, JP, LG, EG, EH, JH, RH, STS, TM, JM) contributed to the interpretation of data. JM drafted the manuscript and EH, TD, STS, and JH contributed significantly to the preparation. All the authors critically revised the manuscript and gave final approval, and agree to be accountable for all aspects of the work, ensuring both its integrity and accuracy.

Competing interests

The authors declare that they have no competing interests.

Author details

[1]Department of Medicine, Drammen Hospital, Vestre Viken Health Trust, Dronninggata 41, 3004 Drammen, Norway. [2]Morbid Obesity Centre, Vestfold Hospital Trust, Tønsberg, Norway. [3]Department of Endocrinology, Morbid Obesity and Preventive Medicine, Institute of Clinical Medicine, University of Oslo, Oslo, Norway. [4]Department of Medicine, Vestfold Hospital Trust, Tønsberg, Norway. [5]Centre for Clinical Heart Research, Department of Cardiology, Oslo University Hospital Ullevål, Oslo, Norway. [6]Faculty of Medicine, University of Oslo, Oslo, Norway. [7]Department of Medicine, Drammen Hospital Trust, Drammen, Norway. [8]Department of Cardiology, Oslo University Hospital Rikshospitalet, Oslo, Norway. [9]Linneus University, Kalmar, Sweden. [10]Department of Behavioural Sciences in Medicine and Faculty of Medicine, University of Oslo, Oslo, Norway.

References

1. Gregg EW, Cheng YJ, Narayan KM, Thompson TJ, Williamson DF. The relative contributions of different levels of overweight and obesity to the increased prevalence of diabetes in the United States: 1976-2004. Prev Med. 2007;45:348–52.
2. Donahoe SM, Stewart GC, McCabe CH, Mohanavelu S, Murphy SA, Cannon CP, Antman EM. Diabetes and mortality following acute coronary syndromes. JAMA. 2007;298:765–75.
3. Sabanayagam C, Liew G, Tai ES, Shankar A, Lim SC, Subramaniam T, Wong TY. Relationship between glycated haemoglobin and microvascular complications: is there a natural cut-off point for the diagnosis of diabetes? Diabetologia. 2009;52:1279–89.
4. Singer DE, Nathan DM, Anderson KM, Wilson PW, Evans JC. Association of HbA1c with prevalent cardiovascular disease in the original cohort of the Framingham heart study. Diabetes. 1992;41:202–8.
5. Hayward RA, Reaven PD, Wiitala WL, Bahn GD, Reda DJ, Ge L, McCarren M, Duckworth WC, Emanuele NV, Investigators V. Follow-up of glycemic control and cardiovascular outcomes in type 2 diabetes. N Engl J Med. 2015;372:2197–206.
6. Fox CS, Golden SH, Anderson C, Bray GA, Burke LE, de Boer IH, Deedwania P, Eckel RH, Ershow AG, Fradkin J, et al. Update on prevention of cardiovascular disease in adults with type 2 diabetes mellitus in light of recent evidence. Diabetes Care. 2015;38:1777–803.
7. American Diabetes Association. Classification and Diagnosis of Diabetes. Diabetes Care. 2017;40:S11–s24.
8. American Diabetes Association. Standards of medical care in diabetes-2011. Diabetes Care. 2011;34 Suppl 1:S11–S61.
9. Huang Y, Cai X, Mai W, Li M, Hu Y. Association between prediabetes and risk of cardiovascular disease and all cause mortality: systematic review and meta-analysis. BMJ. 2016;355:i5953.
10. Gillies CL, Abrams KR, Lambert PC, Cooper NJ, Sutton AJ, Hsu RT, Khunti K. Pharmacological and lifestyle interventions to prevent or delay type 2 diabetes in people with impaired glucose tolerance: systematic review and meta-analysis. BMJ. 2007;334:299.
11. Aikens JE. Prospective associations between emotional distress and poor outcomes in type 2 diabetes. Diabetes Care. 2012;35:2472–8.
12. Aghili R, Polonsky WH, Valojerdi AE, Malek M, Keshtkar AA, Esteghamati A, Heyman M, Khamseh ME. Type 2 diabetes: model of factors associated with glycemic control. Can J Diabetes. 2016;40:424–30.
13. Fisher L, Mullan JT, Arean P, Glasgow RE, Hessler D, Masharani U. Diabetes distress but not clinical depression or depressive symptoms is associated with glycemic control in both cross-sectional and longitudinal analyses. Diabetes Care. 2010;33:23–8.
14. Munkhaugen J, Sverre E, Peersen K, Gjertsen E, Gullestad L, Moum T, Otterstad JE, Perk J, Husebye E, Dammen T. The role of medical and psychosocial factors for unfavourable coronary risk factor control. Scand Cardiovasc J. 2015;50:1–32.
15. Statistics Norway. https://www.ssb.no/befolkning/statistikker/flytting (Accessed 25 Apr 2017) and http://cvdnor.b.uib.no/files/2013/08/CVDNOR-Data-and-Quality-Report1.pdf (Date of origination: July, 2013. Accessed 25 May 2016).
16. Peersen K, Munkhaugen J, Gullestad L, Dammen T, Moum T, Otterstad JE. Reproducibility of an extensive self-report questionnaire used in secondary coronary prevention. Scand J Public Health. 2017;45:269–76.
17. Kurtze N, Rangul V, Hustvedt BE, Flanders WD. Reliability and validity of self-reported physical activity in the Nord-Trøndelag health study: HUNT 1. Scand J Public Health. 2008;36:52–61.

18. Okwechime IO, Roberson S, Odoi A. Prevalence and predictors of pre-diabetes and diabetes among adults 18 years or older in Florida: a multinomial logistic modeling approach. PLoS One. 2015;10:e0145781.
19. Kirk JK, Bell RA, Bertoni AG, Arcury TA, Quandt SA, Goff DC Jr, Narayan KM. Ethnic disparities: control of glycemia, blood pressure, and LDL cholesterol among US adults with type 2 diabetes. Ann Pharmacother. 2005;39:1489–501.
20. Ibanez B, James S, Agewall S, Antunes MJ, Bucciarelli-Ducci C, Bueno H, Caforio ALP, Crea F, Goudevenos JA, Halvorsen S, et al. 2017 ESC guidelines for the management of acute myocardial infarction in patients presenting with ST-segment elevation. Eur Heart J. 2018;39:119–77.
21. Anderson JL, Adams CD, Antman EM, Bridges CR, Califf RM, Casey DE Jr, Chavey WE 2nd, Fesmire FM, Hochman JS, Levin TN, et al. 2012 ACCF/AHA focused update incorporated into the ACCF/AHA 2007 guidelines for the management of patients with unstable angina/non-ST-elevation myocardial infarction. J Am Coll Cardiol. 2013;61:e179–347.
22. Marfella R, Rizzo MR, Siniscalchi M, Paolisso P, Barbieri M, Sardu C, Savinelli A, Angelico N, Del Gaudio S, Esposito N, et al. Peri-procedural tight glycemic control during early percutaneous coronary intervention up-regulates endothelial progenitor cell level and differentiation during acute ST-elevation myocardial infarction: effects on myocardial salvage. Int J Cardiol. 2013;168:3954–62.
23. Lenzen M, Ryden L, Ohrvik J, Bartnik M, Malmberg K, Scholte Op Reimer W, Simoons ML. Diabetes known or newly detected, but not impaired glucose regulation, has a negative influence on 1-year outcome in patients with coronary artery disease. Eur Heart J. 2006; 27:2969–74.
24. Norhammar A, Malmberg K, Diderholm E, Lagerqvist B, Lindahl B, Ryden L, Wallentin L. Diabetes mellitus: the major risk factor in unstable coronary artery disease even after consideration of the extent of coronary artery disease and benefits of revascularization. J Am Coll Cardiol. 2004;43:585–91.
25. Grundy SM, Cleeman JI, Daniels SR, Donato KA, Eckel RH, Franklin BA, Gordon DJ, Krauss RM, Savage PJ, Smith SC Jr, et al. Diagnosis and management of the metabolic syndrome: an American Heart Association/ National Heart, Lung, and Blood Institute scientific statement. Circulation. 2005;112:2735–52.
26. Creager MA, Luscher TF, Cosentino F, Beckman JA. Diabetes and vascular disease: pathophysiology, clinical consequences, and medical therapy: part I. Circulation. 2003;108:1527–32.
27. Balestrieri ML, Rizzo MR, Barbieri M, Paolisso P, D'Onofrio N, Giovane A, Siniscalchi M, Minicucci F, Sardu C, D'Andrea D, et al. Sirtuin 6 expression and inflammatory activity in diabetic atherosclerotic plaques: effects of incretin treatment. Diabetes. 2015;64:1395–406.
28. Iannaccone M, Quadri G, Taha S, D'Ascenzo F, Montefusco A, Omede' P, Jang IK, Niccoli G, Souteyrand G, Yundai C, et al. Prevalence and predictors of culprit plaque rupture at OCT in patients with coronary artery disease: a meta-analysis. Eur Heart J Cardiovasc Imaging. 2016;17:1128–37.
29. Marfella R, Ferraraccio F, Rizzo MR, Portoghese M, Barbieri M, Basilio C, Nersita R, Siniscalchi LI, Sasso FC, Ambrosino I, et al. Innate immune activity in plaque of patients with untreated and L-thyroxine-treated subclinical hypothyroidism. J Clin Endocrinol Metab. 2011;96:1015–20.
30. Marfella R, Sardu C, Calabrò P, Siniscalchi M, Minicucci F, Signoriello G, Balestrieri ML, Mauro C, Rizzo MR, Paolisso G, et al. Non-ST-elevation myocardial infarction outcomes in patients with type 2 diabetes with non-obstructive coronary artery stenosis: effects of incretin treatment. Diabetes Obes Metab. 2018;20:723–9.
31. Gaede P, Lund-Andersen H, Parving HH, Pedersen O. Effect of a multifactorial intervention on mortality in type 2 diabetes. N Engl J Med. 2008;358:580–91.
32. Ofori SN, Kotseva K. Comparison of treatment outcomes in patients with and without diabetes mellitus attending a multidisciplinary cardiovascular prevention programme (a retrospective analysis of the EUROACTION trial). BMC Cardiovasc Disord. 2015;15:11–7.
33. Peersen K, Munkhaugen J, Gullestad L, Liodden T, Moum T, Dammen T, Perk J, Otterstad JE. The role of cardiac rehabilitation in secondary prevention after coronary events. Eur J Prev Cardiol. 2017;24:1360–8.
34. Roy T, Lloyd CE. Epidemiology of depression and diabetes: a systematic review. J Affect Disord 2012;142 Suppl:S8–21.
35. Deschenes SS, Burns RJ, Graham E, Schmitz N. Prediabetes, depressive and anxiety symptoms, and risk of type 2 diabetes. A community-based cohort study. J Psychosom Res. 2016;89:85–90.
36. Murphy BM, Elliott PC, Higgins RO, Le Grande MR, Worcester MU, Goble AJ, Tatoulis J. Anxiety and depression after coronary artery bypass graft surgery: most get better, some get worse. Eur J Cardiovasc Prev Rehabil. 2008;15:434–40.
37. Wong EM, Afshar R, Qian H, Zhang M, Elliott TG, Tang TS. Diabetes distress, depression and glycemic control in a Canadian-based specialty care setting. Can J Diabetes. 2017;41:362–5.
38. Morin CM, LeBlanc M, Daley M, Gregoire JP, Merette C. Epidemiology of insomnia: prevalence, self-help treatments, consultations, and determinants of help-seeking behaviors. Sleep Med. 2006;7:123–30.
39. Zhu B, Hershberger PE, Kapella MC, Fritschi C. The relationship between sleep disturbance and glycaemic control in adults with type 2 diabetes: an integrative review. J Clin Nurs. 2017;26:4053–64.
40. Tan X, van Egmond L, Chapman CD, Cedernaes J, Benedict C. Aiding sleep in type 2 diabetes: therapeutic considerations. Lancet Diabetes Endocrinol. 2017;6:60–8.
41. Khan MS, Aouad R. The effects of insomnia and sleep loss on cardiovascular disease. Sleep Med Clin. 2017;12:167–77.
42. Engeda J, Mezuk B, Ratliff S, Ning Y. Association between duration and quality of sleep and the risk of pre-diabetes: evidence from NHANES. Diabet Med. 2013;30:676–80.
43. Kowall B, Lehnich AT, Strucksberg KH, Fuhrer D, Erbel R, Jankovic N, Moebus S, Jockel KH, Stang A. Associations among sleep disturbances, nocturnal sleep duration, daytime napping, and incident prediabetes and type 2 diabetes: the Heinz Nixdorf recall study. Sleep Med. 2016;21:35–41.
44. Wandell PE, Carlsson A, Steiner KH. Prevalence of diabetes among immigrants in the Nordic countries. Curr Diabetes Rev. 2010;6:126–33.
45. Kumar BN, Selmer R, Lindman AS, Tverdal A, Falster K, Meyer HE. Ethnic differences in SCORE cardiovascular risk in Oslo, Norway. Eur J Cardiovasc Prev Rehabil. 2009;16:229–34.
46. Wilkinson E, Waqar M, Sinclair A, Randhawa G. Meeting the challenge of diabetes in ageing and diverse populations: a review of the literature from the UK. J Diabetes Res. 2016;2016:8030627. Epub 2016 Oct 17
47. Kotseva K, Wood D, De Bacquer D, De Backer G, Ryden L, Jennings C, Gyberg V, Amouyel P, Bruthans J, Castro Conde A, et al. EUROASPIRE IV: a European Society of Cardiology survey on the lifestyle, risk factor and therapeutic management of coronary patients from 24 European countries. Eur J Prev Cardiol. 2016;23:636–48.
48. Gyberg V, De Bacquer D, De Backer G, Jennings C, Kotseva K, Mellbin L, Schnell O, Tuomilehto J, Wood D, Ryden L, et al. Patients with coronary artery disease and diabetes need improved management: a report from the EUROASPIRE IV survey. Cardiovasc Diabetol. 2015;14:133.
49. WHO Guidelines Approved by the Guidelines Review Committee. Use of Glycated Haemoglobin (HbA1c) in the Diagnosis of Diabetes Mellitus: Abbreviated Report of a WHO Consultation. Geneva: World Health Organization; 2011.

Whole-exome sequencing identifies R1279X of *MYH6* gene to be associated with congenital heart disease

Ehsan Razmara[1] and Masoud Garshasbi[1,2*]

Abstract

Background: Myosin VI, encoded by *MYH6*, is expressed dominantly in human cardiac atria and plays consequential roles in cardiac muscle contraction and comprising the cardiac muscle thick filament. It has been reported that the mutations in the *MYH6* gene associated with sinus venosus atrial septal defect (ASD type III), hypertrophic (HCM) and dilated (DCM) cardiomyopathies.

Methods: Two patients in an Iranian family have been identified who affected to Congenital Heart Disease (CHD). The male patient, besides CHD, shows that the thyroglossal sinus, refractive errors of the eye and mitral stenosis. The first symptoms emerged at the birth and diagnosis based on clinical features was made at about 5 years. The family had a history of ASD. For recognizing mutated gene (s), whole exome sequencing (WES) was performed for the male patient and variants were analyzed by autosomal dominant inheritance mode.

Results: Eventually, by several filtering processes, a mutation in *MYH6* gene (NM_002471.3), c.3835C > T; R1279X, was identified as the most likely disease-susceptibility variant and then confirmed by Sanger sequencing in the family. The mutation frequency was checked out in the local databases. This mutation results in the elimination of the 660 amino acids in the C-terminal of Myosin VI protein, including the vital parts of the coiled-coil structure of the tail domain.

Conclusions: Our study represents the first case of Sinus venosus defect caused directly by *MYH6* stop codon mutation. Our data indicate that by increase haploinsufficiency of myosin VI, c.3835C > T mutation with reduced penetrance could be associated with CHD.

Keywords: *MYH6*, Congenital heart disease, ASD type III, Nonsense mutation, WES

Background

Congenital Heart Defects (CHDs) are one of the major causes of death due to congenital malformations and show some of the more preponderant malformations among live births. It has been revealed that both familial and sporadic forms of CHDs result from mutations in several genes based on human cases and animal models [1, 2]. Based on targeted deletions studies in mice, it has been suggested that there are more than five hundred genes involved in heart disorders (Mouse Genome Informatics (http://www.informatics.jax.org)) [3]. CHDs treat greatly as a complex trait and to date, the number of familial cases has distinguished by the Mendelian segregation of single-gene mutations are so few [4].

Both inherited and non-inherited factors account for congenital heart disease (CHD). The incidence of CHD approximately is 0.4–0.6% live births and real prevalence is about 4% [5, 6]. Our knowledge about CHD's causes and mechanisms remains restricted in spite of the advances in diagnosis and interventions. With development of whole exome/genome sequencing more CHD causing genes possibly will be clarified which will increase our insight into the genetic causes of CHD.

Numerous epidemiological studies have suggested a genetic component of CHD etiology. Approximately, 25% of CHD cases occur as a complex trait with related defects in other organs as a sporadic malformative association, Mendelian syndrome or chromosomal abnormality [7]. The rest

* Correspondence: masoud.garshasbi@modares.ac.ir
[1]Department of Medical Genetics, Faculty of Medical Sciences, Tarbiat Modares University, Tehran, Iran
[2]Department of Medical Genetics, DeNA laboratory, Tehran, Iran

of cases occur as isolated defects and both sporadic and familial cases that showing Mendelian patterns of inheritance, have been reported [8, 9]. To date, several diseases associated with *MYH6* mutations such as hypertrophic (HCM), dilated cardiomyopathy (DCM) and atrial septal defect (ASD) have been reported [10]. ASD is categorized as the second most common CHD and accounts for 10% of all cardiac malformations [11]. Around 80% of persistent small ASDs close spontaneously during infancy or childhood, but the large one could cause serious defects such as congestive heart failure, pulmonary vascular disease and etc. [12]. There are various types of ASD; ASD type III — sinus venosus atrial septal defect— is caused by mutations in *MYH6* [13]. It has not been identified any correlation between the stop codon mutations of *MYH6* and ASD type III but in the present study, we could detect this correlation.

In the present study, we checked out a clinically characterized family with a history of congenital heart disease. In this family, we observed an obvious autosomal-dominant inheritance with reduced penetrance ($K = 50\%$). We identified a novel nonsense mutation in *MYH6*, NM_002471.3 c.3835C > T; R1279X, by WES of the patient in SH1190831 family and then this mutation was confirmed by Sanger sequencing.

Methods

Patients and clinical evaluations

The study protocol was approved by the local medical ethics committee of Tarbiat Modares University, Tehran, Iran. Written informed consents were obtained from all individuals. All of the patient's clinical information and the medical histories were collected at the Department of Medical Genetics, *DeNA* Laboratory, Tehran, Iran.

We enrolled 5 members of this family in our study (two affected, two unaffected and one carrier) (Table 1). Subjects were adjusted by meticulous medical records including a complete physical examination, a 12-lead Echocardiogram (ECG), Ultrasonic cardiogram (UCG) and other relevant features such as PR, QRS interval, QT, QTc duration and QRS axis were measured. QRS axis was presumed as normal when its value was measured between -30° and $+90^{\circ}$ and was classified abnormal when out of this range. The normal range of ECG was performed based on the individual ages. For adults, a PR interval above 210 ms and an increased above 100 ms of QRS interval were thought-out prolonged [14].

DNA extraction

Genomic DNA was isolated from peripheral blood of the family members by the *ROCHE* DNA Extraction Kit (Cat. No. 11814770001). DNA concentration was measured by Thermo Scientific™ Nanodrop 2000 (Thermo Fisher Scientific, Wilmington, DE, USA).

NGS study

Exome capturing and high throughput sequencing (HTS) was performed on the proband (III:1). The Nextera Rapid Capture Exome kit with 340,000 probes designed against the human genome was utilized to enrich the approximately 37 Mb (214,405 exons) of the Consensus Coding Sequences (CCS) from fragmented genomic DNA. Due to limitations of the method, not all exons were fully covered and all of the pathogenic variants cannot be totally excluded. An overall coverage of 98.19% was achieved, with 2188 missing base pairs (a coding region including ±2 bp). At the next step, an end to end in-house bioinformatics pipelines including base calling, primary filtering of low-quality reads and probable artifacts, and annotation of variants were applied.

The reads were aligned to the NCBI human reference genome (gh19/NCBI37.1) with SNP & Variation Suite version 8.0 (SVS v8.0) and DNASTAR Lasergene12 (DNASTAR Inc., Madison, Wisconsin USA). Small indel detection was used with the Unified Genotyper tool from GATK tools in Galaxy online database (http://

Table 1 Clinical and Electrocardiographic Features in Members of SH1190831 Family

Member	status	Age range(year)	Symptoms	Clinical ECG diagnosis	QRS axis	Heart Rate Beats/ min	Electrocardiography			Mutation
							RA (mm)	RV (mm)	LVEF (%)	
III.1[a,b]	P	7-11	ASD type III, Thyroglossal Sinus, Mitral Stenosis, Refractive Errors Of The Eye	RBBB	− 58°	75	29	34	63	WT/p.R1279X
II.2	P	57–61	sinus venosus atrial septal defect (ASD type III)	RBBB	−65°	88	35	33	59	WT/p.R1279X
II.3	H	36–40	Asymptomatic	ND	+ 42°	93	26	32	67	WT/WT
II.4	H	43–47	Asymptomatic	ND	+ 43°	85	31	30	64	WT/p.R1279X
II.5	H	40–44	Asymptomatic	ND	+ 42°	83	23	28	66	WT/WT

NA Not Detected, *ASD* Atrial Septal Defect, *RBBB* Right Bundle Branch Block, *P* Patient, *H* Healthy
[a]Whole exome sequence is applied to this individual
[b]Index case

www.usegalaxy.org). The missense, nonsense, silent, and indel mutations rates were estimated by Galaxy online tool and finally were confirmed by Ivariantguide® (https://www.advaitabio.com).

Because of the Autosomal dominant nature of the mutation, for the first step, we assumed that the variant (s) should be transferred in heterozygote manner, so we excluded the homozygote variants and then several filtering steps were applied to prioritize all variants: 1) Variants in dbSNP132 (https://www.ncbi.nlm.nih.gov/projects/SNP) and 1000 Genomes Project (http://www.1000genomes.org) with allele frequencies more than 1% were excluded. 2) The rest of variants underwent further exclusion in Exome Sequencing Project (ESP) (http://evs.gs.washington.edu/EVS) and Exome Aggregation Consortium (ExAC) database. 3) The intragenic, intronic, UTRs regions and synonymous variants were excluded from later analysis. 4) The SIFT (http://sift.jcvi.org/), Provean (http://provean.jcvi.org) and Mutation Taster (http://www.mutationtaster.org) were used to predict variants pathogenicity (Table 2).

All suspected pathogenic variants were checked out in HGMD (http://www.hgmd.cf.ac.uk) and ClinVar (https://www.ncbi.nlm.nih.gov/clinvar). Finally, based on family pedigree, autosomal dominant inheritance pattern and clinical information were used to evaluate identified variants. Based on the clinical information, specific attention has been paid to the 42 genes known Congenital Heart Diseases. ConSurf (http://www.consurf.tau.ac.il) database was applied to provide evolutionary conservation profile for Myosin VI protein and showing the staple role of the mutation (Fig. 2c). As well as, frequency of the mutation was checked out based on the local database (http://www.iranome.ir); all information related to the In-silico prediction such as conservation, allele frequency, and damaging prediction were depicted in Table 2.

Mutation validation and co-segregation analysis

Sanger sequencing in forward and reverse directions was performed to validate the candidate variants found in WES and then segregation analyses were performed in the family. The primers were designed by Primer3.0 (http://bioinfo.ut.ee/primer3-0.4.0) web-based server (Table 3). We checked out the lack of SNPs in the genomic region corresponding to the 3′ ends of primers by looking through the dbSNP database. The primers specificity was checked by the in-silico-PCR tool in UCSC genome browser and Primer blast of NCBI genome browser and finally, the PCR was utilized in standard conditions and then the polymerase chain reaction (PCR) products were sequenced by ABI 730XL, using the conventional capillary system, and then the Sequences were analyzed by Genome Compiler online tool (http://www.genomecompiler.com/) to identify the alternations.

Results

Clinical features

We identified two patients — the female and the male patients— in an Iranian family. The female patient had sinus venosus atrial septal defect, although the male patient manifested other symptoms, as well as ASD type III, such as thyroglossal sinus to refractive errors of the eye and mitral stenosis. The proband (III.1), a male was between the age range of 12–16, affected with ASD and Thyroglossal sinus. Both parents were assessed for the relevant clinical features but we could not detect any relevant symptoms. Physical examination demonstrated ASD in the patients (Table 1). The family history examination clarified that the patient II2 has the same condition. The II.4 sample, in spite of carrying the mutation, indicated no obvious phenotype implying the reduced penetrance in this condition. All family members were recruited for further physical examination and all gathered records have been reported in Table 1.

Genetic analysis

It is postulated that the pedigree may represent an autosomal dominant inheritance with reduced penetrance. To elucidate the underlying genetic cause (s), genomic DNA was obtained from the patient and analyzed by whole exome sequencing (WES). R1279X mutation was confirmed by Sanger sequencing (Fig. 1b).

The detected SNVs and deletion/insertions were analyzed by several filtering methods. 66,109 variants were found in the exome of the proband after alignment and SNV calling. After several exclusion processes by using of dbSNP132, 1000 Genomes Project, Exome Sequencing Project (ESP), and ExAc databases, thirteen variants were identified and then prioritized by patients' phenotype. Eventually, with the patient's phenotypes, only one relevant variant was identified that shared by two affected and one carrier family members (II2, III1, II4) but not observed in other healthy parent or normal control (II5).

In the same statement, of the 1187 variants, 13 were ranked using three database tools (Provean, Mutation Taster, Sift) and finally, among the thirteen variants, a unique variant was opted as a pathogenic mutation of this

Table 2 Several online databases that used to confirm the pathogenicity of the R1279X mutation in *MYH6* gene

Mutation Taster	EXAC	SIFT	1000 Genome	Iranome	PROVEAN
Damaging	Not reported	Damaging	Not reported	Not reported	Damaging

Table 3 Sequences of the primers used to confirm the mutation by Sanger sequencing

Patient ID	Gene	Variant	Primers
SH1190831	*MYH6*	c.3835C > T (p.R1279X)	F 5'-CACACTCACCCTTCCTGTCT-3' R 5'-CTGAAATGAGGGGCTTGTGG-3'

unique family based on patient's phenotype by utilizing CentoMD (https://www.centogene.com) and ClinVar. (https://www.ncbi.nlm.nih.gov/clinvar/) (Fig. 1c).

Samples from the available members of the SH1190831 family were subjected to Sanger sequencing to confirm the candidate variant of *MYH6* gene.

To find the main cause of CHD in the proband by known genetic mutation (s), based on proband phenotype, we especially focused on the 42 genes that have critical roles in CHD etiology and revised our strategies with a filter of pertinent variants in these genes (Additional file 1: Table S1). The single patient analysis concentrated on the possibility of a known causative gene that underlies CHD.

Discussion

Atrial septal defect (ASD), a persistent interatrial communication, is one of the common congenital abnormalities occurring in various forms consists of ostium secundum (ASD type II, ~ 75% of cases), ostium primum (ASD type I, 15–20%), sinus venosus (ASD type III, 5–10%), and rarely, coronary sinus defects [15]. ASDs, based on the defected gene, have been classified into several groups. The mutations in various genes have been associated with atrial septal defects, for instance, mutations in *NKX2–5*, *GATA4*, *TBX5*, and *MYH6* [16].

It has been identified that there are at least 35 classes of molecular motors into the myosin superfamily that move along actin filaments [17]. Several studies have described various functions for Myosin VI such as membrane trafficking, endocytosis, organizing and stabilizing the actin cytoskeleton and playing a material role in inner-ear hair cells [18–20]. Myosin VI is the merely class of myosin that known to move toward the minus-end of actin filaments. Intuitively, dimerization of the myosin can expand its movement along actin

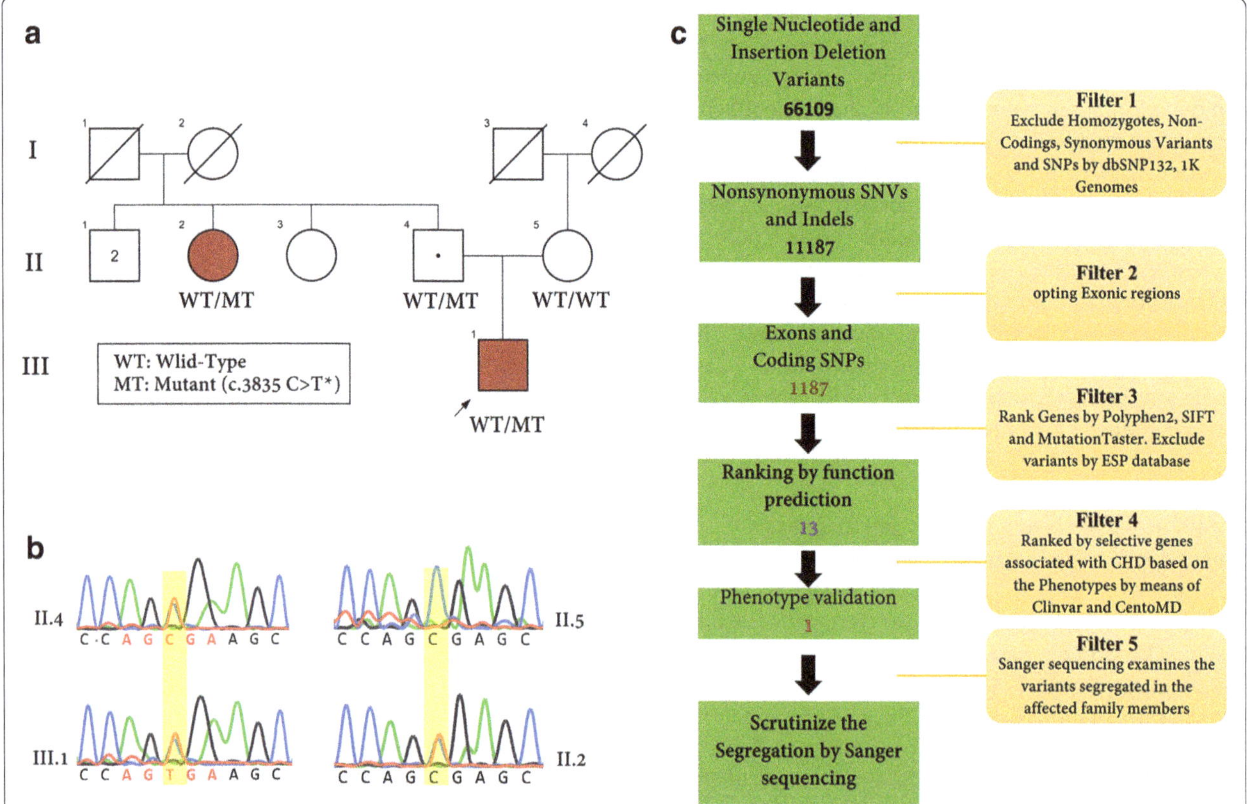

Fig. 1 Pedigree, chromatograms and filtering procedures in the SH1190831 family. **a** Pedigree of SH1190831 family is comprised of three generations. The squares and circles indicate males and females, respectively. The arrow appoints the proband of the family. The mutation, c.3835C > T in *MYH6*, has been demonstrated that segregated in this family. **b** Sequence chromatogram showing heterozygote state of the nucleotide sequence of *MYH6 in* c.3835C > T. **c** Schematic representation of filtering strategies that applied in this research. The filtering process was applied according several strategies which are demonstrated in the schematic representation. For more investigation, we reevaluated the filtering steps by regard to this fact that the disease could be engendered by autosomal recessive; however, we could not detect any relevant variants according to this supposition

filament but it must be noticed that the Myosin VI does not contain a well-defined coiled-coil dimerization domain, suggesting that myosin-VI does not form a constitutive dimer on its own. The *MYH6* gene encodes Myosin heavy chain, α isoform (MHC-α) in human Myosin VI [21]. This protein has several important domains such as head domain, IQ domain, cargo-binding domain, tail domain and etc. (Fig. 2). The tail domain involves two distinct section: Coiled-coil domain and globular domain. It has been identified that the tail domain has a staple role in interacting with the target, especially uncoated vesicles [22].

NGS and particularly whole exome sequencing techniques have been developed into a robust and cost-effective tool to identify the new variants or genes for rare Mendelian unknown disorders [23–25]. This technique has been used in genetic diagnostics helping to increase the clinical and mutational spectrum of known and unknown diseases [26, 27]. But sometimes it is so difficult to distinguish between pathogenic and benign mutations [28, 29]. Several filtering strategies have been developed to exclude variants that are implausible to cause disease.

In this study, we utilized the WES technique to identify a nonsense mutation at nucleotide 3835 of *MYH6* gene. This mutation is located at the extremely conserved region in *MYH6* gene in Primates, Myosin heavy chain-α isoform (MHC-α), and it is presumed to result in a truncated protein that is associated with Cardiomyopathy and ASD type 3 (OMIM: 614089, 613,251). Previously, it has been reported that the mutations in *MYH6* are associated with late-onset hypertrophic cardiomyopathy, atrial septal defects and sick sinus syndrome [14, 30]. There are numerous reports on the association of *MYH6* mutations and CHD [31].

In the present study, we identified a nonsense variant, c.3835C > T, R1279X, by whole exome sequencing in the coiled-coil region or tail domain of *MYH6* gene. This

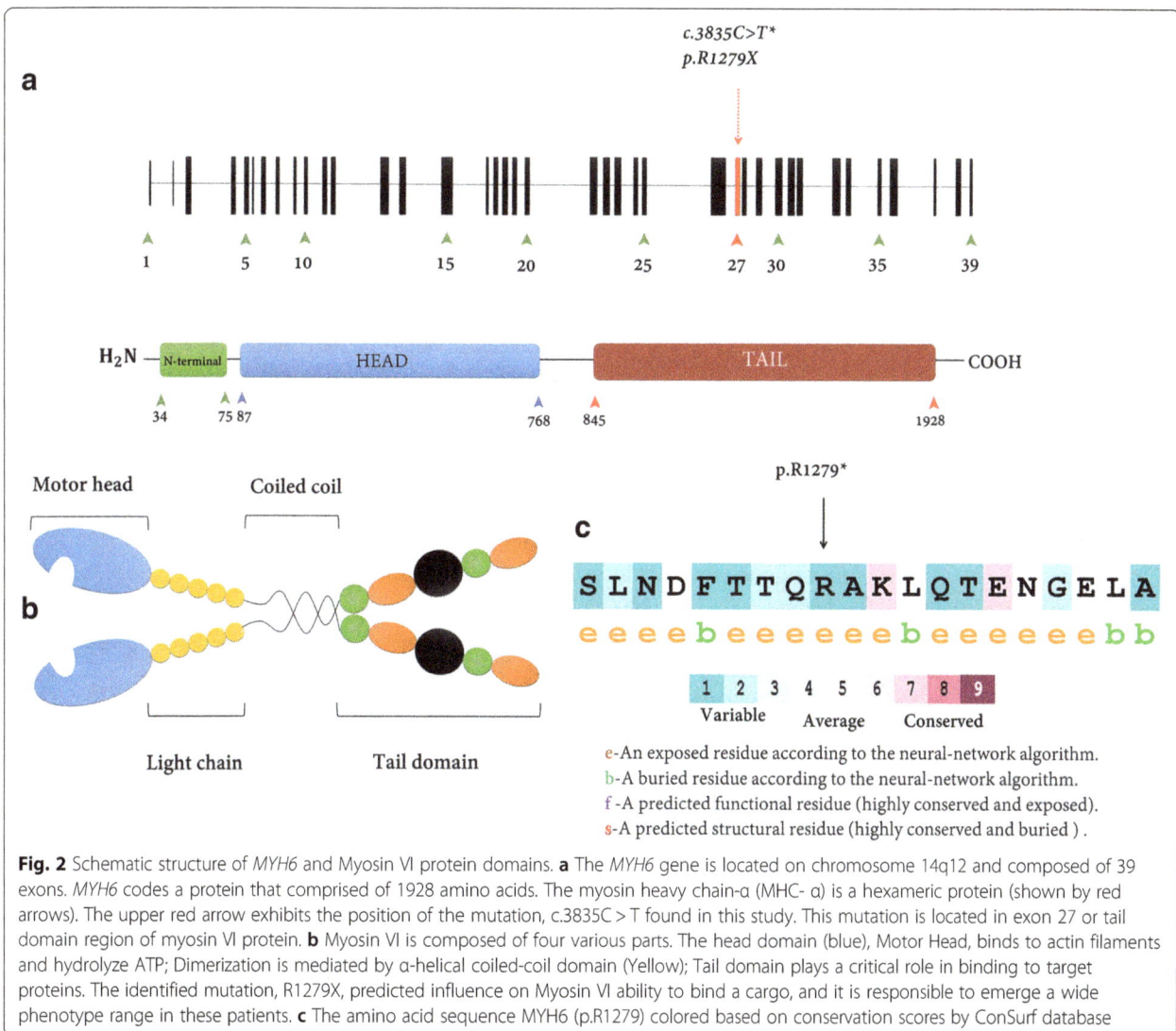

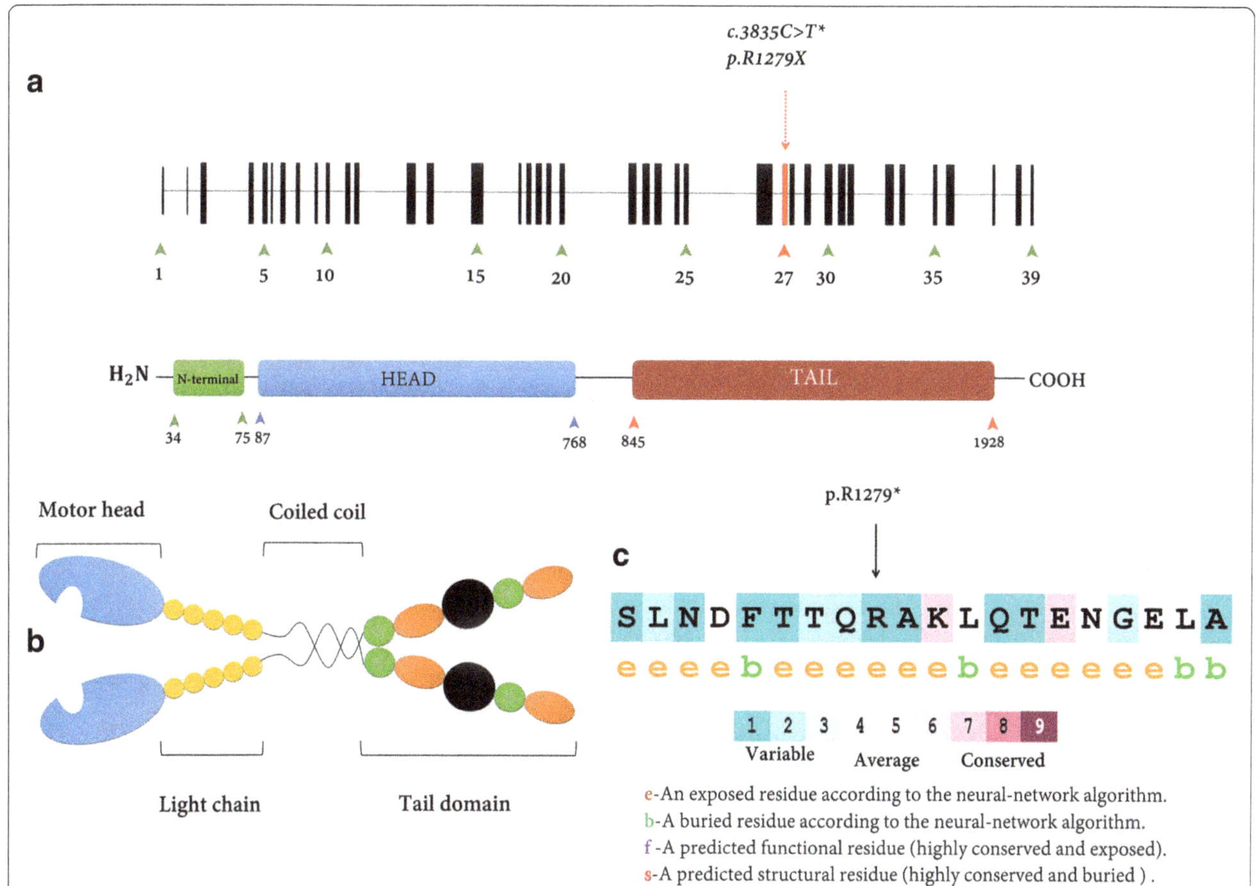

Fig. 2 Schematic structure of *MYH6* and Myosin VI protein domains. **a** The *MYH6* gene is located on chromosome 14q12 and composed of 39 exons. *MYH6* codes a protein that comprised of 1928 amino acids. The myosin heavy chain-α (MHC- α) is a hexameric protein (shown by red arrows). The upper red arrow exhibits the position of the mutation, c.3835C > T found in this study. This mutation is located in exon 27 or tail domain region of myosin VI protein. **b** Myosin VI is composed of four various parts. The head domain (blue), Motor Head, binds to actin filaments and hydrolyze ATP; Dimerization is mediated by α-helical coiled-coil domain (Yellow); Tail domain plays a critical role in binding to target proteins. The identified mutation, R1279X, predicted influence on Myosin VI ability to bind a cargo, and it is responsible to emerge a wide phenotype range in these patients. **c** The amino acid sequence MYH6 (p.R1279) colored based on conservation scores by ConSurf database

region mediates interaction with cargo molecules or other myosin subunits. After several staple filtering and annotation processes, to predict whether the variant was deleterious or not, we utilized several databases such as SIFT, Mutation Taster, and Provean. We also analyzed intronic, synonymous, nonsense, missense and frameshift indel changes to predict whether those changes could affect splicing process by influencing on donor or acceptor splice sites, with mutation taster and Neutral Network Splice (NNSplice version 0.9).

It has been illustrated that the reduced penetrance could take the Centre stage in increasing prevalence atrial septal defects in familial form. According to the Sanger sequencing results, the mother of the patient, II.4, is a carrier for R1279X mutation. It could be justified by reduced penetrance. This phenomenon can make genetic counseling more challenging because of the difficult interpretation of a person's family medical history and prediction the risk of passing a genetic condition to offspring.

R1279X mutation could increase the truncated proteins in the cell and, as a result, cell should prevent this process by Nonsense-mediated decay response (NMD response) which is increasingly appreciated as one of the central mechanisms of RNA surveillance, with a big deal role not only in physiological control of gene expression but also in modulating defects and acquired genetic diseases. NMD could confront the cells with reduced amounts of the protein which has known haploinsufficiency (i.e., reduced amounts of protein due to a mutant or null allele) [32]. In nutshell, NMD must be considered when the functional effect of the premature termination codon (PTC). It has been identified that the haploinsufficiency has a staple role in the pathogenesis of cardiovascular diseases [33, 34]. Based on the nonsense mutation influence on proteins, we propose haploinsufficiency as a predicted mechanism of pathogenesis of c.3835C > T, R1279X mutation in the patients, but more studies need to uncover the exact mechanism of CHD pathogenicity.

Our result indicates that this nonsense mutation (R1279X) in *MYH6* might be the genetic cause of congenital heart disease. Our study confirms that the *MYH6* gene has an important role in heart functions but we recommend the applying animal modeling to scrutinize the distinctive role of this mutation.

Conclusions

For the first time, we identified a nonsense mutation, c.3835C > T, R1279X, in *MYH6* gene as a possible cause of CHD in an Iranian family. This finding will increase our knowledge about the aetiology of this rare condition by effective clarification of the causative gene mutations and will enhance the mutational spectrum of CHD and should consider in the diagnosis of these diseases.

Abbreviations

ASD: Atrial septal defect; CCS: Consensus Coding Sequences; CHD: Congenital Heart Disease; DCM: dilated cardiomyopathies; ECG: 12-lead Echocardiogram; ESP: Exome Sequencing Project; HCM: hypertrophic cardiomyopathies; HTS: high throughput sequencing; UCG: Ultrasonic cardiogram; WES: Whole-Exome sequencing

Acknowledgements

We thank the family for their participation in this study. We are especially grateful to the staffs of DeNA laboratory for helping us in this research and additionally, we appreciate supports from Dr. Elika Esmaeilzadeh and Dr. Farveh Ehya, Tarbiat Modares University, Tehran, Iran. This research received no specific grant from any funding agency, commercial or not for profit sectors.

Authors' contributions

Conceived and designed the experiments: MG Conducted the experiments: MG, ER Analysed the data: ER Contributed reagents/materials/analysis tools: MG, ER Wrote the paper: ER, MG. All authors read and approved the final manuscript.

Competing interests

The authors declare that they have no competing interests.

References

1. Calcagni G, Digilio MC, Sarkozy A, Dallapiccola B, Marino B. Familial recurrence of congenital heart disease: an overview and review of the literature. Eur J Pediatr. 2007;166(2):111–6.
2. Fahed AC, Gelb BD, Seidman J, Seidman CE. Genetics of congenital heart disease: the glass half empty. Circ Res. 2013;112(4):707–20.
3. Ghosh TK, Granados-Riveron JT, Buxton S, Setchfield K, Loughna S, Brook JD. Studies of genes involved in congenital heart disease. Journal of Cardiovascular Development and Disease. 2014;1(1):134–45.
4. El Malti R, Liu H, Doray B, Thauvin C, Maltret A, Dauphin C, Gonçalves-Rocha M, Teboul M, Blanchet P, Roume J. A systematic variant screening in familial cases of congenital heart defects demonstrates the usefulness of molecular genetics in this field. Eur J Hum Genet. 2016;24(2):228.
5. Pierpont ME, Basson CT, Benson DW, Gelb BD, Giglia TM, Goldmuntz E, McGee G, Sable CA, Srivastava D, Webb CL. Genetic basis for congenital heart defects: current knowledge. Circulation. 2007;115(23):3015–38.
6. Wren C, Irving CA, Griffiths JA, O'Sullivan JJ, Chaudhari MP, Haynes SR, Smith JH, Hamilton JL, Hasan A. Mortality in infants with cardiovascular malformations. Eur J Pediatr. 2012;171(2):281–7.
7. Gill HK, Splitt M, Sharland GK, Simpson JM. Patterns of recurrence of congenital heart disease: an analysis of 6,640 consecutive pregnancies evaluated by detailed fetal echocardiography. J Am Coll Cardiol. 2003;42(5):923–9.
8. Robert E. In: Ferencz C, Rubin JD, Loffredo C, Magee CA, editors. Epidemiology of congenital heart disease: the Baltimore-Washington infant study, 1981–1989 (perspectives in pediatric cardiology series, volume 4), vol. 376. Armonk, New York: Futura Publishing Company, Inc; 1993. $75. In.: Pergamon; 1994.
9. Ferencz C, Neill CA, Boughman JA, Rubin JD, Brenner JI, Perry LW. Congenital cardiovascular malformations associated with chromosome abnormalities: an epidemiologic study. J Pediatr. 1989;114(1):79–86.
10. Carniel E, Taylor MR, Sinagra G, Di Lenarda A, Ku L, Fain PR, Boucek MM, Cavanaugh J, Miocic S, Slavov D. α-Myosin heavy chain. Circulation. 2005; 112(1):54–9.
11. Qm Z, Xj M, Jia B, Gy H. Prevalence of congenital heart disease at live birth: an accurate assessment by echocardiographic screening. Acta Paediatr. 2013;102(4):397–402.
12. Nyboe C, Olsen MS, Nielsen-Kudsk J, Hjortdal V. Atrial fibrillation and stroke in adult patients with atrial septal defect and the long-term effect of closure. Heart. 2015;0:1-6.heartjnl-2014-306552.

13. Ouyang P, Saarel E, Bai Y, Luo C, Lv Q, Xu Y, Wang F, Fan C, Younoszai A, Chen Q. A de novo mutation in NKX2. 5 associated with atrial septal defects, ventricular noncompaction, syncope and sudden death. Clin Chim Acta. 2011;412(1):170–5.
14. Posch MG, Waldmuller S, Müller M, Scheffold T, Fournier D, Andrade-Navarro MA, De Geeter B, Guillaumont S, Dauphin C, Yousseff D. Cardiac alpha-myosin (MYH6) is the predominant sarcomeric disease gene for familial atrial septal defects. PLoS One. 2011;6(12):e28872.
15. Martin SS, Shapiro EP, Mukherjee M. Atrial septal defects – clinical manifestations, Echo assessment, and intervention. Clinical Medicine Insights Cardiology. 2014;8(Suppl 1):93–8.
16. Geva T, Martins JD, Wald RM. Atrial septal defects. Lancet. 2014;383(9932): 1921–32.
17. Odronitz F, Kollmar M. Drawing the tree of eukaryotic life based on the analysis of 2,269 manually annotated myosins from 328 species. Genome Biol. 2007;8(9):R196.
18. Frank DJ, Noguchi T, Miller KG. Myosin VI: a structural role in actin organization important for protein and organelle localization and trafficking. Curr Opin Cell Biol. 2004;16(2):189–94.
19. Mermall V, McNally JG, Miller KG. Transport of cytoplasmic particles catalysed by an unconventional myosin in living Drosophila embryos. Nature. 1994;369(6481):560–2.
20. Buss F, Arden SD, Lindsay M, Luzio JP, Kendrick-Jones J. Myosin VI isoform localized to clathrin-coated vesicles with a role in clathrin-mediated endocytosis. EMBO J. 2001;20(14):3676–84.
21. Tanigawa G, Jarcho JA, Kass S, Solomon SD, Vosberg H-P, Seidman J, Seidman CE. A molecular basis for familial hypertrophic cardiomyopathy: an αβ cardiac myosin heavy chain hybrid gene. Cell. 1990;62(5):991–8.
22. Hasson T. Myosin VI: two distinct roles in endocytosis. J Cell Sci. 2003; 116(17):3453–61.
23. Ng SB, Buckingham KJ, Lee C, Bigham AW, Tabor HK, Dent KM, Huff CD, Shannon PT, Jabs EW, Nickerson DA. Exome sequencing identifies the cause of a mendelian disorder. Nat Genet. 2010;42(1):30–5.
24. Yang Y, Muzny DM, Reid JG, Bainbridge MN, Willis A, Ward PA, Braxton A, Beuten J, Xia F, Niu Z. Clinical whole-exome sequencing for the diagnosis of mendelian disorders. N Engl J Med. 2013;369(16):1502–11.
25. Razmara EBF, Esmaeilzadeh-Gharehdaghi E, Almadani N, Garshasbi M. The first case of NSHL by direct impression on EYA1 gene and identification of one novel mutation in MYO7A in the Iranian families. Iran J Basic Med Sci. 2018;21:6–9.
26. Churko JM, Mantalas GL, Snyder MP, Wu JC. Overview of high throughput sequencing technologies to elucidate molecular pathways in cardiovascular diseases. Circ Res. 2013;112(12):1613–23.
27. Sanders SJ, Murtha MT, Gupta AR, Murdoch JD, Raubeson MJ, Willsey AJ, Ercan-Sencicek AG, DiLullo NM, Parikshak NN, Stein JL. De novo mutations revealed by whole-exome sequencing are strongly associated with autism. Nature. 2012;485(7397):237–41.
28. Bamshad MJ, Ng SB, Bigham AW, Tabor HK, Emond MJ, Nickerson DA, Shendure J. Exome sequencing as a tool for Mendelian disease gene discovery. Nat Rev Genet. 2011;12(11):745–55.
29. Landstrom A, Ackerman MJ. The Achilles' heel of cardiovascular genetic testing: distinguishing pathogenic mutations from background genetic noise. Clinical Pharmacology & Therapeutics. 2011;90(4):496–9.
30. Ching Y-H, Ghosh TK, Cross SJ, Packham EA, Honeyman L, Loughna S, Robinson TE, Dearlove AM, Ribas G, Bonser AJ. Mutation in myosin heavy chain 6 causes atrial septal defect. Nat Genet. 2005;37(4):423–8.
31. Weismann CG, Gelb BD. The genetics of congenital heart disease: a review of recent developments. Curr Opin Cardiol. 2007;22(3):200–6.
32. Holbrook JA, Neu-Yilik G, Hentze MW, Kulozik AE. Nonsense-mediated decay approaches the clinic. Nat Genet. 2004;36(8):801.
33. Marston S, Copeland ON, Jacques A, Livesey K, Tsang V, McKenna WJ, Jalilzadeh S, Carballo S, Redwood C, Watkins H. Evidence from human myectomy samples that MYBPC3 mutations cause hypertrophic cardiomyopathy through haploinsufficiency. Circ Res. 2009;105(3):219–22.
34. Cattin M-E, Bertrand AT, Schlossarek S, Le Bihan M-C, Skov Jensen S, Neuber C, Crocini C, Maron S, Lainé J, Mougenot N. Heterozygous Lmna delK32 mice develop dilated cardiomyopathy through a combined pathomechanism of haploinsufficiency and peptide toxicity. Hum Mol Genet. 2013;22(15):3152–64.

7

Effect of serum electrolytes within normal ranges on QTc prolongation: a cross-sectional study

Yintao Chen[1], Xiaofan Guo[1], Guozhe Sun[1], Zhao Li[1], Liqiang Zheng[2] and Yingxian Sun[1*]

Abstract

Background: Many previous clinical studies have reported that prolongation of the QT interval corrected for heart rate (QTc) is associated with an increased risk of sudden cardiac death and all-cause mortality. This study aimed to explore associations between serum electrolytes and QTc prolongation in the north-eastern Chinese rural general population.

Methods: We performed a cross-sectional study including 10,334 (4820 men and 5514 women) from the general population aged ≥35 years in the Liaoning Province from 2012 to 2013. Anthropometric measurements, laboratory examinations and self-reported lifestyle factor information, echocardiography and electrocardiogram were collected by trained personnel. The associations between serum electrolytes and QTc prolongation were tested using multiple linear regression and logistic regression analyses.

Results: The mean QTc interval were 415.6 ± 18.8 and 470.1 ± 23.1 ms in normal group and QTc prolongation group respectively. The prevalence of QTc prolongation increased significantly with a decrease in serum potassium and an increase in magnesium. Stepwise multiple linear regression showed that age, hypertension, waist circumference were prominently positive associated with QTc interval both in male and female population. But serum potassium was significantly inversely associated with QTc interval. Serum magnesium and calcium also showed a positive relationship with QTc interval. Furthermore, multiple logistic regression found that lower quartile of serum potassium had higher risk for QTc prolongation, especially in female population (Q2 vs. Q4: OR: 1.54, 95%CI: 1.01–2.35; Q1 vs. Q4: OR: 2.02, 95%CI: 1.36–3.01). In addition, the higher serum magnesium increased the risk of QTc prolongation, which was significantly only in male population.

Conclusions: In present Chinese rural general population, even with normal range, a decrease in serum potassium and an increase in serum magnesium are important risk factors for QTc prolongation.

Keywords: QTc prolongation, Electrocardiography, Serum electrolytes, Serum potassium

* Correspondence: yxsun@cmu.edu.cn
[1]Department of Cardiology, The First Hospital of China Medical University, Shenyang 110001, People's Republic of China
Full list of author information is available at the end of the article

Background

Many previous studies have concluded that prolongation of the QT interval corrected for heart rate (QTc) is associated with an increased risk of sudden cardiac death, arrhythmias and all-cause mortality [1–3]. At present, an electrocardiogram showing QTc prolongation is an important indicator for treatment and medication in clinical practice [4]. Many epidemiological risk factors for QTc prolongation have previously been reported, including older age, sex hormones and electrolyte disturbances [5–7]. Disturbances in serum electrolytes might induce or facilitate clinical arrhythmias by interacting with abnormal myocardial tissue, and this could even occur in a bundle of normal cardiac tissue. Furthermore, strong evidences has been found that identified hypokalaemia as a risk factor for QTc prolongation [8], and the dietary intake of potassium has also been independently associated with the QTc interval [9]. The same clinical studies also found that the concentrations of sodium, calcium and magnesium influence the QTc interval [7, 10, 11]. Therefore, electrolyte abnormalities might be an early sign of arrhythmia, including QTc prolongation. However, most of the relevant studies recruited participants from clinical patients, such as patients undergoing haemodialysis [10], patients with chronic kidney disease [12] or patients receiving psychotropic drugs treatment [13], who usually suffer from disturbances in serum electrolytes, and the number of participants was restricted to hundreds. Studies of the associations between serum electrolytes and QTc prolongation in a large sample from a Chinese general population have been rare. The characteristics of the general population and the above groups of patients are quite different which might result in very different conclusions, and the former population generally has normal levels of serum electrolytes. This present study aimed to explore associations between serum electrolytes and QTc prolongation in the north-eastern Chinese rural general population, which have not previously been reported to the best of our knowledge.

Methods

Study population

The detailed methods used in this study have been previously published [14]. A multi-stage, stratified randomly cluster-sampling scheme was adopted to build a representative sample of men and women in Liaoning Province that is located in Northeast China. From January 2012 to August 2013, we invited all the eligible permanent residents aged ≥35 years from each village to attend the study. Finally, 11,956 participants (85.3%) agreed and completed the present study. The study was approved by the Ethics Committee of China Medical University (Shenyang, China). All procedures were performed in accordance with the ethical standards. Written consent was obtained in all participants after they had been informed of the objectives, benefits, medical items and confidentiality agreement of personal information. If the participants were illiterate, we obtained the written informed consents from their proxies.

In present study, only participants with a complete set of data regarding the variables analyzed in the study were included, the exclusion criteria includes: recent use (two weeks before) of diuretics or diuretics-containing traditional Chinese medicine ($n = 1056$), recent use of unspecified antihypertensive drugs ($n = 353$), recent use of antipsychotics ($n = 9$), eGFR < 60 mL/min/1.73 m2 ($n = 241$), making a final sample size of 10,334 (4820 men and 5514 women).

Data collection and measurements

The data collection and measurement methods used in this study have been previously described [14]. Data on demographic characteristics, lifestyle risk factors, dietary habits and any medicines used in previous 2 weeks were collected during a single visit by cardiologists and trained nurses using a standard questionnaire by a face-to-face interview. All eligible investigators must attend the organized training sessions in advance to maintain the importance of standardization and the study procedures. A strict test was administered after this training sessions, and only those who scored perfectly on the test could become investigators. During data collection, our inspectors received further instruction and support from a subcommittee for quality control of central steering committee.

The participants were advised to avoid caffeinated beverages and exercise for at least 30 min before the measurement. After a rest period of at least 5 min, blood pressure was measured three times at intervals of 2 min using a standardized automatic electronic sphygmomanometer (HEM-907; Omron, Japan). The mean of three measurements of blood pressure was calculated and used in all analyses. Hypertension was defined as a systolic blood pressure of 140 mmHg or greater, a diastolic blood pressure of 90 mmHg or greater, or self-reported current treatment for hypertension with antihypertensive medication [15].

Fasting blood samples were collected in the morning after at least 12 h of fasting for all participants. Blood samples were obtained from an antecubital vein into vacutainer tubes containing EDTA. Blood chemical analyses were performed at a central, certified laboratory. Serum electrolytes, fasting plasma glucose (FPG), lipid profiles, serum creatinine (SCr), and uric acid were analyzed enzymatically on an autoanalyzer (Olympus, Kobe, Japan). All laboratory equipment was calibrated and blinded duplicate samples were used. Diabetes mellitus was diagnosed according to the WHO criteria:

FPG ≥ 7 mmol/L (126 mg/dL) and/or being on treatment for diabetes [16]. Dyslipidemia was defined according to the National Cholesterol Education ProgramThird Adult Treatment Panel (ATP III) criteria [17]. High total cholesterol (TC) was defined as TC ≥ 6.21 mmol/L (240 mg/dL). Low high density lipoprotein cholesterol (HDL-c) was defined as HDL-c < 1.03 mmol/L (40 mg/dL). High low density lipoprotein cholesterol (LDL-c) was defined as LDL-C ≥ 4.16 mmol/L (160 mg/dL). High triglyceride (TG) was defined as ≥2.26 mmol/L (200 mg/dL). The estimated glomerular filtration rate (eGFR) was estimated using the Chronic Kidney Diesease Epidemiology Collaboration (CKD-EPI) equation [18].

The method and standard of echocardiography measurements has been published by our previous article [19]. Left ventricular end-diastolic internal dimension (LVIDd), interventricular septal thickness (IVSd), posterior wall thickness (PWTd) were used to estimate the Left ventricular mass (LVM) by the Devereux's formula according to the American Society of Echocardiography simplified cubed equation [20]. $LVM = 0.8 \times [1.04\{(IVSTd + PWTd + LVIDd)^3 - LVIDd^3\}] + 0.6$ g. Left ventricular mass index was obtained after that LVM was divided by $height^{2.7}$. And left ventricular hypertrophy (LVH) was diagnosed using the following defining criteria [21]: > 48 $g/m^{2.7}$ and 44 $g/m^{2.7}$ for men and women respectively.

Twelve-lead resting, ten-second ECGs were performed on all participants by well-trained cardiologists using an ECG machine (MAC 5500; GE Healthcare, Little Chalfont, Buckinghamshire, UK). All ECGs were standard resting ECGs (25 mm/second paper speed and 10 mm/mV amplitude). After capturing images, QTc intervals were calculated and recorded automatically by the MUSE Cardiology Information System (version 7.0.0; GE Healthcare), the error of which determined by an automatic algorithm was less than ±20 ms. The accuracy was 99.98%, and the sensitivity was 99.62% [22]. In present study, Fridericia's formula ($QTc = QT/RR^{1/3}$) was used to correct the QT interval [23]. Prolonged QTc was defined according to the national guidelines, which recommended cut points of 450 milliseconds or longer in male and 460 milliseconds or longer in female [24].

Statistical analysis

Continuous variables were expressed as mean values and standard deviation (SD), whereas categorical variables were described as frequencies and percentages. Comparisons between variables were analyzed by t-test or chi-square test as appropriate. The associations between serum electrolytes and prolonged QTc interval were tested using Pearson correlation, multiple linear regression and logistic regression analyses, with standard regression coefficient (β), odds ratio (OR) and 95% confidence intervals (CIs) calculated. All statistical analyses were performed using SPSS version 22.0 software (IBM Corp., Armonk, NY, USA), and $P < 0.05$ indicated statistical significance.

Results

The population characteristics by QTc prolongation were showed in Table 1 and Additional file 1: Table S1. The prevalence of QTc prolongation in total participants was 4.1%. Participants with QTc prolongation were more likely to be older, higher WC, FPG, TC, HDL-C, LDL-C, blood pressure (SBP and DBP), $LVMI_{ht2.7}$, serum calcium and serum magnesium, but lower eGFR and mean serum potassium ($P < 0.05$). The mean QTc interval were 415.6 ± 18.8 and 470.1 ± 23.1 ms in normal group and QTc prolongation group respectively.

Considered the gender difference for QTc prolongation, the different prevalence in male and female grouped by quartiles of electrolytes was analyzed (Fig. 1). Both in male and female, the prevalence of QTc prolongation was increasing significantly with a decrease in the concentration of serum potassium, which was opposite to serum total calcium in female and magnesium in total sample. And the prevalence of QTc prolongation was high to 5.7% in female population with lowest quartile of serum potassium. It seemed that both lower and higher serum sodium would increase the prevalence of QTc prolongation.

Stepwise multiple linear regression was used to analysis the risk factors of QTc prolongation (Table 2). Lots of potential risk factors were included in the regression model, and it was showed that age, hypertension, waist circumference were prominently positive associated with QTc interval in both male and female population. But serum potassium was significantly inversely associated with QTc interval in both male and female. Serum magnesium and calcium also showed a positive relationship with QTc interval. But diabetes and serum uric acid was more positive relevant for QTc prolongation just in male. And serum sodium did not show significant association with QTc interval, which was removed from the regression model finally.

Furthermore, multiple logistic regression (Table 3) was used to explore the relationships between serum electrolytes and QTc prolongation. It was found that lower quartile of serum potassium had higher risk for QTc prolongation, especially in female population (Q2 vs. Q4: OR: 1.54, 95%CI: 1.01–2.35; Q1 vs. Q4: OR: 2.02, 95%CI: 1.36–3.01). In addition, the higher serum magnesium also increased the risk of prolonged QTc in total population and male population. Compared with the lowest quartile of sodium, only the quartile 3 showed negative association with QTc prolongation in male participants (OR: 0.47, 95%CI: 0.28–0.80). But calcium didn't show any statistically positive association with QTc prolongation.

Table 1 Characteristics in population with or without QTc prolongation

Variables	Normal QTc	QTc prolongation	*P* value
n (%)	9913 (95.9)	421 (4.1)	
Age, years	52.9 ± 10.2	58.6 ± 11.0	< 0.001
Gender(%)			
Male	4631 (46.7)	189 (44.9)	0.463
Female	5282 (53.3)	232 (55.1)	
Race (Han) (%)	9390 (94.7)	393 (93.3)	0.219
Current smoking (%)	3546 (35.8)	150 (35.6)	0.953
Current drinking (%)	2303 (23.2)	110 (26.1)	0.169
Physical activity (%)			
Low	2766 (27.9)	134 (31.8)	0.212
Moderate	6590 (66.5)	264 (62.7)	
Heavy	557 (5.6)	23 (5.5)	
Body mass index (kg/m2)	24.6 ± 3.6	24.9 ± 3.5	0.132
waist circumference (cm)	81.9 ± 9.7	83.8 ± 9.5	< 0.001
Diet score	2.3 ± 1.1	2.3 ± 1.1	0.451
LDL-cholesterol, mmol/L	2.9 ± 0.8	3.0 ± 0.8	0.004
HDL-cholesterol, mmol/L	1.4 ± 0.4	1.5 ± 0.4	0.002
Triglycerides, mmol/L	1.6 ± 1.5	1.6 ± 1.3	0.741
Total cholesterol (mmol/L)	5.2 ± 1.1	5.3 ± 1.1	0.017
Fasting glucose, mmol/L	5.8 ± 1.6	6.1 ± 2.2	0.06
Systolic blood pressure, mmHg	139.2 ± 22.0	152.8 ± 27.6	< 0.001
Diastolic blood pressure, mmHg	81.2 ± 11.3	83.9 ± 13.8	< 0.001
Estimated GFR (mL/min/1.73m^2)	94.3 ± 14.3	92.0 ± 13.9	0.001
Serum uric acid, mmol/L	287.4 ± 82.0	293.0 ± 84.5	0.176
Serum sodium, mmol/L	141.2 ± 2.2	141.4 ± 2.4	0.124
Serum potassium, mmol/L	4.2 ± 0.3	4.1 ± 0.4	< 0.001
Serum calcium, mmol/L	2.32 ± 0.1	2.34 ± 0.1	< 0.001
Serum magnesium, mmol/L	0.8 ± 0.1	0.9 ± 0.1	0.022
LVMI$_{ht2.7}$, g/m$^{2.7}$[a]	39.2 ± 28.3	43.1 ± 12.5	0.005
QTc Fredericia, ms	415.6 ± 18.8	470.1 ± 23.1	< 0.001
QRS duration> 120 ms	117 (1.2)	67 (15.9)	< 0.001

Values are mean (SD) unless otherwise indicated. *P*-values represent the result of standard T test or Pearson chi-square test to detect differences between the groups. The echocardiography measurements were showed in Additional file 1: Table S1

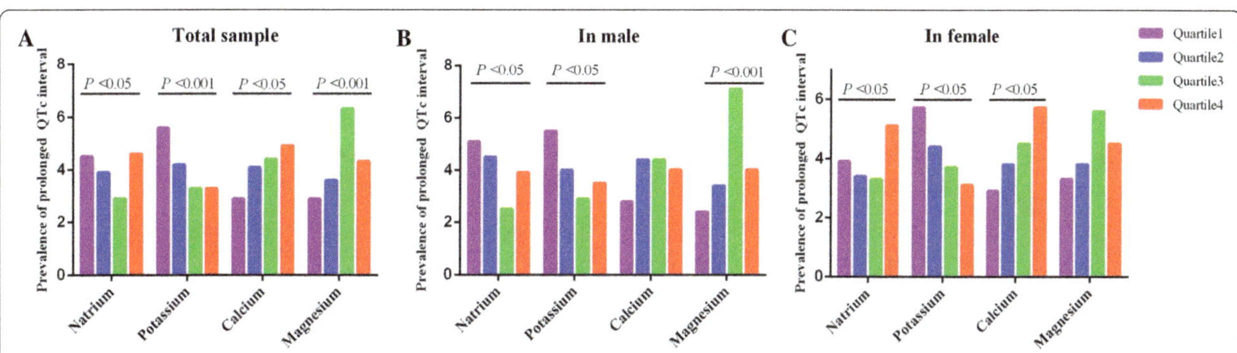

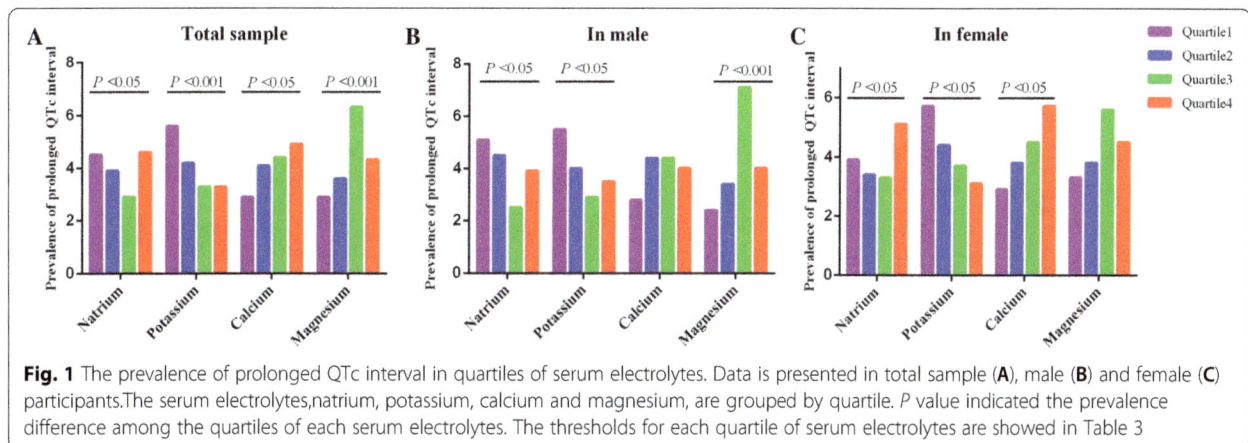

Fig. 1 The prevalence of prolonged QTc interval in quartiles of serum electrolytes. Data is presented in total sample (**A**), male (**B**) and female (**C**) participants.The serum electrolytes,natrium, potassium, calcium and magnesium, are grouped by quartile. *P* value indicated the prevalence difference among the quartiles of each serum electrolytes. The thresholds for each quartile of serum electrolytes are showed in Table 3

Table 2 Stepwise multiple linear regression for associations between coronary risk factors and QTc interval

	Male			Female		
Variables	Coef[a]	SE[b]	beta[c]	Coef[a]	SE[b]	beta[c]
Age (per 10 years)	4.98	0.35	0.25	1.82	0.38	0.08
current smoking (yes/no)	1.55	0.60	0.04	3.60	0.80	0.06
waist circumference	0.20	0.03	0.09	0.23	0.03	0.10
Hypertension	5.58	0.63	0.13	3.34	0.64	0.08
Diabetes (yes/no)	2.66	1.04	0.04	–	–	–
Estimated GFR	0.09	0.03	0.06	0.09	0.03	0.06
Serum uric acid	0.01	0.004	0.05	–	–	–
Serum calcium	5.77	2.44	0.04	10.72	2.34	0.07
Serum potassium	−7.76	0.85	−0.13	−6.44	0.88	−0.10
Serum magnesium	20.23	3.87	0.08	9.93	2.28	0.06
$LVMI_{ht2.7}$	–	–	–	0.03	0.01	0.04

The short dashes meaned that the variable was removed by the stepwise process, and there were other adjusted variables including dietscore, current drinking, BMI, physical activity, dyslipidaemia, and serum sodium which also removed from all the models finally. [a] unstandardized coefficient, [b]standard error, [c]standardized beta. , and the *P* <0.05 for all β values in the table

Discussion

It has been observed that electrolyte disturbances may trigger or facilitate clinical arrhythmias that might result in sudden death, even in a bundle of normal cardiac tissue [25]. Previous clinical studies found that changes in the QTc interval were inversely associated with levels of serum potassium and magnesium after dialysis [13] and a low Ca^{2+} concentration in the dialysate [10]. QTc prolongation has also been considered to increase the risk of ventricular arrhythmia and sudden death in clinical patients affected by acquired or genetic long QT syndrome [10], which is also presented in the healthy population [26]. However, studies that reported the association between serum electrolytes and the QTc prolongation in a general population have been rare. In the present general population, in contrast to previous patient groups, stepwise linear regression showed that QTc prolongation had a positive relationship with serum magnesium and calcium, and a prominent negative relationship with of serum potassium in both male and female sbjects. However, after adjustment for other factors, multiple logistic regression only found a significant inverse association between serum potassium and QTc

Table 3 Multiple logistic regression for associations between quartiles of serum electrolytes and QTc prolongation

		Total sample			Male			Female		
	Thresholds (mmol/L)	OR	Lower	Upper	OR	Lower	Upper	OR	Lower	Upper
Serum sodium										
Quartile1	<140.0	Reference			Reference			Reference		
Quartile2	140.0-140.9	0.89	0.63	1.24	0.84	0.53	1.34	1.00	0.61	1.65
Quartile3	141.0-141.9	*0.61**	*0.43**	*0.87**	*0.47**	*0.28**	*0.80**	0.83	0.50	1.37
Quartile4	≥ 142.0	0.83	0.62	1.11	0.67	0.44	1.03	1.11	0.72	1.72
Serum potassium										
Quartile1	<4.00	*1.72**	*1.30**	*2.28**	*1.67**	*1.10**	*2.54**	*2.02**	*1.36**	*3.01**
Quartile2	4.00-4.19	1.32	0.98	1.78	1.19	0.77	1.85	*1.54**	*1.01*	*2.35*
Quartile3	4.20-4.39	1.04	0.76	1.43	0.85	0.53	1.37	1.27	0.83	1.95
Quartile4	≥ 4.40	Reference			Reference			Reference		
Serum Calcium										
Quartile1	<2.24	Reference			Reference			Reference		
Quartile2	2.24-2.32	1.30	0.94	1.79	1.60	0.99	2.60	1.09	0.70	1.70
Quartile3	2.33-2.41	1.28	0.92	1.78	1.41	0.85	2.34	1.19	0.76	1.86
Quartile4	≥ 2.42	1.30	0.92	1.83	1.16	0.68	1.99	1.40	0.89	2.22
Serum magnesium										
Quartile1	<0.80	Reference			Reference			Reference		
Quartile2	0.80-0.83	1.33	0.91	1.95	1.83	0.97	3.46	1.13	0.70	1.83
Quartile3	0.84-0.89	*1.88**	*1.20**	*2.93**	*4.06**	*2.00**	*8.22**	1.05	0.58	1.91
Quartile4	≥ 0.90	*1.55**	*1.06**	*2.26**	*2.47**	*1.32**	*4.64**	1.21	0.74	1.96

All the serum electrolytes were adjusted by each other in the same model. The other adjustment factors included age, serum uric acid, body mass index, waist circumference, race, diet score, current smoking, current drinking, physical activity, eGFR, hypertension, dyslipidaemia, diabetes and LVH

OR odds ratio

**P* < 0.05

prolongation in both male and female subjects, and a positive association between serum magnesium and QTc prolongation in male subjects alone. Regarding the general population in the present study, the first quartile cut-off for serum potassium (4 mmol/L) was much higher than the clinical diagnostic threshold for hypokalaemia (3.5 mmol/L), and the prevalence of hypokalaemia in this population was only 0.9% ($n = 95$). The prevalences of hyperkalaemia (0.2%, $n = 21$, > 5.3 mmol/L) and hypermagnesemia (0.1%, $n = 6$, > 1.28 mmol/L) were even lower. Hence, the vast majority of the participants who were examined had normal levels of serum potassium and magnesium. However, we also found that even when the ranges were normal, a decrease in serum potassium and an increase in serum magnesium increased the risk of QTc prolongation in the present general population.

It is well known that the QTc interval is regulated or affected by dysfunction of the cardiac autonomic nervous system [27]. The sympathetic and parasympathetic nervous systems control the force of heart contractions by influencing calcium channels and control the heart rate via potassium channels, as well as controlling atrioventricular transduction [28]. It has previously been reported that two-pore-domain-potassium (K2P) channels are also expressed in the autonomic nervous system, where they might be important modulators of neuronal excitability [29]. In addition, as the most abundant intracellular cation, potassium is the key determinant of the resting membrane potential. The potassium gradient and the concentration of other electrolytes could modulate potassium currents, which might result in abnormal electrocardiographic findings [25]. Thus, serum potassium could influence the QTc interval directly by modulating potassium currents or indirectly by affecting cardiac the autonomic nervous system.

One important characteristic of this general population is that nearly half of the population suffered from hypertension. They also lived in north-eastern China, which is an area with a high dietary sodium intake. It has previously been reported that individuals with hypertension displayed QTc prolongation or QTc dispersion [30]. Some researchers have postulated that sympathetic predominance and chronic anxiety could increase QTc prolongation in a hypertensive population. In accordance with previous studies, we also found a significantly positive association between hypertension and QTc prolongation. Because of the relatively poor economic conditions of the present rural population, these hypertensive patients usually selected diuretics or traditional Chinese medicines (containing diuretics) for treatment, which might result in electrolyte disturbance including low serum potassium, and thus increase the risk of QTc prolongation. In particular for the male population with hypertension, a decrease serum potassium within the normal range was also a risk indicator. More attention should be paid during antihypertensive therapy.

In clinical studies, the risk of QTc prolongation could be decreased by potassium supplementation in patients with hypokalaemia, or by an appropriate increase in the concentration of potassium in the dialysate in patients undergoing heamodialysis [10]. However, in the general population, the vast majority of participants had normal levels of serum electrolytes. It would be inappropriate to suggest that they take potassium supplements to reduce the risk of QTc prolongation, which might lead to another risk status, namely, hyperkalaemia. Previous studies found that a low dietary potassium intake was independently associated with QTc prolongation [9], and a significantly higher incidence of cardiovascular disease and mortality [31]. Hence, it might be advisable to consume foods rich in potassium to reduce the risk of QTc prolongation.

A previous study reported that the duration of the post-dialysis QTc interval was inversely correlated with the change in magnesium levels after dialysis [11], which was established on the basis of single-factor analysis in 50 patients with end-stage renal disease who were undergoing regular hemodialysis. However, another study reported that lower levels of serum magnesium were related to a less pronounced increase in the QTc interval in patients with aneurysmal subarachnoid haemorrhage [32]. However, in this study, we found a positive relationship between serum magnesium and QTc prolongation in the general population without eGFR < 60 mL/min/1.73m^2. The clinical observational studies had limited sample sizes and more selection bias, which might be the causes of the difference in the results. The results of our study indicated that an increase of serum magnesium within the normal range might also increase the risk of QTc prolongation in the male population.

The major limitation of the study was a cross-sectional analysis which only made assessment of associations possible and couldn't determine the causal effect. Second, the ECG examination was taken at one occasion only. The confounding effects of systematic error in measurement and morphology of QT intervals could not be ruled out. And due to large population, in this study the analysis has been done from computer measured QTc interval which in several studies have shown differences with manually measured QTc. Third, serum electrolytes were measured only once that might be affected by other confounding factors including dietary intake of electrolytes and urinary electrolyte excretion. But this population was a large sample general population which decreased the selection bias and provided more informative reference values.

Conclusions

In conclusions, the prevalence of QTc prolongation is significantly higher in participants with lower serum potassium and higher magnesium. In present Chinese rural general population, even with normal range, a decrease in serum potassium and an increase in serum magnesium are important risk factors for QTc prolongation. Thus, causes of reducing serum potassium should be paid more attention, especially for female individuals. And the positive association between serum magnesium and QTc prolongation in male population needs more studies to elucidate.

Abbreviations

BMI: Body mass index; ECGs: Electrocardiograph; eGFR: Estimated glomerular filtration rate; FPG: Fasting plasma glucose; HDL-c: High density lipoprotein cholesterol; LDL-c: Low density lipoprotein cholesterol; LVH: Left ventricular hypertrophy; LVM: Left ventricular mass; QTc: Corrected-QT interval; SCr: Serum creatinine; TC: Total cholesterol; TG: Triglyceride; WC: Waist circumference

Acknowledgements

The authors thank Yonghong Zhang, Liying Xing and Guowei Pan for their assistance.

Funding

This study was supported by National Science and Technology Support Program of China (grant number 2012BAJ18B02) and Liaoning Research Center for Translational Medicine of Cardiovascular Disease (grant number 2014225017).

Authors' contributions

YS and LZ designed research; XG, GS, and ZL conducted research and acquired the data; YC and XG analyzed data; YC wrote the article; XG and GS critically revised the manuscript for important intellectual content; YC and YS had primary responsibility for final content. All authors read and approved the final manuscript.

Competing interests

The authors declare that they have no competing interests.

Author details

[1]Department of Cardiology, The First Hospital of China Medical University, Shenyang 110001, People's Republic of China. [2]Department of Clinical Epidemiology, Library, Shengjing Hospital of China Medical University, Shenyang, Liaoning, China.

References

1. Straus SM, Kors JA, De Bruin ML, van der Hooft CS, Hofman A, Heeringa J, Deckers JW, Kingma JH, Sturkenboom MC, Stricker BH, et al. Prolonged QTc interval and risk of sudden cardiac death in a population of older adults. J Am Coll Cardiol. 2006;47(2):362–7.
2. Dekker JM, Schouten EG, Klootwijk P, Pool J, Kromhout D. Association between QT interval and coronary heart disease in middle-aged and elderly men. The Zutphen Study. Circulation. 1994;90(2):779–85.
3. Okin PM, Devereux RB, Howard BV, Fabsitz RR, Lee ET, Welty TK. Assessment of QT interval and QT dispersion for prediction of all-cause and cardiovascular mortality in American Indians: the strong heart study. Circulation. 2000;101(1):61–6.
4. Ambhore A, Teo SG, Bin Omar AR, Poh KK. Importance of QT interval in clinical practice. Singap Med J. 2014;55(12):607–11. quiz 612
5. Mangoni AA, Kinirons MT, Swift CG, Jackson SH. Impact of age on QT interval and QT dispersion in healthy subjects: a regression analysis. Age Ageing. 2003;32(3):326–31.
6. Rautaharju PM, Zhou SH, Wong S, Calhoun HP, Berenson GS, Prineas R, Davignon A. Sex differences in the evolution of the electrocardiographic QT interval with age. Can J Cardiol. 1992;8(7):690–5.
7. Michishita R, Shono N, Kasahara T, Tsuruta T. Association between maximal oxygen uptake and the heart rate corrected-QT interval in postmenopausal overweight women. J Atheroscler Thromb. 2009;16(4):396–403.
8. Vandael E, Vandenberk B, Vandenberghe J, Willems R, Foulon V. Risk factors for QTc-prolongation: systematic review of the evidence. Int J Clin Pharm. 2017;39(1):16–25.
9. Michishita R, Ishikawa-Takata K, Yoshimura E, Mihara R, Ikenaga M, Morimura K, Takeda N, Yamada Y, Higaki Y, Tanaka H, et al. Influence of dietary sodium and potassium intake on the heart rate corrected-QT interval in elderly subjects. J Nutr Sci Vitaminol. 2015;61(2):138–46.
10. Genovesi S, Dossi C, Vigano MR, Galbiati E, Prolo F, Stella A, Stramba-Badiale M. Electrolyte concentration during haemodialysis and QT interval prolongation in uraemic patients. Europace. 2008;10(6):771–7.
11. Alabd MA, El-Hammady W, Shawky A, Nammas W, El-Tayeb M. QT interval and QT dispersion in patients undergoing hemodialysis: revisiting the old theory. Nephron Extra. 2011;1(1):1–8.
12. Sherif KA, Abo-Salem E, Panikkath R, Nusrat M, Tuncel M. Cardiac repolarization abnormalities among patients with various stages of chronic kidney disease. Clin Cardiol. 2014;37(7):417–21.
13. Wenzel-Seifert K, Wittmann M, Haen E. QTc prolongation by psychotropic drugs and the risk of torsade de pointes. Deutsch Arztebl Int. 2011;108(41):687–93.
14. Chen Y, Yu S, Chen S, Guo X, Li Y, Li Z, Sun Y. The Current Situation of Hypertension among Rural Minimal Assurance Family Participants in Liaoning (China): A Cross-Sectional Study. International journal of environmental research and public health. 2016;13(12):E1199.
15. Chobanian AV, Bakris GL, Black HR, Cushman WC, Green LA, Izzo JL Jr, Jones DW, Materson BJ, Oparil S, Wright JT Jr, et al. The seventh report of the joint National Committee on prevention, detection, evaluation, and treatment of high blood pressure: the JNC 7 report. Jama. 2003;289(19):2560–72.
16. Fedaration WHOaID. Definition and diagnosis of diabetes mellitus and intermediate hyperglycemia. In: Report of a WHO/IDF Consultation Geneva. Switzerland: World Health Organization; 2006.
17. Expert Panel on Detection, Evaluation, and Treatment of High Blood Cholesterol in Adults: Executive Summary of The Third Report of The National Cholesterol Education Program (NCEP) Expert Panel on Detection, Evaluation, And Treatment of High Blood Cholesterol In Adults (Adult Treatment Panel III). JAMA. 2001;285(19):2486–497.
18. National Kidney Foundation: K/DOQI clinical practice guidelines for chronic kidney disease: evaluation, classification, and stratification. American journal of kidney diseases: the official journal of the National Kidney Foundation. 2002;39(2 Suppl 1):S1–266.
19. Sun GZ, Ye N, Chen YT, Zhou Y, Li Z, Sun YX. Early repolarization pattern in the general population: prevalence and associated factors. Int J Cardiol. 2017;230:614–8.
20. Devereux RB, Alonso DR, Lutas EM, Gottlieb GJ, Campo E, Sachs I, Reichek N. Echocardiographic assessment of left ventricular hypertrophy: comparison to necropsy findings. Am J Cardiol. 1986;57(6):450–8.

21. Li T, Yang J, Guo X, Chen S, Sun Y. Geometrical and functional changes of left heart in adults with prehypertension and hypertension: a cross-sectional study from China. BMC Cardiovasc Disord. 2016;16:114.
22. Li Z, Guo X, Liu Y, Sun G, Sun Y, Guan Y, Zhu G, Abraham MR. Relation of heavy alcohol consumption to QTc interval prolongation. Am J Cardiol. 2016;118(8):1201–6.
23. Fridericia LS. Die systolendauer im elektrokardiogramm bei normalen menschen und bei herzkranken. Acta Med Scand. 1920;53:469–86.
24. Rautaharju PM, Surawicz B, Gettes LS, Bailey JJ, Childers R, Deal BJ, Gorgels A, Hancock EW, Josephson M, Kligfield P, et al. AHA/ACCF/HRS recommendations for the standardization and interpretation of the electrocardiogram: part IV: the ST segment, T and U waves, and the QT interval: a scientific statement from the American Heart Association Electrocardiography and Arrhythmias Committee, Council on Clinical Cardiology; the American College of Cardiology Foundation; and the Heart Rhythm Society: endorsed by the International Society for Computerized Electrocardiology. Circulation. 2009;119(10):e241–50.
25. El-Sherif N, Turitto G. Electrolyte disorders and arrhythmogenesis. Cardiol J. 2011;18(3):233–45.
26. Schouten EG, Dekker JM, Meppelink P, Kok FJ, Vandenbroucke JP, Pool J. QT interval prolongation predicts cardiovascular mortality in an apparently healthy population. Circulation. 1991;84(4):1516–23.
27. Dekker JM, Feskens EJ, Schouten EG, Klootwijk P, Pool J, Kromhout D. QTc duration is associated with levels of insulin and glucose intolerance. The Zutphen Elderly Study. Diabetes. 1996;45(3):376–80.
28. Myslivecek J. Current views on receptors for mediators of the autonomic nervous system of the heart. Casopis Lekaru Ceskych. 2001;140(14):423–6.
29. Cadaveira-Mosquera A, Perez M, Reboreda A, Rivas-Ramirez P, Fernandez-Fernandez D, Lamas JA. Expression of K2P channels in sensory and motor neurons of the autonomic nervous system. J Mol Neurosci. 2012;48(1):86–96.
30. Saadeh AM, Jones JV. Predictors of sudden cardiac death in never previously treated patients with essential hypertension: long-term follow-up. J Hum Hypertens. 2001;15(10):677–80.
31. Umesawa M, Iso H, Date C, Yamamoto A, Toyoshima H, Watanabe Y, Kikuchi S, Koizumi A, Kondo T, Inaba Y, et al. Relations between dietary sodium and potassium intakes and mortality from cardiovascular disease: the Japan collaborative cohort study for evaluation of Cancer risks. Am J Clin Nutr. 2008;88(1):195–202.
32. van den Bergh WM, Algra A, Rinkel GJ. Electrocardiographic abnormalities and serum magnesium in patients with subarachnoid hemorrhage. Stroke. 2004;35(3):644–8.

Predictive value of left atrial appendage lobes on left atrial thrombus or spontaneous echo contrast in patients with non-valvular atrial fibrillation

Fan Wang†, Mengyun Zhu†, Xiaoyu Wang†, Wei Zhang†, Yang Su, Yuyan Lu, Xin Pan, Di Gao, Xianling Zhang, Wei Chen, Yawei Xu, Yuxi Sun* and Dachun Xu*

Abstract

Background: Left atrial appendage morphology has been proved to be an important predictor of left atrial thrombus (LAT) and left atrial spontaneous echo contrast (LASEC) and stroke in patients with non-valvular atrial fibrillation (NVAF). However, the relation between left atrial appendage (LAA) lobes and LAT or LASEC is still unknown. The aim of this study is to investigate the correlation between the number of left atrial appendage lobes and LAT/LASEC in patients with NVAF.

Methods: This monocentric cross-sectional study enrolled 472 consecutive patients with non-valvular atrial fibrillation, who had transthoracic echocardiography (TTE) and transesophageal echocardiography (TEE) prior to cardioversion or left atrial appendage closure (LAAC) from July 2009 to August 2015 in department of cardiology of Shanghai Tenth People's Hospital. Patients who had significant mitral or aortic valve disease, previous cardiac valvular surgery and other complicated cardiac diseases were excluded. Individuals were divided into two groups:the LAT/LASEC group (16.95%), which comprised patients with LAT or LASEC, as confirmed by TEE; and a negative control group (83.05%).Baseline overall group characterization with demographic, clinical, laboratory data and echocardiographic parameters, alongside with information on medication was obtained for all patients. Subgroup analysis with line chart was applied for exploring the association between LAA lobes and LAT/LAESC. Receptor-operating curves (ROC) were used to test the value of LA anteroposterior diameter detected by different echocardiography methods predicting LAT or LASEC. Multivariable logistic regression analysis was used to investigate independent predictors of LAT/LASEC.

(Continued on next page)

* Correspondence: zhggsmlsyx@163.com; 1158009156@qq.com
†Fan Wang, Mengyun Zhu, Xiaoyu Wang and Wei Zhang contributed equally to this work.
Department of Cardiology, Shanghai Tenth People's Hospital, Tongji University School of Medicine, NO. 301 Middle Yanchang Road, Shanghai 200072, China

(Continued from previous page)

Results: Among 472 patients, 23 (4.87%) had LA/LAA thrombus and 57 (12.1%) had LA spontaneous echo contrast. Compared to the negative group, patients in LAT/LASEC group had higher CHA_2DS_2-VASc score (3.79 ± 1.75 vs 2.65 ± 1.76, $p < 0.001$), larger LAD (measured by TTE, 48.1 ± 7.7 vs 44.6 ± 6.5, $P < 0.001$; measured by TEE, 52.2 ± 6.2 vs 46.7 ± 7.1, $P < 0.001$), lower left upper pulmonary venous flow velocity (LUPVFV) (0.54 ± 0.17 m/s vs 0.67 ± 0.26 m/s, CI 95% 0.05–0.22, $P = 0.003$), more left atrial appendage lobes (1.67 ± 0.77 vs 1.25 ± 0.50, $p < 0.001$). There was a good discriminative capacity for LAD detected by TTE (area under the curve (AUC), 0.67, CI 95% 0.61–0.73, $p < 0.001$) and LAD detected by TEE (AUC, 0.73, CI 95% 0.67–0.79, $p < 0.001$). The subgroup analysis based on gender and different LAA lobes yielded similar results (male group: $p < 0.001$;female group: $p = 0.004$) that the number of LAA lobes were significantly associated with LA thrombus or SEC. In multivariable logistic regression analysis, both the number of LAA lobes (odds ratio: 2.37; CI 95% 1.37–4.09; $p = 0.002$) and the persistent AF (odds ratio: 3.57; CI 95% 1.68–7.57; $p = 0.001$) provided independent and incremental predictive value beyond CHA_2DS_2-VASc score.

Conclusion: The number of LAA lobes is an independent risk factor and has a moderate predictive value for LAT/LASEC among NVAF patients in China.

Keywords: Left atrial appendage, Left atrial Thrombus, Left atrial spontaneous echo contrast, Atrial fibrillation

Background

Atrial fibrillation (AF) is one of the most commonly observed arrhythmias in clinical practice with an incidence of 0.77% in China and approximately 1.5–2.0% in the developed world. This arrhythmia is associated with a five-fold risk of stroke, and 20–30% of all strokes are due to AF, thus a higher mortality compared with those without AF [1–3]. Actually, over 90% of embolic stroke was caused by thrombi that originating from left atrial appendage (LAA) [4, 5]. LAA was described as a long, narrow, tubular, wavy, hooked structure with different lobes and a narrow junction and crenellated lumen [6, 7], creating a favorable condition for thrombosis, especially under the situation of AF. Thus it is of great importance to identify the thrombi or signs indicating thrombi formation in LAA. Presence of thrombus, spontaneous echo contrast (SEC) in LA/LAA, or decreased LAA emptying velocity has been reported as markers of thromboembolic risk in non-valvular atrial fibrillation (NVAF) [8–10]. Thrombus was defined as a hyperechogenic non-muscular and non-endocardial mass detected by more than one plane axis during transesophageal echocardiography (TEE), and SEC was defined as smoke-like material with a characteristic swirling motion that persisted throughout the cardiac cycle [11, 12].Actually, the severity of LASEC quantified by different semi-quantitative assessments has been proven to be associated with stroke events in patients with NVAF. It's reported that denser LASEC was accompanied by a higher risk of LAA thrombus formation in patients with NVAF [13–15].However, in our study, we don't pay attention to semi-quantitative methods of LASEC which are largely influenced by the experience of the operator. We look LAA thrombus as the densest LASEC. The presence of at least one of them was designated left atrial abnormality.

Remarkably, it is observed that even in patients with AF, the incidence of AF associated stroke varied widely, ranging from 1 to 20% annually [4]. One possible mechanism behind may be that the incidence of thrombi formation in LAA with different anatomical characteristics, i.e., LAA morphology and number of LAA lobes, varied. Now it is recognized that there were four LAA macroscopic morphologies, including cactus LAA, chicken wing LAA, windsock LAA and cauliflower LAA [5, 16–21]. Several recent studies have demonstrated that different LAA morphologies obtained by Cardiac CT or MRI are closely correlated with LASEC, transient ischaemic attacks (TIA) and strokes in patients with AF [16–21]. However, the relationship between LAA lobes and markers of thromboembolic risk (decreased LAA flow velocity, LASEC, LA thrombus) has not been fully characterized in patients with NVAF. Therefore, the aim of this study is to examine whether the number of left atrial appendage lobes could influence the development of left atrial thrombus (LAT) or left atrial spontaneous echo contrast (LASEC) in patients with NVAF.

Methods

Study design

We studied 472 patients with all types of non-vavular AF. Left atrial thrombus and spontaneous echo contrast were analyzed by 2D-TEE and classified into two groups (LAT or LASEC positive group and negative group). Simultaneously, LAA lobes were counted during TEE procedure. Then, univariate analysis was performed using the Student's t-test and chi-square test. Predictors from univariate analysis were used for obtaining logistic regression models that could determine the relative importance of independent predictors of LAAT and LASEC [22].

Enrollment

This single-center cross-sectional study enrolled patients undergoing TTE and TEE prior to catheter ablation or left atrial appendage closure (LAAC) during a non-valvular AF episode. A total of 472 consecutive participants (males, 57.4%; mean age, 66.1 ± 10.8 years) who were hospitalized at Department of Cardiology of Shanghai Tenth People's Hospital of Tongji University from July 2009 to August 2015 were referred to our center. AF was identified by an electrocardiogram and met the diagnostic criteria used in 2011 ACCF/AHA/HRS Guidelines for the management of patients with AF [1]. Exclusion criteria included: [i] moderate or severe mitral stenosis; [ii] severe mitral regurgitation; [iii] severe aortic stenosis; [iv] prosthetic mitral or aortic valves; [v] patients with unsuitable images for accurate assessment of TEE surrogate markers of stroke; [vi] congenital heart disease (i.e. atrial septal defect, ventricular septal defect, et al...); [vii] any contraindication to TEE (i.e. esophageal obstruction, esophageal varices, et al); [vii] poor image quality. Then all of these patients were stratified into two subgroups based on with or without LAT or LASEC.

Initial data collection

All individuals were subjected to thorough history taking and full clinical evaluation. Patient gender, age, heart rate, systolic blood pressure (SBP), diastolic blood pressure (DBP), type of AF, duration of AF, CHA_2DS_2-VASc score, antiplateletdrugs or anticoagulant drugs, antiarrhythmic drugs, as well as history of congestive heart failure, hypertension, diabetes mellitus, previous stroke, vascular disease and other related diseases, were recorded. CHA_2DS_2-VASc score were calculated with 1 point assigned for a history of congestive heart failure, hypertension, 74 years ≥ age ≥ 65 years, female, diabetes mellitus and vascular disease and 2 points assigned for age ≥ 75 years, a history of stroke or transient ischemic attack (TIA), the maximum score is 9. Specifically, previous stroke also included lacunar infarction.

Echocardiographic data

Doppler echocardiography was performed using commercially available equipment (Vivid 9 system, General Electric, Horten, Norway) and a variable frequency phased-array transducer. Complete M-mode, two-dimensional, spectral- and color-Doppler images were used to obtain the following measurements: left atrial diameter (LAD), left ventricular end systolic diameter (LVESD), left ventricular end diastolic diameter (LVEDD), interventricular septal thickness (IVST), left ventricular posterior wall thickness (LVPWT), left ventricular ejection fraction (LVEF), pulmonary artery pressure (PAP). All measurements were taken according to the recommendations of the American Society of Echocardiography. Left ventricular ejection fractions were derived from biplane apical 2 and 4-chamber views using the modified Simpson's rule algorithm [23, 24].

TEE images were acquired with a 6 T phased array multiplane transoesophageal probe (Fig. 1a). LA and LAA were imaged in different tomographic planes from 0° to 180° to detect the presence of thrombusor SEC. LA thrombus was diagnosed by the presence of an echo-dense mass in left atrium or LAA (Fig. 1b), distinct from bulky pectinate muscles [25] (Fig. 1c). Left atrial spontaneous echocardiographic contrast (LASEC) as prethrombotic state having strong correlation with the occurrence of stroke was defined as a pattern of characteristic dynamic smoke-like swirling echoes in LA or LAA (Fig. 1d), distinct from a white noise artifact in the atrial cavity [26]. A pulsed Doppler sample was used to assess the Left atrial appendage flow velocities (LAAFV) [23]. Maximum emptying and filling velocities were estimated from an average of five well-defined emptying and filling waves. Left upper pulmonary venous flow velocity (LUPVFV) was assessed with a pulsed Doppler sample placed 1-2 cm into the left upper pulmonary vein proximal to where it enters the left atrium and at an angle as parallel as possible to the direction of the blood flow from the short-axis view obtained by advancing the TEE transducer to approximately 30 cm from the incisors [27, 28]. In addition, LAD was also obtained by TEE in the 45° plane.

Classification of left atrial appendage lobes

The definition of a lobe includes following criteria: [i] a visible outpouching part demarcated by an external crease from the body of LAA; [ii] the inner diameter was at least 2-mm; [iii] the direction of lobe could be opposite with the main tubular body of LAA; [iv] the anatomic plane was occasionally but not necessarily lain in a same anatomic plane than the main tubular body; [v] the LAA had at least one lobe [29, 30]. Figure 2 showed the morphology of a LAA, the distinct protrusion parts represent lobes. All relevant measurements during TEE and TTE, LAT, LASEC and LAA lobes were confirmed by two experienced cardiologists, who were blinded to the study.

Statistical analysis

All statistical analyses were performed by SPSS for Windows version 22 (SPSS Inc., Chicago, IL). All continuous data are presented as the mean ± SD and were compared using Student's t-test and one-way analysis of variance (ANOVA) test for two-level and multiple level grouping variables, respectively. Categorical variables are described as count and percent and were compared using Pearson's chi-square test (or Fisher's exact test whenever needed). Then sub-analysis based on gender and different numbers of LAA lobes was used to explore the

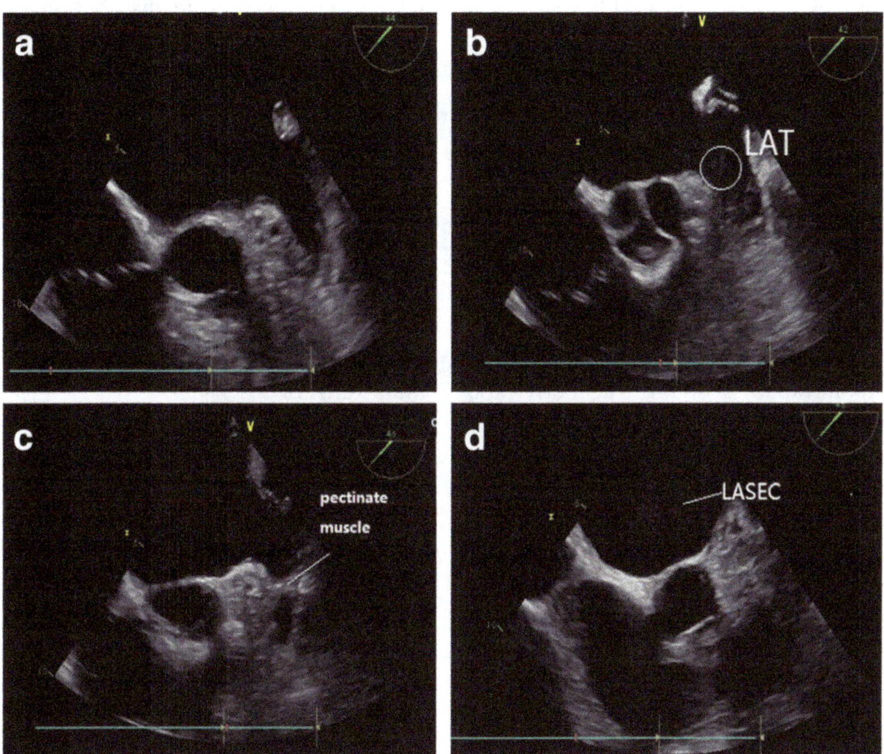

Fig. 1 Echo-pattern of LA or LAA thrombosis. The LAA regions are illustrated in a 2D TEE view (45-degree plane). **a** A normal image of left atrium and left atrial appendage (LAA) with one lobe. **b** A mass of thrombus about 9 × 11 mm^2 in the left atrium near the LAA orifice. **c** A thick pectinate muscle within the LAA cavity, distinct from LAA thrombus. **d** Left atrial spontaneous echo contrast (LASEC) presents as smoke-like swirling echoes

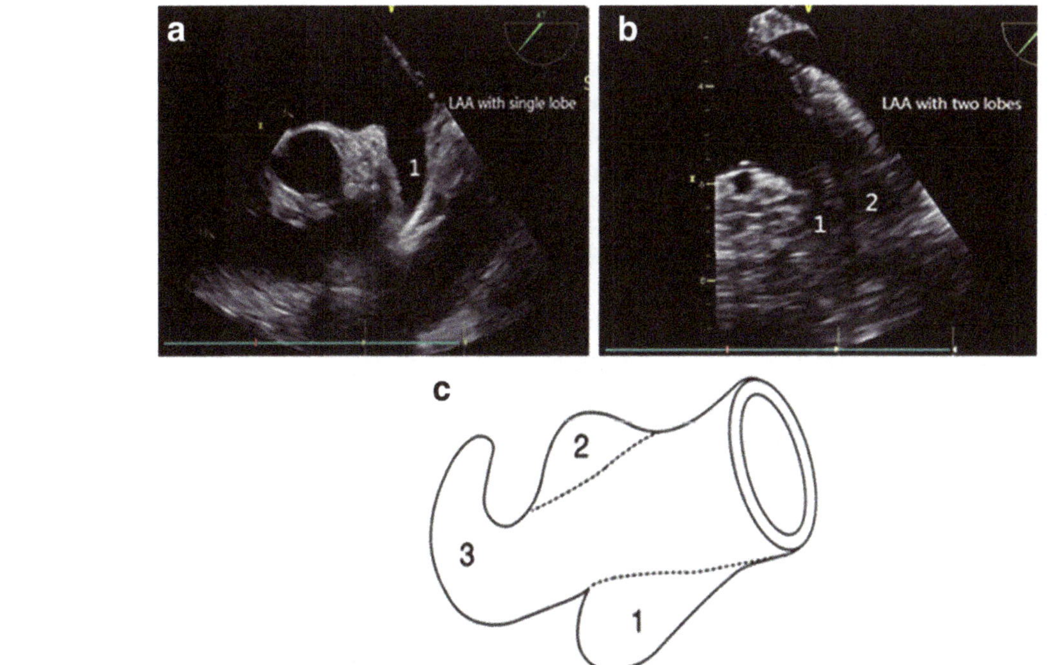

Fig. 2 Ultrasound images of LAA with different lobes by TEE. **a** LAA with one wide and deep lobe, composed by a tubular body and a blind-ending sac. **b** LAA with double lobes having shorts shape. **c** Diagram of a left atrial appendage (LAA) shows lobes (1, 2, and 3)

correlation between LAA lobes and LAT/LASEC, the same as LUPVFV. The receiver operating characteristic (ROC) curve was used to discriminate the power of the LA anteroposterior diameter measured by TTE and TEE in identifying TEE surrogate markers of stroke (LA/LAA thrombus, LASEC) [23]. Comparisons of areas under ROC curves (AUC) were performed between the two measurements, using z-test. Finally, a multivariable logistic regression analysis model was used to identify the significant independent correlates of LAT or LASEC. All potentialco-founders were put into the model on the basis of known clinical relevance or statistically significant association observed in univariate analyses. The odds ratio (OR) and 95% confidence interval (CI) of OR for thrombosis were computed. All tests were 2-sided, and a P value < 0.05 was considered statistically significant.

Results

Study population

Baseline characteristics of 472 patients were shown in Table 1. LAT or LASEC were found in 80 patients (16.95%, LAT: $n = 23$; LASEC: $n = 57$) by TEE examination. As shown in the table, patients with LAT or LASEC were significantly older but with nearly equal heart rate, systolic blood pressure (SBP), diastolic blood pressure (DBP) and without significant predilection for gender. The percentage distribution of prior congestive heart failure, diabetes, hypertension and previous vascular disease were significantly different between 2 patient groups, more in LAT/LASEC group. Simultaneously, patients with thrombosis had a longer duration of AF and more previous stroke events compared to patients without thrombosis; but these differences were statistically insignificant. In addition, persistent AF during hospitalization was more frequent and CHA_2DS_2-VASc score as expected, significantly higher in patients with LAT/LASEC.

Laboratory examinations and echocardiographic characteristics

These patients' baseline laboratory examinations and echocardiographic characteristics were shown in Table 2. There were no significant differences between 2 groups in platelets, ALT, AST, serum creatinine, BUN, D-dimer, and it was the same with LVESD, LVEDD, LVPWT, LAAFV and PFO by TTE. However, patients with LAT/LASEC had lower hemoglobin level (130.7 ± 13.1 vs 134.0 ± 18.6, $P = .049$), larger LA anteroposterior diameter measured by TTE (48.1 ± 7.7 vs 44.6 ± 6.5, $P < .001$) or TEE (52.2 ± 6.2 vs 46.7 ± 7.1, P < .001), slightly thicker ventricular septal (10.7 ± 3.0 vs 9.8 ± 1.7, $P = .018$), lower LVEF (60.3 ± 9.3 vs 63.5 ± 8.8, $P = .005$), higher pulmonary artery pressure (30.9 ± 9.8 vs 28.1 ± 8.2, $P < .011$),

Table 1 Baseline characteristics of included patients with and without LAT/LASEC

	Total (n = 472)	LAT /LASEC group (n = 80)	Non-LAT/LASEC group (n = 392)	P value
Clinical characteristics				
Age(yrs)	66.1 ± 10.8	70.2 ± 9.6	65.3 ± 10.8	< 0.001*
Male (n, %)	271 (57.4%)	40 (50.0%)	231(58.9%)	0.154
HR	86.5 ± 21.8	86.8 ± 18.9	86.4 ± 22.3	0.895
SBP	134.1 ± 18.8	137.0 ± 21.7	133.4 ± 18.1	0.136
DBP	78.7 ± 11.7	79.3 ± 13.1	78.6 ± 11.3	0.642
Persistent AF (n, %)	154 (32.6%)	44 (55.0%)	107 (27.3%)	< 0.001*
Duration of symptoms (months)	45.0 ± 70.4	56.6 ± 76.1	42.4 ± 69.0	0.131
Congestive heart failure (n, %)	73 (15.5%)	24 (30%)	49 (12.5%)	0.003*
Hypertension (n, %)	277 (58.7%)	63 (78.8%)	214 (54.6%)	< 0.001*
Diabetes mellitus (n, %)	77 (16.3%)	20 (25.0%)	57 (14.5%)	0.065
Previous stroke (n, %)	119 (25.2%)	26 (32.5%)	93 (23.7%)	0.174
Vascular disease (n, %)	133 (28.2%)	32 (40.0%)	101 (25.8%)	0.045*
CHA2DS2-VASc score	2.86 ± 1.81	3.79 ± 1.75	2.65 ± 1.76	< 0.001*
Antiplatelet and Anticoagulant drugs				
Aspirin	142 (30.1%)	15 (18.8%)	127 (32.4%)	0.033*
Warfarin	187 (39.6%)	37 (46.3%)	150 (38.3%)	
Dabigatran	47 (10.0%)	13 (32.5%)	34 (8.7%)	
Rivaroxaban	2 (0.42%)	0	2 (0.51%)	

Values are mean ± standard deviation, or number (%)

LAT left atrial thrombus, *LASEC* left atrial appendage spontaneous echo contrast, *AF* atrial fibrillation, *HR* heart rate, *SBP* systolic blood pressure, *DBP* diastolic blood pressure. *P < 0.05

Table 2 Laboratory examinations and echocardiographic characteristics of thrombosis group and control group

	Total ($n = 472$)	LAT /LASEC group ($n = 80$)	Non-LAT/LASEC group ($n = 392$)	P value
Laboratory examinations				
Hb (g/l)	133.8 ± 17.8	130.7 ± 13.1	134.0 ± 18.6	0.049*
Plt (*10^9/l)	186.9 ± 61.6	183.0 ± 54.3	187.7 ± 63.2	0.576
ALT(U/L)	28.6 ± 61.0	22.6 ± 21.1	30.0 ± 66.7	0.361
AST(U/L)	29.7 ± 75.7	24.1 ± 13.8	30.9 ± 83.9	0.508
sCr (mmol/l)	81.3 ± 25.0	85.7 ± 24.8	80.2 ± 25.0	0.102
BUN (mmol/l)	6.3 ± 2.1	5.7 ± 1.7	6.2 ± 2.1	0.167
D-Dimer	0.53 ± 1.67	0.48 ± 0.43	0.54 ± 1.62	0.700
Transthoracic echocardiographic parameters				
LAD (mm)	45.2 ± 6.8	48.1 ± 7.5	44.6 ± 6.5	< 0.001*
LVESD (mm)	30.6 ± 5.6	31.6 ± 5.3	30.4 ± 5.6	0.092
LVEDD (mm)	47.4 ± 5.0	47.5 ± 5.1	47.3 ± 4.5	0.755
IVsT (mm)	9.96 ± 1.98	10.67 ± 3.00	9.79 ± 1.67	0.018*
LVPWT (mm)	9.58 ± 1.60	10.26 ± 2.44	9.42 ± 1.33	0.418
LVEF (%)	63.0 ± 9.0	60.3 ± 9.3	63.5 ± 8.8	0.005*
Pulmonary artery pressure (mmHg)	28.6 ± 8.5	30.9 ± 9.8	28.1 ± 8.2	0.011*
Transesophageal echocardiographic parameters				
LAD (mm)	47.6 ± 7.3	52.2 ± 6.2	46.7 ± 7.1	< 0.001*
Lobes of Left atrial appendage	1.32 ± 0.58	1.67 ± 0.77	1.25 ± 0.50	<0.001*
1 (n, %)	289 (61.2%)	47 (41.3%)	242 (78.3%)	< 0.001*
2 (n, %)	83 (17.6%)	25 (31.3%)	58 (18.8%)	
> = 3 (n, %)	17 (3.6%)	8 (10.0%)	9 (2.9%)	
LUPVFV (m/s)	0.63 ± 0.24	0.54 ± 0.17	0.67 ± 0.26	0.03*
LAAFV (m/s)	0.35 ± 0.19	0.31 ± 0.13	0.37 ± 0.20	0.217
PFO (n, %)	33 (7.0%)	7 (8.8%)	26 (6.6%)	0.532

Values are mean ± standard deviation, or number (%)

LAT left atrial thrombus, *LASEC* left atrial appendage spontaneous echo contrast, *AF* atrial fibrillation, *Hb* hemoglobin, *PLT* platelets, *ALT* glutamate pyruvate transaminase, *AST* glutamicoxaloacetic transaminase, *sCr* serum creatinine, *BUN* blood urea nitrogen, *LAD* left atrial diameter, *LVESD* left ventricular end systolic diameter, *LVEDD* left ventricular end diastolic diameter, *IVST* Interventricular septal thickness, *LVPWT* left ventricular posterior wall thickness, *LVEF* left ventricular ejection fraction, *LAAFV* left atrial appendage flow velocity, *PFO* Patent foramen ovale. *$P < 0.05$

more LAA lobes (1.67 ± 0.77 vs 1.25 ± 0.50, $P < .001$) and lower LUPVFV (0.54 ± 0.17 m/s vs 0.67 ± 0.26 m/s, $P < .011$). Importantly, both T-test and Chi-Square test showed that LAA lobes of patients with LAT/LASEC were significantly more than other patients (Table 2).

LA anteroposterior diameter measurements for identifying LAT/LASEC on TEE

ROC analysis demonstrated that a cut-off value of anteroposterior LAD with 44.5 mmby TTEcould predict the presence of LAT/LASEC. At this level, sensitivity was 76.3% and specificity was 51.2%, Area under the curve (AUC) = 0.67 (CI 95% 0.61–0.73, $p < 0.001$). The value of LAD by TEE with a sensitivity of 72.2% and a specificity of 63.6% was 48.5 mm, AUC = 0.73 (CI 95% 0.67–0.79, $p < 0.001$) (Fig. 3 and Table 3). Thus, LAD by TTE and TEE showed a moderately high discriminatory power of the prediction of LAT/LASEC. However, ROC curve comparison for these two measurements revealed anteroposterior LAD by TEE provided greater predicative value than TTE with a significant difference (difference in AUC = 0.06 ± 0.03,Z = 1.99,$P < 0.05$).

Correlation between the number of LAA lobes and prevalence of LAT/LASEC

In our study, distribution of LAA lobes number was from 1 to 4, consistent with previous studies [9]. The most frequent LAA (61.2%) was a single lobe. The number of double and multiple lobes LAA types was 83 (17.6%) and 17 (3.6%). According to ANOVA, patients showed typical differences in LA thrombosis by TEE depending on LAA lobes number: among patients with LAT/LASEC by TEE, the average number of LAA lobes was 1.67 ± 0.77, compared with 1.25 ± 0.50 among patients with non-LAT/

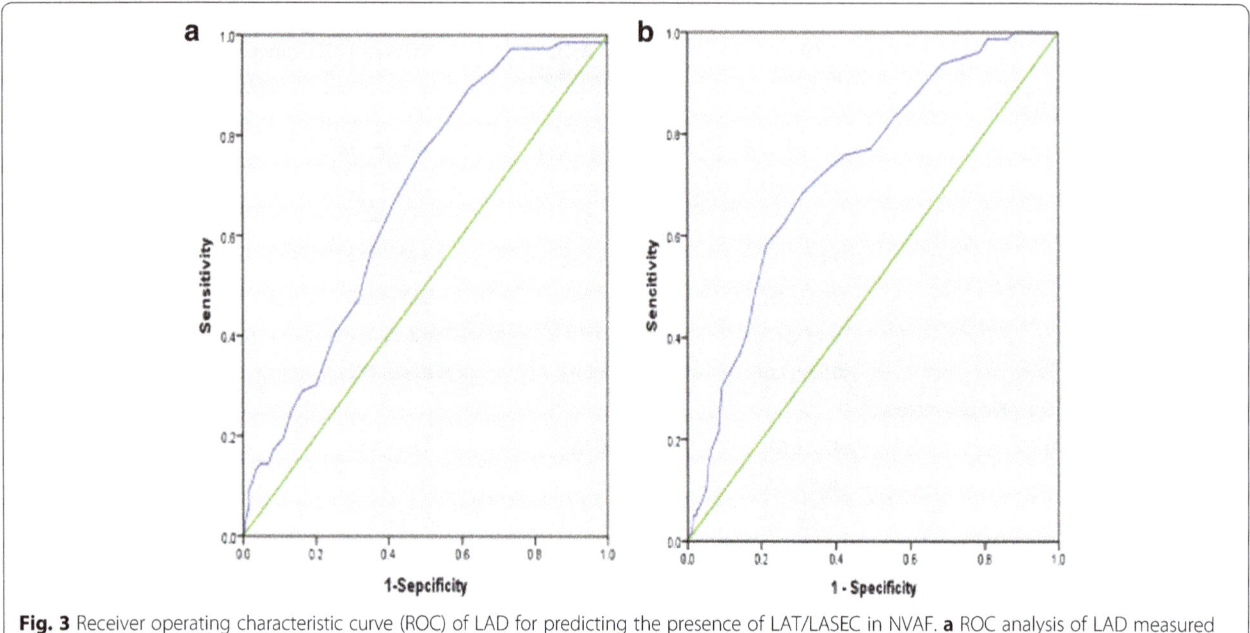

Fig. 3 Receiver operating characteristic curve (ROC) of LAD for predicting the presence of LAT/LASEC in NVAF. **a** ROC analysis of LAD measured by TTE for identifying LAT/LASEC; **b** ROC analysis of LAD measured by TEE for identifying LAT/LASEC

LASEC ($P < 0.001$) (Table 2). Moreover, LAT/LASEC incidence rate increased from single lobe to double and further to multiple lobes in sub-analysis in both male ($P <$ 0.001) and female ($P = 0.004$) subgroup (Fig. 4).

The correlation between LUPVFV and prevalence of LAT/LASEC

Overall, 95 patients (66 in LAT/LASEC group and 29 in non-LAT/LASEC group) had been detected LUPVFV by TEE. The average LUPVFV was 0.63 ± 0.24 m/s. According to analysis of variance, LUPVFV decreased in patients with LAT/LASEC, compared with non-thrombosis patients (difference in means 0.13 m/s, 95% CI 0.10–0.22, $P = 0.032$) (Table 2). In sub-analysis, these patients were divided into four grades by quartiles. LAT/LASEC incidence rate decreased from first quartile to last quartile, but did not reached statistical significance in both male ($p = 0.78$) and female ($p = 0.12$) subgroup (Fig. 5).

Independent predictive factors for LAT or LASEC

Multiple candidate clinical predictors and echocardiography measurements were assessed as univariate independent predictors for LAT/LASEC. Our results demonstrated that age, types of AF, LAD on TTE or TEE, antiplatelet or anticoagulation therapy, as well as CHA_2DS_2-VASc score were significantly correlated with the presence of LAT/LASEC (Tables 1 and 2). Multivariate linear regression analysis was performed to determine the relative importance of independent predictors of LAT/LASEC, the number of LAA lobes (single, double, multiple, odds ratio 2.37; 95% CI 1.37–4.09; $P = 0.002$), AF types (paroxysmal, persistent, odds ratio 3.57; 95% CI 1.68–7.57; $P = 0.001$) and antiplatelet or anticoagulation therapy (aspirin, oral coagulation medicine, odds ratio 0.36; 95% CI 0.13–0.96; $P = 0.04$) were independent predictors of LAT/LASEC (Table 4).

Table 3 The area under ROC curve of LAD to predict LAT/LASEC

	AUC	SE	*P* value	95% CI
LAD measured by TTE	0.670	0.030	<.001	0.611–0.730
LAD measured by TEE	0.729	0.029	<.001	0.672–0.787

ROC receiver operating characteristic, *LAD* left atrial anteroposterior diameter, *LAT* left atrial thrombus, *LASEC* left atrial appendage spontaneous echo contrast, *TTE* transthoracic echocardiography, *TEE* transesophageal echocardiography, *AUC* area under ROC curve, *SE* standard error, *CI* confident interval

Discussion

In the present study, we demonstrated that more LAA lobes number were significantly and independently associated with the presence of LAT and LASEC. Another important finding was that patients with LA thrombosis had a lower LUPVFV. To the best of our knowledge, this is the first study to investigate the roles of LAA lobes number and LUPVFV in predicting left atrial stasis markers: LAT or LASEC.

Accumulative data documented that the presence of thrombus or SEC in LAA/LA are strongly associated with thromboembolism and adverse outcomes in NVAF patients [31–33]. Accordingly, TEE was recommended to evaluate the risk of thromboembolism previous to procedures such as cardioversion, catheter ablation or left atrial appendage closure (LAAC) [1, 34, 35]. In our study, the presence of LAT or LASEC was associated

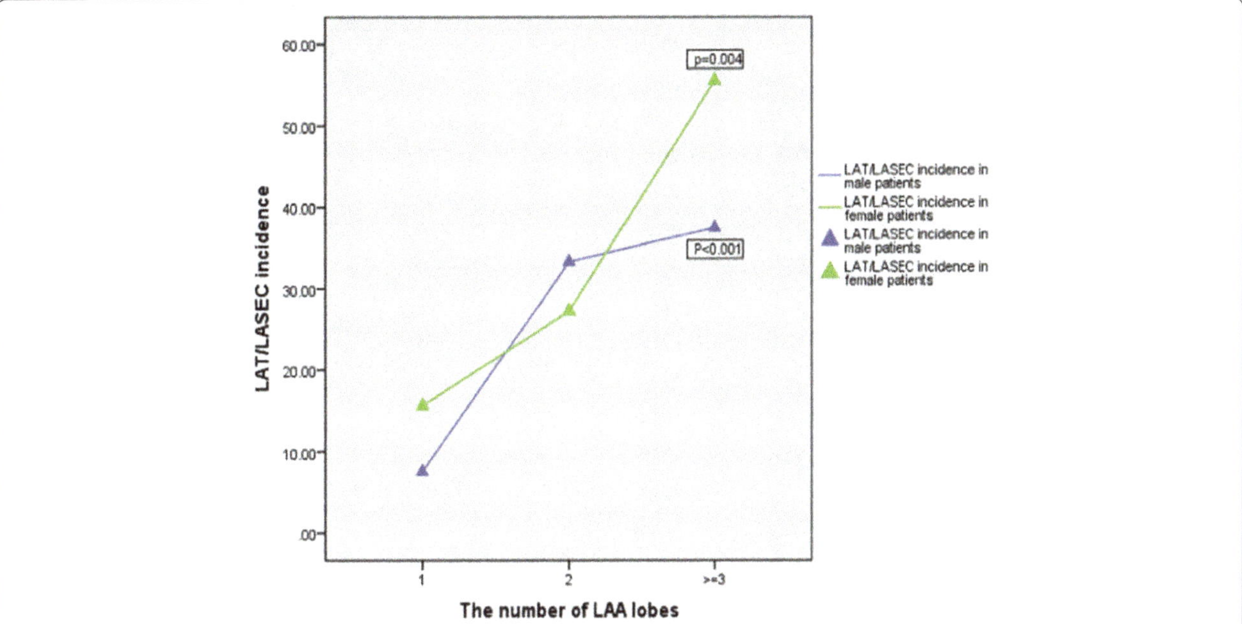

Fig. 4 Correlation between left atrial thrombosis and the number of LAA lobes. According to sub-analysis, LAT/LASEC differs significantly among different numbers of LAA lobes in either male ($P < 0.001$) or female ($P = 0.004$) subgroup. Patients with single lobe LAA show a reduced prevalence of thrombus and SEC during TEE compared with patients with multilobe

with the risk of thromboembolism assessed by CHA_2DS_2-VASc score, due to a higher prevalence of recognized thromboembolic risk factors such as elder, congestive heart failure, vascular disease, hypertension, and diabetes. Furthermore, our results also indicated that LAT or LASEC was closely associated with a larger left atrium, independent of detection methods, such as TTE or TEE, as reported in previous studies [11, 36–38]. However, this association became not significant after adjustment for other potential co-founders. What's

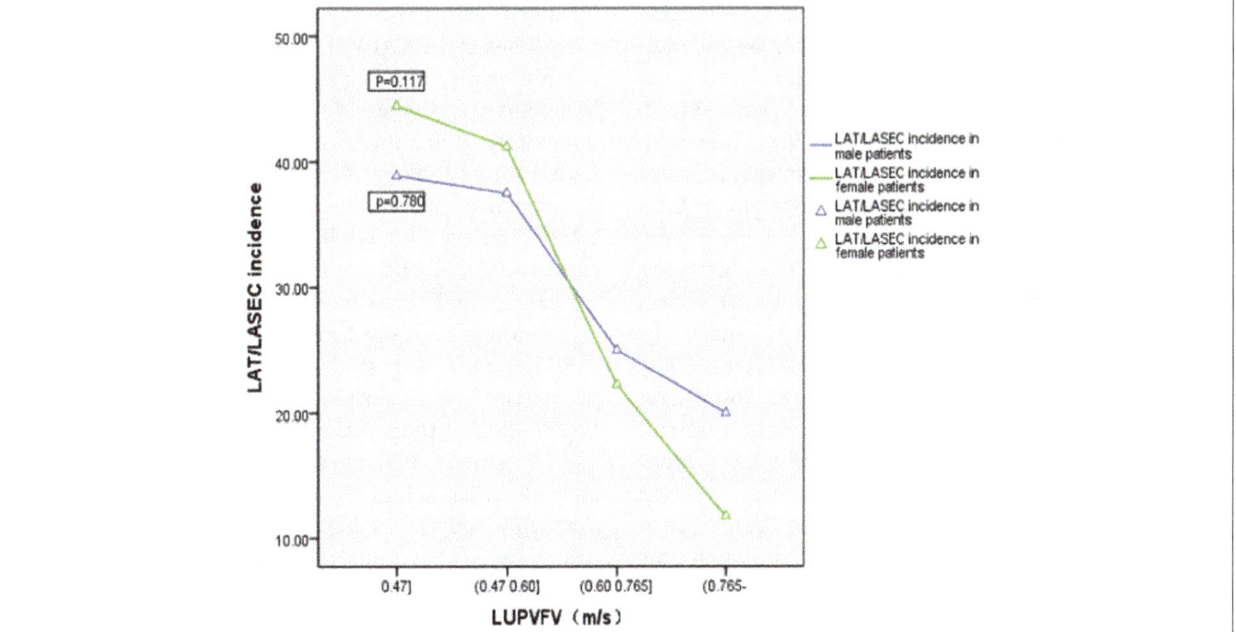

Fig. 5 Correlation between left atrial thrombosis and left upper pulmonary venous flow velocity (LUPVFV).The patients in our study who had been detected LUPVFV during TEE were divided into four groups by quartiles. In sub-analysis, LUPVFV decelerated, and the incidence of LAT/LASEC rose gradually from the last quartile to the first quartile, but did not reached statistical significance in both male ($p = 0.78$) and female ($p = 0.12$) subgroup owing to the small sample size

Table 4 Multivariate logistic regression analysis on predictors of LAT or LASEC in patients with NVAF

	B	S.E.	Wald	df	Sig.	Exp(B)	95%C.I.for Exp(B)	
							Lower	Upper
Sex	.430	.377	1.300	1	.254	1.537	.734	3.215
Age	−.012	.022	.316	1	.574	.988	.947	1.031
HR	.008	.009	.811	1	.368	1.008	.991	1.026
SBP	.007	.011	.498	1	.480	1.008	.987	1.029
DBP	−.011	.017	.463	1	.496	.989	.957	1.021
Persistent AF	1.272	.384	10.975	1	.001	3.566	1.681	7.567
CHA2DS2VASc score	.166	.126	1.733	1	.188	1.180	.922	1.511
Anticoagulation therapy	−1.023	.502	4.157	1	.041	.359	.134	.961
LAD by TTE	.046	.039	1.392	1	.238	1.047	.970	1.130
LAD by TEE	.060	.035	2.949	1	.086	1.061	.992	1.136
The number of LAA lobes	.862	.279	9.566	1	.002	2.367	1.371	4.086
Constant	−10.144	2.573	15.544	1	.000	.000		

LAT left atrial thrombus, *LASEC* left atrial appendage spontaneous echo contrast, *AF* atrial fibrillation, *HR* heart rate, *SBP* systolic blood pressure, *DBP* diastolic blood pressure, *LAD* left atrial diameter, *TTE* transthoracic echocardiography, *TEE* transesophageal echocadiography, *LAA* left atrial appendage

more, our result showed that LAD by TEE provided greater predicted value than by TTE. Although, recent researchers found that LA area in four-chamber view, indexed area-length volumes and diastolic function parameters (E/e' and e' velocity) displayed strong correlation with left atrial stasis markers (LAT, LASEC, LAAFV < 20 cm/s) in patients with non-valvular AF [11, 39], our study limited by missing data couldn't be conducted in these aspects.

Previous studies indicated that the number of lobes was variable, with the prevalence of single lobe ranging from 20 to 42.7%, double lobes from 25.2 to 64.3%, multiple lobes from 26.0 to 35.7% [5, 18, 30]. However, our result showed that patients with a single lobe were in the majority(61.2%), and double lobes 17.9%. These variations may be attributable to the race discrepancy, sample sizes of population and subjective judgment of LAA morphology.

LAA morphology was often classified into four types: (i) Chicken Wing LAA, a main lobe (> 4 cm) with a folded angle under 100°; (ii) Windsock LAA, a main lobe (> 4 cm) with a folded angle over 100°; (iii) Cactus LAA, a main lobe (< 4 cm) with more than two lobes over 1 cm; and (iv) Cauliflower LAA, a main lobe (< 4 cm) with no forked lobes. Such a division of LAA morphology which was originally designed to help practical planning for a transcatheter LAA closure device placement is now widely recognized [40].According to the classification, a Chicken Wing LAA often has only one lobe, sometimes two, while multilobed LAA were more common in NON-Chicken Wing patients. A large number of studies reported an association between LAA morphologies and the risk of TIA and stroke, Chicken Wing LAA had a highest LAA emptying flow velocity and a lowest risk of TIA and stroke [16, 18]. These studies documented that LAA emptying flow and LAAFV decreased in multilobed LAA [18], whereas LAAFV was associated with thrombus formation and stroke, regarded as a predictor of LA thromboembolism [20, 41].Thus, our results support the findings of previous studies: patient with complicated morphology (like non-chicken LAA) had more commonly multilobed LAA, lower LAAFV and was more likely to develop thrombus and SEC than patient with a single lobe LAA. Further research should explore the correlation between LAA lobes and LAAFV.

Additionally, it is generally believed that Chicken Wing LAA is similar to Windsock LAA, and it is also difficult to differentiate Cactus LAA from Cauliflower LAA by morphology. Therefore, such category method is subjective and conflicting. However, the number of LAA lobes by TEE is objective and easy to test, while cardiac CT and MRI are expensive and deleterious, thus we can apply TEE to acquire the number of LAA lobes and examine LAT and LASEC simultaneously.

Additionally, our study documented that left upper pulmonary venous flow velocity (LUPVFV) decreased in LAT/LASEC group. LUPVFV can reflect LA pressure and LV diastolic filling pressure (E/e'), which are important influential factors for LAAFV [27, 42]. Consequently, the combined use of LUPVFV and LAA lobes number can provide additional clinical implications for risk stratification.

Study limitations

This study has several limitations. First, this study is a single-center study with a relatively small sample. Second, the retrospective design of the study is an additional limitation. Large-scale studies with long-term follow-up are warranted to evaluate the predictive value of LAA lobes for stroke. Third, we investigated a relatively low risk population reflected by a mean CHA_2DS_2-VASc score of 2.86. Additionally, the rate of anticoagulation therapy among these patients was high (80.1%), which may affect the rate of LAT and LASEC and thromboembolic events. Thus, our findings could not be adapted to a high-risk AF population.

Conclusion

More left atrial appendage lobes are associated with significantly higher risk of left atrial thrombus or left atrial spontaneous echo contrast in patients with non-valvular atrial fibrillation. Therefore, the number of LAA lobes is an independent risk factor and has a moderate predictive value for LAT/LASEC among NVAF patients in China.

Abbreviations

AF: Atrial fibrillation; CT: Computer tomography; LA: Left atrium; LAA: Left atrial appendage; LAAC: Left atrial appendage closure; LAAFV: Left atrial appendage flow velocity; LAD: Left atrial diameter; LASEC: Left atrial spontaneous echo contrast; LAT: Left atrial thrombus; LUPVFV: Left upper pulmonary venous flow velocity; LV: Left ventricle; LVEF: Left ventricular ejection fraction; MRI: Magnetic resonance imaging; NVAF: Non-valvular atrial fibrillation; TEE: Transesophageal echocardiography; TIA: Transient ischemic attack; TTE: Transthoracic echocardiography

Funding

This work was supported by the National Natural Science Foundation of China (81270194). The funders had no role in study design, data collection and analysis, decision to publish, or preparation of the manuscript.

Authors' contributions

DX and YS2 conceived the study, FW, MZ, YS1, WZ, XP and DG acquired the data, FW and MZ performed and analyzed all echocardiograms, DX, FW and YS2 performed statistical analyses, DX, FW, YS2 and MZ drafted the manuscript, YW, WZ, YS2 and WC helped to draft the manuscript, and revised the manuscript critically for important intellectual content, XW, YL, YS1, XP, DG, XZ and YX revised the manuscript critically for important intellectual content. All authors read, revised and accepted the final version of the manuscript. All authors read and approved the final manuscript.

Competing interests

The authors have declared that they have no competing interests.

References

1. Fuster V, Rydén LE, Cannom DS, Crijns HJ, Curtis AB, Ellenbogen KA, Halperin JL, Kay GN, Le Huezey JY, Lowe JE, et al. 2011 ACCF/AHA/HRS focused updates incorporated into the ACC/AHA/ESC 2006 Guidelines for the management of patients with atrial fibrillation: a report of the American College of Cardiology Foundation/American Heart Association Task Force on Practice Guidelines developed in partnership with the European Society of Cardiology and in collaboration with the European Heart Rhythm Association and the Heart Rhythm Society. J Am Coll Cardiol. 2011;57(11): e101–98.
2. Wilke T, Groth A, Mueller S, Pfannkuche M, Verheyen F, Linder R, Maywald U, Bauersachs R, Breithardt G. Incidence and prevalence of atrial fibrillation: an analysis based on 8.3 million patients. Europace. 2013;15(4):486–93.
3. Knecht S, Wilton SB, Haissaguerre M. The 2010 update of the ESC guidelines for the management of atrial fibrillation. Circ J. 2010;74(12):2534–7.
4. Furie KL, Goldstein LB, Albers GW, Khatri P, Neyens R, Turakhia MP, Turan TN, Wood KA. Oral antithrombotic agents for the prevention of stroke in Nonvalvular atrial fibrillation: a science advisory for healthcare professionals from the American Heart Association/American Stroke Association. Stroke. 2012;43(12):3442–53.
5. Beigel R, Wunderlich NC, Ho SY, Arsanjani R, Siegel RJ. The left atrial appendage: anatomy, function, and noninvasive evaluation. JACC Cardiovasc Imaging. 2014;7(12):1251–65.
6. Sharma S, Devine W, Anderson RH, Zuberbuhler JR. The determination of atrial arrangement by examination of appendage morphology in 1842 heart specimens. Br Heart J. 1988;60(3):227–31.
7. Tuccillo B, Stümper O, Hess J, van Suijlen RJ, Bos E, Roelandt JR, Sutherland GR. Transoesophageal echocardiographic evaluation of atrial morphology in children with congental heart disease. Eur Heart J. 1992;13(2):223–31.
8. Zabalgoitia M, Leonard A, Blackshear JL, Safford R, Baker VS. Transesophageal echocardiographic correlates of thromboembolism in high-risk patients with nonvalvular atial fibrillation.The Stroke Prevention in Atrial Fibrillation Investigators Committee on Echocardiographyr. Ann Intern Med. 1998;128(8):639–47.
9. Fatkin D, Kelly RP, Feneley MP. Relations between left atrial appendage blood flow velocity, spontaneous echocardiographic contrast and thromboembolic risk in vivo. J Am Coll Cardiol. 1994;23(4):961–9.
10. Zabalgoitia M, Halperin JL, Pearce LA, Blackshear JL, Asinger RW, Hart RG. Transesophageal echocardiographic correlates of clinical risk of thromboembolism in nonvalvular atrial fibrillation. Stroke prevention in atrial fibrillation III investigators. J Am Coll Cardiol. 1998;31(7):1622–6.
11. Watson T, Shantsila E, Lip GY. Mechanisms of thrombogenesis in atrial fibrillation: Virchow's triad revisited. Lancet. 2009;373(9658):155–66.
12. Thambidorai SK, Murray RD, Parakh K, Shah TK, Black IW, Jasper SE, Li J, Apperson-Hansen C, Asher CR, Grimm RA, et al. Utility of transesophageal echocardiography in identification of thrombogenic milieu in patients with atrial fibrillation (an ACUTE ancillary study). Am J Cardiol. 2005;96(7):935–41.
13. Klein AL, Murray RD, Black IW, Chandra S, Grimm RA, DSa DA, Leung DY, Miller D, Morehead AJ, Vaughn SE, et al. Integrated backscatter for quantification of left atrial spontaneous echo contrast. J Am Coll Cardiol. 1996;28(1):222–31.
14. Fatkin D, Feneley MP. Qualitative or quantitative assessment of spontaneous echo contrast? J Am Coll Cardiol. 1997;29(1):222–4.
15. Bernhardt P, Schmidt H, Hammerstingl C, Omran H. Patients with atrial fibrillation and dense spontaneous echo contrast at high risk a prospective and serial follow-up over 12 months with transesophageal echocardiography and cerebral magnetic resonance imaging. J Am Coll Cardiol. 2005;45(11):1807–12.
16. Di Biase L, Santangeli P, Anselmino M, Mohanty P, Salvetti I, Gili S, Horton R, Sanchez JE, Bai R, Mohanty S, et al. Does the left atrial appendage morphology correlate with the risk of stroke in patients with atrial fibrillation? Results from a multicenter study. J Am Coll Cardiol. 2012;60:531–8.
17. Vargas-Barrón J, Espinola-Zavaleta N, Roldán FJ, Romero-Cárdenas A, Keirns C, Vázquez-Antona C. Transesophageal echocardiographic diagnosis of thrombus in accessory lobes of the left atrial appendage. Echocardiography. 2000;17(7):689–91.
18. Petersen M, Roehrich A, Balzer J, Shin DI, Meyer C, Kelm M, Kehmeier ES. Leftatrial appendage morphology is closely associated with specific echocardiographic flow pattern in patients with atrial fibrillation. Europace. 2015;17(4):539–45.
19. Khurram IM, Dewire J, Mager M, Maqbool F, Zimmerman SL, Zipunnikov V, Belnart R, Marine JE, Spragg DD, Berger RD, et al. Relationship between left atrial appendage morphology and stroke in patients with atrial fibrillation. Heart Rhythm. 2013;10(12):1843–9.
20. Fukushima K, Fukushima N, Kato K, Ejima K, Sato H, Fukushima K, Saito C, Hayashi K, Arai K, Manaka T, et al. Correlation between left atrial appendage morphology and flow velocity in patients with paroxysmal atrial fibrillation. Eur Heart J Cardiovasc Imaging. 2016;17(1):59–66.
21. Sakr SA, El-Rasheedy WA, Ramadan MM, El-Menshawy I, Mahfouz E, Bayoumi M. Association between left atrial appendage morphology evaluated by trans-esophageal echocardiography and ischemic cerebral stroke in patients with atrial fibrillation. Int Heart J. 2015;56(3):329–34.
22. Providência R, Faustino A, Paiva L, Fernandes A, Barra S, Pimenta J, Trigo J, Botelho A, Leitão-Marques AM. Mean platelet volume is associated with the presence of left atrial stasis in patients with non-valvular atrial fibrillation. BMC Cardiovasc Disord. 2013;13:40.

23. Faustino A, Providência R, Barra S, Paiva L, Trigo J, Botelho A, Costa M, Gonçalves L. Which method of left atrium size quantification is the most accurate to recognize thromboembolic risk in patients with non-valvular atrial fibrillation? Cardiovasc Ultrasound. 2014;12:28.
24. Schiller NB, Acquatella H, Ports TA, Drew D, Goerke J, Ringertz H, Silverman NH, Brundage B, Botvinick EH, Boswell R, et al. Left ventricular volume from paired biplane two-dimensional echocardiography. Circulation. 1979;60(3): 547–55.
25. Beppu S, Park YD, Sakakibara H, Nagata S, Nimura Y. Clinical features of intracardiac thrombosis based on echocardiographic observation. Jpn Circ J. 1984;48(1):75–82.
26. Beppu S, Nimura Y, Sakakibara H, Nagata S, Park YD, Izumi S. Smoke-like echo in the left atrial cavity in mitral valve disease: its features and significance. J Am Coll Cardiol. 1985;6(4):744–9.
27. Li Y, Yuan LJ, Cao TS, Duan YY, Jia HP, Liu J. Effects of respiration on pulmonary venous flow and its clinical applications by Doppler echocardiography. Echocardiography. 2009;26(2):150–4.
28. Abdalla IA, Murray RD, Lee JC, White RD, Thomas JD, Klein AL. Does rapid volume loading during transesophageal echocardiography differentiate constrictive pericarditis from restrictive cardiomyopathy? Echocardiography. 2002;19(2):125–34.
29. Üçerler H, İkiz ZA, Özgür T. Human left atrial appendage anatomy and overview of its clinical significance. Anadolu Kardiyol Derg. 2013;13(6): 566–72.
30. Veinot JP, Harrity PJ, Gentile F, Khandheria BK, Bailey KR, Eickholt JT, Seward JB, Tajik AJ, Edwards WD. Anatomy of the normal left atrial appendage: a quantitative study of age-related changes in 500 autopsy hearts: implications for echocariographic examination. Circulation. 1997; 96(9):3112–5.
31. Singer DE, Albers GW, Dalen JE, Go AS, Halperin JL, Manning WJ. Antithrombotic therapy in atrial fibrillation. The sixth ACCP conference on antithrombotic and thrombolytic therapy. Chest. 2004;126(3):429S–56S.
32. Lip GY, Lane D, Van Walraven C, Hart RG. Additive role of plasma von Willebrand factor levels to clinical factors for risk stratification in patients with atrial fibrillation. Stroke. 2006;37(9):2294–300.
33. Zabalgoitia M, Halperin JL, Pearce LA, Blackshear JL, Asinger RW, Hart RG. Transesophageal echocardiographic correlates of thromboembolism in high-risk patients with nonvalvular atrial fibrillation. J Am Coll Cardiol. 1998; 31(7):1622–6.
34. Camm AJ, Kirchhof P, Lip GY, Schotten U, Savelieva I, Ernst S, Van Gelder IC, Al-Attar N, Hindricks G, Prendergast B, et al. Guidelines for the management of atrial fibrillation: the task force for the management of atrial fibrillation of the European Society of Cardiology (ESC). Eur Heart J. 2010;31(19):2369–429.
35. Wunderlich NC, Beigel R, Swaans MJ, Ho SY, Siegel RJ. Percutaneous interventions for left atrial appendage exclusion options, assessment, and imaging using 2D and 3D echocardiography. JACC Cardiovasc Imaging. 2015;8(4):472–88.
36. Osranek M, Bursi F, Bailey KR, Grossardt BR, Brown RD, Kopecky SL, Tsang TS, Seward JB. Left atrial volume predicts cardiovascular events in patients originally diagnosed with lone atrial fibrillation: three-decade follow-up. Eur Heart J. 2005;26(23):2556–61.
37. Leung DY, Boyd A, Arnold H, Chi C, Thomas L. Echocardiographic evaluation of left atrial size and function: current understanding, pathophysiologic correlates, and prognostic implications. Am Heart J. 2008;156(6):1056–64.
38. Tang R, Dong J, Shang M, Du X, Yan X, Long D, Yu R, Wu J, Bai R, Liu N, et al. Impact of left atrium size on left atrial thrombus in patients with non-valvular persistent atrial fibrillation. Zhonghua Yi Xue Za Zhi. 2015;95(14): 1083–7.
39. Doukky R, Garcia-Sayan E, Patel M, Pant R, Wassouf M, Shah S, D'Silva O, Kehoe RF. Impact of diastolic function parameters on the risk for left atrial appendage Thrombus in patients with Nonvalvular atrial fibrillation: a prospective study. J Am Soc Echocardiogr. 2016;29(6):545–53.
40. Wang Y, Di Biase L, Horton RP, Nguyen T, Morhanty P, Natale A. Left atrial appendage studied by computed tomography to help planning for appendage closure device placement. J Cardiovasc Electrophysiol. 2010; 21(9):973–82.
41. Handke M, Harloff A, Hetzel A, Olschewski M, Bode C, Geibel A. Left atrial appendage flow velocity as a quantitative surrogate parameter for thromboembolic risk: determinants and relationship to spontaneous echocontrast and thrombus formation--a transesophageal echocardiographic study in 500 patients with cerebral ischemia. J Am Soc Echocardiogr. 2005;18(12):1366–72.
42. Alnabhan N, Kerut EK, Geraci SA, McMullan MR, Fox E. An approach to analysis of left ventricular diastolic function and loading conditions in the echocardiography laboratory. Echocardiography. 2008;25(1):105–16.

9

Tailored nurse-led cardiac rehabilitation after myocardial infarction results in better risk factor control at one year compared to traditional care: a retrospective observational study

Halldora Ögmundsdottir Michelsen[1,2*], Marie Nilsson[1], Fredrik Schersten[1], Ingela Sjölin[1,2], Alexandru Schiopu[1,2] and Margret Leosdottir[1,2]

Abstract

Background: Cardiac rehabilitation improves prognosis after an acute myocardial infarction (AMI), however, the optimal method of implementation is unknown. The aim of the study was to evaluate the effect of individually-tailored, nurse-led cardiac rehabilitation on patient outcomes.

Method: This single-centre retrospective observational study included 217 patients (62 ± 9 years, 73% men). All patients attended cardiac rehabilitation including at least two follow-up consultations with a nurse. Patients receiving traditional care ($n = 105$) had a routine cardiologist consultation, while for those receiving tailored care ($n = 112$) their need for a cardiologist consultation was individually evaluated by the nurses. Regression analysis was used to analyse risk factor control and hospital readmissions at one year.

Results: Patients in the tailored group achieved better control of total cholesterol (− 0.1 vs + 0.4 mmol/L change between baseline (time of index event) and 12–14-month follow-up, ($p = 0.01$), LDL cholesterol (− 0.1 vs + 0.2 mmol/L, $p = 0.02$) and systolic blood pressure (− 2.1 vs + 4.3 mmHg, p = 0.01). Active smokers, at baseline, were more often smoke-free at one-year in the tailored group [OR 0.32 (0.1–1.0), $p = 0.05$]. There was a no significant difference in re-admissions during the first year of follow-up. In the tailored group 60% of the patients had a cardiologist consultation compared to 98% in the traditional group ($p < 0.001$). The number of nurse visits was the same in both groups, while the number of telephone contacts was 38% higher in the tailored group ($p = 0.02$).

Conclusion: A tailored, nurse-led cardiac rehabilitation programme can improve risk factor management in post-AMI patients.

Keywords: Cardiac rehabilitation, Secondary prevention, Acute myocardial infarction, Cardiovascular risk factors, Nurse-led care

* Correspondence: halldora.michelsen@med.lu.se
[1]Department of Coronary Disease, Skåne University Hospital, Inga Marie Nilsson gata 47, Malmö, Sweden
[2]Department of Clinical Sciences Malmö, Faculty of Medicine, Lund University, Box 117, SE-221 00 Lund, Sweden

Background

Patients with established coronary artery disease are at high risk for recurrent coronary events and other comorbidities related to cardiovascular disease (CVD) [1]. According to Swedish national registries, 18% of acute myocardial infarction (AMI) survivors suffer a second CVD event in the first year and approximately 50% of major coronary artery disease events occur in those with a previous hospital discharge diagnosis of AMI [2]. Effective secondary prevention (SP), aiming to reduce the impact of the established disease, administered through cardiac rehabilitation (CR), a medically supervised program designed to improve cardiovascular health, can reduce this risk and improve prognosis [3–9]. In the most recent prevention guidelines from the European Society of Cardiology (ESC), SP at specialized prevention centres for patients who have suffered an acute coronary event is given the highest recommendation (IA) [10]. It is advocated that patients are offered comprehensive programmes that focus on CVD risk factor management addressing both somatic and psychosocial factors, with special emphasis on the benefits of exercise-based CR [10].

Currently there is a consensus that SP is an integral part of treatment after AMI. Its core components are well identified, and current guidelines recommend a multidisciplinary approach to an overall CVD risk reduction [10, 11]. An individual, patient-tailored risk reduction programme is generally advocated, and studies have previously suggested that it is more efficient [9, 12, 13] and cost-effective [14]. However, several factors such as the optimal length and the cumulative benefits of various components of the CR programme remain unclear [7, 10, 11]. This provided incentive to reorganize our CR programme towards a prolonged individually tailored nurse-led programme where patients need for consultation with a cardiologist was individually evaluated. The aim of this change was to provide the most appropriate and effective post-AMI care and prioritize cardiologist resources. The study, then, evaluated whether the change benefitted AMI survivors in terms of better CVD risk factor management and lower hospital readmission rates.

Methods

The study was a single-centre retrospective observational study comparing a tailored nurse-led CR programme to traditional care.

Study group, data collection and documentation

A total of 217 consecutive patients with AMI admitted to the coronary care unit (CCU) at Skane University Hospital in Malmö during a 14-month period (2013–2015) and who were registered in the Swedish web-system for Enhancement and Development of Evidence-based care in Heart Disease Evaluated According to Recommended Therapies (SWEDEHEART) registry, were included in the study. SWEDEHEART is a nationwide registry that records baseline characteristics, treatments, follow-up and outcome data of consecutive patients with AMI admitted to CCUs in Sweden [15].

SWEDEHEART contains several sub-registries; including a registry for acute care and a registry for CR. The registry for CR only includes patients under 75 years of age, making age ≥ 75 an exclusion criteria in our study [16]. Documentation in SWEDEHEART starts at the time of AMI and continues at two separate follow-up visits at 6–10 weeks and 12–14 months after the index event. Information is collected using standardized forms which includes all parameters listed in Table 1.

The study group was divided by a timeline. The first half of the included patients ($n = 105$) received traditional care, while the latter half of the patients ($n = 112$) received tailored, nurse-led CR.

The follow-up visits (applies to both traditional care and tailored nurse-led care)

Work routines within the CR programme at Skane University Hospital at the time of the study were based on the ESC prevention guidelines from 2012 [17]. The CR team consisted of specialized cardiac nurses, physiotherapists, a counsellor and a supervising cardiologist. The rehabilitation team had daily meetings to discuss patient cases. The patient's follow-up sessions with a nurse were focused on lifestyle, biometric risk factors and medication adherence (see Table 1). Main targets for healthy lifestyles were smoking cessation, physical exercise and diet and weight management in the case of overweight/obesity. Counselling and educational material on healthy food choices were given according to the 2012 Nordic Nutrition Recommendations [18] and the ESC prevention guidelines [17]. Plasma glucose, haemoglobin A1c (HbA1c) and plasma lipids samples were drawn at two seprate nurse visits and analysed at the Clinical Biochemistry department of Skane University Hospital Malmö with accredited methods. Blood pressure was measured (mmHg) with a manual sphygmomanometer after a 5-min rest with patient in sitting position. If blood pressure control or lipid control was inadequate medication was titrated by the nurse, in cooperation with the treating cardiologist. Weight was measured (kg) in light indoor clothing.

At the time of the study the follow-up visits with a physiotherapist included an individual consultation a few weeks after discharge which included an endurance test on a stationary bicycle, followed by a total of eight physiotherapist-led group training sessions at the hospital. Exercise training consisted of organized, individualized exercise-based training containing both fitness training and muscular resistance training equivalent to 12–16 at Borg's perceived exertion scale [19]. Additional

Table 1 Study parameters, definitions, targets and measurements

Parameter	Definition	Target	Measurement
Smoking	Active smoker yes/no	Smoking cessation	Self-reported
Exercise training	Reaching target for exercise training	Fitness training 20–60 min at least three times a week and muscular resistance training at least two times a week equivalent 12–16 at Borg's perceived exertion scale [19]	Participation in hospital-based exercise training, verified by hospital records
Physical activity	Reaching target for physical activity	Any physical activity at least 30 min per day corresponding a brisk walk	Self-reported
Overweight	BMI ≥ 25 kg/m2	Weight loss with target BMI <25 kg/m2	Height in m and weight in kg measured at follow-up visits
Hypertension	SBP ≥140 mmHg DBP ≥90 mmHg	SBP < 140 mmHg DBP < 90 mmHg	With a manual sphygmomanometer with subject in sitting position after 5 min of rest
Blood lipids (mmol/L) above therapeutic goal	TC ≥ 4.5	TC < 4.5	Fasting blood samples (plasma): TC, LDL, HDL, TG
	LDL ≥ 1.8	LDL < 1.8	
	HDL ≤ 1.0	HDL > 1.0 (men)	
	HDL ≤ 1.2	HDL > 1.2 (women)	
	TG ≥ 1.7	TG < 1.7	
Cardioprotective medication	ACEi/ARB, β-blocker, antiplatelet- and lipid-lowering medication	Maximum adherence to treatment	Self-reported
Hospital readmission	Readmission due to CVD	Avoidance	Hospital records

BMI Body mass index, *SBP* systolic blood pressure, *DBP* diastolic blood pressure, *TC* total cholesterol, *TG* triglycerides, *LDL* low density lipoprotein, *HDL* high density lipoprotein, *CVD* cardiovascular disease

home-based exercise training as well as daily physical activity were promoted. During the follow-up sessions the patients were asked how many days during the last week they had performed any physical activity at least 30 min per day corresponding to a brisk walk.

Traditional care

Post-AMI traditional care consisted of a follow-up visit with a nurse at 6–10 weeks after hospital discharge. This first follow-up visit included registry data collection and registration in SWEDEHEART. Following was a standard consultation with cardiologist at three months, after which patients were routinely referred to primary care. More complicated cases and patients with persisting symptoms, however, remained in the care of the CR out-patient unit at the hospital. At 12–14 months, all patients had an additional visit with a nurse, the main reason being the second registration in SWEDEHEART but also for controlling risk factors and offering lifestyle counselling as described above.

Tailored, nurse-led care

Before discharge, patients in the tailored, nurse-led group received a standardized letter explaining the follow-up protocol emphasizing that their primary contacts after hospital discharge would be a nurse and physiotherapist. The letter also explained that their need for a cardiologist consultation would be evaluated by the nurse. Furthermore, the letter stated that the patients would remain in the care of the CR team at the hospital until the second nurse visit at 12–14 months, after which patients would be referred to primary care.

As in traditional care all patients in the tailored group were offered a first follow-up visit with a nurse at 6–10 weeks after hospital discharge. Patients with remaining significant stenosis after culprit intervention, reduced left ventricular function (ejection fraction < 35%) as measured by echocardiography at the time of index event, remaining or recurring symptoms after the index intervention, and having undergone coronary artery bypass grafting (CABG) were automatically scheduled for a consultation with a cardiologist at approximately 3 months post-AMI. Also, patients who did not fit the criteria but either themselves asked for a follow-up visit with a cardiologist or the nurse assessed such a need were also scheduled for a cardiologist consultation.

Unlike traditional care, no patient was referred to primary care until after the second follow-up nurse visit at 12–14 months. Patients were encouraged to contact the CR team at the hospital if they had any questions concerning their heart disease or in the case of new cardiac symptoms – issues which in the traditional group were routinely referred to primary care after the cardiologist consultation at three months post-AMI. In addition, all patients in the tailored, nurse-led group received a letter from the nurse at approximately 6–8 months, promoting healthy lifestyles. At the same time new laboratory measures of lipids and blood glucose were performed. In the case of deranged laboratory values, patients were subsequently contacted by a nurse by telephone.

Information and consent

In accordance with Swedish law, all patients are informed verbally about data registration in the SWEDEHEART registry and the right to get their data erased from the registry upon request. During the 14-month study period none of the patients that were included in the study requested to get their data erased from the registry.

The Regional Ethical Review Board at Lund University approved the study (Dnr 2016/494).

Follow-up and outcome

The pre-specified primary outcomes were comparative delta values for continuous risk factors obtained at the first and second follow-up visits with the nurse. These included systolic and diastolic blood pressure, body mass index (BMI), low density lipoprotein (LDL), high density lipoprotein (HDL) and total cholesterol and triglycerides. Smoking and self-reported physical activity, were compared by direct measures performed at the 12–14-month visit.

Secondary outcomes were the number of follow-up visits and telephone consultations with a nurse or cardiologist and hospital re-admittance rates during the first year post-AMI.

Statistical methods

Baseline characteristics were described with means (± standard deviations) and percentages, using independent samples T-test and chi-square test to assess significance.

A multivariable linear regression analysis using backward selection was used to compare outcome measures between the groups for continuous variables, adjusting for age, gender, BMI, participation in an exercise training programme, comorbidities including previous coronary heart disease and diabetes mellitus, and cardioprotective medication (platelet inhibitors, Angiotensin converting enzyme inhibitors (ACEi), Angiotensin II receptor blockers (ARBs), β-blockers, statins and ezetimibe). Logistic regression analysis, adjusting for the same variables, was used to compare outcome measures between groups for categorical variables. To minimize the confounding effect of any differences between the groups at baseline, for continuous variables, delta values were calculated between the first and second follow-up rather than comparing crude measurements at 12–14 months only. However, as the 6–10-week variable for self-reported physical activity was confounded by the fact that the patients in the tailored nurse-led group more frequently participated in hospital-based exercise training at that time, the actual 12–14-month follow-up variable was used (not delta). All data was analysed by using the SPSS 23.0 statistical software package (SPSS Inc., Chicago, IL).

Results

Baseline characteristics

Baseline characteristics (at the time of the index event) are shown in Table 2. No patient was lost to follow-up. Except for baseline total cholesterol, there were no significant differences between the groups.

Patients in the tailored group had a higher participation rate in hospital-based exercise training during follow-up (74% vs 61%, $p = 0.04$). Self-reported use of cardioprotective medication at one year was similar between the two groups apart from a higher reported intake of ezetimibe in the tailored group compared to the traditional group (21% vs 10%, p = 0.04) (see Table 3).

Primary end-points

Results from the multivariable analysis for continuous variables are displayed in Table 4. We observed significant reductions in systolic blood pressure, total and LDL cholesterol between the first and second nurse visits favouring the tailored, nurse-led CR group. Active smokers at baseline were more often smoke-free at the 12–14-month follow-up in the tailored nurse-led care group: $n = 25$ out of 40 (63%) vs. $n = 18$ out of 43 (42%); OR 0.32 (CI 0.1–1.0), $p = 0.05$ whereas self-reported physical activity was lower (1.3 *(±2.1)* vs 1.9 (±2.3) days during the last week performing at least 30 min of moderate physical activity, $p = 0.04$).

Secondary end-points

In the tailored nurse-led group 34% of patients were scheduled for a follow-up visit with a cardiologist in accordance with the predefined criteria. In addition, 29 patients were, after an individual evaluation by the CR teams nurse, scheduled for a follow-up visit with a cardiologist. Thus, in total, 60% ($n = 67$ out of 112) of the patients had at least one cardiologist consultation during the follow-up period. In the traditional care group 98% of the patients had a scheduled consultation with a cardiologist ($n = 103$ out of 105, p for difference < 0.001). Two patients in the traditional care group preferred their follow-up to be with a privately practicing cardiologist (i.e. not working at the CR unit), both patients having a previous history of CVD. Of all the patients in the tailored care group who were assessed not to be in need for a cardiologist consultation, only one patient asked to see a cardiologist. The number of nurse visits was the same (2.4 visits/patient in the tailored group vs 2.6 visits/patient/year in the traditional group, $p = 0.30$), while telephone contacts with the CR team increased by 38% (5.8 vs 4.1 telephone contacts/patient/year, $p = 0.02$) in the tailored care group.

Table 2 Baseline characteristics

	Traditional care	Tailored nurse-led care	*P*-value
Number of patients:	105	112	
Demographics:			
• Men	*n* = 57, 71%	*n* = 83, 74%	0.67
• Age, years	61.7 (±9.1)	61.8 (±8.0)	0.10
Risk factors:			
• Diabetes Mellitus	*n* = 33, 31%	*n* = 21, 19%	0.10
• Active smoker	*n* = 43, 41%	*n* = 40, 36%	0.35
• SBP, mmHg	149.9 (±32.2)	153.7 (±24.2)	0.33
• DBP, mmHg	87.1 (±17.3)	87.4 (±15.2)	0.90
• BMI, kg/m2	27.3 (±4.5)	27.9 (±4.5)	0.37
• Total cholesterol, mmol/L	5.0 (±1.2)	4.6 (±1.0)	0.01
• LDL, mmol/L	3.0 (±1.2)	2.7 (±0.9)	0.45
• HDL, mmol/L	1.2 (±0.4)	1.2 (±0.4)	0.19
• TG, mmol/L	1.8 (±1.3)	1.5 (±0.7)	0.07
LVEF at the time of index event			
• Normal (≥50%)	*n* = 68, 65%	*n* = 88, 79%	0.09
• Mildly decreased (40–49%)	*n* = 20, 19%	*n* = 17, 15%	
• Moderately decreased (30–39%)	n = 8, 8%	n = 4, 4%	
• Severely decreased (≤29%)	n = 3, 3%	n = 0	
History of cardiovascular disease:			
AMI, PCI or CABG	*n* = 19, 18%	*n* = 22, 20%	0.83
Type of myocardial infarction			
• NSTEMI	*n* = 74, 70%	*n* = 73, 65%	0.40
• STEMI	*n* = 31, 30%	*n* = 38, 34%	0.49
Number of vessels affected			
• No significant stenosis	n = 7, 16%	n = 4, 10%	0.44
• 1–2 affected vessels	*n* = 23, 51%	*n* = 27, 64%	
• 3 affected vessels or left main stenosis	*n* = 15, 33%	n = 11, 26%	
In-hospital treatment:			
• PCI	*n* = 81, 77%	*n* = 85, 76%	0.62
• CABG	*n* = 12, 11%	n = 20, 18%	0.25
Pharmacological treatment at hospital discharge:			
• Platelet inhibitors	n = 105, 100%	*n* = 111, 99%	0.33
• Statins	*n* = 104, 99%	*n* = 110, 98%	0.97
• Ezetimibe	n = 1, 1%	n = 1, 1%	0.62
• ACEi or ARB	n = 103, 98%	n = 103, 92%	0.06
• B-blockers	*n* = 91, 87%	*n* = 96, 86%	0.62

Numbers presented as numbers (n) and percentages (%) or means (±SD) and *p*-values for difference
SBP systolic blood pressure, *DBP* diastolic blood pressure, *BMI* body mass index, *LDL* low density lipoprotein, *HDL* high density lipoprotein, *TG* triglycerides, *LVEF* left ventricular ejection fraction, *PCI* percutaneous coronary intervention, *CABG* coronary artery bypass grafting, *NSTEMI* non-ST elevation myocardial infarct, *STEMI* ST elevation myocardial infarct, *ACEi* angiotensin converting enzyme inhibitor, *ARB* angiotensin II receptor blocker

There was a non-significant trend towards more re-admissions due to cardiovascular causes (angina, AMI, heart failure and stroke) in the traditional group: $n = 10$ out of 105 (9.5%) vs. $n = 4$ out of 112 (3.6%) in the tailored nurse-led group; OR 2.8 (CI 0.8–9.3), $p = 0.1$. Out of readmissions in the tailored nurse-led group all four were due

Table 3 Pharmacological treatment and participation in exercise training reported at the 12–14-month visit

	Traditional care	Tailored nurse-led care	*P*-value
Pharmacological treatment:			
• Platelet inhibitors	*n* = 93, 89%	*n* = 102, 91%	0.54
• Statins	*n* = 92, 88%	n = 102, 91%	0.41
• Ezetimibe	n = 11, 10%	n = 23, 21%	0.04
• ACEi or ARB	n = 91, 87%	n = 96, 86%	0.84
• B-blocker	*n* = 78, 74%	n = 85, 76%	0.98
Participation in exercise training	*n* = 64, 61%	n = 83, 74%	0.04

Numbers presented as numbers (n) and percentages (%)and p-values for difference
ACEi angiotensin converting enzyme inhibitor, *ARB* angiotensin II receptor blocker

to angina and no patients were readmitted due to AMI, heart failure or stroke ($n = 0$ out of 112 (0.0%) vs. $n = 8$ out of 105 (7.6%) $p = 0.003$).

Discussion

In this study we compared two groups of AMI survivors who received either traditional post-AMI care or tailored, nurse-led CR. In the tailored group the patients' main contact at the CR clinic was a nurse and the need to have a post-AMI follow-up visit with a cardiologist was individually evaluated. In addition, a letter from the nurse promoting healthy lifestyles, and laboratory measures of lipids and blood glucose were performed at approximately 6–8 months. Finally, patients in the tailored group were not referred to primary care until after the 12–14-month follow-up visit with a nurse. The prolonged care did not lead to an increased number of visits to a nurse, and cardiologist visits were fewer. However, the number of telephone contacts increased.

We observed a significantly better control of total and LDL cholesterol and systolic blood pressure between baseline and at 12–14-months in the tailored group compared to the traditional group after adjusting for use of cardioprotective medication, prior CVD, diabetes and participation in exercise training. This, in turn, can reduce the relative risk for repeated CVD events [20, 21]. There was also a significant increase in smoking cessation rates at 12–14 months follow-up in the tailored group and a significantly higher participation rate in the hospital-based exercise training programme. The tailored group had less self-reported physical activity, which can be confounded by the higher participation in the exercise training programme. There was a non-significant trend towards fewer re-admissions due to cardiovascular causes during the first year post-AMI in the tailored group. Our findings suggest that offering tailored nurse-led CR may have a beneficial effect on outcomes as compared to the traditional type of care where patients receive a standardized, one-for-all follow-up.

Despite the acknowledged importance of CR, patients are not reaching their therapeutic goals [4]. The ideal method of implementation remains unclear and consequently the exemplary rehabilitation programme has yet to be designed [4, 7, 10, 17, 22, 23]. Suggested reasons for patients not reaching preventive goals include CR programmes commonly relying on short-term interventions,

Table 4 Risk factors at first (6–10 weeks) and second (12–14 months) follow-up visits and the difference (delta values) there between for patients receiving traditional and tailored nurse-led care, respectively

	Traditional care			Tailored, nurse-led care			
	First visit	Second visit	Difference (delta value)	First visit	Second visit	Difference (delta value)	P for difference
SBP (mmHg)	129.2 (±18.5)	133.5 (±21.0)	+4.3 (±20.3)	132.8 (±20.2)	130.7 (±15.1)	−2.4 (±16.0)	0.01
DBP (mmHg)	79.8 (±10.6)	79.9 (±10.3)	+ 0.1 (±11.6)	81.7 (±10.0)	79.1 (±8.9)	−2.6 (±9.3)	0.18
BMI (kg/m^2)	27.8 (±4.6)	26.2 (±3.8)	−0.5 (±1.5)	30.7 (±2.5)	28.3 (±3.9)	−0.1 (±1.8)	0.15
Total cholesterol (mmol/L)	3.5 (±0.68)	3.8 (±0.98)	+ 0.4 (±1.0)	3.6 (±0.83)	3.6 (±0.93)	−0.1 (±0.8)	0.02
LDL (mmol/L)	1.6 (±0.59)	1.8 (±0.91)	+ 0.2 (±0.9)	1.8 (±0.66)	1.6 (±0.70)	−0.1 (±0.7)	0.02
HDL (mmol/L)	1.2 (±0.40)	1.4 (±0.43)	+ 0.1 (±0.3)	1.2 (±0.41)	1.3 (±0.43)	+ 0.1 (±0.2)	0.06
TG (mmol/L)	1.36 (±0.82)	1.35 (±0.92)	−0.01 (±0.8)	1.35 (±0.75)	1.31 (±0.79)	−0.04 (±0.7)	0.59

Numbers presented as means (±SD) and p-values for difference. Adjusted for age, gender, previous heart disease, diabetes mellitus, BMI, participation in exercise training, and cardioprotective medication at 12–14-months
SBP systolic blood pressure, *DBP* diastolic blood pressure, *BMI* body mass index, *LDL* low density lipoprotein, *HDL* high density lipoprotein, *TG* triglycerides

being rigid in design, and not being adequately implemented [4, 24–26]. The reorganization of the CR programme at our clinic was designed to increase programme flexibility and to optimize utilization of the team's qualifications. As such, the primary patient responsibility lies with the nurses, while cardiologist resources focus on high-risk patients.

The decision of having the CR programme coordinated by nurses was based on evidence that nurse-led programmes can improve lifestyle, risk factor control and quality of life [8, 9, 27, 28]. EUROACTION was a multicentre study that demonstrated significant benefits of a nurse-led CR programme. The study showed that patients who participated in a nurse-led study model showed improvement in risk factor management and lifestyle changes as compared to standard care [9]. Another example is the RESPONSE trial, a study that randomized post-AMI patients to a 6 month CR programme with either traditional- or nurse-led care [8]. At 12–14 months post-AMI patients in the nurse-led group had better risk factor control, fewer hospital readmissions and emergency department visits as well as a 17% lower predicted risk ratio of mortality when compared to the control group. Our study results are in line with EUROACTION and RESPONSE trial results, confirming the benefits and safety of nurse-led SP programmes with an interdisciplinary approach. However, these studies included multiple follow-up nurse visits which requires resources. Our study model is easily applicable since patients, even though, remaining in the care the CR team under a 12–14-month period had two follow-visits with a nurse and the need for a consultation with a cardiologist is individually assessed and, thus, resources were prioritised.

Apart from receiving a nurse-led programme, patients in the tailored group remained in the care of the CR clinic for 12–14 months post-AMI while patients in the traditional group were routinely referred to primary care three months post-AMI. European guidelines recommend a follow-up time in an outpatient setting of at least 8–12 weeks post-AMI while advocating an even more flexible model with a preferred follow-up time of at least one year [11].

EUROASPIRE III and IV which are multinational surveys on CVD prevention, demonstrated that most patients at high CVD risk being treated in the primary care setting do not reach predefined preventive therapeutic and lifestyle goals [4, 24, 29]. Surveys done among primary care physicians in Europe show a lack of use of evidence-based prevention guidelines for reasons like time constraints, lack of perceived usefulness, inadequate knowledge and preference for using own experience [10, 30]. This may partly account for the difference in risk factor control between the two study groups.

The availability and utilization of CR varies. Previous studies, based in the United States, have shown that CR is highly under-utilized, with under half and as low as 13.9% of patients receiving CR [31, 32]. It has also been shown that certain patient groups are significantly less likely to receive CR. These include older individuals and women, with sex-differences increasing with age, as well as, non-whites, and patients with comorbidities (including congestive heart failure, previous stroke, diabetes mellitus, or cancer) [31–33]. However, since Swedish health-care is tax-funded, ensuring equal access to all, irrespective of income, this is less of an issue [34].

Strengths and limitations

The study was a retrospective observational study where no patient was lost on follow-up. The changes in follow-up structure evaluated in the study were simple and of low cost. They should thus be easy to replicate at other CR centres.

To our advantage, approximately 75% of all Swedish AMI survivors, < 75 years of age, admitted to CCU units around the country, attend CR. However, certain subgroups are overrepresented in the group of non-attenders, especially those with comorbidities, possibly limiting the generalisability of our findings [34].

The study only included AMI survivors under the age of 75 years, thus limiting applicability to other patient and age groups. As there were several differences between tailored and traditional care (i.e. decreased number of cardiologist visits, increased number of telephone contacts, a letter and laboratory measures at 6–8 months and longer time of follow-up) it is impossible to draw any conclusions as to which component of the tailored care resulted in better outcomes.

In our study, patients in the tailored group had a higher participation rate in hospital-based exercise training during follow-up. Exercise training is a core component of a CR programme [11, 17] and it has been shown to lead to improved prognosis and decreased hospital admissions for patients with CVD [35–37]. As such, even though participation in an exercise program was adjusted for in our analysis, a residual confounding effect cannot be ruled out. Also, at the time of the study information on home-based exercise training in the SWEDEHEART registry was not available, causing a possible bias.

Possible external effects such as changes in operations of local primary care centres could have affected the study results, since the groups were divided by a timeline. Possible factors such as behavioural or psychological status, as well as socioeconomic status could have interfered with participation in the CR programme on an individual level. Also, use of ezetimibe increased during the study period, possibly creating a bias even though adjustments were made in the multivariable analyses. In addition, some of the primary end-points were self-reported and were not collected in an otherwise verifiable fashion.

Conclusion

In conclusion, we showed that providing a tailored, nurse-led CR programme resulted in improvements in lifestyle and risk factor management, supporting the advantages of a tailored, multidisciplinary CR programme.

Abbreviations

ACEi: Angiotensin converting enzyme inhibitor; AMI: Acute myocardial infarction; ARB: Angiotensin II receptor blocker; BMI: Body mass index; CABG: Coronary artery bypass grafting; CCU: Coronary care unit; CR: Cardiac rehabilitation; CVD: Cardiovascular disease; ESC: European Society of Cardiology; HDL: High density lipoprotein; LDL: Low density lipoprotein; SP: Secondary prevention; SWEDEHEART: The Swedish web-system for Enhancement and Development of Evidence-based care in Heart Disease Evaluated According to Recommended Therapies

Funding

Governmental funding of clinical research within the NHS (National Health Services), Sweden, as well as, support from the Department of Cardiology, Skane University Hospital, Malmo, Sweden.

Authors' contributions

ML planned the study. ML, MN and IS organized the work routines for the study model. FS approved the study and the reorganization of the CR unit. HÖM and ML analyzed and interpreted the patient data. AS gave feedback on data interpretation and the manuscript. All authors read and approved the final manuscript.

Competing interests

The authors declare that they have no competing interests.

References

1. Piepoli MF, Corra U, Dendale P, Frederix I, Prescott E, Schmid JP, et al. Challenges in secondary prevention after acute myocardial infarction: a call for action. Eur J Prev Cardiol. 2016;23(18):1994–2006.
2. Jernberg T, Hasvold P, Henriksson M, Hjelm H, Thuresson M, Janzon M. Cardiovascular risk in post-myocardial infarction patients: nationwide real world data demonstrate the importance of a long-term perspective. Eur Heart J. 2015;36(19):1163–70.
3. Chow CK, Jolly S, Rao-Melacini P, Fox KA, Anand SS, Yusuf S. Association of diet, exercise, and smoking modification with risk of early cardiovascular events after acute coronary syndromes. Circulation. 2010;121(6):750–8.
4. Kotseva K, Wood D, De Bacquer D, De Backer G, Ryden L, Jennings C, et al. EUROASPIRE IV: a European Society of Cardiology survey on the lifestyle, risk factor and therapeutic management of coronary patients from 24 European countries. Eur J Prev Cardiol. 2016;23(6):636–48.
5. Estruch R, Ros E, Salas-Salvado J, Covas MI, Corella D, Aros F, et al. Primary prevention of cardiovascular disease with a Mediterranean diet. N Engl J Med. 2013;368(14):1279–90.
6. Wilson K, Gibson N, Willan A, Cook D. Effect of smoking cessation on mortality after myocardial infarction: meta-analysis of cohort studies. Arch Intern Med. 2000;160(7):939–44.
7. Rauch B, Davos CH, Doherty P, Saure D, Metzendorf MI, Salzwedel A, et al. The prognostic effect of cardiac rehabilitation in the era of acute revascularisation and statin therapy: a systematic review and meta-analysis of randomized and non-randomized studies - the cardiac rehabilitation outcome study (CROS). Eur J Prev Cardiol. 2016;23(18):1914–39.
8. Jorstad HT, Alings AM, Liem AH, von Birgelen C, Tijssen JG, de Vries CJ, et al. RESPONSE study: randomised evaluation of secondary prevention by outpatient nurse SpEcialists: study design, objectives and expected results. Neth Heart J. 2009;17(9):322–8.
9. Wood DA, Kotseva K, Connolly S, Jennings C, Mead A, Jones J, et al. Nurse-coordinated multidisciplinary, family-based cardiovascular disease prevention programme (EUROACTION) for patients with coronary heart disease and asymptomatic individuals at high risk of cardiovascular disease: a paired, cluster-randomised controlled trial. Lancet. 2008;371(9629):1999–2012.
10. Piepoli MF, Hoes AW, Agewall S, Albus C, Brotons C, et al. 2016 European Guidelines on cardiovascular disease prevention in clinical practice: The Sixth Joint Task Force of the European Society of Cardiology and Other Societies on Cardiovascular Disease Prevention in Clinical Practice (constituted by representatives of 10 societies and by invited experts): Developed with the special contribution of the European Association for Cardiovascular Prevention & Rehabilitation (EACPR). Eur J Prev Cardiol. 2016; 23(11):NP1–NP96.
11. Piepoli MF, Corra U, Adamopoulos S, Benzer W, Bjarnason-Wehrens B, Cupples M, et al. Secondary prevention in the clinical management of patients with cardiovascular diseases. Core components, standards and outcome measures for referral and delivery: a policy statement from the cardiac rehabilitation section of the European Association for Cardiovascular Prevention & Rehabilitation. Endorsed by the Committee for Practice Guidelines of the European Society of Cardiology. Eur J Prev Cardiol. 2014;21(6):664–81.
12. Giannuzzi P, Temporelli PL, Marchioli R, Maggioni AP, Balestroni G, Ceci V, et al. Global secondary prevention strategies to limit event recurrence after myocardial infarction: results of the GOSPEL study, a multicenter, randomized controlled trial from the Italian cardiac rehabilitation network. Arch Intern Med. 2008;168(20):2194–204.
13. McAlister FA, Lawson FM, Teo KK, Armstrong PW. Randomised trials of secondary prevention programmes in coronary heart disease: systematic review. BMJ. 2001;323(7319):957–62.
14. Anderson L, Thompson DR, Oldridge N, Zwisler AD, Rees K, Martin N, et al. Exercise-based cardiac rehabilitation for coronary heart disease. Cochrane Database Syst Rev. 2016;1:CD001800.
15. Hagström E, Nilsson L, Hambreus K. Swedeheart Annual report. Huddinge, 141 86 Stockholm: Karolinska University Hospital 2015. Report No.: ISSN: 2000–1843.
16. RIKS-HIA. 2016. [Available from: http://www.ucr.uu.se/swedeheart/start-riks-hia].
17. Perk J, De Backer G, Gohlke H, Graham I, Reiner Z, Verschuren M, Albus C, Benlian P, Boysen G, Cifkova R, Deaton C, Ebrahim S, Fisher M, Germano G, Hobbs R, Hoes A, Karadeniz S, Mezzani A, Prescott E, Ryden L, Scherer M, Syvänne M, Scholte op Reimer WJ, Vrints C, Wood D, Zamorano JL, Zannad F. European Guidelines on cardiovascular disease prevention in clinical practice (version 2012): the Fifth Joint Task Force of the European Society of Cardiology and Other Societies on Cardiovascular Disease Prevention in Clinical Practice (constituted by representatives of nine societies and by invited experts). Eur J Prev Cardiol. 2012;19(4):585–667.
18. Nordic Council of Ministers. Nordic Nutrition Recommendations 2012: Integrating nutrition and physical activity. 5 ed. Copenhagen: Nordisk Ministerråd; 2014. p. 627.
19. Borg G. Perceived exertion as an indicator of somatic stress. Scand J Rehabil Med. 1970;2(2):92–8.
20. Law MR, Morris JK, Wald NJ. Use of blood pressure lowering drugs in the prevention of cardiovascular disease: meta-analysis of 147 randomised trials in the context of expectations from prospective epidemiological studies. BMJ. 2009;338:b1665.
21. Cholesterol Treatment Trialists Collaboration, Fulcher J, O'Connell R, Voysey M, Emberson J, Blackwell L, et al. Efficacy and safety of LDL-lowering therapy among men and women: meta-analysis of individual data from 174,000 participants in 27 randomised trials. Lancet. 2015; 385(9976):1397–405.

22. Giannuzzi P, Temporelli PL, Maggioni AP, Ceci V, Chieffo C, Gattone M, et al. GlObal secondary prevention strategiEs to limit event recurrence after myocardial infarction: the GOSPEL study. A trial from the Italian cardiac rehabilitation network: rationale and design. Eur J Cardiovasc Prev Rehabil. 2005;12(6):555–61.
23. Giannuzzi P, Saner H, Bjornstad H, Fioretti P, Mendes M, Cohen-Solal A, et al. Secondary prevention through cardiac rehabilitation: position paper of the working group on cardiac rehabilitation and exercise physiology of the European Society of Cardiology. Eur Heart J. 2003;24(13):1273–8.
24. Kotseva K, Wood D, De Backer G, De Bacquer D, Pyorala K, Keil U, et al. EUROASPIRE III: a survey on the lifestyle, risk factors and use of cardioprotective drug therapies in coronary patients from 22 European countries. Eur J Cardiovasc Prev Rehabil. 2009;16(2):121–37.
25. Kotseva K, Wood D, De Backer G, De Bacquer D, Pyorala K, Keil U, et al. Cardiovascular prevention guidelines in daily practice: a comparison of EUROASPIRE I, II, and III surveys in eight European countries. Lancet. 2009;373(9667):929–40.
26. Jackson L, Leclerc J, Erskine Y, Linden W. Getting the most out of cardiac rehabilitation: a review of referral and adherence predictors. Heart. 2005;91(1):10–4.
27. Campbell NC. Secondary prevention clinics: improving quality of life and outcome. Heart. 2004;90(Suppl 4):iv29–32. discussion iv9–40
28. Campbell NC, Ritchie LD, Thain J, Deans HG, Rawles JM, Squair JL. Secondary prevention in coronary heart disease: a randomised trial of nurse led clinics in primary care. Heart. 1998;80(5):447–52.
29. Kotseva K, De Bacquer D, De Backer G, Ryden L, Jennings C, Gyberg V, et al. Lifestyle and risk factor management in people at high risk of cardiovascular disease. A report from the European Society of Cardiology European Action on secondary and primary prevention by intervention to reduce events (EUROASPIRE) IV cross-sectional survey in 14 European regions. Eur J Prev Cardiol. 2016;23(18):2007–18.
30. Dallongeville J, Banegas JR, Tubach F, Guallar E, Borghi C, De Backer G, et al. Survey of physicians' practices in the control of cardiovascular risk factors: the EURIKA study. Eur J Prev Cardiol. 2012;19(3):541–50.
31. Suaya JA, Shepard DS, Normand SL, Ades PA, Prottas J, Stason WB. Use of cardiac rehabilitation by Medicare beneficiaries after myocardial infarction or coronary bypass surgery. Circulation. 2007;116(15):1653–62.
32. Witt BJ, Jacobsen SJ, Weston SA, Killian JM, Meverden RA, Allison TG, et al. Cardiac rehabilitation after myocardial infarction in the community. J Am Coll Cardiol. 2004;44(5):988–96.
33. Sanghavi M, Gulati M. Sex differences in the pathophysiology, treatment, and outcomes in IHD. Curr Atheroscler Rep. 2015;17(6):511.
34. Bäck M, Ekström M, Hagström E, Leosdottir M. Swedeheart Annual report 2017. Huddinge, 141 86 Stockholm: Karolinska University Hospital 2018. Report No.: ISSN: 2000-1843.
35. Anderson L, Taylor RS. Cardiac rehabilitation for people with heart disease: an overview of Cochrane systematic reviews. Cochrane Database Syst Rev. 2014;12:CD011273.
36. Grazzi G, Mazzoni G, Myers J, Codeca L, Pasanisi G, Napoli N, et al. Improved walking speed is associated with lower hospitalisation rates in patients in an exercise-based secondary prevention programme. Heart. 2016;102(23):1902–8.
37. Kavanagh T, Hamm LF, Beyene J, Mertens DJ, Kennedy J, Campbell R, et al. Usefulness of improvement in walking distance versus peak oxygen uptake in predicting prognosis after myocardial infarction and/or coronary artery bypass grafting in men. Am J Cardiol. 2008;101(10):1423–7.

10

Pulmonary vein anatomy variants as a biomarker of atrial fibrillation – CT angiography evaluation

M. Skowerski[2], I. Wozniak-Skowerska[1], A. Hoffmann[1], S. Nowak[1], T. Skowerski[2*], M. Sosnowski[3], A. M. Wnuk-Wojnar[1] and K. Mizia-Stec[1]

Abstract

Background: It has been suggested that changes in pulmonary veins (PV) and left atrium (LA) anatomy may have an influence on initiating atrial fibrillation (AF) and the effectiveness of pulmonary vein isolation (PVI) in patients (pts) with atrial fibrillation.

The aim of the study was to assess anatomy abnormalities of the PV and LA in the patients with the history of AF and compare it with the control group(CG).

Methods: The multi-slice tomography (MSCT) scans were performed in 224 AF pts. before PVI (129 males, mean age 59 ± 9 yrs). The CG consisted of 40 pts. without AF (26 males, age 45 ± 9 yrs). LA and PV anatomy were evaluated. Diameters of PV ostia were measured in two directions: anterior-posterior (AP) and superior-inferior (SI) automatically using Vitrea 4.0.

Results: Pulmonary veins anatomy variants were observed more frequently in the atrial fibrillation group - 83 pts. (37%) vs 6 pts. (15%) in CG; 9% (21 pts) left common ostia (CO), 2% (5 pts) right CO, 19% (42 pts) additional right PV (APV), (1.8%) 4 pts. APV left, 8% right early branching (EB) and 3.5% left EB. The LA diameter differed significantly in AF vs CG group (41.2 ± 6 mm vs 35 ± 4.2 mm, $p < 0.0001$) respectively.

Conclusions: The anomalies of pulmonary vein anatomy occurred more often in pts. with AF. They can be defined as an image biomarkers of atrial fibrillation. Right additional (middle) pulmonary vein was the most important anomaly detected in AF patients as well as enlargered diameters of the LA and PV ostia.

Keywords: Atrial fibrillation, Pulmonary vein isolation, CT angiography

Background

Atrial fibrillation (AF) is a frequently occurring arrhythmia that impairs the life functioning, is associated with the increasing medical supervision, the risk of other diseases and pharmacological therapy complications. Pulmonary vein isolation (PVI) over the last decade has become the most demanded method for AF treatment. Even with experience in ablation, knowledge of left atrial anatomy and pulmonary vein anatomy is necessary [1]. A detailed visualization of the left atrium (LA) and pulmonary vein (PV) anatomy can be obtained by several different imaging methods including transesophageal or intracardiac echocardiography, rotational angiography, multislice computed tomography (MSCT) or three-dimensional gadolin-enhanced magnetic resonance. The MSCT is one of the most common and objective methods [2–5]. Anatomic varations of left atrium such as common ostia, additional pulmonary vein or early branching are common and previously described.

Some authors suggest that those anomalies may play a significant role in the pathophysiology of atrial fibrillation and even increase its prevalence [4, 6]. The safety and effectiveness of PVI in patients with AF is still under intensive clinical investigation [5, 7]. Therefore, the purpose of this study was to evaluate the occurrence of anatomy anomalies of PV and the left atrium using

* Correspondence: tskowerski@gmail.com
[2]Department of Cardiology, School of Health Sciences, Medical University of Silesia, Katowice, Poland
Full list of author information is available at the end of the article

MSCT scans performed in patients with AF and compare the results with no history of AF (control group).

Methods

Study population

A total of 271 pts. are analyzed in this paper. The study population (AF group) consisted of 224 patients (129 males, mean age 59 ± 9 yrs., range 22–74 yrs) with the history of paroxysmal and/or persistent symptomatic non-valvular AF referred to our hospital for qualification for PVI. The study was approved by the ethics committee and conformed to the Declaration of Helsinki. An informed written consent was obtained from every patient enrolled in the study. All the patients from the study group had well documented episodes of AF using Holter ECG and/or surface ECG. MSCT images were performed for LA and PV visualization. Exclusion criteria involved: history of congenital heart diseases, left ventricular systolic dysfunction (LV EF < 35%), hemodynamically significant valvular heart diseases. The subjects who underwent PVI were also excluded from the study.

The control group (CG) consisted of 40 pts. (26 males, mean age 45 ± 9 yrs) with no history of AF. MSCT scans were performed due to the symptoms of suspected pathologies in a coronary artery disease and/or aortic disease, which were finally excluded. The clinical characteristics of the study population and the control group are presented in Table 1.

Seven patients were excluded from the study due to rare anomalies that are described in the results.

MSCT of PVs

Multislice computed tomography (MSCT) scans were performed in all patients with a 64-slice Toshiba Multislice Aquilion System (Toshiba Medical System, Japan). Retrospective electrocardiographic gating was performed to minimize cardiac motion artifacts.

Non-ionic contrast material (Ultravist 370, Schering AG) was injected in the antebrachial vein (120 ml in three phases, phase one-70 ml, flow 5.0 ml/s-100% contrast, phase two- 30 ml the same flow-60% contrast and 40% saline, phase three-20 ml, 4.0 ml/s flow-100% saline, by means of a dual-head power injector-Injector CT2, Medtron, Germany).

Table 1 Baseline characteristics of AF patients and CG

	AF (n = 224)	CG (n = 40)
Age (years)	59 ± 9	47 ± 8
Gender (M/F)	129/95	16/15
Hypertension	140 (63%)	17 (53%)
BMI > 25	152 (68%)	14 (45%)
DM	23 (10%)	0
MI	15 (7%)	0
Stroke	11 (5%)	0
LVEF ECHO (%)	54 ± 9	60 ± 5

MI, myocardial infarction, *DM* diabetes mellitus, *BMI* body mas index

Data sets were subsequently analyzed on Vitrea post-processing workstation (Vital Images) using 2-D and 3-D viewing modes. Electrocardiographically gated datasets were reconstructed automatically at different time of the R-R cycle length to approximate end-diastole phase of the cardiac cycle. Additional reconstruction windows were constructed after the examination of datasets if motion artifacts were present. Scans were analyzed by consensus of two observers. Images were evaluated using 0.5 mm thin-slab maximum intensity projections (MIP) and curved multiplanar reconstructions (cMPR).

LA diameters were measured with the maximal anterior-posterior distance in the oblique-sagittal view. The PV anatomy was assessed - the number of PV, common ostia and the branching pattern. The diameters of PV ostia were measured in two directions (anterior-posterior (AP) and superior-inferior (SI)). We defined the anomalies as follows in accordance with previous publications [3, 6, 8]:

- Additional pulmonary vein (APV) was defined as an extra PV up to pattern of 4 PVs.
- Common ostia (CO) was defined when the distance between the virtual border of the LA and the bifurcation of both PVs was 0.5 cm or less.
- Early branching (EB) was specified as the bifurcation of the PV within 1 cm of origin from the LA.
- Venous ostium index (VOI) determined the ovality shape of ostia and was calculated by dividing MSCT measurements in the AP and the SI directions. When the ratio approaches 1.0 the ostium is more rounded, when it deviates from 1.0 the shape is more oval.

Endoluminal views were routinely rendered and allowed a precise visualisation of the pulmonary vein ostia, pulmonary vein orientation, distance to the first branch, geometry of pulmonary vein branches and common ostia.

Statistical analysis

The baseline clinical parameters and the results of parametric data were compared using the two-sample t-tests for normally distributed continuous variables between AF and CG group (Student's t-test or Wilcoxon matched paired test). The Chi-square test was used to analyze nonparametric data. All of the text and table results are expressed as means ± standard deviation (SD) from the mean or a number (percentage). Statistical evaluation was performed using the software Statistica ver. 8.0 Stat

Soft Pl. *P* value < 0.05 was considered statistically significant.

Results

LA dimension

The mean value (measured in CT) of the LA size was significantly larger in AF group vs CG group (41.2 ± 6 mm vs 35.4 ± 4 mm, $p < 0.0001$). Twenty six (11.6%) of AF pts. had LA larger than 50 mm, in comparison to CG, were no pts. had LA so enlarged.

Anatomical anomalies

All data are presented in Table 2. The typical anatomical pattern of the pulmonary vein described as two right and two left PVs was observed more often in CG than in AF group – 34 pts. (85%) vs 150 pts. (67%) pts.; $p < 0.05$.

PV anatomy anomalies – additional pulmonary veins, common ostia or early branching were found more frequently in the AF group – 83 pts. (37%) as compared to the CG – 6 pts. (15%); p < 0.05.

Forty two (18.7%) pts. from AF group had additional right PV (APV), contrary to the CG where no APVs were observed. The mean diameter of APV's was significantly smaller than the mean diameter of main veins (AP 7.2 ± 1.6 mm, SI 7.3 ± 1.8 mm vs AP 14.7 ± 3.0 mm, SI 17.4 ± 2.4 mm, $p < 0.0001$).

We recognized two types of common ostia of PVs:

- a long trunk CO with more than 20 mm distance between the left atrium and the bifurcation (5 AF pts., 0 CG pts)
- a short trunk CO – less than 20 mm distance between the left atrium and the bifurcation (21 AF pts., 6 CG pts).

The mean size of common ostia in AF patients was significantly larger than the diameter of main veins (AP 16.7 ± 4.2 mm, SI 24.5 ± 5.5 mm, p < 0.0001). There was a trend towards left-sided single ostia especially in AF patients.

There was no difference in the occurrence of early branching (EB) in AF - 5% (11 pts) as compared to CG - 5% (2 pts).

Table 2 Results: comparison of anatomical anomalies in AF patients and CG pts.

		AF (n = 224)	CG (n = 40)	p
LA CT (mm)		41.2 ± 6	35.4 ± 4	< 0.0001
Additional PV	right	42 (18.7%)	0	< 0.05
	left	4 (1.8%)	0	0.45
Common ostium	right	5 (2%)	2 (6.4%)	0.13
	left	21 (9%)	4 (12,9%)	0.5
Other anomalies		6 (2.7%)	0	

In the study group some other anomalies were discovered:

- two additional PVs (right sided) - 1 pt. (Fig. 1);
- two additional PVs on the left and right side – 1 pt.;
- single left PV – 1 pt. (Fig. 2);
- and left common ostia with a right additional PV (middle PV) - in 2 pts. (Fig. 3);
- abnormality of PV localization: all four left PVs were close to each other on the backside of LA (Fig. 4).

Pulmonary vein ostia

The AP and SI diameters of the PV ostia were significantly larger in the atrial fibrillation group than in the control group - results are shown in Table 3. In both groups the mean ostial diameter of the superior PV was larger than that of the inferior PV.

The venous ostium index (VOI) calculated for each PV proves the oval shape of most of them. Only the VOI of the right inferior pulmonary vein (RIPV) did differ between the groups ($p < 0.005$). Table 4 presents the VOI ratios.

Incidental findings

We also found rare anomalies in 7 pts. with AF – they were excluded from the analysis but we find it worth presenting. Partially anomalous pulmonary venous return was observed in 2 pts., atrial septal defect with anomalous insertion right upper PV into the right atrium - in 1 pt., and anomalous insertion of the middle meningeal vein into the right upper pulmonary vein - in 1 pt. One patient had right atrial diverticulum and 1 pt. left atrial diverticulum with a clot. No other clots were found in the LA. Right atrial myxoma localised in the interatrialis septum was diagnosed in 1 pt.

Discussion

Several researchers, cardiologists, radiologists and surgeons studied the anatomy of LA and PV because of a variety of endovascular and surgical techniques used for invasive therapy of patients with AF [2–7].

This study once again proves the existence of significant differences in anatomy of LA and PV in AF patients in comparison with healthy individuals [2, 3]. This study presents a significantly larger group of pts. (224 pts) with AF than our previous publication [8] (82 pts) and other previously published papers – Bittner et al. [9] (166 pts. with AF.), Kubala et al. [7] 118 pts. with AF. Also the number of PV anomalies is greater than in other studies. [7–10]. In reference to Chen (710 pts. with AF, 710 pts. CG) et al. [11] our study is consistent with the dimensions of PVs - larger PVs in AF group, in contrast to our findings in Chen's study the occurrence of PV variants did not differ between the groups. On the

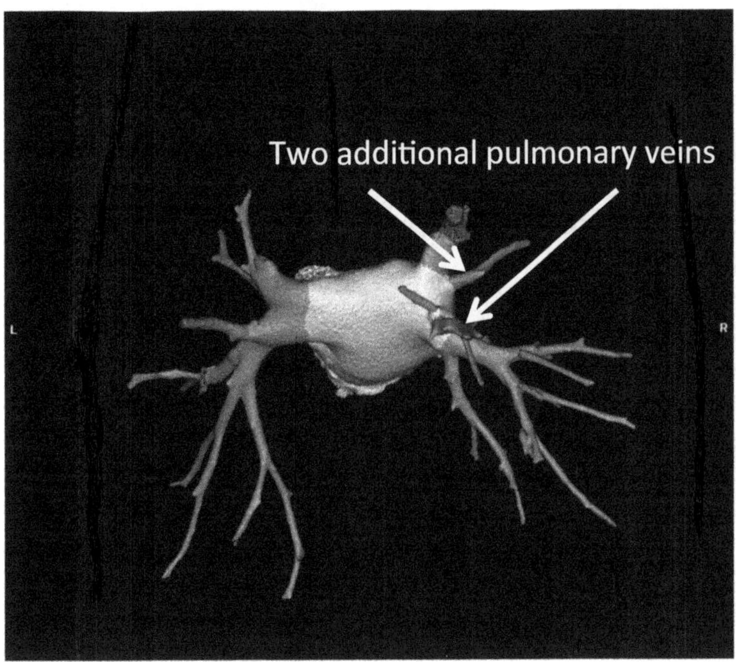

Fig. 1 Computed tomography scan with three-dimensional reconstruction of pulmonary veins and the left atrium. The arrow indicates an additional pulmonary vein

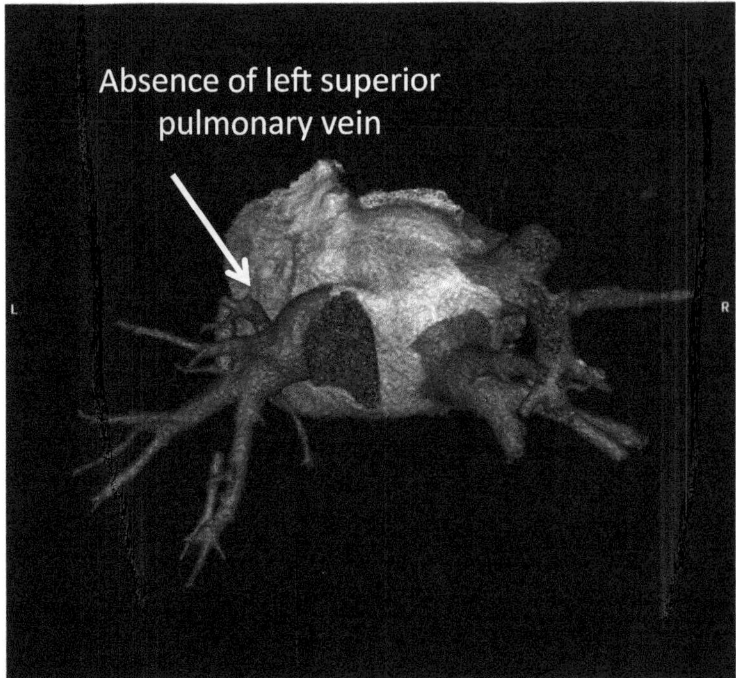

Fig. 2 Three-dimensional reconstruction of pulmonary veins and left atrium. Arrow indicates a common truncus of the left pulmonary vein

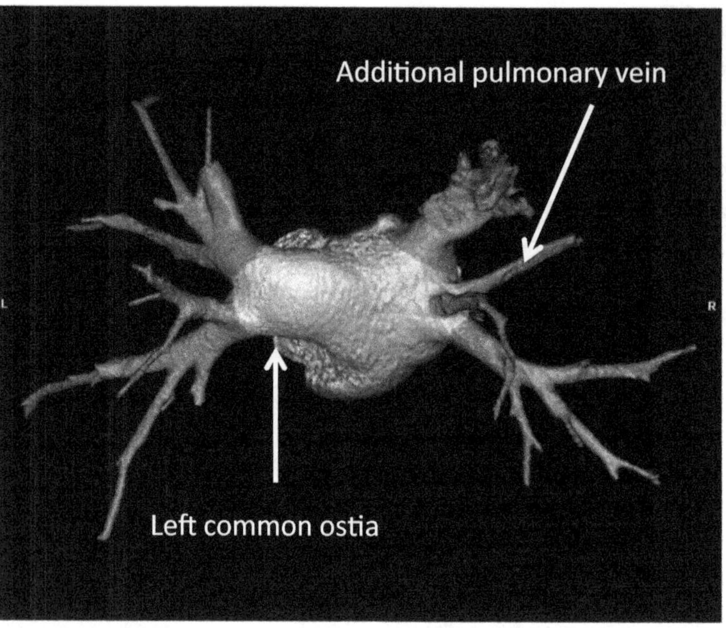

Fig. 3 Left common ostia with right additional PV (middle PV)

other hand one of the most extensive studies describing PV anatomy by Tekbas et al. shows the prevalence of PV abnormalities only in 26 (3,3%) out of 783 patients without atrial fibrillation [12].

The VOI ratio defining the shape of the pulmonary vein ostium is useful information for the operator - some research suggest it may define the method of ablatoin (cry ablation vs radio-frequency), predict the outcome and the complications (such as PV occlusion) [13].

Prior studies have proven that MSCT and cardiac magnetic resonance (CMR) are appropriate, non-invasive, widely available tools for describing LA anatomy and PV

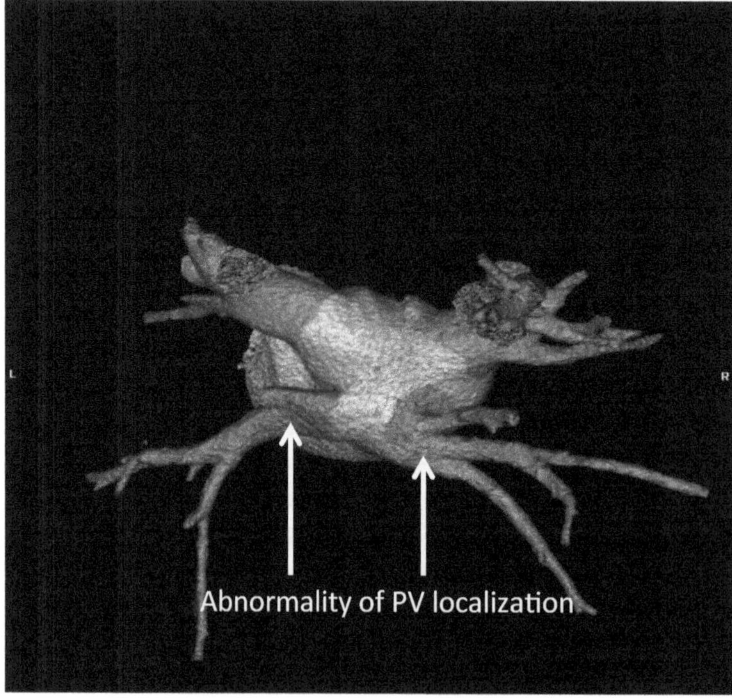

Fig. 4 Abnormality of PV localization: all (4) PVs left were close to each other on the posterior wall of LA

Table 3 Comparison results of SI and AP diameters of typical pattern 4 PVs in AF patients and CG (mean ± SD)

Pulmonary veins	AF ($n = 224$)	CG ($n = 40$)	p
SI in mm			
RSPV	18.5 ± 2.0	14.8 ± 2.9	< 0.0001
RIPV	16.8 ± 1.9	13.9 ± 3.4	< 0.0001
LSPV	18.2 ± 2.6	15.1 ± 2.3	< 0.0001
LIPV	16.1 ± 3.1	13.7 ± 2.7	< 0.0001
AP in mm			
RSPV	16.5 ± 3.0	13.7 ± 2.9	< 0.0001
RIPV	15.2 ± 2.1	13.6 ± 3.4	< 0.0001
LSPV	14.7 ± 2.7	12.0 ± 2.5	< 0.0001
LIPV	12.4 ± 4.3	10.3 ± 3.7	< 0.001

RSPV right superior pulmonary vein, *RIPV* right inferior pulmonary vein, *LSPV* left superior pulmonary vein, *LIPV* left inferior pulmonary vein
AF (+): right superior vs. right inferior PV - SI $p < 0.0001$, AP $p < 0.02$
left superior vs. left inferior PV - SI $p < 0.0001$, AP $p < 0.0001$,
GC: right superior vs. right inferior PV - SI $p < 0.005$, AP NS,
left superior vs left inferior PV - SI $p < 0.05$, AP $p < 0.05$

attachments in the patients qualified for the ablation procedure [2–16]. Moreover, CMR images allow for non-invasive therapy stratification using the atrial wall tissue characterization map for fibrosis assessment. It seems to be a good predictor for procedural outcome [2–10]. Although it has to be noticed that nowadays the left atrial model reconstruction with imaging by the electroanatomical mapping system is more often performed before the ablation procedure and CT/CMR imaging is not necessary to achieve good results and/or minimize complications [17, 18]. Thus it doesn't change the significance of our findings.

Similarly to previous observations [2, 3, 8, 19–21] the data collected confirm larger diameters of LA, superior and inferior PVs in patients with AF. We want this study to underline the complexity of anatomical changes that may trigger AF.

It has been suggested that those anomalies may affect the results of pulmonary vein ablation [7, 8, 22–24]. Kubala et al. describes a superior clinical outcome in patients with typical 4 PV pattern in comparison with the patients with the left CO [7]. Sohns et al. analyzed 138 pts. and proved the impact of PV anatomy on AF recurrence after PVI [24]. Mulder's et al. study was not conclusive - he presented only statistical trends of the relation between PV anatomy and PVI efficacy [10].

Table 4 VOI ratio in AF patients and CG (mean ± SD)

VOI	AF *(n = 224)*	CG *(n = 40)*	p
RSPV	0.93 ± 0.2	0.94 ± 0.2	NS
RIPV	0.91 ± 0.1	1.02 ± 0.2	< 0.005
LSPV	0.83 ± 0.2	0.81 ± 0.2	NS
LIPV	0.79 ± 0.2	0.75 ± 0.2	NS

RSPV right superior pulmonary vein, *RIPV* right inferior pulmonary vein, *LSPV* left superior pulmonary vein, *LIPV* left inferior pulmonary vein

In contrast, a few studies state the opposite [25], eg. a recent paper by Heeger et al. analizes the outcome of PVI using cryoballoon in 74 pts. with left common ostia PV; he found the efficacy of PVI equal in the study and the control group, although in some cases the presence of left CO of PV required a different PVI technique [26].

The lack of decisive opinion on PV anatomy calls for carrying out more studies with larger groups. The full recognition of AF pathophysiology, LA and PV anatomy and remodelling are essential for optimalization of AF treatment strategies.

It should be noted that rare pathological findings were observed in pts. with AF initially qualified for PVI. The precise left atrium visualization helped us to properly qualify the patient for ablation and avoid procedural complications.

Anatomical anomalies of LA and PV may potentially increase the periprocedural complications and affect PVI efficacy [27]. We consider identifying anatomy anomalies as an important factor that may change the operator's approach and modify the therapeutic strategy.

The main limitation of this paper is the number of patients in the control group.

Conclusions

The anomalies of pulmonary vein anatomy occur more often in pts. with atrial fibrillation. They can be defined as an image biomarkers of atrial fibrillation. The right additional pulmonary vein was the most common anomaly detected in AF patients as well as enlarged diameters of the LA and PV ostia. The differences of pulmonary veins anatomy apply not only to the number of PVs but also to the localization and shape of PV's ostia.

Abbreviations

AF: Atrial fibrillation; APV: Additional pulmonary vein; CG: Control group; CMR: Cardiac magnetic resonanse; CO: Common ostia; EB: Early branching; ECG: Electrocardiogram; MSCT: Multi-slice computer tomography; PTS: Patients; PVI: Pulmonary vein isolation; SD: Standart deviation; VOI: Venous ostium index

Funding

The authors received no specific funding for this work.

Authors' contributions

MS1 conceived the idea for the study, supervised it, analyzed the CT scans and wrote the manuscript with IWS. AH and SN helped with CT scans evaluation. TS created the data base, drafted the article and performed the statistical analysis. MS2, AMWW and KMS revised the article. All authors were involved in data collection. All authors edited and approved the final version of the manuscript.

Competing interests
The authors declare that they have no competing interests.

Author details
[1]First Department of Cardiology, School of Medicine in Katowice, Medical University of Silesia, Katowice, Poland. [2]Department of Cardiology, School of Health Sciences, Medical University of Silesia, Katowice, Poland. [3]Unit of Noninvasive Cardiovascular Diagnostics, Medical University of Silesia, Katowice, Poland.

References
1. Calkins H, Kuck KH, Cappato R et al. 2012 HRS/EHRA/EACS expert consensus statement on catheter and surgical ablation of atrial fibrillation: recommendations for patient selection, procedural techniques, patients management and follow-up, definitions, endpoints and research trial design: a report of the Heart Rhythm Society (HRS) task force on catheter and surgical ablation of atrial fibrillation. Heart Rhythm; 2012 9: 632–696.
2. Kato R, Lickfett L, Meininger G, et al. Pulmonary vein anatomy in patients undergoing catheter ablation of atrial fibrillation. Circulation. 2003;107:2004–10.
3. Jongbloed M, Bax J, Lamb H, et al. Multislice computed tomography versus intracardiac echocardiography to evaluate the pulmonary veins before radiofrequency catheter ablation of atrial fibrillation. J Am Coll Cardiol. 2005;45:43–50.
4. Tekbas G, Ekici F, Tekbas E, et al. Evaluation of pulmonary vein variations in the middle pulmonary lobe with 64-slice multidetector computed tomography. Eur Rev Med Pharmacol Sci. 2011;15(12):1395–400.
5. Yokokawa M, Olgun H, Sundaram B, et al. Impact of preprocedural imaging on outcomes of catheter ablation in patients with atrial fibrillation. J Interv Card Electrophysiol. 2012;34(3):255–62.
6. Akiba T, Mirikawa T, Inagaki T, et al. A new classification for right top pulmonary vein. Ann Thorac Surg. 2013 Apr;95(4):12277–30.
7. Kubala M, Hermida JS, Nadij G, et al. Normal pulmonary veins anatomy is associated with better AF-free survival after cryoablation as compared to atypical anatomy with common left pulmonary vein. Pacing Clin Electrophysiol. 2011;34(7):837043.
8. Woźniak-Skowerska I, Skowerski M, Wnuk-Wojnar A, et al. Comparison of pulmonary veins anatomy in patients with and without atrial fibrillation: analysis by multislice tomography. Int J Cardiol. 2011;146(2):181–5.
9. Bittner A, Monnig G, Vagt A, et al. Pulmonary vein variants predispose to atrial fibrillation: a case-control study using multislice enhanced computed tomography. Europace. 2011;13:1394–400.
10. Mulder AAW, Wijffels MCEF, Wever EFD, et al. Pulmonary vein anatomy and long-term outcome after multi-electrode pulmonary vein isolation with phased radiofrequency energy for paroxysmal atrial fibrillation. Europace. 2011;13:1557–61.
11. Chen J, Yang Z, Xu H, et al. Assessments of pulmonary vein and left atrial anatomical variants in atrial fibrillation patients for catheter ablation with cardiac CT. Eur Radiol. 2017;27:660–70.
12. Tekbas G, et al. Evaluation of pulmonary vein variations and anomalies with 64 slice multi detector computed tomography. Wien Klin Wochenschr. 2012;124:3–10.
13. Baran J, Piotrowsk R, Sikorska A, et al. Impact of pulmonary vein ostia anatomy on efficacy of cryoballoon ablation for atrial fibrillation. Heart Beat Journal. 2016;1:65–70. https://doi.org/10.24255/hbj/68162.
14. Tekbas G, Gumus H, Onder H, et al. Evaluation of pulmonary vein variations and anomalies with 64 slice multi detector computed tomography. Wiener klinische Wochenscgrift. 2012;124:3–10.
15. Manghat NE, Mathias HC, Kakani N, et al. Pulmonary venous evaluation using electrocardiogram-gated 64-detector row cardiac CT. Br J Radiol. 2012;85(1015):965–71.
16. Schafer D, Meyer C, Bullens R, et al. Limited angle C-arm tomography and segmentation for quidance of atrial fibrillation ablation procedures. Med Imae Comput Assist Interv. 2012;15:634–41.
17. De Potter T, Bardhaj G, Viggiano A, et al. Rotational angiography as a Periprocedural imaging tool in atrial fibrillation ablation. Arrhythm Electrophysiol Rev. 2014;3(3):173–6.
18. Bonso A, Fantinel M, Scalchi G, et al. Left atrial model reconstruction in atrial fibrillation ablation: reliability of new mapping and complex impedance systems. Europace. 2016;
19. Marom E, Herdon J, Kim YH, et al. Variations in pulmonary venous drainage to the left atrium implication for radiofrequency ablation. Radiology. 2004; 230:824–9.
20. Thai WE, Wai B, Lin K, et al. Pulmonary venous anatomy imaging with low-dose, prospectively ECG-triggered, high-pitch 128-slice dual-source computed tomography. Circ Arrhythm Electrophysiol. 2012;5(3):521–30.
21. Ratajczak P, Sławińska A, Martynowska-Rymer I, et al. Anatomical evaluation of the pulmonary veins and the left atrium using computed tomography before catheter ablation: reproducibility of measurements. Pol J Radiol. 2016;81:228–32.
22. Tsao HM, Wu MH, Yu WC, et al. Role of right middle pulmonary vein in patients with paroxysmal atrial fibrillation. J Cardiovasc Electrocardiol. 2001; 12:1353–7.
23. Streb W, Jarski P, Przybylski R, et al. Right atrial diverticulum in an adult person. Kardiol Pol. 2007;65:1090–3.
24. Sohns C, Sohns JM, Bergau L, et al. Pulmonary vein anatomy predicts freedom from atrial fibrillation using remote magnetic navigation for circumferential pulmonary vein ablation. Europace. 2013;15:1136–42.
25. Dennis W, Tops LF, Delgado V, et al. Effect of pulmonary vein anatomy and left atrial dimensions on outcome of circumferential radiofrequency catheter ablation for atrial fibrillation den Uijl. American Journal of Cardiology. 2011;107:243–9.
26. Heeger C, Tscholl V, Wissner E, et al. Acute efficacy, safety, and long-term clinical outcomes using the second-generation cryoballoon for pulmonary vein isolation in patients with a left common pulmonary vein: a multicenter study. Heart Rhythm. 2017;14:1111–8.
27. Sorgente A, Chierchia G, De Battista C, et al. Pulmonary vein ostium shape and orientation as possible predictors of occlusion in patients with drug-refractory paroxysmal atrial fibrillation undergoing cryoballoon ablation. Europace. 2011;13:205–12.

11

INvestigation on Routine Follow-up in CONgestive HearT FAilure Patients with Remotely Monitored Implanted Cardioverter Defibrillators SysTems (InContact)

Claudius Hansen[1*], Christian Loges[2], Karlheinz Seidl[3], Frank Eberhardt[4], Herbert Tröster[5], Krum Petrov[6], Gerian Grönefeld[7], Peter Bramlage[8], Frank Birkenhauer[9] and Christian Weiss[10]

Abstract

Background: In heart failure (HF) patients with implantable cardioverter defibrillators (ICD) or cardiac resynchronisation therapy defibrillators (CRT-D), remote monitoring has been shown to result in at least non-inferior outcomes relative to in-clinic visits. We aimed to provide further evidence for this effect, and to assess whether adding telephone follow-ups to remote follow-ups influenced outcomes.

Methods: InContact was a prospective, randomised, multicentre study. Subjects receiving quarterly automated follow-up only (telemetry group) were compared to those receiving personal physician contact. Personal contact patients were further divided into those receiving automated follow-up plus a telephone call (remote+phone subgroup) or in-clinic visits only.

Results: Two hundred and ten patients underwent randomisation (telemetry $n = 102$; personal contact $n = 108$ [remote+phone: $n = 53$; visit: $n = 55$]). Baseline characteristics were comparable between groups and subgroups. Over 12 months, 34.8% of patients experienced deterioration of their Packer Clinical Composite Response, with no significant difference between the telemetry group and personal care ($p > 0.999$), remote+phone ($p = 0.937$) or visit ($p = 0.940$) patients; predefined non-inferiority criteria were met. Mortality rates (5.2% overall) were comparable between groups and subgroups ($p = 0.832/p = 0.645$), as were HF-hospitalisation rates (11.0% overall; $p = 0.605/p = 0.851$). The proportion of patients requiring ≥1 unscheduled follow-up was nominally higher in telemetry and remote +phone groups (42.2 and 45.3%) compared to the visit group (29.1%). Overall, ≥ 1 ICD therapy was delivered to 15.2% of patients.

Conclusion: In HF patients with ICDs/CRT-Ds, quarterly remote follow-up only over 12 months was non-inferior to regular personal contact. Addition of quarterly telephone follow-ups to remote monitoring does not appear to offer any clinical advantage.

Keywords: Heart failure, Implantable cardioverter defibrillator, Cardiac resynchronisation therapy defibrillator, Remote monitoring, Packer heart failure clinical composite response

* Correspondence: hansen@hgz-goettingen.de
[1]Herz- und Gefäßzentrum am Krankenhaus Neu-Bethlehem, Humboldtallee 6, 37073 Göttingen, Germany
Full list of author information is available at the end of the article

Background

Heart failure (HF) represents a substantial health burden, affecting approximately 26 million people on a global scale and accounting for 1–2% of all hospitalisations in Europe and America [1]. In patients with HF that cannot be effectively managed through medication alone, an implantable cardioverter defibrillator (ICD) or cardiac resynchronisation therapy defibrillator (CRT-D) is commonly indicated [2, 3].

Remote monitoring (RM) of implanted devices has been shown to have a number of advantages over exclusive in-clinic follow-up [4]. Firstly, it facilitates assessment of treatment regimens and optimisation of device functionality without the need for regular outpatient visits [4–6]. This reduces healthcare costs, issues surrounding appointment scheduling, and transportation costs for patients living in remote areas [7], and has been suggested to result in better adherence to follow-up [8]. Secondly, RM may encourage patients to take more responsibility for their own health status, and provide constant peace-of-mind that their device is functioning as intended [9, 10]. Indeed, RM can provide invaluable data for the early identification of clinically important irregularities, such as low battery output, device/lead faults, arrhythmias, and atrial fibrillation [11–14]. This has been demonstrated not only to allow timely prevention of clinical emergencies and mortality, but also to reduce the incidence of inappropriate device interventions [4, 6, 14–21]. Thus, the frequency of cardiovascular hospitalisation and long-term healthcare resource expenditure may be reduced [20, 22–24].

Given the available evidence, the Heart Rhythm Society (HRS) currently recommends that, where possible, use of remote care systems to monitor and interrogate implantable cardiac devices should be used in place of regular in-clinic visits, with a face-to-face evaluation taking place at least once every 12 months [11]. However, the value of supporting remote follow-ups with additional telephone contact has not yet been assessed.

In the present analysis, we aimed to provide more evidence that quarterly automated follow-ups are non-inferior to follow-ups which involve personal physician contact in HF patients with recently implanted ICD/CRT-D devices over 12 months. Secondly, we aimed to determine whether the type of physician contact affected outcomes. Of particular interest was whether the addition of quarterly physician telephone calls to remote follow-ups improved outcomes relative to both automated follow-ups only and traditional in-clinic visits.

Methods

INvestigation on Routine Follow-up in CONgestive HearT FAilure Patients With Remotely Monitored Implanted Cardioverter Defibrillators SysTems (InContact) was a prospective, randomised, multicentre study conducted at 17 sites across Germany (see center list at end of article). The first patient was enrolled in February 2010 and study completion occurred in March 2014. The protocol was approved by the relevant ethics committees and the study was carried out in accordance with the Declaration of Helsinki 1964 and its amendments. All patients provided written informed consent.

Patients and study groups

Only patients with ICD/CRT-D implantation indications consistent with guidelines (new device, generator replacement, or upgrade) were eligible for the present study. Additional inclusion criteria were: age ≥ 18 and < 80 years; ejection fraction ≤35%; New York Heart Association (NYHA) class I-III; and sufficient home infrastructure to support the use of a Merlin@home™ transmitter. Patients were excluded from the study if they had second-degree Mobitz type II or third-degree atrioventricular block; severe renal insufficiency; a life expectancy < 12 months; were pregnant; or were participating in a simultaneous study with an active therapy arm. Patients who had experienced a myocardial infarction or undergone a coronary angiology in the 3 months prior to enrolment were also excluded.

Following ICD/CRT-D implantation, patients were randomised in a 1:1 ratio into two study arms: those who were to receive quarterly personal contact with a physician (personal contact group) plus RM, and those who were to receive quarterly automated follow-up via Merlin.net only (telemetry group). Personal contact patients were further randomised into two subgroups: quarterly personal telephone calls with a physician/supporting nurse (remote+phone group), or quarterly in-clinic visits only (visit group). All of these groupings applied to the 12-month period between the first and thirteenth month after implantation. Regardless of study group, daily automatic alarm checks were activated for all patients throughout the study period.

Study visits and documentation

A full medical history was taken for each patient prior to the day of ICD/CRT-D implantation (baseline). Prior to hospital discharge (PHD), quality of life (QoL) was assessed using the Minnesota Living with Heart Failure Questionnaire (MLHFQ; a self-administered, disease-specific questionnaire composed of 21 items, each with a 6-point scale [0 = no impact of HF on QoL, 5 = a great deal of impact]) [25]. The correct installation of the Merlin@home™ transmitter was verified within the first month post-intervention. Patients were provided with appropriate information on how to use their transmitter device. Quarterly scheduled sessions and device checks were set up by the clinic.

All patients attended an in-clinic visit 1 month (± 14 days) and 13 months (± 30 days) after ICD/CRT-D implantation, at which their Packer Heart Failure Clinical Composite Response score (Packer score) was determined, medication recorded, and QoL (MLHFQ) assessed. ICD/CRT-D function was then assessed for all patients at 4 and 7 months (± 14 days), either remotely or during the in-clinic appointment (visit group only). An optional follow-up was also carried out at 10 months. Adverse events and ICD/CRT-D measurements were recorded at each time point. Neither in-clinic or telephone interviews were pre-scripted, but were based around the discussion of device data.

Outcome measures

The primary outcome measure was the proportion of patients with a worse Packer score at 13 months relative to their status at 1 month [26]. This composite outcome measure was determined via a stepwise assessment including the following parameters: HF-related death or hospitalisation (worse); deterioration of NYHA class or self-assessed health (worse); improved NHYA class or self-assessed health (improved); none of the above (unchanged).

Secondary outcome measures included the rates of all-cause mortality, HF-hospitalisations, and arrhythmias over the same 12-month period. The number of unscheduled (in-clinic, telephone-based or remote) follow-ups, the proportion of all follow-ups that had disease-relevant findings, and the number of delivered/appropriate ICD therapies were also documented. Changes in QoL between PHD, 1 and 13 months were assessed.

Statistical analysis

The sample size calculation was based on a non-inferiority hypothesis, with a 15% margin for the occurrence of packer endpoint score deterioration at 13-month follow-up assumed. Pre-set values were 5% for the significance level and 80% for the power. A required sample size of 186 patients with complete datasets was calculated for a 1:1 (subgroups: 2:1:1) randomised design. After considering rates of drop out and incomplete data sets (predicted at approximately 20% overall), a total of 210 patients were planned for recruitment.

For continuous variables, a t-test, Wilcoxon signed-rank test or Mann-Whitney U-test were used for two-way comparisons and a Kruskal-Wallis test for three-way comparisons. A chi-square test (or Fisher's exact test in the case of frequencies < 5%) was used for comparing categorical variables. In cases where more than two subgroups were compared and the comparison was significant, Pairwise comparisons of the groups were carried out and p-values were adjusted using the Bonferroni method. To test for the non-inferiority of telemetry compared to personal contact, the 95% confidence interval (CI) for the difference in the proportions of patients with a worsened Packer outcome at 13-month follow-up was calculated. Where the lower bound of this 95% CI exceeded -0.15, automated follow-up was considered non-inferior to personal contact.

Results

The 210 patients initially enrolled in the study were randomised into either the telemetry ($n = 102$; 49%) or personal contact ($n = 108$; 51%) group (Fig. 1). Those in the personal contact group were further randomised into the remote+phone ($n = 53$; 25%) or visit ($n = 55$; 26%) subgroups.

Baseline characteristics

Baseline characteristics were similar between all groups and subgroups (Table 1). Overall, patients had a mean age of 63.8 years, were predominantly male (84.3%), and had a mean NYHA class of 2.3 ± 0.7 [median 2; range 1–3; 42.9% NYHA III]. The majority had ischemic cardiac disease (59.0%).

Beta-blockers were the most commonly prescribed cardiac drug at baseline (92.9%), followed by amiodarone (11.4%). Only 6.7% of patients were not receiving any HF medication. Diuretics were being taken by 83.8% of the study population, angiotensin-converting enzyme inhibitors by 79.5%, spironolactone by 54.8%, and angiotensin II receptor blockers by 16.2%.

The majority of patients received their ICD in a primary prevention setting (84.8%). The most frequently implanted device was a single chamber ICD (51.4%), followed by a CRT-D (32.4%) and dual-chamber ICD (16.2%). A DF-4 connecter was implanted in 71.4% of cases. The most common ICD model was Fortify (36.2%) followed by Current + (18.1%) and Unify (12.4%). All other models were used at a frequency of < 7%.

Outcomes at 13 months

Of the patients enrolled, 184 were available for the primary endpoint analysis, 92 (90.2%) in the telemetry and 92 (85.2%) in the personal contact group (remote +phone: 44 patients, 83.0%; visit: 48 patients, 87.3%).

Primary endpoint: Packer heart failure clinical composite response

Overall, 34.8% of patients had a worse Packer score at 13 months relative to 1 month, with 15.2% remaining unchanged and 50.0% experiencing an improvement. This distribution was not significantly different between telemetry and personal care group ($p = 0.855$) or telemetry, remote+phone and visit groups/subgroups ($p = 0.967$) (Fig. 2).

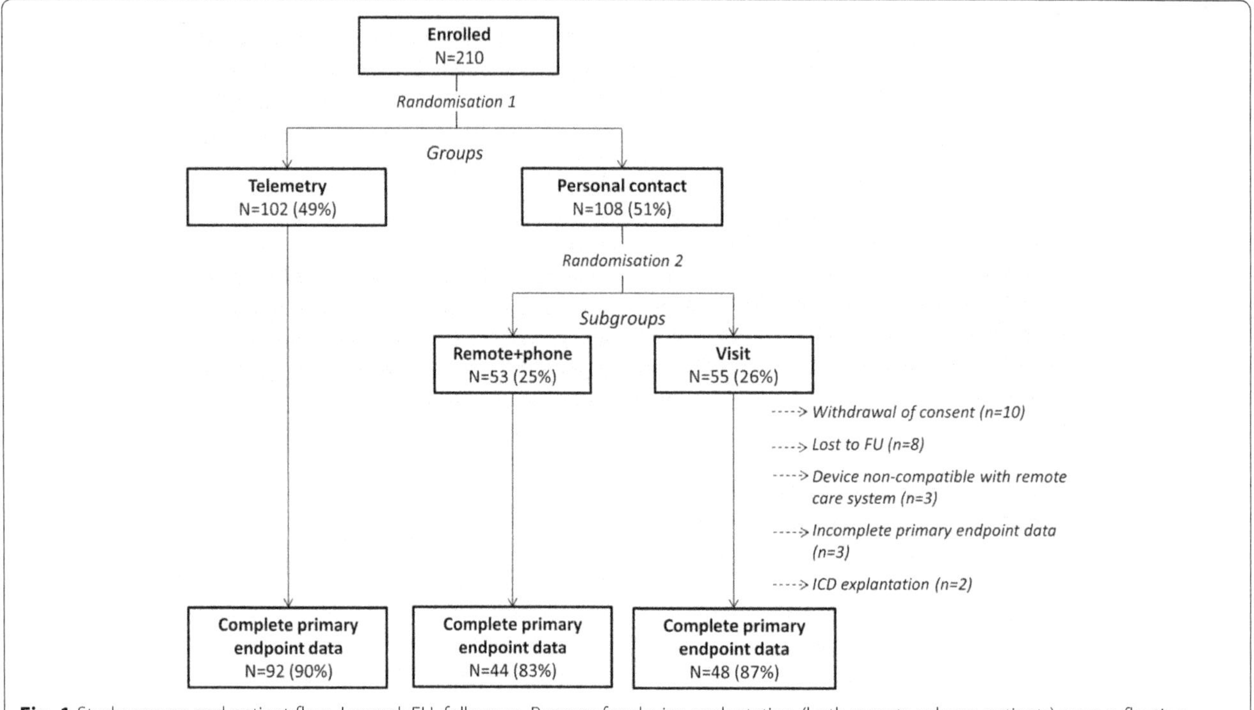

Fig. 1 Study groups and patient flow. Legend: FU, follow-up. Reasons for device explantation (both remote+phone patients) were a floating structure at the atrial electrode and successful heart transplantation

When considering only the proportion of patients with a worse packer score, no significant difference was detected between the telemetry compared to personal care group ($p > 0.999$). As the difference between means was 0.000 and the 95% CI (– 1.1376 to 0.1376) lower limit greater than the predefined non-inferiority delta (– 0.15), non-inferiority of telemetry compared to personal follow up was concluded. Furthermore, no significant difference was found when comparing the telemetry group to the remote+phone subgroup ($p = 0.937$), the telemetry group to the visit subgroup ($p = 0.940$), or the remote+phone and visit subgroups ($p = 0.894$).

Mortality and HF-hospitalisation

During the course of the study, mortality rates were comparable between telemetry and personal contact groups (4.9% vs. 5.6%, $p = 0.832$), and telemetry, remote +phone and visit groups (4.9% vs. 7.5% vs. 3.6%, respectively; $p = 0.645$) (Table 2). Of the 11 deaths which occurred during the course of the study, 4 were from cardiac origin (HF and coronary artery disease), 4 were from non-cardiac origin, and 3 were of "unclear" origin. The origin of death was "unclear" in three of five patients (60%) in the telemetry group compared to none of six (0%) in either of the personal contact groups.

HF-hospitalisation occurred at similar rates in the telemetry and personal contact groups (9.8% vs. 12.0%, $p = 0.605$) (Table 2). This was also the case when comparing telemetry, remote+phone and visit groups/subgroups (9.8% vs. 11.3% vs. 12.7%, $p = 0.851$).

Follow-ups

Overall, 100 patients (47.6%) had at least one relevant finding from at least one ICD/CRT-D follow-up, with no significant differences between the telemetry and personal contact groups ($p = 0.693$) or telemetry, remote +phone and visit groups/subgroups ($p = 0.789$) (Table 3). Again, findings were predominantly medical (82 patients; 39.0% overall), with only 35 patients found to have ICD-related technical findings (16.7% overall). This trend was consistent across all groups and subgroups.

In total, 219 unscheduled follow-ups (102 in-clinic; 106 remote; 11 telephone-based) occurred in 83 patients over a mean period of 369.8 ± 114.7 days. The proportion of patients with at least one unscheduled follow-up was nominally higher in the telemetry compared to personal contact group (42.2% vs. 37.0%, $p = 0.448$), and in the telemetry and remote+phone groups (42.2 and 45.3%) compared to the visit group (29.1%, $p = 0.171$) (Fig. 3). The proportion of patients with physician-initiated unscheduled follow-ups was also nominally higher in telemetry and remote+phone groups (28.4 and 32.1% vs. 18.2%), though did not reach statistical significance. The unscheduled follow-up was considered reasonable in 75.0 and 77.8% of cases in the telemetry and personal contact groups ($p = 0.631$), and 79.6 and 75.6% of remote+phone and visit subgroups (p

Table 1 Baseline characteristics

	Telemetry	Personal contact			*p*-value (telemetry vs. personal contact)	*p*-value (telemetry vs. remote + phone vs. visit)
	(N = 102) n (%) / mean ± SD	All (*N* = 108) n (%) / mean ± SD	Remote + phone (*N* = 53) n (%) / mean ± SD	Visit (*N* = 55) n (%) / mean ± SD		
Age (years)	62.5 ± 12.2	65.1 ± 10.1	64.7 ± 9.1	65.4 ± 11.1	0.192	0.312
Female (%)	17 (16.7)	16 (14.8)	7 (13.2)	9 (16.4)	0.712	0.844
Disease parameters						
LVEF (%)	28.2 ± 7.1	28.3 ± 8.9	29.7 ± 10.8	26.9 ± 6.5	0.368	0.562
NYHA class (mean ± SD)	2.4 ± 0.6	2.3 ± 0.7	2.3 ± 0.7	2.3 ± 0.7	0.524	0.804
NYHA class (median)	2 (range 1–3)	2 (range 1–3)	2 (range 1–3)	2 (range 1–3)		
NYHA I	7.8	12.0	13.2	10.9		
NYHA II	48.0	46.3	43.4	49.1		
NYHA III	44.1	41.7	43.4	40.0		
Cardiac disease type					0.834	0.357
None (%)	0 (0.0)	1 (0.9)	1 (1.9)	0 (0.0)		
Ischemic (%)	58 (56.9)	66 (61.1)	30 (56.6)	36 (65.5)		
Non-ischemic (%)	41 (40.2)	38 (35.2)	19 (35.8)	19 (34.5)		
Other (%)	3 (2.9)	3 (2.8)	3 (5.7)	0 (0.0)		
ICD indication					0.861	0.508
Primary prevention	86 (84.3)	92 (85.2)	43 (81.1)	49 (89.1)		
Secondary prevention	16 (15.7)	16 (14.8)	10 (18.9)	6 (10.9)		
Cardiac medication						
None	5 (4.9)	9 (8.3)	4 (7.5)	5 (9.1)	0.319	0.578
Class 2 (beta-blockers)	96 (94.1)	99 (91.7)	49 (92.5)	50 (90.9)	0.491	0.751
Class 4	1 (1.0)	1 (0.9)	1 (1.9)	0 (0.0)	1.0	0.744
Amiodarone	12 (11.8)	12 (11.1)	5 (9.5)	7 (12.7)	0.882	0.856
Cardiac medication						
Diuretics	87 (85.3)	89 (82.4)	43 (81.1)	46 (83.6)	0.570	0.800
ACE inhibitors	81 (79.4)	86 (79.6)	38 (71.7)	48 (87.3)	0.969	0.134
ARB	18 (17.6)	16 (14.8)	10 (18.9)	6 (10.9)	0.578	0.456
Spironolactone	54 (53.5) [a]	61 (56.5)	28 (52.8)	33 (60.0)	0.661	0.686
Device type					0.320	0.313
ICD Single Chamber	57 (55.9)	51 (47.2)	27 (50.9)	24 (43.6)		
ICD Dual Chamber	13 (12.7)	21 (19.4)	12 (22.6)	9 (16.4)		
CRT-D	32 (31.4)	36 (33.3)	14 (26.4)	22 (40.0)		
DF-4 connector	73 (71.6)	77 (71.3)	36 (67.9)	41 (74.5)	0.965	0.748
MLHFQ score PHD	33.6 ± 22.0	33.3 ± 22.0	33.7 ± 24.7	33.0 ± 19.3	0.861	0.976
MLHFQ score at 1 M	24.0 ± 20.3	21.8 ± 19.3	22.8 ± 23.7	20.9 ± 14.2	0.543	0.631

LVEF left ventricular ejection fraction, *NYHA* New York Heart Association, *ICD* implantable cardioverter-defibrillator, *ACE* angiotensin-converting enzyme, *ARB* angiotensin II receptor blockers, *CRT-D* cardiac resynchronization therapy implantable cardioverter-defibrillator, *MLHFQ* Minnesota Living with Heart Failure Questionnaire, *PHD* pre-hospital discharge, *1 M* 1 month

[a] Data was missing for 1 patient

= 0.797 also vs. telemetry group) (Table 3). However, only 51.1% yielded findings, with this proportion nominally higher in the visit subgroup (64.4%) compared to the telemetry (45.8%) and remote+phone (51.9%) group/subgroup ($p = 0.104$). Findings of a medical nature were generally more common than technical findings (35.2% vs. 9.6%, overall). System revisions were required in six patients (5.9%) in the telemetry group (three

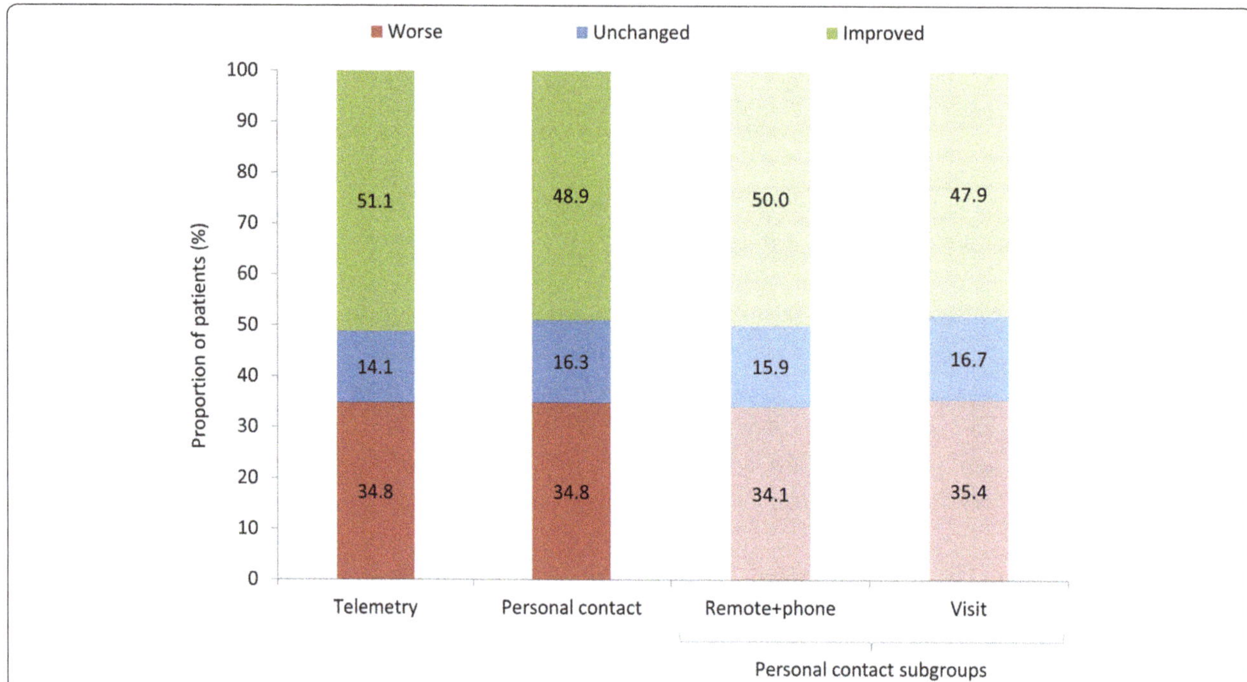

Fig. 2 Change in Packer score at 13 months vs. 1 month. Legend: Proportions are relative to the number of patients in each group/subgroup with all relevant data available (telemetry: $n = 92$; personal contact: $n = 92$ including remote+phone: $n = 44$ and visit: $n = 48$). The distribution of the type of change in Packer score (worse, unchanged or improved) was not significantly different between telemetry vs. personal care ($p = 0.855$) or telemetry vs. remote+phone vs. visit groups/subgroups ($p = 0.967$)

dislodgements, one myocardial perforation, one planned placement of an epicardial left ventricular lead, and one anticipated perforation of device through skin) and one patient (0.9%) in the personal contact (remote+phone) group (dislodgement and myocardial perforation; $p = 0.059$) (Table 3).

Arrhythmias and ICD therapies

Stored tachycardias occurred in 22.9% of the population, with no significant differences between groups ($p = 0.579$) or subgroups ($p = 0.899$) (Table 2). Rates of ventricular fibrillation/tachycardia and supraventricular tachycardia (SVT) were statistically comparable between telemetry and personal contact groups (19.6% vs. 15.7%, $p = 0.462$; and 17.6% vs. 10.2%, $p = 0.117$, respectively). The same was true for subgroup comparisons.

Overall, at least one ICD therapy was delivered to 32 patients (15.2%) during follow-up, with ATP therapy given to 14.3% and shock to 8.6% of all patients. These trends were consistent across groups and subgroups.

Functional status and quality of life

Overall, NYHA class worsened by a mean of 0.08 ± 0.672 between 1 and 13 months (median 2, range 1–3), with no significant differences found for group ($p = 0.888$) or subgroup ($p = 0.912$) comparisons (Table 2). NYHA class worsened in 24.0%, was unchanged in 59.6% and improved in 16.4% of the total population, again without significant differences in distribution between groups ($p = 0.639$) or subgroups ($p = 0.715$).

The overall mean change in MLHFQ score between PHD and 13 months was − 9.38, with a mean increment of 1.64 between 1 and 13 months. This trend was consistent across all groups and subgroups, with no significant differences detected (Table 2).

Discussion

We aimed to compare the outcomes of HF patients receiving quarterly automated ICD/CRT-D follow-up compared to those receiving personal physician follow-up at the same intervals over 12 months. We further explored the impact of the type of physician contact on outcomes. Given its prior absence in the literature, the effect of adding telephone follow-up to remote follow-up was of particular interest. We found that comparable proportions of the different follow-up groups/subgroups experienced a worsening of their Packer score over the course of the study. The same was true for rates of mortality, HF-hospitalisation, unscheduled follow-ups, and inappropriate ICD therapy. Taking into account the robust comparability of baseline characteristics, our data suggest that a 12-month follow-up programme via a fully automated system is non-inferior to a programme involving regular physician contact. Furthermore, the

Table 2 Secondary outcomes: Packer sub-items, cardiac parameters, and QoL

	Telemetry (*N* = 102) n (%) / mean ± SD	Personal contact			p-value (telemetry vs. personal contact)	p-value (telemetry vs. remote + phone vs. visit)
		All (*N* = 108) n (%) / mean ± SD	Remote + phone (N = 53) n (%) / mean ± SD	Visit (N = 55) n (%) / mean ± SD		
Packer sub-items						
Death	5 (4.9)	6 (5.6)	4 (7.5)	2 (3.6)	0.832	0.645
Cardiac	1 (20.0)	3 (50.0)	2 (50.0)	1 (50.0)	0.259	0.292
Non-cardiac	1 (20.0)	3 (50.0)	2 (50.0)	1 (50.0)		
Origin unclear	3 (60.0)	0 (0.0)	0 (0.0)	0 (0.0)		
HF-hospitalisation[b]	10 (9.8)	13 (12.0)	6 (11.3)	7 (12.7)	0.605	0.851
NYHA class at 13 M vs. 1 M[a]					0.639	0.715
Worse	22 (25.3)	19 (22.6)	7 (17.9)	12 (26.7)		
Unchanged	49 (56.3)	53 (63.1)	27 (69.2)	26 (57.8)		
Improved	16 (18.4)	12 (14.3)	5 (12.8)	7 (15.6)		
Change in NYHA class at 13 M vs. 1 M[a]	−0.07 ± 0.71	−0.10 ± 0.63	−0.8 ± 0.62	−0.11 ± 0.65	0.888	0.912
Self-assessment[c]						
Worse	8 (9.2)	10 (11.8)	6 (15.0)	4 (8.9)	0.582	0.564
Unchanged	24 (27.6)	21 (24.7)	9 (22.5)	12 (26.7)		
Improved	55 (63.2)	54 (63.5)	25 (62.5)	29 (64.4)	0.966	0.982
Cardiac events						
Stored tachycardia[d]	25 (24.5) / 4.8 ± 15.6	23 (21.3) / 2.2 ± 9.0	11 (20.8) / 1.0 ± 4.5	12 (21.8) / 3.5 ± 11.8	0.579 / 0.431	0.850 / 0.680
VT/VF[d]	20 (19.6) 2.1 ± 9.1	17 (15.7) 1.3 ± 6.7	8 (15.1) 0.8 ± 3.7	9 (16.4) 1.8 ± 8.7	0.462 / 0.409	0.752 0.689
SVT[d]	18 (17.6) 2.8 ± 11.4	11 (10.2) 1.0 ± 5.4	4 (7.5) 0.2 ± 1.0	7 (12.7) 1.7 ± 7.5	0.117 0.097	0.216 0.180
Cardiac decompensations	9 (8.8)	9 (8.3)	5 (9.4)	4 (7.3)	0.899	0.915
QoL						
Change in MLHFQ score at 13 M vs. PHD	−8.4 ± 20.3	−10.5 ± 21.6	−12.1 ± 22.7	−9.1 ± 20.8	0.472	0.724
Change in MLHFQ score at 13 M vs. 1 M	0.7 ± 16.8	2.7 ± 20.5	3.0 ± 22.2	2.4 ± 19.1	0.666	0.837

NYHA New York Heart Association, *13 M* 13 months, *HF* heart failure, *VF* ventricular fibrillation, *VT* ventricular tachycardia, *SVT* supraventricular tachycardia, *MLHFQ* Minnesota Living with Heart Failure Questionnaire, *PHD* pre-hospital discharge, *1 M* 1 month

[a]Data based on non-missing values ($n = 171$)

[b]Data based on non-missing values ($n = 174$)

[c]Data based on non-missing values ($n = 172$)

[d]Percentage of patients / number of tachycardia events

addition of telephone follow-ups to quarterly automated follow-ups appears not to produce a clinical advantage, though further corroboratory data would be instructive.

Packer heart failure clinical composite response

Change in Packer score was used as a primary assessment criterion as it is considered to provide a clinically meaningful overview of HF status, encompassing changes in both disease parameters and risk of major clinical events [26, 27]. However, it has been employed in only a few RM studies to date. The 664-patient IN-TIME study used this endpoint to demonstrate that telemonitoring plus standard care resulted in 8.3% fewer patients deteriorating over 12 months compared to those receiving standard care only ($p = 0.013$) [16]. While this did not address the question of whether remote follow-up alone can replace physician follow-up, it did suggest the advantage of combining RM plus personal contact over exclusive face-to-face assessment.

In terms of studies assessing the value of entirely remote follow-ups, only the 16-month EVOLVO study appears to have employed the Packer composite endpoint [28]. This study compared 99 patients exclusively receiving remote follow-up with 101 receiving in-clinic

Table 3 Secondary outcomes: follow-ups between months 1 and 13

	Telemetry (N = 102) n (%) / mean ± SD	Personal contact			p-value (telemetry vs. personal contact)	p-value (telemetry vs. remote +phone vs. visit)
		All (N = 108) n (%) / mean ± SD	Remote+phone (N = 53) n (%) / mean ± SD	Visit (N = 55) n (%) / mean ± SD		
FU duration (days)	372.8 ± 100.3	366.9 ± 127.5	349.9 ± 147.8	384.0 ± 102.0	0.689	0.490
Unscheduled FUs						
No. of FUs /patient	1.2 ± 2.6	0.9 ± 1.8	1.0 ± 1.7	0.8 ± 2.0	0.550	0.285
Total number	120	99	54	45		
Considered reasonable	90 (75.0)	77 (77.8%)	43 (79.6)	34 (75.6)	0.631	0.797
With findings	55 (45.8)	57 (57.6)	28 (51.9)	29 (64.4)	0.084	0.104
Medical	40 (33.3)	37 (37.4)	17 (31.5)	20 (44.4)	0.534	0.335
Technical	9 (7.5)	12 (12.1)	9 (16.7)	3 (6.7)	0.249	0.126
All FUs						
Patients with relevant findings at ≥1 FU	50 (49.0)	50 (46.3)	26 (49.1)	24 (43.6)	0.693	0.789
Medical	42 (41.2)	40 (37.0)	19 (35.8)	21 (38.2)	0.539	0.803
Technical	16 (15.7)	19 (17.6)	11 (20.8)	8 (14.5)	0.711	0.642
Patients with ICD therapy at ≥1 FU	17 (16.7)	15 (13.9)	7 (13.2)	8 (14.5)	0.576	0.839
ICD shock	9 (8.8)	9 (8.3)	4 (7.5)	5 (9.1)	0.899	0.792
ATP therapy	16 (15.7)	14 (13.0)	7 (13.2)	7 (12.7)	0.573	0.851
System revisions						
Patients requiring ≥1	6 (5.9)	1 (0.9)	1 (1.9)	0 (0)	0.059	0.141
Mean per patient	0.06 ± 0.02	0.01 ± 0.10	0.02 ± 0.14	0.00 ± 0.00	0.046	0.118

FU follow-up, *ICD* implanted cardioverter-defibrillator, *ATP* anti-tachycardia pacing

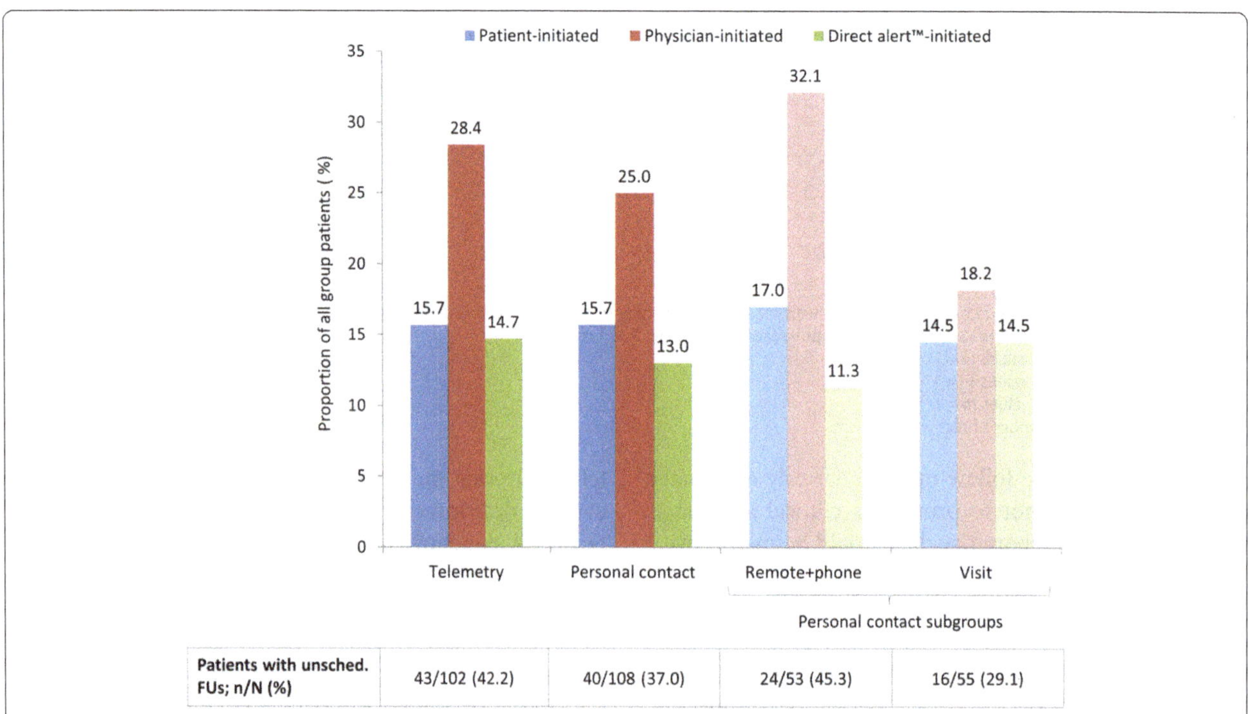

Fig. 3 Unscheduled follow-ups between 1 and 13 months. Legend: unsched., unscheduled; FU, follow-up. The percentages displayed in the table and graph are proportional to the total number of patients within the respective group/subgroup that had ≥1 unscheduled follow-up. The three initiation types are not exclusive and any one patient may be represented by multiple bars. The distribution of initiation types was not significantly different between telemetry vs. personal care or telemetry vs. remote+phone vs. visit groups/subgroups. Follow-ups could be in-house or remote

follow-up only, and found no significant difference in the proportion of patients with a worse Packer score at 16 months relative to baseline (34% vs. 44%, respectively). Concurrently, 35% of all patients in the present study were found to have experienced a deterioration in Packer score between 1 and 13 months, with this applying to a comparable proportion of telemetry and personal contact (including visit) patients. Furthermore, the non-inferiority of the entirely remote approach was statistically indicated according to the predefined criteria. Thus, our data support previous findings that automated follow-up regimes are non-inferior to in-clinic follow-up regimes in terms of composite response. In addition, our data go further, indicating for the first time that addition of a telephone call to quarterly remote follow-ups may not provide any significant advantage over RM alone. In light of this, current HRS guidelines appear to be appropriate [11], though further validation of our findings in larger-scale studies is required.

Mortality

There was no difference in all-cause mortality at 12 months in the telemetry compared to the visit group (4.9% vs. 3.6%, respectively). This is in line with other randomised control trials (RCTs), such as the MORE-CARE (9.2% vs. 7.9%, $p = 0.594$) and TELECART (7.9% vs. 8.9%, $p = 0.54$) studies and a large-scale meta-analysis comparing RM to outpatient follow-up (odds ratio [OR] 0.83, 95% CI 0.58–1.17, $p = 0.285$) [17]. Conversely, several observational studies have identified lower mortality rates in patients receiving telemonitoring compared to those followed up in-house [15, 18]. Perhaps the most convincing of these is ALTITUDE, which compared 10,272 matched ICD and CRT-D patients with or without remote network follow-up over 5 years post-implant [15]. The risk of death was found to be halved by application of RM (ICD: hazard ratio [HR] 0.56, 95% CI 0.47–0.67, $p < 0.001$; CRT-D; HR 0.45, 95% CI 0.39–0.53, $p < 0.001$); however, follow-up modality was decided by the treating physician based on device availability and logistics, introducing a probable bias. Furthermore, patients may receive more rigorous assessment in the context of a RCT, resulting in a higher quality of in-house care provision. Regardless of the cause, it is important to note that findings from RCTs, however robust, may not directly translate into a real-world context. This should be taken into consideration when reflecting upon the finding that there was no significant difference in mortality rates between telemetry and remote+phone groups, even when stratified by cause of death. While our analysis was explorative, this once more indicates that addition of telephone contact to remote follow-up may not be advantageous for reducing fatalities, at least in the context of an RCT. Of interest is the finding that the cause of death was "unclear" in 60% of telemetry patients compared to none of the personal contact patients, suggesting that the availability of certain information may be lost through entirely remote management. Nonetheless, further investigation of the present findings through real-world observational registries may be informative.

HF-hospitalisations

No significant differences were found between groups or subgroups with respect to the frequency of HF-hospitalisations. Again, this was consistent with previous findings from RCTs, including CONNECT and EVOLVO [14, 28–30]. These studies reported annual rates ranging from 0.39–0.50 cardiovascular hospitalisations per patient, with no difference between RM and in-clinic groups ($p = 0.99$ and $p = 0.464$ for each study, respectively) [14, 28]. Furthermore, a recently published meta-analysis pooling data from 7 RCTs found no significant reduction in the odds of hospitalisation with RM compared to standard care (OR 0.83; 95% CI 0.63–1.10; $p = 0.196$) [17]; however, it should be noted that this referred to hospitalisation for all-causes. Nonetheless, the apparent lack of impact of telephone contact in addition to remote follow-up on HF-hospitalisation rates in the present study is unsurprising.

Interestingly, observational studies have consistently associated telemetry with a reduction in hospitalisation frequency [12, 23, 24]. Again, this discrepancy is likely due to socioeconomic and geographical bias reflective of real-world trends and applications. Thus, evaluating the effect of RM plus telephone follow-up on HF-hospitalisation rates in a real-world setting may prove interesting. Of note, observational studies have also linked RM to a shorter duration of hospitalisation episodes and lower associated costs [12, 23, 24], with one analysis specifically identifying a reduction in cardiovascular hospitalisation expenditure as the key driver for the cost savings associated with RM [23]. Though these parameters were beyond the scope of the present analysis, they should be borne in mind for future studies evaluating the value of telephone contact as an adjunct to RM.

Unscheduled follow-ups

Though not reaching statistical significance, the proportion of patients who had at least one unscheduled follow-up in the present study was approximately 15% higher in the telemetry and remote+phone groups compared to the visit group. This appears to have been largely driven by more frequent physician-initiated follow-ups. A higher yearly rate of additional follow-ups in remotely monitored patients compared to those regularly attending in-clinic appointments was also noted in TRUST (0.78 vs. 0.50 visits/person/year, $p = 0.009$),

CONNECT (2.24 vs. 1.95 visits/person/year, $p = 0.099$), EuroEco (0.95 vs. 0.62 visits/person/year, $p = 0.005$), and MORE-CARE (IRR 2.80, 95% CI 2.16–3.63, $p < 0.001$) studies [13, 14, 29, 30]. In addition, a recent meta-analysis reported RM to be associated with a non-significant trend towards greater odds of experiencing an unscheduled follow-up (OR 1.29; 95% CI 0.99–1.67, $p = 0.061$) [17]. This trend may be representative of physicians feeling less confident about their patient's conditions when not meeting them on a regular basis and thus being more likely to initiate unscheduled contact. However, such contact was not necessarily required in all cases, with findings at an unscheduled follow-up nominally less frequent in the telemetry and remote +phone groups compared to the visit group. Given that remote+phone and telemetry patients cited "perceived clinical symptoms" as the reason for patient-initiated unscheduled follow-up significantly more frequently than visit patients (16.7 and 5.8% vs. 2.2%, $p = 0.002$), insecurity in those unable to meet face-to-face with their treating physician on a regular basis may also have contributed. Taken together, our data may indicate that neither telemetry nor telephone contact can replace in-clinic visits for instilling confidence in patients and physicians alike, though the present study was not specifically designed to identify such an effect.

System revisions were more common in the telemetry compared to the personal contact group. A similar trend was reported by the TRUST trial, with home monitoring found to result in a greater rate of in-person system revisions compared to conventional monitoring (29.9% vs. 14.5% at 100 days; $p = 0.018$) [31, 32]. While TRUST authors attribute this finding to the earlier detection of technical issues using RM, this explanation is less applicable to the present study, given that RM and direct alerts were activated for all patients. Thus, the reason for this imbalance remains illusive and merits further exploration.

Arrhythmias and ICD therapies

There were no significant differences between groups and subgroups with respect to cardiac decompensations or number of stored tachycardias. Similarly, a study by Marcantoni et al. designed particularly to explore the effect of RM on supraventricular and ventricular arrhythmias also found no difference in incidence when comparing patients followed remotely to those followed in the clinic [19]. However, the study did report a reduction in associated events in the RM group, explained as due to the earlier detection and pre-emptive treatment of such arrhythmias.

ICD therapy (shock or ATP) is associated with an increased risk of mortality and HF deterioration, regardless of its appropriacy [33, 34]. This is thought to be partly due to the negative inotropic consequences of the therapy, which may result in a significant reduction in cardiac index [35–37]. Consequently, avoidance of inappropriate therapy is paramount. In the present study, approximately 15% of patients received ICD therapy over 12 months, with no notable differences across groups or subgroups. This is consistent with the majority of previously published studies [6, 15, 17, 21].

Quality of life

It has been suggested that RM can reduce the inconvenience of attending in-clinic visits and anxiety between follow-ups, resulting in a positive effect on QoL [10]. However, most studies have found it to have no effect on QoL [5, 29], with the exception of the EVOLVO study [28]. Although MLHFQ score fell by approximately 9 points between PHD and 13 months in the present study, indicating an overall improvement in QoL, a minor deterioration between months 1 and 13 occurred in all groups. This deterioration was marginally smaller in the remote +phone group, though this effect was not significant due to the large within-group variations (demonstrated by very large standard deviations). Our data are thus in line with previous evidence that neither automated remote follow-up nor personal contact appear to be superior for improving MLHFQ-measured patient QoL.

Limitations

This was a prospective, randomised multicentre study in Germany with patients being monitored using the Merlin@home™ system. We regard this, together with the possible use of different ICD/CRT-D devices, as a particular strength of the study. However, our findings may not be generalizable to patients using other RM systems. In addition, while we endeavoured to ensure consecutive enrolment, this was not always possible; as such, we cannot guarantee the elimination of selection bias. Furthermore, the relevance of medical and technical findings was determined at the physician's discretion, potentially leading to subjectivity bias. Nevertheless, randomisation ensured that any one physician was treating both RM and personal contact patients, likely resulting in a reasonably uniform impact of such bias across groups and subgroups. Finally, limited patient numbers may have prevented detection of small but significant effects owing to insufficient statistical power. Indeed, initial sample size calculations were performed based on between-group comparisons, with subgroup comparisons thus being suboptimally powered. As such, large-scale observational studies would be informative.

Conclusions

In HF patients with recently implanted ICDs/CRT-Ds, entirely automated remote follow-up is non-inferior to follow-up with personal contact over a period of 12 months. Furthermore, the addition of a telephone call to quarterly automated follow-ups does not appear to be beneficial for improving outcomes, though further studies are necessary to corroborate this finding. Nevertheless, the present study provides additional evidence in support of the safe and effective replacement of regular physician contact with fully-automated follow-up in this patient population.

Center list - Germany

Herz-und Gefäßzentrum am Krankenhaus Neu-Bethlehem Göttingen gGmbH, 37,073 Göttingen; Städtisches Klinikum Lüneburg gGmbH, 21,339 Lüneburg; SLK-Kliniken Heilbronn GmbH Klinikum am Plattenwald, 74,177 Bad Friedrichshall; Klinikum Ingolstadt GmbH, 85,049 Ingolstadt; Evangelisches Krankenhaus Kalk, 51,103 Köln; Marienhospital Stuttgart, 70,199 Stuttgart; Klinikum Sindelfingen-Böblingen gGmbH, 71,065 Sindelfinden; Asklepios Klinik Barmbek, 22,307 Hamburg; Kardiologische Gemeinschaftspraxis am Park Sanssouci, 14,471 Potsdam; Segeberger Kliniken GmbH, 23,795 Bad Segeberg; Kardiologische Praxis – Partnergesellschaft, 71,634 Ludwigsburg; Asklepios Klinik Bad Oldesloe, 23,843 Bad Oldesloe; Evangelisches Krankenhaus Bielefeld gGmbH, 33,617 Bielefeld; Marienhaus Klinikum St. Elisabeth-Krankenhaus, 56,564 Neuwied; Asklepios Klinik St. Georg, 20,099 Hamburg; Universitätsklinikum Essen (AöR), 45,122 Essen; Praxis Dr. med. Balbach / Ruppert, 72,622 Nürtingen.

Abbreviations

ACE: Angiotensin converting enzyme; ARB: Angiotensin receptor blocker; ATP: Antitachycardia pacing; CI: Confidence interval; CRT-D: Cardiac resynchronisation therapy defibrillator; FU: Follow up; HF: Heart failure; HRS: Heart Rhythm Society; ICD: Implantable cardioverter defibrillator; LVEF: Left ventricular ejection fraction; MLHFQ: Minnesota Living with Heart Failure Questionnaire; NYHA: New York Heart Association; PHD: Pre-hospital discharge; QoL: Quality of life; RM: Remote monitoring; SD: Standard deviation; SVT: Supraventricular tachycardia; VF: Ventricular fibrillation; VT: Ventricular tachycardia

Acknowledgements

The authors would like to express their sincere thanks to Rita Omega Ella (Abbott – St. Jude Medical) for providing statistical supervision.

Funding

Abbott (formerly St. Jude Medical; Eschborn, Germany) funded the study. The sponsor was involved in the design of the study, the data collection, the analysis and interpretation of the data and during the revision of the manuscript.

Authors' contributions

Conception: CH, CL, KS, FH, HT, KP, GG, PB, FB; Design: CH, CL, KS, FH, HT, KP, GG, PB, FB; Acquisition: CH, CL, KS, FH, HT, KP, GG, PB, FB, CW; Interpretation of data: CH, CL, KS, FH, HT, KP, GG, PB, FB, CW; Drafting the work: CH, PB; Critical revision for important intellectual content: CL, KS, FH, HT, KP, GG, FB, CW; Final approval: CH, CL, KS, FH, HT, KP, GG, PB, FB, CW; Agrees to be accountable: CH, CL, KS, FH, HT, KP, GG, PB, FB, CW. All authors read and approved the final manuscript.

Competing interests

Peter Bramlage has received honoraria relevant to this topic. Frank Birkenhauer is an employee of Abbott. The other authors have no competing interest to declare.

Author details

[1]Herz- und Gefäßzentrum am Krankenhaus Neu-Bethlehem, Humboldtallee 6, 37073 Göttingen, Germany. [2]SLK-Kliniken Heilbronn Klinikum am Plattenwald, Bad Friedrichshall, Germany. [3]Klinikum Ingolstadt, Ingolstadt, Germany. [4]Evangelisches Krankenhaus Kalk, Köln, Germany. [5]Marienhospital Stuttgart, Stuttgart, Germany. [6]Kreiskliniken Böblingen Standort Sindelfingen, Sindelfingen, Germany. [7]Asklepios Klinik Barmbek, Hamburg, Germany. [8]Institut für Pharmakologie und Präventive Medizin, Cloppenburg, Germany. [9]Abbott - St. Jude Medical GmbH, Eschborn, Germany. [10]Städtisches Klinikum Lüneburg gGmbH, Lüneburg, Germany.

References

1. Ambrosy AP, Fonarow GC, Butler J, Chioncel O, Greene SJ, Vaduganathan M, et al. The global health and economic burden of hospitalizations for heart failure: lessons learned from hospitalized heart failure registries. J Am Coll Cardiol. 2014;63(12):1123–33.
2. Yancy CW, Jessup M, Bozkurt B, Butler J, Casey DE Jr, Drazner MH, et al. ACCF/AHA guideline for the management of heart failure: a report of the American College of Cardiology Foundation/American Heart Association Task Force on Practice Guidelines. J Am Coll Cardiol. 2013;62(16):e147–239.
3. Ponikowski P, Voors AA, Anker SD, Bueno H, Cleland JG, Coats AJ, et al. ESC Guidelines for the diagnosis and treatment of acute and chronic heart failure: The Task Force for the diagnosis and treatment of acute and chronic heart failure of the European Society of Cardiology (ESC). Developed with the special contribution of the Heart Failure Association (HFA) of the ESC. Eur J Heart Fail. 2016;18(8):891–975.
4. Bertini M, Marcantoni L, Toselli T, Ferrari R. Remote monitoring of implantable devices: should we continue to ignore it? Int J Cardiol. 2016; 202:368–77.
5. Mabo P, Victor F, Bazin P, Ahres S, Babuty D, Da Costa A, et al. A randomized trial of long-term remote monitoring of pacemaker recipients (the COMPAS trial). Eur Heart J. 2012;33(9):1105–11.
6. Osmera O, Bulava A. The benefits of remote monitoring in long-term care for patients with implantable cardioverter-defibrillators. Neuro Endocrinol Lett. 2014;35(Suppl):140–8.
7. Fauchier L, Sadoul N, Kouakam C, Briand F, Chauvin M, Babuty D, et al. Potential cost savings by telemedicine-assisted long-term care of implantable cardioverter defibrillator recipients. Pacing Clin Electrophysiol. 2005;28(Suppl 1):S255–9.
8. Varma N, Michalski J, Stambler B, Pavri BB. Superiority of automatic remote monitoring compared with in-person evaluation for scheduled ICD follow-up in the TRUST trial - testing execution of the recommendations. Eur Heart J. 2014;35(20):1345–52.
9. Heidbuchel H, Lioen P, Foulon S, Huybrechts W, Ector J, Willems R, et al. Potential role of remote monitoring for scheduled and unscheduled evaluations of patients with an implantable defibrillator. Europace. 2008; 10(3):351–7.
10. Jung W, Rillig A, Birkemeyer R, Miljak T, Meyerfeldt U. Advances in remote monitoring of implantable pacemakers, cardioverter defibrillators and cardiac resynchronization therapy systems. J Interv Card Electrophysiol. 2008;23(1):73–85.
11. Slotwiner D, Varma N, Akar JG, Annas G, Beardsall M, Fogel RI, et al. HRS expert consensus statement on remote interrogation and monitoring for cardiovascular implantable electronic devices. Heart Rhythm. 2015;12(7):e69–100.
12. Dario C, Delise P, Gubian L, Saccavini C, Brandolino G, Mancin S. Large controlled observational study on remote monitoring of pacemakers and implantable cardiac defibrillators: a clinical, economic, and organizational evaluation. Interact J Med Res. 2016;5(1):e4.
13. Varma N, Epstein AE, Irimpen A, Schweikert R, Love C. Efficacy and safety of automatic remote monitoring for implantable cardioverter-defibrillator follow-up: the Lumos-T safely reduces Routine office device follow-up (TRUST) trial. Circulation. 2010;122(4):325–32.

14. Crossley GH, Boyle A, Vitense H, Chang Y, Mead RH. The CONNECT (clinical evaluation of remote notification to reduce time to clinical decision) trial: the value of wireless remote monitoring with automatic clinician alerts. J Am Coll Cardiol. 2011;57(10):1181–9.
15. Saxon LA, Hayes DL, Gilliam FR, Heidenreich PA, Day J, Seth M, et al. Long-term outcome after ICD and CRT implantation and influence of remote device follow-up: the ALTITUDE survival study. Circulation. 2010;122(23):2359–67.
16. Hindricks G, Taborsky M, Glikson M, Heinrich U, Schumacher B, Katz A, et al. Implant-based multiparameter telemonitoring of patients with heart failure (IN-TIME): a randomised controlled trial. Lancet. 2014;384(9943):583–90.
17. Parthiban N, Esterman A, Mahajan R, Twomey DJ, Pathak RK, Lau DH, et al. Remote monitoring of implantable cardioverter-defibrillators: a systematic review and meta-analysis of clinical outcomes. J Am Coll Cardiol. 2015; 65(24):2591–600.
18. Akar JG, Bao H, Jones PW, Wang Y, Varosy PD, Masoudi FA, et al. Use of remote monitoring is associated with lower risk of adverse outcomes among patients with implanted cardiac defibrillators. Circ Arrhythm Electrophysiol. 2015;8(5):1173–80.
19. Marcantoni L, Toselli T, Urso G, Pratola C, Ceconi C, Bertini M. Impact of remote monitoring on the management of arrhythmias in patients with implantable cardioverter-defibrillator. J Cardiovasc Med (Hagerstown). 2015;16(11):775–81.
20. De Simone A, Leoni L, Luzi M, Amellone C, Stabile G, La Rocca V, et al. Remote monitoring improves outcome after ICD implantation: the clinical efficacy in the management of heart failure (EFFECT) study. Europace. 2015; 17(8):1267–75.
21. Guedon-Moreau L, Lacroix D, Sadoul N, Clementy J, Kouakam C, Hermida JS, et al. A randomized study of remote follow-up of implantable cardioverter defibrillators: safety and efficacy report of the ECOST trial. Eur Heart J. 2013; 34(8):605–14.
22. Ladapo JA, Turakhia MP, Ryan MP, Mollenkopf SA, Reynolds MR. Health care utilization and expenditures associated with remote monitoring in patients with implantable cardiac devices. Am J Cardiol. 2016;117(9):1455–62.
23. Ricci RP, Vicentini A, D'Onofrio A, Sagone A, Rovaris G, Padeletti L, et al. Economic analysis of remote monitoring of cardiac implantable electronic devices: results of the health economics evaluation registry for remote follow-up (TARIFF) study. Heart Rhythm. 2017;14(1):50–7.
24. Piccini JP, Mittal S, Snell J, Prillinger JB, Dalal N, Varma N. Impact of remote monitoring on clinical events and associated health care utilization: a nationwide assessment. Heart Rhythm. 2016;13(12):2279–86.
25. Rector ST, Kubosh JNC. Patients' self-assessment of their congestive heart failure. Part 2: content, reliability and validity of a new measure, the Minnesota living with heart failure questionnaire. Heart Failure. 1987;3:198–209.
26. Packer M. Proposal for a new clinical end point to evaluate the efficacy of drugs and devices in the treatment of chronic heart failure. J Card Fail. 2001;7(2):176–82.
27. Vardas PE, Auricchio A, Blanc J-J, Daubert J-C, Drexler H, Ector H, et al. Guidelines for cardiac pacing and cardiac resynchronization therapy. Eurospace. 2007;9(10):959–98.
28. Landolina M, Perego GB, Lunati M, Curnis A, Guenzati G, Vicentini A, et al. Remote monitoring reduces healthcare use and improves quality of care in heart failure patients with implantable defibrillators: the evolution of management strategies of heart failure patients with implantable defibrillators (EVOLVO) study. Circulation. 2012;125(24):2985–92.
29. Heidbuchel H, Hindricks G, Broadhurst P, Van Erven L, Fernandez-Lozano I, Rivero-Ayerza M, et al. EuroEco (European health economic trial on home monitoring in ICD patients): a provider perspective in five European countries on costs and net financial impact of follow-up with or without remote monitoring. Eur Heart J. 2015;36(3):158–69.
30. Boriani G, Da Costa A, Quesada A, Ricci RP, Favale S, Boscolo G, et al. Effects of remote monitoring on clinical outcomes and use of healthcare resources in heart failure patients with biventricular defibrillators: results of the MORE-CARE multicentre randomized controlled trial. Eur J Heart Fail. 2017;19(3):416–25.
31. Varma N, Epstein AE, Schweikert R, Michalski J, Love CJ. Role of automatic wireless remote monitoring immediately following ICD implant: the Lumos-T reduces Routine office device follow-up study (TRUST) trial. J Cardiovasc Electrophysiol. 2016;27(3):321–6.
32. Varma N, Michalski J, Epstein AE, Schweikert R. Automatic remote monitoring of implantable cardioverter-defibrillator lead and generator performance: the Lumos-T safely RedUceS RouTine office device follow-up (TRUST) trial. Circ Arrhythm Electrophysiol. 2010;3(5):428–36.
33. Sweeney MO, Sherfesee L, DeGroot PJ, Wathen MS, Wilkoff BL. Differences in effects of electrical therapy type for ventricular arrhythmias on mortality in implantable cardioverter-defibrillator patients. Heart Rhythm. 2010;7(3):353–60.
34. Poole JE, Johnson GW, Hellkamp AS, Anderson J, Callans DJ, Raitt MH, et al. Prognostic importance of defibrillator shocks in patients with heart failure. NEJM. 2008;359(10):1009–17.
35. Tokano T, Bach D, Chang J, Davis J, Souza JJ, Zivin A, et al. Effect of ventricular shock strength on cardiac hemodynamics. J Cardiovasc Electrophysiol. 1998;9(8):791–7.
36. Hasdemir CAN, Shah N, Rao AP, Acosta H, Matsudaira K, Neas BR, et al. Analysis of troponin I levels after spontaneous implantable cardioverter defibrillator shocks. J Cardiovasc Electrophysiol. 2002;13(2):144–50.
37. Yamaguchi H, Weil MH, Tang W, Kamohara T, Jin X, Bisera J. Myocardial dysfunction after electrical defibrillation. Resuscitation 2002; 3:289–96.

12

Impact of clinical presentation and presence of coronary sclerosis on long-term outcome of patients with non-obstructive coronary artery disease

Christine K. Kissel[1,2*], Guanmin Chen[3,4], Danielle A. Southern[3,4], P. Diane Galbraith[1], Todd J. Anderson[1] and for the APPROACH investigators

Abstract

Background: Non-obstructive coronary artery disease (NOCAD) is a common finding on coronary angiography. Our goal was to evaluate the long-term prognosis of NOCAD patients with stable angina (SA).

Methods: The study cohort consisted of 7478 NOCAD patients with normal EF (≥ 50%), and SA who underwent coronary angiography between 1995 and 2012. We compared NOCAD patients (stenosis< 50%) with 10,906 patients with stable obstructive CAD (≥ 50%). The primary endpoint was all-cause mortality. Secondary endpoints included repeat angiography, progressive CAD, and PCI. A second comparison group consisted of 7344 patients with NOCAD presenting with an ACS. Rates of all-cause mortality of NOCAD ACS patients were compared to NOCAD SA patients.

Results: Median follow-up time was 6.5 years. NOCAD patients had a lower risk of all-cause mortality compared to CAD patients (HR CAD vs. NOCAD 1.33 (1.19–1.49); $p < 0.001$). This was driven by patients with normal coronary arteries (HR CAD vs. normal 1.63 (1.36–1.94), $p < 0.001$), whereas patients with minimal disease (> 0% and < 50%) were at similar risk as CAD patients (HR CAD vs. minimal 1.08 (0.99–1.29), $p = 0.06$). In NOCAD patients, the strongest predictors of all-cause mortality were age and minimal disease. SA patients with NOCAD had low rates of repeat angiography (7.3%), future CAD (2.3%) and PCI (1.7%). NOCAD ACS patients had a 41% increase in all-cause mortality risk compared to NOCAD SA patients (HR 1.41 (1.25–1.6), $p < 0.001$).

Conclusions: This study underlines the importance of minimal CAD, as it is not a benign disease entity and portends a similar risk as stable obstructive CAD.

Keywords: Coronary artery disease, Prognosis, Stable angina, Acute coronary syndrome

Background

Non-obstructive coronary artery disease (NOCAD) is a common finding on diagnostic coronary angiograms with rates of up to 50–60% in patients with stable angina (SA) and of about 30% in certain population with acute coronary syndromes (ACS) [1–4]. Symptomatic patients with NOCAD have often been reassured of the innocuousness of the results, and frequently no further preventive measures were taken [5, 6]. The etiology of symptoms in these patients appears to be heterogeneous and prognosis was often deemed favourable. Recently, the conception that NOCAD is a benign disease has been challenged [3, 4, 6, 7]. Jespersen et al. showed a graded increase in major adverse cardiovascular events (MACE) in patients with normal arteries, non-obstructive, and obstructive coronary disease. These findings were confirmed by Maddox et al. who demonstrated an increase of all-cause mortality and MI rate from non-obstructive to obstructive CAD by extent of vessel distribution in a cohort of mostly male veterans presenting for an elective coronary angiogram

* Correspondence: Christine.Kissel@gmail.com
[1]Department of Cardiac Sciences and Libin Cardiovascular Institute of Alberta, Cumming School of Medicine, University of Calgary, Calgary, AB, Canada
[2]Department of Cardiology, University Heart Center, University Hospital Zurich, Rämistrasse 100, CH-8091 Zürich, Switzerland
Full list of author information is available at the end of the article

[7]. One of the first study groups who followed NOCAD patients systematically was the WISE study group (Women's Ischemia Syndrome Evaluation). WISE primarily examined women, who were found to have cardiac syndrome X, i.e. chest pain of an ischemic origin and NOCAD. The authors demonstrated a high rate of all-cause mortality rate (18% in 10 years), and high rates of repeat angiogram (19%) in women with NOCAD and SA [3]. In contrast, the Swedish Coronary Angiography and Angioplasty Registry (SCAAR) registry demonstrated a low all-cause mortality of 0.3–0.4% in NOCAD patients with SA at 2 years [2], hereby raising the question about contemporary, long-term all-cause mortality in NOCAD.

Furthermore, it is well known that presentation with an ACS with obstructive CAD portends an increased mortality risk. Previous studies addressed ACS patients with NOCAD, which is also termed myocardial infarction with non-obstructive coronary arteries (MINOCA), but study size was either small or patients were followed only in the short-term [8–12].

Our aim was therefore to evaluate prognosis and its predictors in a large, contemporary population of patients of both sexes with NOCAD. We also sought to investigate whether presentation with an ACS leads to a worse prognosis compared to stable NOCAD patients.

Methods

Data source and collection

Eligible subjects included all adults over the age of 18 years undergoing their first cardiac catheterization between January 1, 1995 to March 31, 2012, registered in the Alberta Provincial Project for Outcome Assessment in Coronary Heart Disease (APPROACH©) database [13]. APPROACH is a prospective cohort of all adults undergoing cardiac catheterization in Alberta, Canada. APPROACH contains detailed patient information, as well as specifics on coronary anatomy and therapeutic interventions. Data were entered at time of catheterization and are routinely enhanced by merging the clinical registry data to administrative records.

Data collection included e.g. sociodemographic characteristics, comorbidities and risk factors, disease specific variables (e.g. indication for procedure, angina status), and medications at time of catheterization. Angiography results including coronary anatomy, extent of coronary stenosis, and LV ejection fraction (EF) were also recorded [13]. The degree of stenosis was visually assessed by the angiographer with no quantitative measurement. Subsequent angiographies and revascularization procedures are also collected.

APPROACH and this protocol were approved in accordance with the Declaration of Helsinki by the Institutional Ethics Review Board of the University of Calgary. Patients signed informed consent to allow data collection, clinical follow-up, and anonymous data reporting.

Study population

Normal coronaries, minimal disease (i.e. coronary sclerosis) and significant obstructive disease were defined as 0%, > 0 and < 50% and ≥ 50% luminal narrowing in any epicardial coronary artery, respectively. The NOCAD cohort consisted of those with normal coronary arteries or minimal disease. We identified patients with a normal EF (≥50%) who presented with either SA or an ACS.

Stable angina (SA) was defined as Canadian Cardiovascular Society (CCS) class 1, 2 or 3 angina with inclusion of clinically stable patients with atypical chest pain. ACS was defined as unstable angina or non–ST-elevation MI or ST-elevation MI in accordance to universal myocardial infarction criteria.

Patients with an EF below 50% or prior percutaneous coronary intervention (PCI) or coronary artery bypass grafting (CABG) were excluded, as well as patients with significant valvular disease, or left main disease, or referrals for pre- or post-transplant work-up, evaluation of heart failure, congenital heart disease, or serious arrhythmia. Patients with incomplete data were likewise excluded. The rate of incomplete data was low (3.7%).

The main study group consisted of patients with NOCAD (coronary stenosis < 50%) presenting with SA ($n = 7478$). Comparison Group I contained patients with significant CAD (≥ 50% stenosis) who presented with SA ($n = 10{,}906$). Comparison Group II included patients with NOCAD presenting with an ACS ($n = 7344$).

Outcomes

The primary end-point was all-cause mortality with the primary efficacy analysis consisting of a comparison between CAD and NOCAD patients with SA. Follow-up all-cause mortality was ascertained through semi-annual linkage to the Alberta Bureau of Vital Statistics. The survival time from the date of first catheterization was calculated using the date of death. The survival time was censored if the patient was still alive on 31 March 2012. Secondary endpoints were development of obstructive CAD (≥ 50% stenosis on subsequent angiograms), repeat angiogram, and future PCI in NOCAD patients. Any patient who had a second angiogram during the follow-up period was counted once as having had a repeat angiogram.

Statistical methods

Summary statistics for categorical variables presented include counts and percentage, and for continuous variables include mean and standard deviation. The difference for categorical variables between NOCAD and CAD was tested by Chi-square test; and the difference for continuous variables were evaluated by student's t-test. Cox's proportional hazard regression model was used to compare all-cause mortality between CAD and NOCAD. The crude hazard ratio (HR) and adjusted HR with their 95% confidence intervals were estimated. In the multivariable-adjusted model, we adjusted the HRs for age, diabetes mellitus (DM), and hypertension. The analyses for Cox's proportional hazard regression model were stratified by the groups of NOCAD and its subgroups of normal coronaries, and minimal disease (> 0 and < 50%), as well as obstructive CAD. We estimated HRs between NOCAD and CAD patients, stratified by coronary status, and between NOCAD patients presenting with SA or an ACS.

Moreover, Cox's proportional hazard regression models were used to investigate predictors for all-cause mortality among patients with NOCAD. Pre-specified variables for the univariate Cox regression model included age over 55 years, presence of DM, positive stress test, abnormal baseline ECG, hypertension, or previous or current smoking, as well as having undergone more than two angiograms for the same condition.

Factors, which showed a significant association with increased mortality in the univariate analysis, were entered in the multivariate regression model using a stepwise method. To explore the effect of sex, we included this factor in our analyses, independently of the significance level in the univariate model. We conducted these analyses for NOCAD patients with SA. All statistical analyses were performed using statistical software SAS (Version 9.3, Institute Inc., Cary, NC).

Results

During the study period, there were 141,004 patients in the APPROACH registry with 70.2% men and 29.8% women. For reasons previously described, we excluded 92,126 patients, leaving a population of 48,878 subjects with normal EF. Figure 1 shows that of the normal EF group, 7478 subjects had NOCAD presenting with SA. In the NOCAD subgroup, the percentage of women was substantially higher than the total APPROACH population (48.5%). NOCAD was found in 40.7% of all patients presenting with SA, whereas the rate for NOCAD in patients presenting with an ACS was 24.1% (Fig. 1). The median follow-up time was 6.5 years, the maximum was 13.5 years.

Baseline characteristics of NOCAD population with SA

NOCAD patients were significantly younger, were more likely to be female and had significantly lower rates of cardiovascular risk factors compared to CAD patients. A similar picture emerged when patients with normal coronary arteries were compared to patients with minimal disease (Additional file 1: Table S1). At the time of catheterization, medication use was higher in the CAD population (Table 1).

Comparison of all-cause mortality of NOCAD versus CAD patients

The crude all-cause mortality at 10 years occurred in 5.3% and 9.8% of stable patients with NOCAD and CAD, respectively ($p < 0.001$). SA patients with NOCAD had a lower risk of all-cause mortality than patients with CAD after adjustment for basic risk factors (Table 2). However, when the NOCAD population was divided in patients with completely normal coronary arteries and

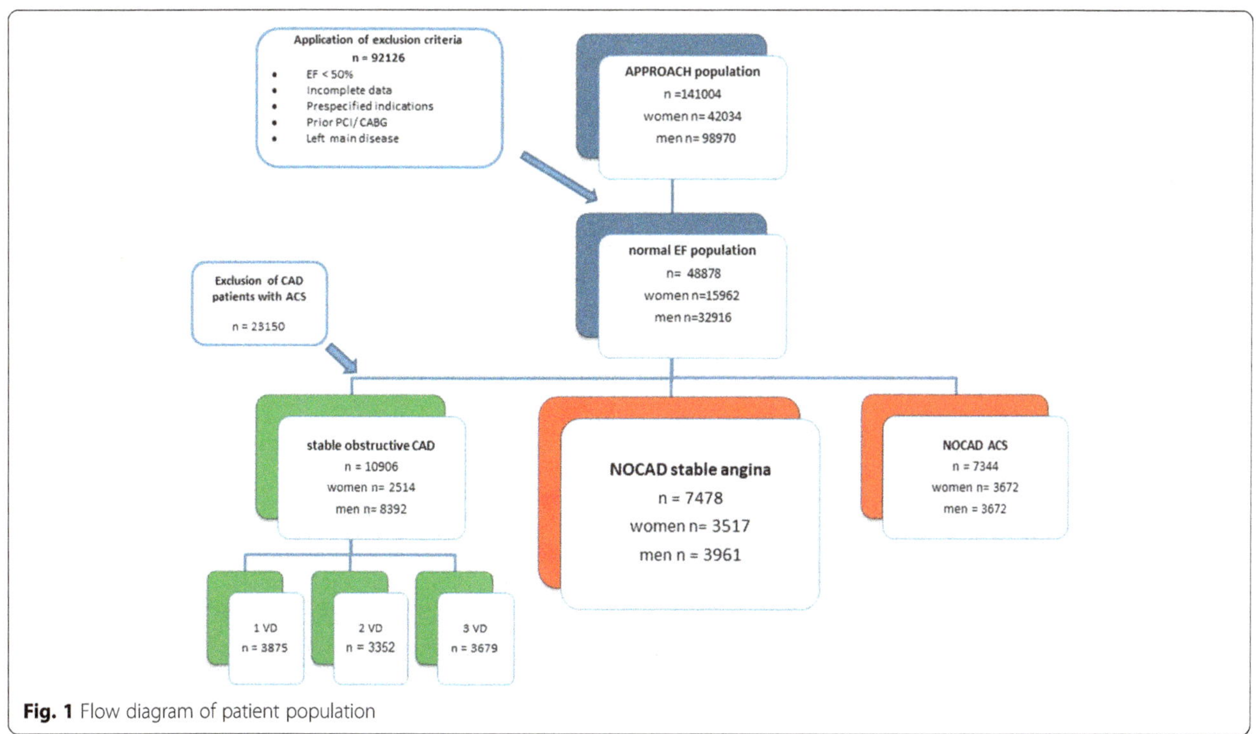

Fig. 1 Flow diagram of patient population

Table 1 Comparison of Baseline Characteristics of Stable Angina Patients: NOCAD versus CAD

	NOCAD ($n = 7478$)	CAD ($n = 10{,}906$)	*p*-value*
Age, mean years	58.8 ± 10.9	64.0 ± 10.2	< 0.001
Female (%)	3517 (47%)	2514 (23.1%)	< 0.001
EF calculated ($n = 2599$)	64.9 ± 7.5	63.7 ± 12.6	< 0.001
Normal coronary arteries	49.4%	N/A	N/A
Cardiovascular risk factors:			
Hypertension (%)	60.4	72.1	< 0.001
Dyslipidemia (%)	65.6	79.2	< 0.001
Diabetes mellitus (%)	16.8	26.6	< 0.001
Smoker- current/ previous (%)	52.5	61.6	0.04
Current smoker (%)	17.7	18.9	< 0.001
Positive family history (%)	29.6	29.1	0.47
Medications at time of cath:			
Aspirin	5286/7159 (73.8%)	8940/10555 (84.7%)	< 0.001
P2Y12 Inhibitor	480/6878 (7%)	1105/10078 (11.0%)	< 0.001
Beta-blockers	3561/7060 (50.4%)	6626/10423 (63.6%)	< 0.001
Statins	3285/6926 (47.4%)	6681/10048 (66.5%)	< 0.001
Calcium channel blockers	1269/6911 (18.4%)	2343/10115 (23.2%)	< 0.001
ACE-inhibitor	1957/6969 (28.1%)	3983/10429 (38.2%)	< 0.001
Long acting nitrates	867/6862 (12.6%)	1716/ 10,043 (7.1%)	< 0.001
Insulin	193/5760 (3.4%)	445/8442 (5.3%)	< 0.001

*for comparison NOCAD vs. CAD

patients with minimal disease, the latter appeared to have a similar risk as CAD patients (Table 2). Patients with completely normal coronary arteries had a lower risk compared to patients with CAD. The Kaplan Meier survival curves between NOCAD (normal, minimal), and obstructive CAD adjusted for age, hypertension, and diabetes are depicted in Fig. 2.

When NOCAD patients presented with an ACS rather than with SA, they had a 41% increase in mortality risk (NOCAD ACS vs. SA HR 1.41 (1.25–1.6), $p < 0.001$).

Secondary endpoints in NOCAD SA population

Over a median of 6.5 years of follow up, the percentage of subjects with a repeat catheterization was low ($n = 543$ (7.3%)). Simultaneously, progression to obstructive CAD in patients with NOCAD was small ($n = 170$ (2.3%)), as well as the necessity to perform a PCI ($n = 128$ (1.7%)). Overall, patients with a NOCAD had significantly lower rates of cardiac procedures than patients with stable one-vessel CAD ($p < 0.001$).

Independent predictors of primary and secondary endpoints

To determine independent predictors of all-cause mortality in the NOCAD population, we performed a multivariate Cox regression analysis, including pre-specified variables as described in the methods' section. Age above 55 years was the strongest independent predictor of all-cause death (Table 3). Subjects with minimal disease compared with normal coronary arteries were at increased

Table 2 All-cause mortality and adjusted hazard ratios for comparison of CAD patients with NOCAD patients

	Deaths n	Total n	10-year rate (%)	Age, DM, HTN- adjusted HR (95% CI)	*p*-value
NOCAD	398	7478	5.3	1.33 (1.19–1.49)	< 0.001*
normal	132	3691	3.6	1.63 (1.36–1.94)	< 0.001†
minimal	266	3787	7	1.08 (0.95–1.23)	0.06‡
CAD (> 50%)	1068	10,906	9.8	–	–

*: CAD vs. NOCAD; †: CAD vs. normal; ‡: CAD vs. minimal

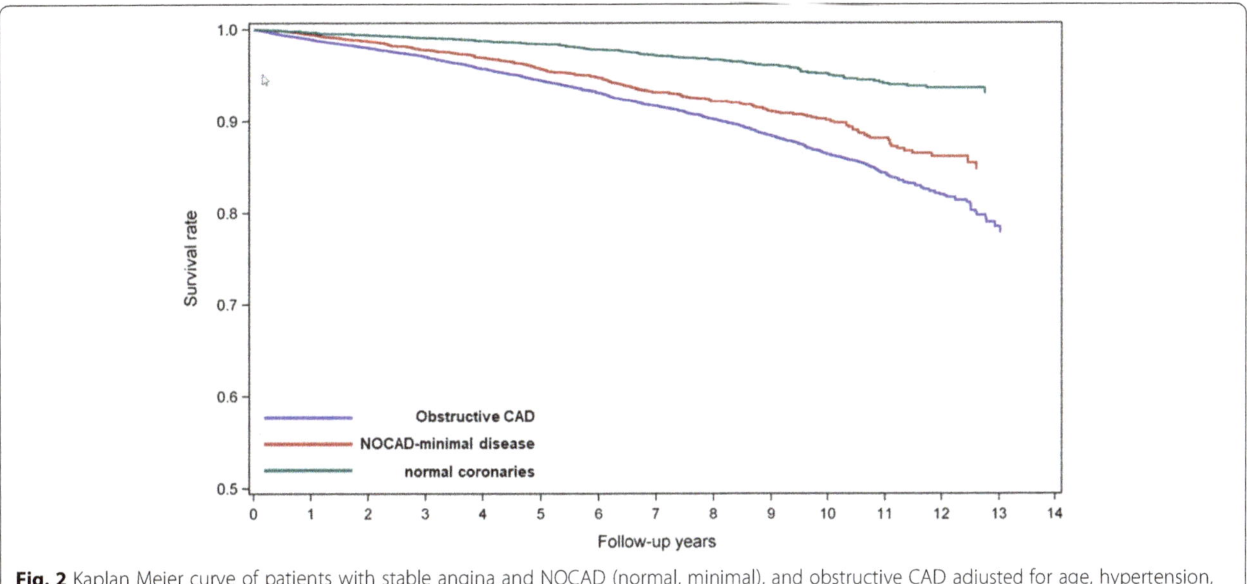

Fig. 2 Kaplan Meier curve of patients with stable angina and NOCAD (normal, minimal), and obstructive CAD adjusted for age, hypertension, and diabetes

risk of death, and this was higher than the risk associated with the presence of diabetes or smoking (Table 3).

Table 4 shows that for the secondary endpoints of future development of obstructive CAD, repeat angiogram, and future PCI, presence of minimal CAD was the strongest independent predictor in all of the three subgroups, followed by DM, and male sex.

Discussion

Our large, contemporary study of SA patients with NOCAD and normal LV-function found several key findings. Patients with NOCAD had favourable long-term rates of repeat angiography, future CAD, and PCI. Nevertheless, patients with minimal disease had a similar risk of all-cause mortality as patients with stable CAD. Finally, NOCAD patients presenting with an ACS, had a 41% increase in all-cause mortality compared with those with a SA presentation.

We were able to demonstrate low rates of repeat angiography for patients with NOCAD. Our rate of repeat catheterization is in line with results reported by others [9, 14]. But this is in contrast to reports from the WISE study cohort, which reported higher rates of repeat angiography of 18–34.5% [15, 16]. The WISE cohort had a high proportion of persistently symptomatic women [16]. Data on persistence of symptoms is unfortunately not available to us. We can only speculate whether our lower rate of repeat catheterization is due to lower rate of persistent symptoms, or an increased awareness of physicians of cardiac syndrome X, and microvascular angina. Further potential explanations might be differences in national/regional practices.

We further showed that NOCAD patients presenting with ACS are at increased risk for all-cause mortality. In daily practice however, the finding of NOCAD on coronary angiography is often regarded as insignificant, even when patients present with an ACS. The cause of ACS in NOCAD patients is often unclear, and a variety of etiologies can account for the findings [12, 17]. It is also well documented that a large number of plaque ruptures occur at the site of non-obstructive lesions that lead to thrombotic occlusion [18, 19]. Some of the ACS patients likely had a plaque rupture but the thrombus was not visible at time of cardiac catheterization anymore. Furthermore, plaque erosion is a potential cause for ACS, which might have been missed in some cases [20]. Since we did not routinely perform intravascular ultrasound or optical coherence tomography (OCT), we do not know the percentage of patients with a plaque rupture or erosion without obvious filling defect. Furthermore, it is known that in symptomatic patients with NOCAD, endothelial dysfunction can lead to signs and symptoms of coronary ischemia and is associated with a worse prognosis [9, 21–23]. We do not have any measures of

Table 3 Independent predictors for all-cause mortality in NOCAD SA patients

Variables	HR (95% CI)	*p*-value
Minimal CAD vs. Normal	1.69 (1.35–2.12)	< 0.001
Age ≥ 55 years vs. Age < 55 years	3.34 (2.48–4.51)	< 0.001
Diabetes mellitus vs. No diabetes	1.5 (1.16–1.94)	0.002
Normal ECG vs. Abnormal	0.67 (0.52–0.87)	0.002
Hypertension vs. No hypertension	1.23 (0.98–1.55)	0.08
Smoker vs. Non-smoker	1.53 (1.23–1.91)	< 0.001
Men vs. Women	1.26 (1.01–1.56)	0.04

Table 4 Independent predictors for repeat angiogram, future PCI, and progression of CAD in NOCAD SA patients

	Repeat angiogram (n = 543)		Future PCI (n = 128)		Future CAD (n = 170)	
Variables	HR (95% CI)	*p*-value	HR (95% CI)	*p*-value	HR (95% CI)	*p*-value
Minimal vs. normal	1.87 (1.53–2.29)	< 0.001	3.78 (2.38–6.01)	< 0.001	3.83 (2.59–5.66)	< 0.001
Age ≥ 55 years vs. age < 55 years	1.41 (1.14–1.75)	0.001	1.15 (0.76–1.75)	0.51	1.52 (1.05–2.2)	0.03
Diabetes mellitus vs. no diabetes	1.64 (1.28–2.1)	< 0.001	3.3 (2.15–5.08)	< 0.001	2.03 (1.34–3.07)	0.001
Normal ECG vs. abnormal	0.8 (0.63–1.01)	0.06	1.13 (0.73–1.75)	0.57	0.61 (0.39–0.94)	0.03
Hypertension vs. no hypertension	1.2 (0.98–1.47)	0.07	1.18 (0.78–1.78)	0.44	1 (0.71–1.4)	0.98
Smoker vs. non-smoker	1.15 (0.94–1.4)	0.18	1.05 (0.7–1.57)	0.82	1.42 (1–2.01)	0.05
Men vs. women	1.42 (1.17–1.74)	< 0.001	2.33 (1.52–3.57)	< 0.001	1.78 (1.25–2.52)	0.001

endothelial function in this study. We can only speculate that coronary endothelial dysfunction led to symptoms and was possibly more pronounced in patients presenting with an ACS, which in turn led to a worse outcome. On the other hand, myocarditis and Takotsubo cardiomyopathy are also potential causes for an ACS- like presentation in patients with NOCAD. Albeit Takotsubo was first described in 1990 in a Japanese publication and has gained worldwide recognition since [24], awareness for Takotsubo was delayed in Western countries and it could well be that some of the earlier inclusions in the APPROACH cohort underdiagnosed Takotsubo. Taken together, patients with NOCAD and ACS likely constitute different etiologies [12, 17]. Given that this patient cohort has a 41% increase in risk, a thorough work-up is warranted to better define the etiology in the individual patient, and to appropriately treat patients according to etiology. In clinical reality, patients with an ACS and NOCAD, and no obvious filling defect, or spasm, often receive less secondary preventive measures [5, 17].

In regard to the increased all-cause mortality risk of patients with minimal disease, our data reinforces results from contemporary studies done by coronary computed tomography angiography (CCTA), which showed that patients with NOCAD had a similar mortality risk as patients with obstructive 1-vessel CAD [25]. Concomitantly, the study confirms a graded increase in risk from normal coronaries to non-obstructive disease to obstructive CAD as reported by angiographic studies, as well as by CCTA studies [4, 5, 15, 25–27]. Recently, Maddox et al. were able to show a graded increase of all-cause mortality and MI rate at 1 year from non-obstructive to obstructive CAD in a large, mostly male, cohort of US veterans who presented for an elective coronary angiogram [5]. Although we did not divide the groups by extent of disease, we were able to confirm an increase in all-cause mortality from normal to coronary sclerosis to obstructive disease in an all-comer population for a longer follow-up period. One of the most important findings of our studies was that patients with minimal disease had a similar HR for all-cause mortality as patients with stable CAD. Minimal disease was an independent predictor of similar strength as DM and smoking in our study. This is in line with several other studies. Recent meta-analyses also confirmed a poorer prognosis of patients with minimal disease compared to patients with normal arteries [28]. Furthermore, Lin et al. demonstrated that the detection of NOCAD improves prediction of mortality beyond conventional risk factor assessment [26].

Overall, data appears to accumulate that the finding of NOCAD is not benign and should prompt consideration of secondary prevention measures as used in subjects with stable obstructive CAD. Large-scale studies are warranted to determine the benefit of such measures.

Limitations

Some limitations apply to this study. Foremost, this was not a randomized controlled trial but a population-based registry study with all its ensued limitations of potential confounding and unmeasured covariates. However, the strength of the APPROACH registry is that it provides a real-world scenario and it captures all deaths and revascularization procedures within the province.

Of note is that APPROACH is a procedure-based registry and not a clinical registry. We cannot exclude a diagnosis, angiogram and/or hospitalization referral bias. However, based on information from an APPROACH ACS registry, it is known that 73.9% of women and 85.1% of men ($p < 0.05$) who present to our region with ACS undergo catheterization. Furthermore, we used multivariable adjustment as strategy to account for baseline differences between patients with NOCAD and CAD. Nevertheless, residual confounding cannot be excluded.

One of the major limitations is that there is no data on the cause of death or cardiovascular death in particular in the APPROACH database. Rehospitalisation rates for ischemia or heart failure, stroke, or quality of life measures are not known for NOCAD patients. Those endpoints have been proven to be of special importance in patients with NOCAD [4, 14, 16]. Nonetheless, data on the hard endpoint of all-cause mortality is robust and of clinical significance. We are also lacking data on long-term medication use or risk factor control. During the long follow-up period from 1995 to 2012, medical management of patients also might have changed. For instance, high dose statin therapy became more common in the early twenty-first century. Also, physicians might have been more prone to use secondary preventive measures in NOCAD over time. A further concern is that it can be difficult to discern normal coronaries from NOCAD. Intravascular ultrasound data, or OCT would have been beneficial but is rarely used for diagnostic angiograms under the specified conditions. Furthermore, grade of stenosis was not assessed in a core lab by quantitative coronary analysis. Therefore, under- or overestimation of stenosis grade cannot be ruled out. In spite of these limitations, our study represents a real-world scenario and is similar to other large-scale registries.

In regard to the study design, one of the main drawbacks is the lack of an asymptomatic, normal control. However, previous studies have shown that there is a graded increase from asymptomatic controls to symptomatic with normal coronary arteries [4].

Conclusion

In conclusion, stable patients with NOCAD have low rates of repeat angiography, future CAD, and PCI. This is reassuring when dealing with and treating these patients. However, subjects with minimal disease should be considered at similar risk as patients with stable, obstructive CAD, which might argue for more aggressive risk factor control in these patients. Also, NOCAD patients presenting with an ACS have a 41% increase in risk for all-cause mortality which might warrant more intensive diagnostic evaluation, treatment, and follow-up.

Abbreviations

ACS: acute coronary syndrome; APPROACH: Alberta Provincial Project for Outcome Assessment in Coronary Heart Disease; CABG: coronary artery bypass grafting; CAD: coronary artery disease; DM: diabetes mellitus; EF: ejection fraction; HR: hazard ratio; HTN: hypertension; NOCAD: non-obstructive coronary artery disease; OCT: optical coherence tomography; PCI: percutaneous coronary intervention; SA: stable angina

Funding

Christine Kissel was supported by the Freiwillige Akademische Gesellschaft, Basel, Switzerland, as well as by a research fellowship award of Eli Lilly Canada Inc..

Authors' contributions

CK Kissel MD: design, analysis and interpretation of data, drafting of manuscript, G Chen MD, PhD: analysis and interpretation of data, DA Southern MSc: acquisition of data, PD Galbraith BN, MSc: conception and acquisition of data, TJ Anderson MD: conception, design, drafting of manuscript

Competing interests

The authors declare that they have no competing interests.

Author details

[1]Department of Cardiac Sciences and Libin Cardiovascular Institute of Alberta, Cumming School of Medicine, University of Calgary, Calgary, AB, Canada. [2]Department of Cardiology, University Heart Center, University Hospital Zurich, Rämistrasse 100, CH-8091 Zürich, Switzerland. [3]O'Brien Institute of Public Health, Cumming School of Medicine, University of Calgary, Calgary, AB, Canada. [4]Department of Community Health Sciences, Cumming School of Medicine, University of Calgary, Calgary, Canada.

References

1. Shaw LJ, Shaw RE, Merz CN, Brindis RG, Klein LW, Nallamothu B, Douglas PS, Krone RJ, McKay CR, Block PC, et al. Impact of ethnicity and gender differences on angiographic coronary artery disease prevalence and in-hospital mortality in the American College of Cardiology-National Cardiovascular Data Registry. Circulation. 2008;117(14):1787–801.
2. Johnston N, Schenck-Gustafsson K, Lagerqvist B. Are we using cardiovascular medications and coronary angiography appropriately in men and women with chest pain? Eur Heart J. 2011;32(11):1331–6.
3. Sharaf B, Wood T, Shaw L, Johnson BD, Kelsey S, Anderson RD, Pepine CJ, Bairey Merz CN. Adverse outcomes among women presenting with signs and symptoms of ischemia and no obstructive coronary artery disease: findings from the National Heart, Lung, and Blood Institute-sponsored Women's ischemia syndrome evaluation (WISE) angiographic core laboratory. Am Heart J. 2013;166(1):134–41.
4. Jespersen L, Hvelplund A, Abildstrom SZ, Pedersen F, Galatius S, Madsen JK, Jorgensen E, Kelbaek H, Prescott E. Stable angina pectoris with no obstructive coronary artery disease is associated with increased risks of major adverse cardiovascular events. Eur Heart J. 2012;33(6):734–44.
5. Maddox TM, Ho PM, Roe M, Dai D, Tsai TT, Rumsfeld JS. Utilization of secondary prevention therapies in patients with nonobstructive coronary artery disease identified during cardiac catheterization: insights from the National Cardiovascular Data Registry Cath-PCI registry. Circ Cardiovasc Qual Outcomes. 2010;3(6):632–41.
6. Pepine CJ, Ferdinand KC, Shaw LJ, Light-McGroary KA, Shah RU, Gulati M, Duvernoy C, Walsh MN, Bairey Merz CN. Committee ACiW: emergence of nonobstructive coronary artery disease: a Woman's problem and need for change in definition on angiography. J Am Coll Cardiol. 2015;66(17):1918–33.
7. Maddox TM, Stanislawski MA, Grunwald GK, Bradley SM, Ho PM, Tsai TT, Patel MR, Sandhu A, Valle J, Magid DJ, et al. Nonobstructive coronary artery disease and risk of myocardial infarction. Jama. 2014;312(17):1754–63.
8. Gehrie ER, Reynolds HR, Chen AY, Neelon BH, Roe MT, Gibler WB, Ohman EM, Newby LK, Peterson ED, Hochman JS. Characterization and outcomes of women and men with non-ST-segment elevation myocardial infarction and nonobstructive coronary artery disease: results from the can rapid risk stratification of unstable angina patients suppress adverse outcomes with early implementation of the ACC/AHA guidelines (CRUSADE) quality improvement initiative. Am Heart J. 2009;158(4):688–94.
9. Ong P, Athanasiadis A, Borgulya G, Voehringer M, Sechtem U. 3-year follow-up of patients with coronary artery spasm as cause of acute coronary syndrome: the CASPAR (coronary artery spasm in patients with acute coronary syndrome) study follow-up. J Am Coll Cardiol. 2011;57(2):147–52.
10. De Ferrari GM, Fox KA, White JA, Giugliano RP, Tricoci P, Reynolds HR, Hochman JS, Gibson CM, Theroux P, Harrington RA, et al. Outcomes among non-ST-segment elevation acute coronary syndromes patients with no angiographically obstructive coronary artery disease: observations from 37,101 patients. Eur Heart J Acute Cardiovasc Care. 2014;3(1):37–45.
11. Pasupathy S, Air T, Dreyer RP, Tavella R, Beltrame JF. Systematic review of patients presenting with suspected myocardial infarction and nonobstructive coronary arteries. Circulation. 2015;131(10):861–70.
12. Agewall S, Beltrame JF, Reynolds HR, Niessner A, Rosano G, Caforio AL, De Caterina R, Zimarino M, Roffi M, Kjeldsen K, et al. ESC working group position paper on myocardial infarction with non-obstructive coronary arteries. Eur Heart J. 2017;38(3):143–53.
13. Ghali WA, Knudtson ML. Overview of the Alberta provincial project for outcome assessment in coronary heart disease. On behalf of the APPROACH investigators. Can J Cardiol. 2000;16(10):1225–30.

14. Humphries KH, Pu A, Gao M, Carere RG, Pilote L. Angina with "normal" coronary arteries: sex differences in outcomes. Am Heart J. 2008;155(2):375–81.
15. Sharaf BL, Pepine CJ, Kerensky RA, Reis SE, Reichek N, Rogers WJ, Sopko G, Kelsey SF, Holubkov R, Olson M, et al. Detailed angiographic analysis of women with suspected ischemic chest pain (pilot phase data from the NHLBI-sponsored Women's ischemia syndrome evaluation [WISE] study angiographic Core Laboratory). Am J Cardiol. 2001;87(8):937–41. A933
16. Johnson BD, Shaw LJ, Pepine CJ, Reis SE, Kelsey SF, Sopko G, Rogers WJ, Mankad S, Sharaf BL, Bittner V, et al. Persistent chest pain predicts cardiovascular events in women without obstructive coronary artery disease: results from the NIH-NHLBI-sponsored Women's Ischaemia syndrome evaluation (WISE) study. Eur Heart J. 2006;27(12):1408–15.
17. Niccoli G, Scalone G, Crea F. Acute myocardial infarction with no obstructive coronary atherosclerosis: mechanisms and management. Eur Heart J. 2015; 36(8):475–81.
18. Libby P, Theroux P. Pathophysiology of coronary artery disease. Circulation. 2005;111(25):3481–8.
19. Stone GW, Maehara A, Lansky AJ, de Bruyne B, Cristea E, Mintz GS, Mehran R, McPherson J, Farhat N, Marso SP, et al. A prospective natural-history study of coronary atherosclerosis. N Engl J Med. 2011;364(3):226–35.
20. Falk E, Nakano M, Bentzon JF, Finn AV, Virmani R. Update on acute coronary syndromes: the pathologists' view. Eur Heart J. 2013;34(10):719–28.
21. Murthy VL, Naya M, Taqueti VR, Foster CR, Gaber M, Hainer J, Dorbala S, Blankstein R, Rimoldi O, Camici PG, et al. Effects of sex on coronary microvascular dysfunction and cardiac outcomes. Circulation. 2014;129(24):2518–27.
22. Ong P, Athanasiadis A, Borgulya G, Mahrholdt H, Kaski JC, Sechtem U. High prevalence of a pathological response to acetylcholine testing in patients with stable angina pectoris and unobstructed coronary arteries. The ACOVA study (abnormal COronary VAsomotion in patients with stable angina and unobstructed coronary arteries). J Am Coll Cardiol. 2012;59(7):655–62.
23. Manganaro A, Ciraci L, Andre L, Trio O, Manganaro R, Saporito F, Oreto G, Ando G. Endothelial dysfunction in patients with coronary artery disease: insights from a flow-mediated dilation study. Clin Appl Thromb Hemost. 2014;20(6):583–8.
24. Templin C, Ghadri JR, Diekmann J, Napp LC, Bataiosu DR, Jaguszewski M, Cammann VL, Sarcon A, Geyer V, Neumann CA, et al. Clinical features and outcomes of Takotsubo (stress) cardiomyopathy. N Engl J Med. 2015; 373(10):929–38.
25. Min JK, Dunning A, Lin FY, Achenbach S, Al-Mallah M, Budoff MJ, Cademartiri F, Callister TQ, Chang HJ, Cheng V, et al. Age- and sex-related differences in all-cause mortality risk based on coronary computed tomography angiography findings results from the international multicenter CONFIRM (coronary CT angiography evaluation for clinical outcomes: an international multicenter registry) of 23,854 patients without known coronary artery disease. J Am Coll Cardiol. 2011;58(8):849–60.
26. Lin FY, Shaw LJ, Dunning AM, Labounty TM, Choi JH, Weinsaft JW, Koduru S, Gomez MJ, Delago AJ, Callister TQ, et al. Mortality risk in symptomatic patients with nonobstructive coronary artery disease: a prospective 2-center study of 2,583 patients undergoing 64-detector row coronary computed tomographic angiography. J Am Coll Cardiol. 2011;58(5):510–9.
27. Wang ZJ, Zhang LL, Elmariah S, Han HY, Zhou YJ. Prevalence and prognosis of nonobstructive coronary artery disease in patients undergoing coronary angiography or coronary computed tomography angiography: a meta-analysis. Mayo Clin Proc. 2017;92(3):329–46.
28. Huang F-Y, Huang B-T, Lv W-Y, Liu W, Peng Y, Xia T-L, Wang P-J, Zuo Z-L, Liu R-S, Zhang C, et al. The prognosis of patients with nonobstructive coronary artery disease versus normal arteries determined by invasive coronary angiography or computed tomography coronary angiography: a systematic review. Medicine. 2016;95(11):e3117.

13

Prevalence and associated factors of ischemic heart disease (IHD) among patients with diabetes mellitus

Boonsub Sakboonyarat* and Ram Rangsin

Abstract

Background: Ischemic Heart Disease (IHD) is the first ranked among most common causes of death involving cardiovascular and other diseases. The information on the prevalence of IHD in Thailand is lacking especially among patients with diabetes mellitus. The objectives of this study were to determine the prevalence of IHD among patients with diabetes mellitus and to determine factors associated with IHD in a nation-wide survey.

Methods: A cross-sectional study to assess national outcomes among patients with diabetes who visited 831 public hospitals in Thailand was conducted in 2013 to evaluate status of care among patients with diabetes aged at least 18 years who received medical treatment in the target hospital for the last 12 months.

Results: A total of 25,902 patients with diabetes were included in this study. IHD was detected among 918 patients (3.54%; 95%CI 3.32–3.77). Multivariate analysis was conducted to determine which factors were most associated with IHD, and the results showed age (AORs 1.05; 95%CI 1.04–1.05), being male (AORs 1.78; 95%CI 1.53–2.07), hypertensive comorbidity (AORs 2.10; 95%CI 1.68–2.62), being in Health Region 4 (AORs 1.93; 95%CI 1.54–2.35), presenting hyperglycemic crisis (AORs 1.53; 95%CI 1.14–2.06) and insulin therapy (AORs 1.40; 95%CI 1.17–1.66) were the highest associated factors for IHD in this population.

Conclusion: Our data emphasized that IHD was a problem among patients with diabetes. Diabetic patients should be regularly assessed for IHD and their risk factors should be better controlled. Moreover, the Ministry of Public Health managers and clinicians should provide further preventative strategies to attenuate cardiovascular disease.

Keywords: Ischemic heart disease, Diabetes mellitus, Nation-wide survey, Prevalence, Associated factors

Background

Ischemic Heart Disease (IHD) is the first ranked and most common cause of death in cardiovascular and overall diseases [1]. The estimated prevalence of IHD among people aged ≥18 years in 2013 was 6.1, 6.4, 5.3 and 3.7% in Caucasian, African, Latino and Asian populations, respectively [1]. The prevalence increased with age and more prevalence was noted among males [2]. One recent study showed that the number of estimated deaths caused by IHD in Southeast Asia increased from 5.73 to 8.14 million from 1990 to 2013 [3]. Prevalence of IHD increased in patients with potential risk factors such as diabetes mellitus [4, 5]. Globally, adults with diabetes total 381 million. The estimated global prevalence of diabetes mellitus among adult populations was 8.3, 9.6, 5.7, 6.8, 8.6 and 6.4% in North American and Caribbean (NAC), African, European, Western Pacific and Thai populations [6]. Diabetes mellitus increases independent risk of IHD approximately 1.5 and 1.7 fold among males and females, respectively [7]. In 2007, a related study conducted among patients with diabetes reported that the age-standardized incidence rate (per 1000 person-years) of first coronary heart disease (CHD) events was 28.8 among males and 23.3 among females [8].

* Correspondence: Boonsub1991@pcm.ac.th
Department of Military and Community Medicine, Phramongkutklao College of Medicine, Bangkok 10400, Thailand

Epidemiological data of IHD in Asian populations has been studied in many countries. From 2007 to 2008, the prevalence of CHD in China was 0.63% [9]. In 2002, the overall prevalence of CHD in India was 8.2% [10]. However, limited information is available regarding the prevalence of IHD in the Thai general population in 1991 was 0.99% [11], especially among patients with major risk factors such as diabetes mellitus. We determined the prevalence of IHD among patients with diabetes mellitus using a nation-wide, cross-sectional survey among patients with diabetes mellitus. The secondary objective of this study was to determine factors associated with IHD.

Methods

Study designs

The data of this study were retrieved from database: An assessment in Quality of Care among Patients Diagnosed with Type2 Diabetes and Hypertension Visiting Ministry of Public Health and Bangkok Metropolitan Administration Hospital in Thailand (Thailand DM/HT) after the permission of the Medical Research Network of the Consortium of Thai Medical Schools (MedResNet).

The Thailand DM/HT evaluation survey was a nation-wide, cross-sectional study aiming to assess outcomes among patients with diabetes visiting public hospitals of the Ministry of Public Health (MoPH), Thailand and private hospitals and clinics in Bangkok was conducted from 2012 to 2013. The main objective of the Thailand DM/HT evaluation survey was to evaluate the status of care and was supported by the Thai National Health Security Office (NHSO).

Subjects

The healthcare system in Thailand can be categorized in two types comprising (1) healthcare under the MoPH and (2) private healthcare such as private clinics and hospitals. All Thais have healthcare coverage schemes such as the universal coverage scheme, social insurance scheme and government officer scheme. These healthcare schemes are supported by the NHSO. All of the hospitals under the MoPH at all levels, i.e., community (district), general (provincial) and regional nationwide and some private clinics in Bangkok were invited to participate in the study.

A stratified two-stage cluster sampling method proportional to the size was used to select national and provincial representative samples of patients with diabetes in Thailand. The stratified sample was drawn from a subset of all MoPH hospitals in Thailand. For Bangkok, the targeted institutes included all hospitals and clinics under the NHSO. The first level (province) comprised 77 strata while the second level constituted hospitals within each province. The second level was categorized in 5 strata by size, i.e., regional center hospital (> 500 beds), provincial general (middle) hospital (200–500 beds), first level one (F1) (90–120 beds), first level two (F2) hospital (60 beds) and first level three (F3) hospital (10–30 beds). All university medical centers were excluded from this study.

Inclusion criteria for this study comprised patients with diabetes aged at least 18 years receiving hospital medical treatment in hospital, drawn using the specified sampling method, during the previous 12 months. Any patient who had participated in a clinical trial was excluded. Those patients may have received trial medication or placebo, influencing the outcome of the study.

Data collection

A total of 833 hospitals under the MoPH were categorized as 33 regional hospitals, 83 general hospitals and 717 first level or community hospitals including the first level one (F1) 73 hospitals, the first level two (F2) 126 hospitals and the first level three (F3) 518 hospitals. All regional and general hospitals were selected, as well as 10% of F1 hospitals, 20% of F3 hospitals and 70% of F3 hospitals. This faction was based on the proportion of patient care provided at the various levels of hospitals. Patients with a diagnosis of diabetes mellitus were randomized and registered at each hospital. A standardized case report form was used to obtain the required information from medical records and was sent to the Thailand DM/HT study of the Medical Research Network of the Consortium of Thai Medical Schools (MedResNet) central data management unit in Nonthaburi. Data were retrieved from patient's medical records, status of diabetes complications and results of laboratory tests.

Measurements

Data collected included demographics, weight, height, body mass index (BMI), waist circumference, smoking behavior, systolic blood pressure (SBP), diastolic blood pressure (DBP), cardiovascular complications such as left ventricular hypertrophy (LVH), diabetic complications such as diabetic retinopathy (DR) and diabetic nephropathy (DN), blood chemistry data including fasting plasma glucose (FPG), hemoglobin A1c (HbA1c), hematocrit (Hct), hemoglobin (Hb), serum creatinine (Cr), uric acid, lipid profile including total cholesterol (TC), triglyceride (TG), high density lipoprotein cholesterol (HDL) and low density lipoprotein cholesterol (LDL), available electrocardiogram (ECG) data and results, history of anti-hyperglycemic and antiplatelet drug use and glomerular filtration rate (GFR) calculated using the epidemiology collaboration formula (EPI). Our study enrolled those patients with diabetes who were diagnosed and received ongoing medical care in a hospital. Hospitals in Thailand normally use the standard diagnosis and treatment following Thai clinical practice guidelines for diabetes and diagnosis and classification of diabetes mellitus using Diabetes Care, 2010. Diabetes mellitus was defined as FPG ≥126 mg/dl and confirmed by repeat testing at a second visit. Fasting is defined as no caloric intake for at least 8 h [12]. IHD was defined as myocardial infraction or history of coronary revascularization. Diagnosis of myocardial infraction was performed using standard criteria including stable angina and acute coronary syndrome, categorized as ST-T segment elevation myocardial infraction, nonST-T segment elevation myocardial infraction and unstable angina.

Statistical analysis

Data were coded and entered in the STATA/MP for Windows, Version 12 (Stata Corp LP, TX). Categorical data were presented as number and percentage. Continuous data were presented as mean and standard deviation (SD). Prevalence was analyzed using descriptive statistics and reported as percentage and 95% confident interval. The chi-square test was used to compare categorical data. Continuous data was compared using the *t*-test. Continuous data were grouped to analyze associated factor using odds ratio (OR). The magnitude of associations was presented as crude ORs with 95% confidence interval. The multivariate analysis was performed using logistic regression analysis and Forward Stepwise (LR) to adjust confounders. Stepwise *p*-value for entry was 0.05, and *p*-value for removal was set at 0.10. The Hosmer-Lemeshow goodness-of-fit of the logistic regression models was performed with *p*-value = 0.494. The complete case analysis and imputation method were used for any missing data. Missing values were imputed based on the means of the complete case. A *p*-value less than 0.05 was considered statistically significant.

Results

Demographic data

A total of 25,902 patients with diabetes mellitus were enrolled in this study from 2012 to 2013. Average age was 60.6 ± 10.5 years, 8076 (32.2%) were male and 17,836 (68.8%) were female. The average diabetes duration of patients was 7.1 ± 4.7 years while the average HbA1c level was 8.0 ± 2.2%. Baseline characteristics of this study are shown in Table 1. One third of participants lived in northeastern Thailand. In all, 62.5% subjects visited community or first level (F1, F2 and F3) hospitals. In this study, patients with hypertension totaled 29.1%. Prevalence of IHD among patients with diabetes was 3.54% (95%CI 3.32–3.77), increased with older age and was more common among males. Fig. 1 shows a bar graph representing IHD prevalence for every 10 years of age separated in male, female and overall.

Associated factors of IHD among patients with diabetes

Additional file 1 shows univariate analysis results regarding factors associated with IHD. Significant associated factors included older age, being male, health region, hospital level, insurance scheme, religion, occupation, GFR, HT comorbidity, HT duration, LVH, LAE, AF, DM duration, DN, DR and insulin, sulfonylurea, thiazolidinedione and aspirin therapy. Because a number of patients had missing values for HbA1c, this may have decreased the statistical power of the complete cases analysis. As a result, we applied imputation to handle the missing value and the results of multivariate analysis after imputation showed similarity to the original independent associations with IHD. Multivariate analysis showed the risk factors of IHD included age, being male, being in Health Region 4, hypertensive comorbidity and insulin therapy (Table 2).

Discussion

Our present nation-wide survey showed the prevalence of IHD among Thai patients with diabetes mellitus was 3.54%. IHD was significantly associated with being male, age, being in Health Region 4, hypertensive comorbidity, presenting hyperglycemic crisis and insulin therapy. To our knowledge, this is the first report on the prevalence and risk factors of IHD among Thai patients with diabetes. The prevalence of IHD was 0.99% among the general population in Thailand reported in 1991 [11]. A related study in Sweden found a much higher prevalence of IHD (21.97%) among patients with diabetes including those aged from 45 to 74 years [13]. In contrast, our study enrolled all patients with diabetes aged from 35 to 97 years. However, when the same age groups as the Swedish study were analyzed, the prevalence of IHD was 2.75%. In the general population, the prevalence of IHD in Caucasian populations is normally higher than that among Asians [1, 7] and diabetes amplifies this morbidity. The present study enrolled patients with diabetes who received medical treatment in MoPH hospitals all over Thailand and public and private clinics in Bangkok under the NHSO. However, these populations did not include patients with diabetes who received medical treatment in health promoting hospitals (HPHs). These HPHs, primary care units of a community hospital, usually provide health care and medication for uncomplicated diabetes cases. The prevalence of IHD in this study may have been overestimated because the diabetic cases in HPHs were not included.

After adjusting for confounding factors by multivariate analysis, only older age, being male, being in Health Region 4, hypertensive comorbidity, presenting hyperglycemic crisis and insulin therapy remained significantly associated with IHD among patients with diabetes. Prevalence of IHD tended to be higher with older age similar to related studies in Sweden [13] and Finland

Table 1 Baseline characteristics of patients (total number of subjects =25,902)

Baseline Variables	*n*	Mean ± SD or number (%)
Gender	25,902	
Female		17,836 (68.8)
Male		8076 (32.2)
Age	25,902	60.6 ± 10.5
Hospital level	25,902	
Regional center		3096 (12)
General provincial		4911 (19)
Community		16,187 (62.5)
Bangkok metropolitan administration		1708 (6.5)
Diabetic duration	25,902	7.1 ± 4.7
Waist circumference	17,488	88.5 ± 10.4
Body mass index (kg/m^2)	24,643	25.5 ± 4.4
Fasting plasma glucose	23,048	154.7 ± 58.4
HbA1c level	20,481	8 ± 2.2
GFR_EPI	15,986	67.2 ± 31
LDL	15,544	108.6 ± 36.8
HDL	14,126	46.9 ± 13.8
Triglyceride	15,548	175.4 ± 110.9
Total cholesterol	14,775	187.7 ± 44.5
Uric acid	4553	6.1 ± 1.8
Smoking	23,806	
Never		21,249 (89.2)
Current Smoker		1036 (4.4)
Ex-smoker		1521 (6.4)
Hypertensive comorbidity	25,902	
No		7527 (29.1)
Yes		18,375 (70.9)

SD standard deviation, *HbA1c* hemoglobinA1c, *GFR_EPI* glomerular infiltration rate calculated by epidemiology collaboration formula, *LDL* low density lipoprotein cholesterol, *HDL* high density lipoprotein cholesterol

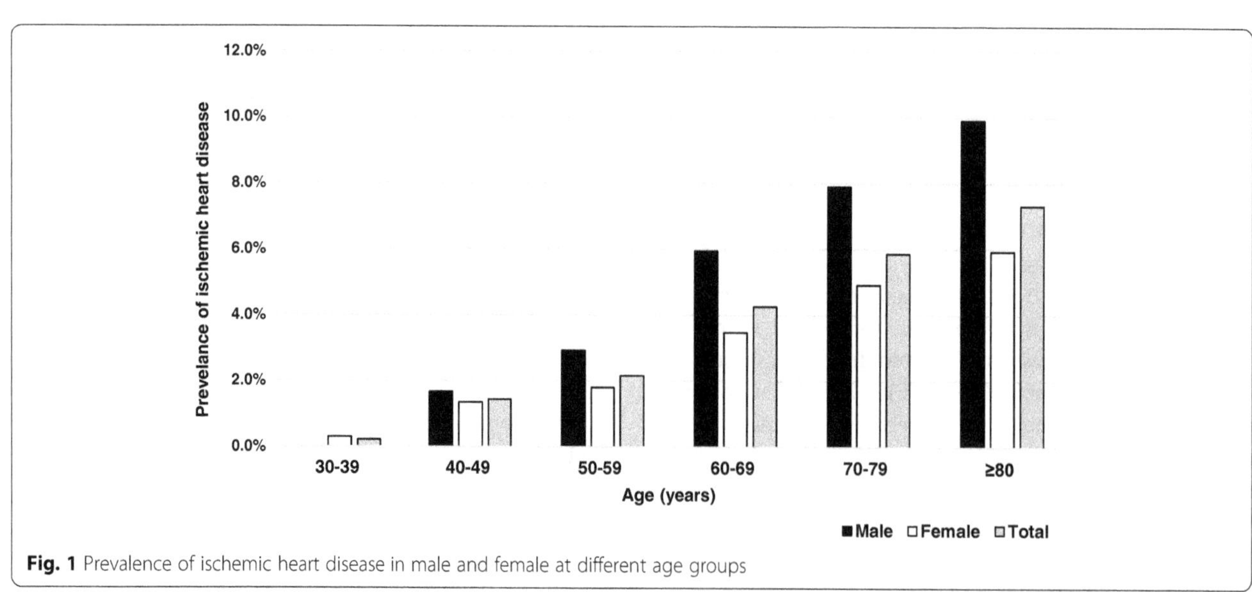

Fig. 1 Prevalence of ischemic heart disease in male and female at different age groups

Table 2 Multivariate logistic regression for factors associated with ischemic heart disease in diabetic patients. (N = 25,902)

Factors	IHD n (%)	No-IHD n (%)	AORs	95% CI
Age (years)	65.9 ± 9.5	60.4 ± 10.5	1.05[b]	(1.04–1.05)
Gender				
Female	523 (3)	17,303 (97)	1	
Male	395 (4.9)	7681 (95.1)	1.78[b]	(1.53–2.07)
Health regions				
Other health regions	774 (3.3)	22,877 (96.7)	1	
The 4th health region	144 (6.4)	2107 (93.6)	1.93[b]	(1.54–2.35)
Hypertensive Comorbidity				
No	129 (1.8)	7398 (98.2)	1	
Yes	789 (4.3)	17,586 (95.7)	2.10[b]	(1.68–2.62)
Hyperglycemic crisis				
No	846 (3.4)	23,680 (96.6)	1	
Yes	72 (5.2)	1304 (94.8)	1.53[a]	(1.14–2.06)
Insulin therapy				
No	659 (3.3)	19,685 (96.7)	1	
Yes	259 (4.7)	5299 (95.3)	1.40[b]	(1.17–1.66)

[a]$p < 0.01$, [b]$p < 0.001$
AORs Adjusted odds ratio for age, gender, health regions, hypertensive comorbidity, duration of diabetes mellitus, hyperglycemic crisis, insulin therapy and HbA1c level, *IHD* Ischemic heart disease, *CI* confidence interval

[14]. Among the elderly, changes occurring in endothelial function include loss of arterial elasticity and reduced arterial compliance, so more vascular aging and degenerative processes lead to atherosclerosis disease [15]. In addition, the endothelium experiences changed arterial function by decreased nitric oxide and increased endothelin causing a pro-coagulant state and promoting vascular smooth muscle growth and exaggerated increased risk of cardiovascular events [16]. Another reason is the elderly often have a low frequency of physical activity. A recent study showed that adults, who were physically active at least twice weekly, had decreased risk of CHD [17, 18].

The result of our study was similar to studies in the US and in western and Asian populations [2, 9, 19–21]. Most studies have found that IHD was more common among males than females [9, 11, 14, 19, 20, 22]. IHD being common among males was probably related to hormonal effects. In the premenopausal period, females' sex-hormones such as estrogen promote increased HDL and decreased LDL causing a cardio-protective effect [23, 24]. However, a related study in Pakistan showed that central adiposity is significantly higher among females compared with males regarding patients with type 2 diabetes mellitus [25]. Consequently, adiposity is positively related to IHD especially among females [26]. Patients presenting more adiposity may lead to IHD by adipocytokines by the inflammatory pathway causing vascular pathology and establishing atherothrombosis [27]. In addition, differing lifestyle or behavioral patterns between male and female indicate males present higher behavioral risks, e.g., from smoking, that predispose cardiovascular events [28].

However, several related studies have shown that higher BMI leads to risk for IHD [29–31]. The results of statistical analysis in this study found that a higher BMI exhibited a trend of dose response effect to IHD, but without significance. One result from the homogeneity in these diabetes populations is being categorized as overweight to obesity. In addition, patients, who have undergone a long duration with diabetes, may lead to presenting higher BMI. These diabetic populations are at greater risk for IHD; however, the duration of diabetes was not significant in the final model of this study.

The present study found that patients with diabetes, who present hypertensive comorbidity, are at increased risk for IHD. Hypertension is related to IHD and can be described by pathophysiology. The neuro-mediators of hypertension including angiotensin II can promote plasminogen activator inhibitor (PAI-1) expression and increased PAI-1 levels inhibiting the function of tissue plasminogen activator (tPA) resulting in increased myocardial infraction. In addition, the hypertensive stage adds extra pressure that can damage the arterial wall making it more vulnerable and building up plaque associated with atherosclerosis [32]. This study showed that hyperglycemic crisis was related to a high prevalence of IHD with an adjusted ORs of 1.53 (95% CI, 1.14–2.06). Acute hyperglycemia can attenuate endothelial function and reduce nitric oxide (NO) bioavailability [33, 34]. These actions promote monocyte and vascular smooth muscle cell migration into the intima and form macrophage foam cells, characterizing the initial morphological changes of atherosclerosis [35]. The study showed that insulin therapy was related to a high prevalence of IHD with an adjusted ORs of 1.40 (95% CI, 1.17–1.66). Insulin is more likely to be used among patients with more severe diabetes mellitus of longer duration and more complications such as chronic kidney disease. Therefore, these patients with insulin therapy have an increased number of cardiovascular events.

We have an explanation why IHD related to Health Region 4 in our study. The study showed this region had the highest prevalence of IHD at 6.4%. Health Region 4 is in central Thailand, a peripheral area near the Bangkok Metropolitan Area, where sufficient public health services are much more available. As a result, more patients can access services creating a higher load of reported cases. In addition, the area, which features several agriculture businesses, has more than enough dietary products combined with inappropriate patient dietary behaviors might have promoted a higher risk of cardiovascular disease. Consequently, the patients with diabetes in this area exhibited higher BMIs on average than others area, resulting in a higher risk for IHD [29, 30]. In addition, the patients with diabetic in Health Region 4 had higher age levels than the patients with diabetes in other areas. Although we adjusted age in the final model, the residual effect of age remained.

The study employed a cross-sectional design, and as such, the results could show only factors associated with IHD. The data presented in this study were obtained in the 2012–2013 Thailand DM/HT study of the NHSO from the Medical Research Network of the Consortium of Thai Medical Schools (MedResNet) central data management system. We were aware of missing data from this observational study. Even though this represented a relatively large sample size of the study population and some data were missing as from the nationwide observational (real life situation) study, the associations between factors and outcomes were able to be presented. In the study, we relied on evidence from medical records to identify ischemic heart disease; therefore, a small proportion of individuals with undiagnosed ischemic heart disease may have been misclassified non-differentially. The effect of misclassification decreases the observed effect size (odds ratio) of the associations (toward null). However, the officers who enter data in each hospital received proper training and verified reviewed medical records. The strength of this study was its nation-wide scope for IHD in a diabetic population. Thus, the finding of the study can be generalized and applied in others diabetic population.

Conclusion

The prevalence of IHD in a diabetic population in this study was 3.54%, higher than the prevalence of IHD in the general population in most related reports. Factors associated with IHD included age, being male, hypertensive comorbidity, being in Health Region 4, presenting hyperglycemic crisis and insulin therapy. Our data emphasized that IHD was a problem among patients with diabetes. Diabetic patients should be regularly assessed for IHD and their risk factors should be better controlled. Moreover, the Ministry of Public Health managers and clinicians should provide further preventative strategies to attenuate cardiovascular disease.

Abbreviations

BMI: body mass index; CI: confident interval; DBP: diastolic blood pressure; FPG: fasting plasma glucose; GFR_EPI: glomerular infiltration rate calculated by epidemiology collaboration formula; Hb: hemoglobin,; HbA1c: hemoglobin A1c; Hct: hematocrit; HDL: high density lipoprotein cholesterol; HT: hypertension; IHD: ischemic heart disease; LDL: low density lipoprotein cholesterol; LVH: left ventricular hypertrophy; MoPH: Ministry of Public Health; NHSO: National Health Security Office ; SBP: systolic blood pressure; SD: standard deviation; TC: total cholesterol; TG: triglyceride

Acknowledgements

The authors wish to thank the entire staff members of the Department of Military and Community Medicine, Phramongkutklao College of Medicine, for their support in completing this study. The authors thank Professor Colonel Mathirut Mungthin for support and for proofreading this manuscript.

Funding

No funding was received.

Authors' contributions

B.S. and R.R. participated in conception, design and statistical analysis; B.S. drafted the manuscripts. Both authors read and approved the final manuscripts.

Competing interests

The authors declare that they have no competing interests.

References

1. Abubakar I, Tillmann T, Banerjee A. Global, regional, and national age-sex specific all-cause and cause-specific mortality for 240 causes of death, 1990–2013: a systematic analysis for the Global Burden of Disease Study 2013. Lancet (London, England). 2015;385(9963):117–71.
2. Mozaffarian D, Benjamin EJ, Go AS, Arnett DK, Blaha MJ, Cushman M, et al. Heart disease and stroke statistics--2015 update: a report from the American Heart Association. Circulation. 2015;131(4):e29–322.
3. Roth GA, Forouzanfar MH, Moran AE, Barber R, Nguyen G, Feigin VL, et al. Demographic and epidemiologic drivers of global cardiovascular mortality. N Engl J Med. 2015;372(14):1333–41.
4. Diabetes mellitus: a major risk factor for cardiovascular disease. A joint editorial statement by the American Diabetes Association; The National Heart, Lung, and Blood Institute; Th e Juvenile Diabetes Foundation International; The National Institute of Diabetes and Digestive and Kidney Diseases; and The American Heart Association. Circulation 1999;100(10): 1132–1133.
5. Grundy SM, Benjamin IJ, Burke GL, Chait A, Eckel RH, Howard BV, et al. Diabetes and cardiovascular disease: a statement for healthcare professionals from the American Heart Association. Circulation. 1999; 100(10):1134–46.
6. Aguiree F, Brown A, Cho NH, Dahlquist G, Dodd S, Dunning T, et al. IDF diabetes atlas. 2013.
7. Wilson PW, D'Agostino RB, Levy D, Belanger AM, Silbershatz H, Kannel WB. Prediction of coronary heart disease using risk factor categories. Circulation. 1998;97(18):1837–47.
8. Avogaro A, Giorda C, Maggini M, Mannucci E, Raschetti R, Lombardo F, et al. Incidence of coronary heart disease in type 2 diabetic men and women: impact of microvascular complications, treatment, and geographic location. Diabetes Care. 2007;30(5):1241–7.
9. Yang ZJ, Liu J, Ge JP, Chen L, Zhao ZG, Yang WY. Prevalence of cardiovascular disease risk factor in the Chinese population: the 2007-2008 China National Diabetes and metabolic disorders study. Eur Heart J. 2012; 33(2):213–20.
10. Krishnan MN. Coronary heart disease and risk factors in India - on the brink of an epidemic? Indian Heart J. 2012;64(4):364–7.
11. Tatsanavivat P, Klungboonkrong V, Chirawatkul A, Bhuripanyo K, Manmontri A, Chitanondh H, et al. Prevalence of coronary heart disease and major cardiovascular risk factors in Thailand. Int J Epidemiol. 1998;27(3):405–9.
12. Diagnosis and classification of diabetes mellitus. Diabetes Care 2010;33 Suppl 1:S62–S69.
13. Wiréhn A-BE, Östgren CJ, Carstensen JM. Age and gender differences in the impact of diabetes on the prevalence of ischemic heart disease: a population-based register study. Diabetes Res Clin Pract. 2008;79(3):497–502.
14. Jousilahti P, Vartiainen E, Tuomilehto J, Puska P. Sex, age, cardiovascular risk factors, and coronary heart disease: a prospective follow-up study of 14 786 middle-aged men and women in Finland. Circulation. 1999;99(9):1165–72.
15. Jani B, Rajkumar C. Ageing and vascular ageing. Postgrad Med J. 2006; 82(968):357–62.
16. GE M, Allen PB, Morgan DR, Hanratty CG, Silke B. Nitric oxide modulation of blood vessel tone identified by arterial waveform analysis. Clin Sci. 2001; 100(4):387–93.
17. Sundquist K, Qvist J, Johansson S-E, Sundquist J. The long-term effect of physical activity on incidence of coronary heart disease: a 12-year follow-up study. Prev Med. 2005;41(1):219–25.
18. Oguma Y, Shinoda-Tagawa T. Physical activity decreases cardiovascular disease risk in women: review and meta-analysis. Am J Prev Med. 2004;26(5):407–18.
19. Ohira T, Iso H. Cardiovascular disease epidemiology in Asia: an overview. Circ J. 2013;77(7):1646–52.
20. Bhatnagar P, Wickramasinghe K, Williams J, Rayner M, Townsend N. The epidemiology of cardiovascular disease in the UK 2014. Heart. 2015; 101(15):1182–9.
21. Sanchis-Gomar F, Perez-Quilis C, Leischik R, Lucia A. Epidemiology of coronary heart disease and acute coronary syndrome. Ann Transl Med. 2016;4(13):256.
22. Ueshima H, Sekikawa A, Miura K, Turin TC, Takashima N, Kita Y, et al. Cardiovascular disease and risk factors in Asia: a selected review. Circulation. 2008;118(25):2702–9.
23. Shahar E, Folsom AR, Salomaa VV, Stinson VL, McGovern PG, Shimakawa T, et al. Relation of hormone-replacement therapy to measures of plasma fibrinolytic activity. Atherosclerosis risk in communities (ARIC) study investigators. Circulation. 1996;93(11):1970–5.
24. Grady D, Rubin SM, Petitti DB, Fox CS, Black D, Ettinger B, et al. Hormone therapy to prevent disease and prolong life in postmenopausal women. Ann Intern Med. 1992;117(12):1016–37.
25. Akhter O, Fiazuddin F, Shaheryar A, Niaz W, Siddiqui D, Awan S, et al. Central adiposity is significantly higher in female compared to male in Pakistani type 2 diabetes mellitus patients. Indian J Endocrinol Metab. 2015;19(1):72.
26. Canoy D. Distribution of body fat and risk of coronary heart disease in men and women. Curr Opin Cardiol. 2008;23(6):591–8.
27. Golia E, Limongelli G, Natale F, Fimiani F, Maddaloni V, Russo PE, et al. Adipose tissue and vascular inflammation in coronary artery disease. World J Cardiol. 2014;6(7):539.
28. Mons U, Muezzinler A, Gellert C, Schottker B, Abnet CC, Bobak M, et al. Impact of smoking and smoking cessation on cardiovascular events and mortality among older adults: meta-analysis of individual participant data from prospective cohort studies of the CHANCES consortium. BMJ (Clinical research ed). 2015;350:h1551.
29. Flint AJ, Rexrode KM, Hu FB, Glynn RJ, Caspard H, Manson JE, et al. Body mass index, waist circumference, and risk of coronary heart disease: a prospective study among men and women. Obesity Res Clinical Practice. 2010;4(3):e171–e81.
30. Collaboration APCS. Body mass index and cardiovascular disease in the Asia-Pacific region: an overview of 33 cohorts involving 310 000 participants. Int J Epidemiol. 2004;33(4):751–8.
31. Joshy G, Korda R, Attia J, Liu B, Bauman A, Banks E. Body mass index and incident hospitalisation for cardiovascular disease in 158 546 participants from the 45 and up study. Int J Obes. 2014;38(6):848.
32. Libby P, Theroux P. Pathophysiology of coronary artery disease. Circulation. 2005;111(25):3481–8.
33. Williams SB, Goldfine AB, Timimi FK, Ting HH, Roddy MA, Simonson DC, et al. Acute hyperglycemia attenuates endothelium-dependent vasodilation in humans in vivo. Circulation. 1998;97(17):1695–701.
34. Low Wang CC, Hess CN, Hiatt WR, Clinical Update GAB. Cardiovascular disease in diabetes mellitus: atherosclerotic cardiovascular disease and heart failure in type 2 diabetes mellitus - mechanisms, management, and Clinical Considerations. Circulation. 2016;133(24):2459–502.
35. Perkins JM, Joy NG, Tate DB, Davis SN. Acute effects of hyperinsulinemia and hyperglycemia on vascular inflammatory biomarkers and endothelial function in overweight and obese humans. Am J Physiol Endocrinol Metab. 2015;309(2):E168–76.

14

Admission homocysteine is an independent predictor of spontaneous reperfusion and early infarct-related artery patency before primary percutaneous coronary intervention in ST-segment elevation myocardial infarction

Jing Li[1*], Ying Zhou[1], Yaowen Zhang[2] and Jingang Zheng[1]

Abstract

Background: Spontaneous reperfusion (SR) and early infarct related artery (IRA) patency before primary percutaneous coronary intervention (PPCI) might bring extra benefit for patients with ST-segment elevation myocardial infarction (STEMI). This study premilinarily screened the independent predictors of SR, and assessed the relationship between SR and plasma homocysteine (HCY).

Methods: The medical records of 998 patients who were diagnosed as STEMI and underwent emergency coronary angiography were retrospectively studied, SR was defined as achievement of TIMI grade 3 flow in the IRA before PCI. The baseline characteristics, clinical manifestations and hematological variables were compared between SR and NSR group. Optimal cutoff point of HCY was calculated with receiving operating characteristics (ROC) analysis, multivariate logistic regression models were used to identify predictors of SR.

Results: 229 (22.95%) patients showed angiographic SR. For HCY, the area under the curve was 0.70 (95% CI: 0.63–0.77, $P = 0.034$), the optimized cut off point was 17.55 μmol/L. Preinfarct angina (95% CI: 1.61–5.65, $P = 0.0005$), plasma C-reactive protein (CRP) level (95% CI: 0.87–0.99, $P = 0.016$) and HCY < 17.55 μmol/L (95% CI: 2.43–8.72, $P < 0.0001$) were found to be independent predictors for SR.

Conclusion: In patients with STEMI, HCY < 17.55 μmol/L, preinfarct angina and plasma CRP level were independent predictors of SR.

Keywords: ST-segment elevation myocardial infarction, Spontaneous reperfusion, Pre-interventional IRA patency, Predictor, Homocysteine

* Correspondence: nami2003@163.com
[1]Department of Cardiology, China-Japan Friendship Hospital, No. 2, Yinghua Road, Beijing 100029, China
Full list of author information is available at the end of the article

Background

Early infarct related artery (IRA) patency and prompt myocardial reperfusion are crucial for improving clinical outcomes in patients with ST-segment elevation myocardial infarction (STEMI) [1], primary percutaneous coronary intervention (PPCI) is the current therapy of choice to achieve IRA patency. Furthermore, outcomes of patients with STEMI undergoing PPCI are closely related to the initial IRA blood flow prior to PPCI [2–4]. In an analysis from the Primary Angioplasty in Myocardial Infarction (PAMI) trials [5], initial thrombolysis in myocardial infarction (TIMI) grade 3 flow derived from spontaneous reperfusion (SR) was associated with improved left ventricular function, decreased adverse cardiovascular events and reduced short and long-term mortality independent of successful PPCI, implying that SR might bring extra benefit of myocardial salvage for STEMI patients before PPCI. Thus the concept of IRA patency was extended to the pre-PPCI phase, to predict and facilitate SR might provide alternative methods for acute risk assessment and tailoring of adjunctive therapies during coronay intervention, predictors of SR might thus provide important prognostic information. However, little has been known about the predictors or clinical biomarkers SR.

Since thrombus formation is the main mechanism of the obstruction of IRA in STEMI [6], and timely spontaneous thrombolysis lead to spontaneous reperfusion [7], factors influencing spontaneous thrombolysis might be able to predict the process of SR.

Homocysteine (HCY) is a sulfur-containing amino acid that functions as a key intermediate in methionine metabolism [8], which is believed to promote atherothrombosis through several mechanism [9], and hyperhomocystenemia (HHCY) (plasma HCY > 10 mmol/L) is currently recognized as a new independent risk factor for atherosclerotic vascualr disease. Furthermore, HHCY is related to impaired formation of the fibrin networkby inducing slower coagulation process and rendering more tightly packed fibrin clots, hence influencing the process of spontaneous thrombolysis [10]. Therefore, we speculated that HCY might be a predictor of early SR in STEMI patients.

In the present study, we aimed to premilinarily screen the clinical predictors of SR and assess the possible relationship between SR and plasma HCY.

Methods

Patient population

This retrospective, single center observational study was based on review of medical records, electrocardiographic analysis and cardiac catheterization films of 998 consecutive patients presenting from January 1,2012 through January 1,2015 to China-JapanFriendshipHospital (Beijing, China) with suspected acute STEMI, who underwent emergency coronary angiography on admission within 12 h of symptom onset and activation of the emergency PCI protocol. Exclusion criteria were: coronary spasm proved to be responsible for STEMI with angiographic SR; left bundle branch block; thrombolytic therapy before arrival to our hospital; and final diagnosis other than STEMI, such as non-ST-segment elevation myocardial infarction (NSTEMI), unstable angina, takotsubo cardiomyopathy and myocarditis.

Diagnosis of STEMI was based on the presence of symptoms of ischemia, increased serum biomarkers (cardiac-specific troponin) and ST-segment elevation≥1 mm in ≥2 contiguous leads [11]. Angiographic SR was defined as achievement of TIMI grade 3 flow in the IRA before PCI (first contrast injection) [6].

Laboratory analysis

In all patients, venous peripheral blood samples were taken on admission for measurement of hematological variables. Samples were obtained in the emergency room or coronary care unit (CCU) before medication, and processed within 30 min from collection, the first dataset was used for analysis if more than one assessment was performed. Blood counts were measured by the BECKMAN COULTER LH780 Hematology analyzer system (USA). Plasma creatinine, uric acid, HCY and C-reactive protein were measured by BECKMAN COULTER Chemistry Analyzer AU5800 (USA). Prothrombin Time and Activated partial thromboplastin time were measured by a STAGO Compact (France). Troponin-I was measured by a BECKMAN Image 800 Analyzer (USA).

In all patients, the left ventricular ejection fraction (LVEF) was measured within 24 h since admitted in emergency room by tracing contours of the LV using the manual biplane Simpson's rule [12](Vivid E9, GE Ultrasound A5, Horten, Norway).

Medication during hospital stay

All patients received a loading dose of 300 mg aspirin and 300-600 mg clopidogrel, and a single subcutaneous bolus of low molecular weight heparin (LMWH) in transit or at the emergency room. 3000 U intravenous heparin was routinely administered in the catheterization room before angiography. An additional dose of (6000 U) and glycoprotein IIb/IIIa antagonist would be adopted if PPCI was necessary. All patients were managed with standard administration of 100 mg aspirin, 75 mg clopidogrel, ß-blockers, ACEI/ARB and statins according to the guidelines for STEMI.

Coronary angiography

All patients received emergency angiography within 12 h of symptom onset using standard techniques. IRA patency referred to those with TIMI grade 3 flow.

Spontaneous reperfusion referred to angiographic SR described in "patient population" section. Time to angiography was defined as the time from onset of ischemic symptoms to the first contrast injection. According to the European Society of Cardiology (ESC) guidelines (2012), primary PCI is defined as PCI in patients with STEMI within 12 h of the onset of chest pain [13].

Statistical analysis

Statistical analyses were performed using SPSS 22.0 software (SPSS Inc., Chicago, USA). Continuous variables were presented as mean ± standard deviation (SD) for normally distributed data, or as median (interquartile range, IQR) for non-normally distributed data, and compared with the Student's T test. Non-parametrics tests were used for non-normally distributed data. Categorical variables were expressed as percentages (%) and compared using the chi-square test.

Optimal cutoff point of HCY was calculated with receiving operating characteristics (ROC) analysis. All P values referred to 2-tailed tests of significance, and $P < 0.05$ was considered significant. HCY was transferred into binary variable according to the cutoff point.

All variables showing significant differences in the univariate comparison were included in the multiple logistic regression analysisto identify predictors of SR. The candidate variables entering multiple logistic regression analysis were: preinfarct angina, previous long-term aspirin medication, uric acid level, CRP level, NLR, PLR and the binary variable of HCY above or below cutoff point. The results were expressed by the odds ratio (OR) and corresponding 95% confidence interval (CI).

Results

Baseline characteristics

Among the 998 STEMI patients enrolled, 229 (22.95%) showed angiographic SR, 156 (68%) of the 229 patients showed ST-segment resolution ≥70% (electrocardiographic SR) before angiography. Distributions of baseline, clinical manifestations and revascularization procedures between patients with SR (SR group) and without SR (NSR group) are shown in Table 1. Multivariate logistic regression models adjusted by age, gender, cardiovascular risk factors, antiplatelet therapy, time to angiography and hematological variables were used to identify predictors of SR.There were no significantly differences in terms of age, gender, family history of myocardial infarction (MI), major cardiovascular risk factors such as current smoker, hypertension, diabetes mellitus, dyslipidemia and chronic renal failure, history of MI, or long-term (>one year) medication of statin between groups. Frequencies of previous long-term aspirin medication and preinfarct angina were higher in the SR group than in the NSR group ($P < 0.05$, respectively). During hospitalization, there were no differences in medication of aspirin, clopidogrel, heparin or GP IIb/IIIa antagonists between the groups. Hematological variables on admission

Table 1 Baseline characteristics of study patients

	SR ($n = 229$)	NSR ($n = 769$)	P Value
Clinical characteristics			
Age(years)	62.13 ± 11.27	61.79 ± 12.86	0.877
Male sex, n (%)	186 (81.22)	636 (82.70)	0.605
Current smokers, n (%)	132 (57.81)	454 (59.11)	0.706
[a]Family history, n (%)	32 (13.97)	89 (11.57)	0.329
Hypertension, n (%)	113 (49.34)	424 (55.14)	0.122
Diabetes, n (%)	46 (20.31)	185 (24.14)	0.211
Stroke, n (%)	25 (10.92)	93 (12.09)	0.628
Dyslipidemia, n (%)	128 (55.89)	414 (53.84)	0.583
Chronic renal failure, n (%)	10 (4.37)	29 (3.77)	0.683
[b]Previous revascularization, n (%)	11 (4.80)	67 (8.71)	0.053
Previous long-term statin, n (%)	36 (15.72)	91 (11.83)	0.121
Previous long-term aspirin, n (%)	57 (24.89)	143 (18.59)	0.037
Preinfarct angina within 1 month, n (%)	143 (62.45)	293 (38.10)	0.001
Time to angiography, hours	5.1[2.7, 7.8]	4.3[2.6, 7.2]	0.212
Clinical manifestations			
SBP, mmHg	124.25 ± 23.07	117.41 ± 21.56	0.018
DBP, mmHg	76.51 ± 12.59	75.44 ± 12.12	0.067
Hear rate, beats/min	67.41 ± 11.1	73.12 ± 14.69	0.021
LVEF, %	58 ± 11	49 ± 10	0.001
Killip2–4, n (%)	50 (21.83)	161(20.93)	0.770
Killip3–4, n (%)	21 (7.86)	87 (10.97)	0.359
IABP use, n(%)	8 (3.49)	80 (10.40)	0.001
Infarct location, n (%)			0.203
Anterior	141 (61.57)	429 (55.79)	
Inferior	78 (34.06)	312 (40.57)	
Lateral	10 (4.37)	28 (3.64)	
Medication of antithrombotic drugs during hospitalization			
Aspirin	229 (100%)	769 (100%)	N/A
Clopidogrel	229 (100%)	769 (100%)	N/A
GP-IIb/IIIa antagonists	44 (19%)	130 (17%)	0.42
Heparin	229 (100%)	769 (100%)	N/A
Revascularization procedures, n (%)			
Primary PCI	145 (63.31)	710 (92.32)	< 0.001
No revascularization	69 (30.13)	59 (7.67)	< 0.001

Data are presented as mean ± SD, IQR or number (percentage)
[a]Family history referred to the history of acute myocardial infarction of the patients' parents, brothers or sisters
[b]PCI or coronary artery bypass grafting

are shown in Table 2. Compared with the NSR group, plasma HCY, CRP, uric acid, NLR and Platelet/lymphocyte ratio (PLR) levels were significantly lower in SR group ($P < 0.05$, for all).

Receiver operating characteristic (ROC) curve analysis of HCY

The value of HCY as predictors of SR was evaluated by means of ROC analysis (Fig. 1).

For HCY, the area under the curve was 0.70 (95% CI: 0.63–0.77, $P = 0.034$). An optimized cutoff point of 17.55 μmol/L showed a sensitivity of 0.53 and specificity of 0.20 for prediction of SR. HCY < 17.55 μmol/L was more common in patients with SR.

HCY was transferred into binary variable according to the cutoff point of 17.55 μmol/L, then HCY ≥17.55 μmol/L and < 17.55 μmol/L as a binary variable, together with pre-infarct angina, CRP and NLR were tested by multiple logistic regression to decide the independent predictors of SR.

Independent predictors of SR in STEMI

Preinfarct angina (95% CI: 1.61–5.65, $P = 0.0005$), plasma C-reactive protein (CRP) level (95% CI: 0.87–0.99, $P = 0.016$) and HCY < 17.55 μmol/L (95% CI: 2.43–8.72, $P < 0.0001$) were found to be independent predictors for SR on multiple logistic regression analysis (Table 3). For these 3 predictors, ROC curve analysis showed the area under the ROC curve was 0.74, 95% CI was 0.68–0.79.

In-hospital and 1-year outcomes

The in-hospital and 1-year clinical outcomes are summarized in Table 4.

Patients with SR showed a significantly better in-hospital course with lower in-hospital mortality. Patients with SR had better preserved heart function, with lower rates of congestive heart failure, pulmonary edema and cardiac shock. Patients with SR also showed a lower rate of malignant cardiac arrhythmia, with lower rates of sustained ventricular tachycardia, primary ventricular fibrillation and asystole. The in-hospital rates of reinfarction were similar between groups.

Patients with SR showed more favorable 1-year outcomes with lower rates of heart failure and mortality. Though patients without SR had more frequently underwent PPCI on IRA, they had statistically similar 1-year rates of reinfarction and ischemia-drived target vessel revascularization compared with patients with SR.

Discussion

Our study showed a 22.95% incidence of angiographic SR in patients with STEMI, similar to the incidence of 14%~ 22% in previous studies [5, 14].

In our study, HCY < 17.55 μmol/L, together with pre-infarct angina and CRP were proved to be independent predictors of SR in STEMI patients; among the 3 predictors, HCY < 17.55 μmol/L showed the most obvious statistical significance.

To the best of our knowledge, this is the first study that investigated the relationship between HCY and pre-PPCI IRA patency in patients with STEMI. Urgent restoration of blood flow in IRA and early myocardial reperfusion is related to improved survival in patients with STEMI [15].This concept was extended to the pre-PCI phase in an analysis from the Primary Angioplasty in

Table 2 Baseline hematological variables of study patients

	SR ($n = 229$)	NSR ($n = 769$)	*P* Value
Mean platelet volume, fL	10.69 ± 1.37	10.74 ± 0.83	0.787
Red cell distribution width, fL	41.4 ± 2.26	41.76 ± 3.04	0.317
Hemocysteine, μmol/L	11.9[9.1, 16.7]	17.8[12.2, 21.8]	<.0001
Peak Troponin-I, ng/mL	8.89[0.76, 15.75]	19.91[8.63, 30.0]	<.0001
Creatinine, umol/mL	81.45[73, 92]	77 [67, 91]	0.101
C-reactive protein,mg/dL	3.48[2.2, 6.35]	5.48[3, 10.1]	0.010
Prothrombin Time, second	13.2[12.6, 13.6]	13.3[12.7, 14.1]	0.159
Activatedpartialthromboplastin time, second	37.85[35.25, 44.65]	40.15[34.8, 48]	0.457
Neutrophil count, × 10^9/L	210.34[184.50, 235.50]	216.38[182.50, 250.0]	0.210
Leukocyte count, ×10^9/L	6.31[4.22, 7.57]	7.13[5.21, 8.47]	0.030
Platelet count, ×10^9/L	2.10[1.5, 2.4]	1.90[1.28, 2.38]	0.080
Neutrophil/lymphocyte ratio	2.86[2.06, 4.18]	3.58[2.58, 5.41]	0.005
Platelet/lymphocyte ratio	108.33[82.7, 138.1]	121.2[90.59, 169.11]	0.053
Creatinine> 108 umol/L, n (%)	14(21.88)	46(22.66)	0.896
Uric acid> 420 mmol/L(male) or > 380(female), n (%)	20(31.25)	33(16.26)	0.009

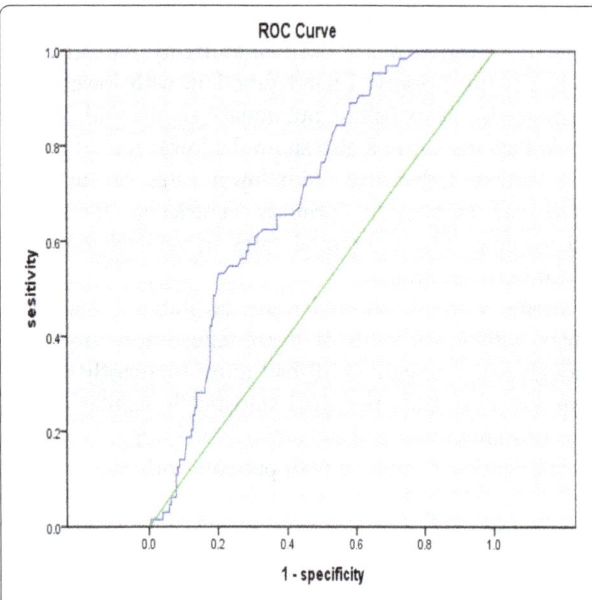

Fig. 1 ROC curve for HCY levels in patients with SR in the baseline angiography. The mean area under the ROC curve was 0.70.

Myocardial Infarction (PAMI) trials [5]. Initial TIMI grade 3 flow remained independently associated with better survival even after adjusting for post-PCI flow. Brener SJ et al. [16] analyzed the combined databases of the Controlled Abciximab and Device Investigation to Lower Late Angioplasty Complications (CADILLAC) and the Harmonizing Outcomes With Revascularization and Stents in Acute Myocardial Infarction (HORIZONS-AMI) trials, suggested that spontaneous reperfusion before PCI might reduce 1-year mortality after primary PCI in STEMI by 39%, even after adjusting for post-PCI TIMI flow. Thus SR could bring extra benefit for the patients with STEMI independent of PPCI. Recognition of non invasive predictors of pre-PPCI SR will provide new treatment information for the very early stage of STEMI, and bring prognostic information.

Because thrombotic occlusion of coronary artery upon a background of atherosclerotic plaque rupture is the ultimate step in the pathogenesis of MI [17], and the fate of an evolving thrombus is largely determined by the balance between coagulating system and fibrinolysis system [18], factors that influence thrombosis and endogenous thrombolysis might play an important role in early SR. The spontaneous lysis of platelet-rich thrombus is

Table 3 Multivariable analysis for the independent predictors of SR

	OR	95% Confidence Interval	*P* Value
Preinfarct angina	3.02	1.61–5.65	0.0005
C-reactive protein	0.92	0.87–0.99	0.016
Hemocysteine< 17.55 μmol/L	4.61	2.43–8.72	< 0.0001

OR Odds ratio

Table 4 In-hospital and 1-year clinical outcomes

Variable	SR (*n* = 229)	NSR (*n* = 769)	*P* Value
In-hospital clinical outcome			
Heart failure, n (%)	13 (5.6)	92 (11.9)	0.006
Pulmonary edema, n (%)	9 (3.9)	69 (9.0)	0.01
Cardiac shock, n (%)	3 (1.3)	39 (5.1)	0.01
Reinfarction, n (%)	6 (2.6)	31 (4.0)	0.32
Primary ventricular fibrillation, n (%)	6 (2.6)	66 (8.6)	0.002
Sustained venticular tachycardia, n (%)	2 (0.8)	34 (4.3)	0.01
High-degree atrioventricular block, n (%)	10 (4.4)	41 (5.3)	0.56
Asystole, n (%)	1 (0.4)	35 (4.6)	0.003
Major bleeding, n (%)	2 (0.9)	12 (3.1)	0.44
All-cause mortality, n (%)	1 (0.4)	21 (2.4)	0.03
1-year clinical outcome			
Reinfarction, n (%)	8 (3.5)	29 (3.8)	0.84
Ischemia-drived target vessel Revascularization, n (%)	25 (10.9)	77 (10.0)	0.69
Heart failure, n (%)	13 (5.6)	107 (13.9)	< 0.001
All-cause mortality, n (%)	2 (0.8)	31 (4.0)	0.02

an important defense mechanism against lasting coronary occlusion, MI could be regarded as a result of the failure of timely spontaneous thrombolysis/fibrinolysis; on the contrary, rapid enhanced endogenous fibrinolysis could spontaneously dissolve thrombus and lead to SR and IRA patency. As a support of the above hypothesis, Christopoulos C et al. [19] reported that patients with STEMI who demonstrated pre-PPCI SR have enhanced endogenous thrombolysis, decreased platelet reactivity and shorter occlusion time in IRA, implying that factors influencing the balance of thrombosis and endogenous thrombolysis might influence the process of SR, and these factors might become potential markers for SR in patients with STEMI. Plasma HCY level is currently a clinical marker of several atherothrombotic vascular disease, and elevated plasma HCY might have some relation with impaired endogenous thrombolysis, therefore, we speculated that HCY could also be a clinical marker of SR.

HCY is a sulfur-containing amino acid that functions as a key intermediate in methionine metabolism. It is produced as a byproduct of methyl-transfer reactions, which are important for the synthesis of DNA, methylated proteins, neurotransmitters and phospholipids [9]. High plasma level of homocysteine, termed as hyperhomocystenemia (HHCY), has been recognized as a biomarker of atherothrombotic vascular disease, overwhelming clinical and epidemiological studies have identified HHCY(> 15 mmol/L) as a new independent risk factor for athroscleroticvascualr disease [20–24].

Furthermore, HHCY is associated with a greater number of diseased arteries and higher severity of coronary diaseases [25], and might be an important predictor for long-term mortality in patients with acute myocardial infarction (MI) [26].

Angiographic findings demonstrated that HHCY was strongly correlated with slow coronary flow (SCF) phenomenon after PCI protocol [27, 28], implying the possible correlation between HHCY and less IRA patency. Current evidence suggests that the microcirculation dysfunction and damage of endothelial cells caused by HCY-induced oxidative stress played an important role in SCF [29–31]. HCY can reduce the basal production of nitric-oxide (NO) in consequence of the emergence of some biochemically active products such as hydrogen peroxide (H_2O_2), superoxide (O_2^-) and hydroxyl radical (HO) [32, 33], and enhance NO degradation by inhibiting the synthesis and activity of NO synthase (NOS), thus lead to decreased bioavailability of NO and impair the endothelium-dependant vasodilation [34]. Therefore, the HHCY-induced endothelial dysfunction might explain the worse initial IRA TIMI flow in patients with STEMI.

It has been reported that total HCY plasma levels are associated with clot permeation and susceptibility to fibrinolysis in coronary artery disease [35]. HHCY has been related to impaired formation of the fibrin network [36, 37]. HCY impairs the fibrinolysis networks by inducing slower coagulation process and rendering more tightly packed fibrin clots [10].Under the influence of HCY, fibrin networks resulted in a more compact structure with shorter, thicker and more branched fibers, these structural properties of fibrin are related to slower spontaneous lysis rate of thrombus, and proved to be less permeable and more resistant to fibrinolysis [38, 39]. Moreover, studies have revealed that mild HHCY (>10umol/L) showed markedly relationship with decreased tissue-type plasminogen activator (t-PA) activity (which is the major activator of fibrinolysis) and impaired spontaneous thrombolysis in STEMI patients [40]. Therefore, HHCY might play a negative role in the process of SR by facilitating thrombus formation towards total occlusion anddecreasing the spontaneous thrombolysis/fibrinolysis in IRA.

Limitations

This is a retrospective, non-randomized design study, we didn't observe the relationship between HCY and mortality, which may help to further evaluate the prognostic value of HCY. However, the aim of the present study was to preliminarily screening the possible non-invasive, easily available marker of SR, it's a new idea to assess the relationship of HCY and SR, and this retrospective study had obtained preliminary results which may be a guide for further investigation to evaluate the predictors of pre-PPCI IRA patency.

Conclusion

The present study showed that in patients with STEMI, preinfarct angina, CRP level, and HCY < 17.55 μmol/L were independent predictors of SR. Elevated plasma level (≥17.55 μmol/L) of HCY was an independent negative predictor of SR. HCY might thus be a useful biomarker to predict early IRA patency in patients with STEMI.

Abbreviations

CRP: C-reactive protein; HCY: Homocysteine; HHCY: Hyperhomocystenemia; IRA: Infarct-related artery; NLR: Neutrophil/lymphocyte ratio; NO: Nitric-oxide; PCI: Percutaneous coronary intervention; PPCI: Primary percutaneous coronary intervention; SCF: Slow coronary flow; SR: Spontaneous reperfusion; STEMI: ST-segment elevation myocardial infarction; TIMI: Thrombolysis in myocardial infarction

Acknowledgements

This research was supported by doctors working in the cardiology department, China-Japan Friendship Hospital in acquisition, analysis and interpretation of data.

Authors' contributions

LJ designed this research, analyzed the clinical data and wrote this manuscript. ZY collected the clinical data and followed up the patients. ZYW did the statistical work. ZJG performed coronary angiography and analyzed all the angiography data. All authors read and approved the final manuscript.

Competing interests

The authors declare that they have no competing interests.

Author details

[1]Department of Cardiology, China-Japan Friendship Hospital, No. 2, Yinghua Road, Beijing 100029, China. [2]Medieco Group Co. Ltd, B901 Building No.20 Hepingxiyuan, Beijing 100029, China.

References

1. Zeymer U, Huber K, Fu Y, et al. Impact of TIMI 3 patency before primary percutaneous coronary intervention for ST-elevation myocardial infarction on clinical outcome: results from the ASSENT-4 PCI study. Eur Heart J Acute Cardiovasc Care. 2012;1(2):136–42.
2. Lekston A, Hudzik B, Szkodzinski J, et al. Spontaneous reperfusion before intervention improves immediate but not long-term prognosis in diabetic

patients with ST-segment elevation myocardial infarction and multivessel coronary artery disease. Cardiol J. 2013;20(4):378–84.
3. Christian TF, Milavetz JJ, Miller TD, Clements IP, Holmes DR, Gibbons RJ. Prevalence of spontaneous reperfusion and associated myocardial salvage in patients with acute myocardial infarction. Am Heart J. 1998;135(3):421–7.
4. Bainey KR, Fu Y, Granger CB, et al. Investigators AA. Benefit of angiographic spontaneous reperfusion in STEMI: does it extend to diabetic patients? Heart. 2009;95(16):1331–6.
5. Stone GW, Cox D, Garcia E, et al. Normal flow (TIMI-3) before mechanical reperfusion therapy is an independent determinant of survival in acute myocardial infarction: analysis from the primary angioplasty in myocardial infarction trials. Circulation. 2001;104(6):636–41.
6. Dewood MA, Spores J, Notske R, et al. Prevalance of total coronary occlusion during the early hours of transmural myocardial infarction. N Engl J Med. 1980; 303(16):897–902.
7. Swan HJ. Acute myocardial infarction: a failure of timely, spontaneous thrombolysis. J Am Coll Cardiol. 1989;13(6):1435–7.
8. Selhub J. Homocysteine metabolism. Annu Rev Nutr. 1999;19:217–46.
9. Welch GN, Loscalzo J. Homocysteine and atherothrombosis. N Engl J Med. 1998;338(15):1042–50.
10. Genoud V, Lauricella AM, Kordich LC, et al. Impact of homocysteine-thiolactone on plasma fibrin networks. J Thromb Thrombolysis. 2014; 38(4):540–5.
11. Thygesen K, Alpert JS, Jaffe AS, Simoons ML, Chaitman BR, White HD, Writing group on the joint ESC/ACCF/AHA/WHF task force for the universal definition of myocardial infarction, et al. Third universal definition of myocardial infarction. Eur Heart J. 2012;33(20):2551–67.
12. Lang RM, Bierig M, Devereux RB, et al. Recommendations for chamber quantification. Eur J Echocardiogr. 2006;7(2):79–108.
13. Task Force on the management of ST segment elevation acute myocardial infarction of the European Society of Cardiology, Steg PG, James SK, Atar D, et al. ESC guidelines for the management of acute myocardial infarction in patients presenting with ST-segment elevation. Eur Heart J. 2012;33(20): 2569–619.
14. Fefer P, Hod H, Hammerman H, et al. Relation of clinically defined spontaneous reperfusion to outcome in ST-elevation myocardial infarction. Am J Cardiol. 2009;103(2):149–53.
15. Investigators TGUSTOA. The effects of tissue plasminogen activator, streptokinase, or both on coronary-artery patency, ventricular function, and survival after acute myocardial infarction. N Engl J Med. 1993;329(22):1615–22.
16. Brener SJ, Mehran R, Brodie BR, et al. Predictors and implications of coronary infarct artery patency at initial angiography in patients with acute myocardial infarction (from the CADILLAC and HORIZONS-AMI trials). Am J Cardiol. 2011; 108(7):918–23.
17. Naghavi M, Libby P, Falk E, et al. From vulnerable plaque to vulnerable patient:a call for new definitions and risk assessment strategies: part II. Circulation. 2003;108(15):1772–8.
18. Bodary PF, Wickenheiser KJ, Eitzman DT. Recent advances in understanding endogenous fibrinolysis: implications for molecular-based treatment of vascular disorders. Expert Rev Mol Med. 2002;4(7):1–10.
19. Christopoulos C, Farag M, Sullivan K, Wellsted D, Gorog DA. Impaired thrombolytic status predicts adverse cardiac events in patients undergoing primary percutaneous coronary intervention. ThrombHaemost. 2017;117(3): 457–70.
20. Ma Y, Li L, Geng XB, et al. Correlation between hyperhomocysteinemia and outcomes of patients with acute myocardial infarction. Am J Ther. 2016; 23(6):e1464–e1468.
21. Wu Y, Huang Y, Hu Y, et al. Hyperhomocysteinemia is an independent risk factor in young patients with coronay artery disease in southern China. Herz 2013; 38(7):779–84.
22. Rasouli ML, Nasir K, Blumenthal RS, Park R, Aziz DC, Budoff MJ. Plasma homocysteine predicts progression of atherosclerosis. Atherosclerosis. 2005;181(1):159–65.
23. Taylor LM Jr, Moneta GL, Sexton GJ, et al. Prospective blinded study of the relationship between plasma homocysteine and progression of symptomatic peripheral arterial disease. J Vasc Surg. 1999;29(1):8–19.
24. Graham IM, Daly LE, Refsum HM, et al. Plasma homocysteine as a risk factor for vascular disease. The European Concerted Action Project JAMA. 1997; 277(22):1775–81.
25. Oudi ME, Aouni Z, Mazigh C, et al. Homocysteine and markers of inflammation in acute coronary syndrome. Exp Clin Cardiol. 2010;15(2):e25–8.
26. Fu Z, Qian G, Xue H, et al. Hyperhomocysteinemia is an independent predictor of long-term clinical outcomes in Chinese octogenarians with acute coronary syndrome. Clin Interv Aging. 2015;10(9):1467–274.
27. Yurtdas M, Özcanl T, Sabri AS, et al. Plasma homocysteine is associated with ischemic findings without organic stenosis in patients with slow coronary flow. J Cardiol. 2013;61(2):138–43.
28. Tang O, Wu J, Qin F. Relationship between methylenetetrahydrofolate reductase gene polymorphism and the coronary slow flow phemonenon. Coron Artery Dis. 2014;25(8):653–7.
29. Sezgin N, Barutcu I, Sezgin AT, et al. Plasma nitric oxide level and its role in slow coronary flow phenomenon. Int Heart J. 2005;46(3):373–82.
30. Sezgin AT, Topal E, Barutcu I, et al. Impaired left ventricle filling in slow coronary flow phenomenon: an echo-doppler study. Angiology. 2005;56(4): 397–401.
31. Tanriverdi H, Evrengul H, Enli Y, et al. Effect of homocysteine-induced oxidative stress on endothelial function in coronary slow-flow. Cardiology. 2007;107(4):313–20.
32. Clarke R, Daly L, Robinson K, et al. Hyperhomocysteinemia: an independent risk factor for vascular disease. N Engl J Med. 1991;324(17):1149–55.
33. Glueck CJ, Show P, Lang JE, Tracy T, Sieve-Smith L, Wang Y. Evidence that homocysteine is an independent risk factor for atherosclerosis in hyperlipidemic patients. Am J Cardiol. 1995;75(2):132–6.
34. Celermajer DS, Sorensen K, Ryalls M, et al. Impaired endothelial function occurs in the systemic arteriesof children with homozygous homocystinuria but not in their heterozygousparents. J Am CollCardiol. 1993;22(3):854–8.
35. Undas A, Brozek J, Jankowski M, Siudak Z, Szczeklik A, Jakubowski H. Plasma homocysteine affects fibrin clot permeability and resistance to lysis in human subjects. Arterioscler Thromb Vasc Biol. 2006;26(6):1397–404.
36. Sauls DL, Wolberg AS, Hoffman M. Elevated plasma homocysteine leads to alterations in fibrin clot structure and stability: implications for the mechanism of thrombosis in hyperhomocysteinemia. J Thromb Haemost. 2003;1(2):300–6.
37. Lauricella AM, Quintana IL, Kordich LC. Effects of homocysteine thiol group on fibrin networks: another possible mechanism of harm. Thromb Res. 2002; 107(1–2):75–9.
38. Quintana IL, Oberholzer MV, Kordich L, Lauricella AM. Impaired fibrin gel permeability by high homocysteine levels. Thromb Res. 2011;127(1):35–8.
39. Lauricella AM, Quintana I, Castañon M, et al. Influence of homocysteine on fibrin network lysis. Blood Coagul Fibrinolysis. 2006;17(3):181–6.
40. Speidl WS, Nikfardjam M, Niessner A, et al. Mild hyperhomocysteinemia is associated with a decreased fibrinolytic activity in patients after ST-elevation myocardial infarction. Thromb Res. 2007;119(3):331–6.

15

Real-world experience comparing two common left atrial appendage closure devices

Christian Fastner[1*], Lea Hoffmann[2], Mohamed Aboukoura[2], Michael Behnes[1], Siegfried Lang[1], Martin Borggrefe[1], Ibrahim Akin[1] and Christoph A. Nienaber[3]

Abstract

Background: The interventional left atrial appendage closure (LAAC) is a guideline-conform alternative to oral anticoagulation (OAC) in non-valvular atrial fibrillation patients with OAC ineligibility. It was aimed to directly compare two contemporary devices in a real-world patient population.

Methods: LAAC was conducted in two centres between 2010 and 2014 as well as between 2014 and 2017, respectively, in a standard fashion based on the specific manufacturer's recommendations. Baseline characteristics, procedural data and event rates during intra-hospital and 6 months follow-up were registered in a retrospective approach, and analysed in device-related groups.

Results: A total of 189 patients presented for LAAC device implantation. Baseline characteristics were mostly evenly distributed. In 148 patients, a Watchman™ device (Boston Scientific, Natick, MA, USA) was successfully implanted, an Amplatzer™ Amulet™ (St. Jude Medical, St. Paul, MN, USA) in 34 patients (96.1 and 97.1%, respectively; $p = 1.00$). Major access site bleedings were more frequent in the Amplatzer™ Amulet™ group (8.9 versus 1.4%; $p = 0.046$). No intra-hospital thromboembolic event was present. During 6 months follow-up, peri-device leaks > 5 mm and thromboembolic events were uncommon (each $p =$ n.s.).

Conclusions: While procedural success was equally high with both contemporary devices, complications during follow-up were rare, and evenly distributed.

Keywords: Atrial fibrillation, Left atrial appendage, Left atrial appendage closure device, Outcome, Comparison

Background

Atrial fibrillation (AF) is the most common cardiac arrhythmia with an age-dependent prevalence from 0.1% among < 55 year olds to 9% in octogenarians [1]. Stroke and systemic embolization are prognostically relevant complications [2]. In patients with an increased risk for thromboembolism under AF, identified by a CHA_2DS_2-VASc score ≥ 2 in men and ≥ 3 in women, systemic oral anticoagulation (OAC) is the guideline conform prophylactic treatment [3]. However, an underuse of these substances is observed in daily practice despite the introduction of non-Vitamin K antagonist oral anticoagulants (NOACs) [4–6]. Typical contraindications for long-term OAC are relevant prior bleedings with a tendency to recidivity, a high predisposition for major bleeding events, other adverse drug reactions, the need for dialysis or the individual patient's refusal [7]. Moreover, some patients suffer from thromboembolic strokes despite adequate OAC [8].

Within the last decade, the interventional left atrial appendage closure (LAAC) was implemented as a prophylactic alternative in all these above-mentioned cases. Currently, it is recommended by the European guidelines on atrial fibrillation (class IIb) in all patients with contraindications to long-term OAC [3]. This locoregional technique rests on the observation that > 90% of all emboli related to non-valvular AF originate from the

* Correspondence: christian.fastner@umm.de
[1]First Department of Medicine, University Medical Centre Mannheim (UMM), Faculty of Medicine Mannheim, University of Heidelberg, European Centre for AngioScience (ECAS), and DZHK (German Centre for Cardiovascular Research) partner site Heidelberg/Mannheim, Theodor-Kutzer-Ufer 1-3, 68167 Mannheim, Germany
Full list of author information is available at the end of the article

left atrial appendage (LAA) [9]. The LAAC with the WATCHMAN™ device (Boston Scientific, Natick, MA, USA) was proven to be non-inferior to long-term OAC for the combined efficacy outcome of stroke, systemic embolization and cardiovascular death in a randomized controlled trial (RCT) [10]. After 3.8 years, the interventional approach was superior to OAC with respect to the combined study endpoint [11]. While the patients in the RCT were anticoagulated for at least 45 days after the procedure, dual antiplatelet agents were shown to be an effective, and safe antithrombotic alternative in all those patients with an absolute contraindication for OAC [12, 13].

Meanwhile, two large registries confirmed efficacy and safety for both common devices, i.e., the WATCHMAN™ device and the AMPLATZER™ Cardiac Plug (St. Jude Medical, St. Paul, MN, USA), in a real-world patient collective [14, 15]. Particularly, the periinterventional complication rates revealed to be much lower than in the initial RCT [14, 16, 17]. Thus, both devices have proven their practical applicability. However, the side-by-side comparison of the two contemporary devices is limited to few data [18]. Based on the assumption that not all the information derived from studies on one device is one-to-one applicable to the other, this study aimed to compare the WATCHMAN™ device to the second-generation AMPLATZER™ Amulet™ regarding patient characteristics, procedural success and complications during follow-up.

Methods

Enrollment

This study is based on retrospective observational registry data from two German centres. Centre 1 (University Hospital Rostock, Rostock, Germany) performed LAAC with the WATCHMAN™ device, centre 2 (University Medical Centre Mannheim, Mannheim, Germany) with the WATCHMAN™ device and the AMPLATZER™ Amulet™. Enrollment period lasted from 2010 to 2014 in centre 1 and from 2014 to 2017 in centre 2. Both centres aimed to include consecutively all LAAC cases to avoid a recruitment bias. Patient characteristics, implantation details including complications and follow-up data was extracted from the original medical documents. The methods were carried out in accordance with the relevant local guidelines and regulations. All protocols were approved by the medical ethics committee of the Faculty of Medicine, University of Rostock, Germany, and the medical ethics committee II of the Faculty of Medicine Mannheim, University of Heidelberg, Germany. Due to the retrospective data acquisition, written informed consent concerning the study was not obtained but all patients consented in the conduction of the procedure beforehand.

Procedure and intra-hospital follow-up

The operators' experience and the conduction of the implantation procedure were comparable in both centres. Specific manufacturer's recommendations were considered. The procedure was performed under conscious sedation, and guided by fluoroscopy, angiography and transoesophageal echocardiography (TOE) in all cases. Device selection in centre 2 was left to the operator's discretion based on preprocedural TOE measurements (orifice and landing zone's diameter, LAA depth, morphology). After device releasing and sheath removal the venous access site was sealed at the discretion of the operator (Z-suture, Perclose ProGlide™ (Abbott, Redwood City, CA, USA)), an arterial access (femoral 5 French sheath), which had been established in some cases, was sealed with manual compression or Angio-Seal™ vascular closure device (Terumo, Shibuya, Japan). Following the procedure, stable device position and potential peri-device leaks were identified by TOE. A thorough clinical examination served to identify neurological or access site complications. In centre 1, postprocedural antithrombotic regimen was individualised, while all patients in centre 2 received acetylsalicylic acid (ASA) lifelong and additional clopidogrel for 6 months.

Mid-term follow-up

In the context of the clinical routine, patients presented 6 months after the procedure for a follow-up visit. A TOE as well as a clinical re-examination were conducted during this visit.

Outcome measures

Successful device implantation was defined in the absence of a relevant peri-device leak, i.e., > 5 mm. A bleeding was categorized as "major bleeding" when the event could be attributed to Bleeding Academic Research Consortium (BARC) definition ≥ type 3. The primary efficacy outcome measure was the absence of stroke and systemic embolization during follow-up, a secondary efficacy outcome measure was successful device deployment. Safety was assessed by the absence of any complication related to the intervention or the postinterventional antithrombotic regimen. Events which could not be traced back to the intervention or the related medical therapy were registered as adverse events.

Statistics

Statistical analyses were performed with SPSS Statistics (IBM, Armonk, NY). Continuous data are presented as means with standard deviation, categorical data as total numbers with group-related percentages. Between the device groups, categorical variables were compared using the chi-squared test or the Fisher's exact test for rare events. The unpaired t-test with Welch correction for unequal variances was applied to compare continuous variables. The statistics were based on the available cases per item. *P* values < 0.05 (two-tailed) were considered statistically significant.

Results

Baseline characteristics

Baseline demographic and clinical characteristics of the study population including risk stratification according to the CHA_2DS_2-VASc and the HAS-BLED scores are displayed in Table 1. A total of 189 patient cases could be included in this registry. Ninety-seven patients were indicated for LAAC in centre 1 and 92 in centre 2. The population presented with a mean CHA_2DS_2-VASc score of 4.4 ± 1.5 ($p = 0.06$ in comparison of both devices) and a mean HAS-BLED score of 3.6 ± 1.1 ($p = 0.12$). 76.7% of patients had a HAS-BLED score ≥ 3 points. In general, baseline characteristics were statistically evenly distributed between the two device groups, except for relevant prior bleeding events, which were significantly more common in patients that received an Amplatzer™ Amulet™ ($p = 0.008$). Consequently, contraindication for long-term OAC was significantly more often defined by a prior bleeding event in the Amplatzer™ Amulet™ group ($p = 0.032$). Irrespective

Table 1 Baseline characteristics

	Watchman™ (*n* = 154)	Amplatzer™ Amulet™ (*n* = 35)	*p* value*	OR (95% CI)
Male, n (%)	105 (68.2)	22 (62.9)	0.55	1.27 (0.58–2.73)
Age [years], mean ± SD	75.2 ± 2.8	77.1 ± 9.7	0.27	–
CHA_2DS_2-VASc score, mean ± SD	4.5 ± 0.1	4.0 ± 1.4	0.06	–
HAS-BLED score, mean ± SD	3.6 ± 0.2	3.7 ± 1.0	0.12	–
HAS-BLED score ≥ 3, *n* (%)	127 (82.5)	33 (94.3)	0.12	3.5 (0.79–15.52)
Type of AF, each *n* (%)				
Paroxysmal	61 (39.6)	17 (48.6)	0.35	0.69 (0.31–1.55)
Persistent	41 (26.6)	4 (11.4)	0.08	3.72 (1.17–13.07)
Permanent	45 (29.2)	14 (40.0)	0.23	0.62 (0.27–1.42)
Unknown	7 (4.5)	0 (0.0)	0.35	–
Congestive heart failure, *n* (%)	47 (30.5)	8 (22.9)	0.42	0.67 (0.28–1.60)
Arterial hypertension, *n* (%)	148 (96.1)	34 (97.1)	1.00	1.38 (0.16–11.84)
Diabetes mellitus, *n* (%)	52 (33.8)	14 (40.0)	0.56	1.31 (0.61–2.79)
Prior cerebrovascular event, each *n* (%)	44 (28.6)	8 (22.9)	0.54	0.74 (0.31–1.76)
Vascular disease, *n* (%)	98 (63.6)	19 (54.3)	0.34	0.68 (0.32–1.43)
Chronic kidney disease, *n* (%)	54 (35.1)	12 (34.3)	1.00	0.97 (0.44–2.10)
Chronic liver disease, *n* (%)	10 (6.5)	4 (11.4)	0.30	1.86 (0.54–6.32)
Prior bleeding, *n* (%)	100 (64.9)	31 (88.6)	**0.008**	4.19 (1.40–12.49)
Bleeding localization, each *n* (%)				
Intracranial	28 (18.2)	6 (17.1)	1.00	1.07 (0.37–3.20)
Gastrointestinal	57 (37.0)	20 (57.1)	**0.036**	0.44 (0.73–1.00)
Muscle	3 (1.9)	0 (0.0)	1.00	–
Skin/mucosal	4 (2.6)	3 (8.6)	0.12	0.28 (0.05–1.70)
Other/unknown	8 (5.2)	2 (5.7)	1.00	0.90 (0.16–6.49)
Indication for LAAC, each *n* (%)				
Prior bleeding	93 (60.4)	28 (80.0)	**0.032**	0.38 (0.14–0.91)
Drug intolerance	25 (16.2)	1 (2.9)	0.05	6.59 (1.12–69.94)
LAA thrombus despite OAC	4 (2.6)	1 (2.9)	1.00	0.91 (0.14–11.39)
Thromboembolic event despite OAC	3 (1.9)	2 (5.7)	0.23	0.33 (0.06–1.92)
Patient's preference	9 (5.8)	0 (0.0)	0.21	–
Other reason	20 (13.0)	3 (8.6)	0.58	1.59 (0.47–5.32)

AF Atrial fibrillation, *CI* Confidence interval, *IQR* Interquartile range, *LAA(C)* Left atrial appendage (closure), *OAC* Oral anticoagulation, *OR* Odds ratio, *SD* Standard deviation

*Fisher's exact or unpaired t-test for the comparison of both groups, $p < 0.05$ indicates statistical significance

of the device group, a prior bleeding event was the most common indication for the intervention (64.0% of the overall population).

Procedural data

Technical success – defined as stable device anchorage and absence of a peri-device leak > 5 mm at the end of the procedure – could be achieved in 96.3% of all patients (p = n.s. between the device groups; Table 2). Four patients of the Watchman™ group were implanted in a second procedure, as they revealed a LAA thrombus during the initial intervention which could be successfully resolved by short-term OAC. Out of the 6 patients without implantation success, 5 had a wide and tub-shaped LAA orifice and neck region which was not providing conditions for adequate device anchorage. In another patient, the LAA thrombus could not be resolved despite proper anticoagulation, and the remaining LAA was too small to implant the device. One implantation failure in the Amplatzer™ Amulet™ group was due to a circulatory collapse and subsequent death in a patient with a highly reduced left ventricular (LV) function.

Both intraprocedurally dislodged Watchman™ devices were successfully snared in the LA cavity, and retrieved through a stable transseptal electrophysiological sheath [19]. In one case, within the same session, a larger Watchman™ device could successfully be implanted.

While all patients were discontinued with OAC in centre 2 after successful device implantation, 94.6% of the successfully implanted patients received dual antiplatelet therapy (DAPT) with ASA and clopidogrel for 6 months in centre 1 as well. Only a small minority of patients received

Table 2 Procedural data and intra-hospital outcome

	Watchman™ (n = 154)	Amplatzer™ Amulet™ (n = 35)	p value*	OR (95% CI)
Successful implantation, n (%)	148 (96.1)	34 (97.1)	1.00	1.38 (0.16–11.84)
Intraprocedural device dislodgement, n (%)	2 (1.3)	0 (0.0)	1.00	0.86 (0.04–18.31)
	Watchman™ (successful n = 148)	Amplatzer™ Amulet™ (successful n = 34)	p value*	OR (95% CI)
Peri-device leak < 5 mm, n (%)	2 (1.4)	0 (0.0)	1.00	0.85 (0.03–18.11)
Access site bleeding, each n (%)	12 (8.1)	6 (17.6)	0.11	0.41 (0.12–1.36)
Minor bleeding	6 (4.1)	2 (5.9)	0.64	1.48 (0.28–7.68)
Major bleeding	2 (1.4)	3 (8.9)	**0.046**	7.07 (1.13–44.09)
Pseudoaneurysm	4 (2.7)	1 (3.0)	1.00	1.09 (0.11–10.01)
Pericardial effusion	12 (8.1)	2 (5.9)	1.00	1.41 (0.27–9.64)
Without hemodynamic impact	7 (4.7)	2 (5.9)	0.68	0.79 (0.14–5.83)
With hemodynamic impact	3 (2.0)	0 (0.0)	1.00	–
Tamponade	2 (1.4)	0 (0.0)	1.00	–
Intra-hospital stroke, n (%)	0 (0.0)	0 (0.0)	1.00	–
Postprocedural device dislodgement, n (%)	1 (0.7)	0 (0.0)	1.00	1.43 (0.06–35.77)
Intra-hospital death, n (%)	1 (0.7)	1 (2.9)	0.34	4.46 (0.27–73.12)
Postprocedural antithrombotic therapy in the first 6 months, each n (%)				
DAPT	140 (94.6)	34 (100.0)	0.36	–
OAC plus clopidogrel	2 (1.4)	0 (0.0)	1.00	–
45 days LMWH plus one antiplatelet agent, DAPT afterwards	6 (4.1)	0 (0.0)	0.60	–

ASA Acetylsalicylic acid, *CI* Confidence interval, *DAPT* Dual antiplatelet therapy, *LMWH* Low molecular weight heparin, *OAC* Oral anticoagulation, *OR* Odds ratio
*Fisher's exact test for the comparison of both groups, $p < 0.05$ indicates statistical significance

anticoagulants after successful LAAC. Six patients were prescribed low molecular weight heparins plus an antiplatelet agent for 45 days followed by DAPT with ASA and clopidogrel for half a year. Additional two patients were treated with phenprocoumon and clopidogrel for 6 months. All patients should continue to receive ASA from month 7 onwards for the rest of their lives.

Postprocedural complications and safety events

Postprocedural major access site bleedings were statistically more common in the Amplatzer™ Amulet™ group ($p = 0.046$; Table 2). All five cases of major bleeding, i.e., bleeding defined by a BARC score ≥ 3, needed blood transfusions, however, none had to be operated. Five pseudoaneurysms were successfully treated by ultrasound-guided compression. Pericardiocentesis was sufficient to resolve 2 pericardial tamponades and 3 hemodynamically relevant pericardial effusions. Nine minor pericardial effusions could be treated conservatively. Heart surgery was needed to retrieve a post-procedurally dislodged Watchman™ device in 1 case.

The above-mentioned peri-procedural death occurred directly after transseptal puncture. Both, air embolism and pericardial tamponade could be ruled out by a thorough analysis of the underlying cause. Rather, deep conscious sedation in connection with a highly-depressed LV function was stated as cause of death. Two more patients died during hospital stay after successful device implantation, however, none of these deaths was linked to the procedure (urosepis and hypokalaemia-induced ventricular fibrillation), and, therefore, termed adverse events. None of the surviving patients developed persistent disability.

Follow-up

One hundred twelve patients in the Watchman™ group (75.7% of the implanted patients) and 30 patients in the Amplatzer™ Amulet™ group (88.2% of the implanted patients) presented at 6 months' follow-up visit (Table 3). One hundred two Watchman™ patients (68.9% of the implanted patients) and 21 Amplatzer™ Amulet™ patients (61.8% of the implanted patients) underwent a TOE examination at follow-up. Meanwhile, device dislodgement in the abdominal aorta was incidentally detected by computed tomography conducted for other reasons in 1 additional patient of the Amplatzer™ Amulet™ group ($p = 1.00$ versus the Watchman™ group), and the device could be successfully retrieved in a catheter-based intervention. In all patients that presented for 6 months' follow-up TOE, the device was detectable in the LAA. Meanwhile, 1 patient of the Watchman™ group with a highly-depressed LV function revealed a LV thrombus 1 months after the implantation which could be resolved by 4 weeks of heparin therapy. The treating physicians decided to prolong the DAPT in a patient whose Watchman™ device was rotated 90° in the LAA, and, therefore, had a peri-device leak > 5 mm to achieve LAA thrombosis nonetheless. Six patients died during follow-up. However, none of these cases could be directly traced to the device implantation nor to the dual antiplatelet therapy. In 1 patient, major bleeding after iatrogenic vascular injury during thoracentesis resulted in haemorrhagic shock and death, however, this was not primarily attributed to the DAPT, but rather to the massive trauma.

Transoesophageal echocardiographic measurements

Table 4 summarizes the TOE measurements of dimensions at baseline and 6 months' follow-up visit of the patients from centre 2. The Watchman™ device was compressed to a significantly higher degree than the Amplatzer™ Amulet™ (77 versus 85%, respectively; $p = 0.015$).

Discussion

This two-centre registry retrospectively analysing a real-world population of non-valvular AF patients that underwent interventional closure of the LAA,

Table 3 Six months follow-up data

	Watchman™ (clinical follow up: $n = 112$; TOE follow-up: $n = 102$)	Amplatzer™ Amulet™ (clinical follow-up: $n = 30$; TOE follow-up: $n = 21$)	p value*	OR (95% CI)
Device detectable in LAA, n (%)	102 (100.0)	21 (100.0)	1.00	–
Peri-device leak < 5 mm, n (%)	14 (13.7)	2 (9.5)	1.00	0.66 (0.13–3.16)
Peri-device leak > 5 mm, n (%)	1 (1.0)	0 (0.0)	1.00	–
Device thrombus, n (%)	4 (4.9)	0 (0.0)	0.59	0.51 (0.02–9.82)
Pericardial effusion, n (%)	2 (2.0)	0 (0.0)	1.00	–
Minor bleeding, n (%)	4 (3.6)	1 (3.3)	1.00	1.07 (0.11–6.24)
Major bleeding, n (%)	6 (5.4)	2 (6.7)	0.68	0.79 (0.13–6.04)
Thromboembolic event, n (%)	1 (0.9)	0 (0.0)	1.00	1.22 (0.04–30.70)
Death, n (%)	4 (3.6)	2 (6.7)	0.61	1.93 (0.33–11.08)

CI Confidence interval, *LAA* Left atrial appendage, *OR* Odds ratio, *TOE* Transoesophageal echocardiography
*Fisher's exact test for the comparison of both groups, $p < 0.05$ indicates statistical significance

Table 4 Transoesophageal echocardiographic measurements

	Watchman™	Amplatzer™ Amulet™	p value*
Baseline TOE			
LAA morphology, each n (%)			0.14
Windsock	22 (38.6)	11 (31.4)	
Cauliflower	16 (28.1)	10 (28.6)	
Chicken wing	14 (24.6)	5 (14.3)	
Cactus	5 (8.8)	9 (25.7)	
LA diameter, mean ± SD	50.6 ± 1.0	48.7 ± 1.4	0.27
LA surface, mean ± SD	24.1 ± 1.2	23.8 ± 1.2	0.83
LAA depth, mean ± SD	29.5 ± 1.1	29.2 ± 1.6	0.87
LAA orifice diameter, mean ± SD			
45°	19.0 ± 0.6	20.5 ± 0.9	0.16
90°	19.6 ± 0.7	20.4 ± 0.9	0.46
135°	20.7 ± 1.2	21.1 ± 1.0	0.82
LAA landing zone diameter, mean ± SD	18.4 ± 0.8	18.6 ± 0.8	0.87
Follow-up TOE			
LA diameter, mean ± SD	48.5 ± 1.4	45.7 ± 2.8	0.37
LA surface, mean ± SD	21.8 ± 1.0	22.4 ± 1.3	0.71
LAA orifice diameter, mean ± SD			
45°	20.0 ± 2.0	24.4 ± 3.5	0.30
90°	22.7 ± 0.8	23.4 ± 1.1	0.57
135°	20.4 ± 2.3	22.5 ± 4.5	0.73
Device diameter post-implantation / initial device diameter, mean ± SD	0.77 ± 0.03	0.85 ± 0.02	**0.015**

LA(A) Left atrial (appendage), *SD* Standard deviation, *TOE* Transoesophageal echocardiography
*Fisher's exact or unpaired t-test for the comparison of both groups, $p < 0.05$ indicates statistical significance; based on the available data of 92 patients from centre 2 with TOE at baseline and 53 patients from centre 2 with TOE at follow-up visit

confirmed excellent efficacy and safety of the interventional approach in both contemporary devices. Regarding relevant outcome parameters, no significant difference was seen in comparison of both devices.

The study collective was both, at high risk for stroke (mean CHA_2DS_2-VASc score 4.4 ± 1.5; $p = 0.06$) and for bleeding events (mean HAS-BLED score 3.6 ± 1.1; $p = 0.12$) which is in line with the European guideline requirements for LAAC [3]. Moreover, the risk profiles were more pronounced than those in the initial approval studies which were conducted in patients eligible for OAC [10, 20], and they certainly reflect the present clinical situation. The baseline characteristics of our collective are in good accordance with those of recently published large registries evaluating outcomes in any one device [14, 16]. Of note, baseline characteristics do not significantly differ between the device groups, facilitating the evaluation of the intervention's impact on outcome parameters, except for the registered rate of prior bleeding events.

Concerning the secondary efficacy outcome measure, success in device deployment (96.3% for both devices; p = n.s.) was comparable high to previously published real-world data (Fig. 1) [14, 16, 18]. Operators in both centres were well trained (≥50 prior implantations each) or were guided by an experienced operator. This is also depicted by the fact, that intra-procedural device dislodgements could be handled within the same intervention without any further harm to the patient. The 4 patients in which procedural success could only be reached after thrombus resolution highlight that boundaries between patients eligible and ineligible for OAC are fluid. Therefore, the long-term ineligibility for OAC might be the guiding principle [3] while short periods of reinitiated anticoagulation may be tolerated by some patients. Besides the classic indication "prior bleeding", ineligibility was also given due to a LAA thrombus and/or thromboembolic event under adequate OAC [21]. Among the cases with "other" indications, the interventional approach is of special interest to AF patients with end-stage renal failure on dialysis as these patients have a tremendously increased stroke risk while they do not seem to profit from medical prophylaxis [22].

The cut-off set for acceptable peri-device leaks is closely linked to the definition of procedural success. Just like in any relevant previous study since the initial PROTECT-AF trial, both centres chose a cut-off of 5 mm as for

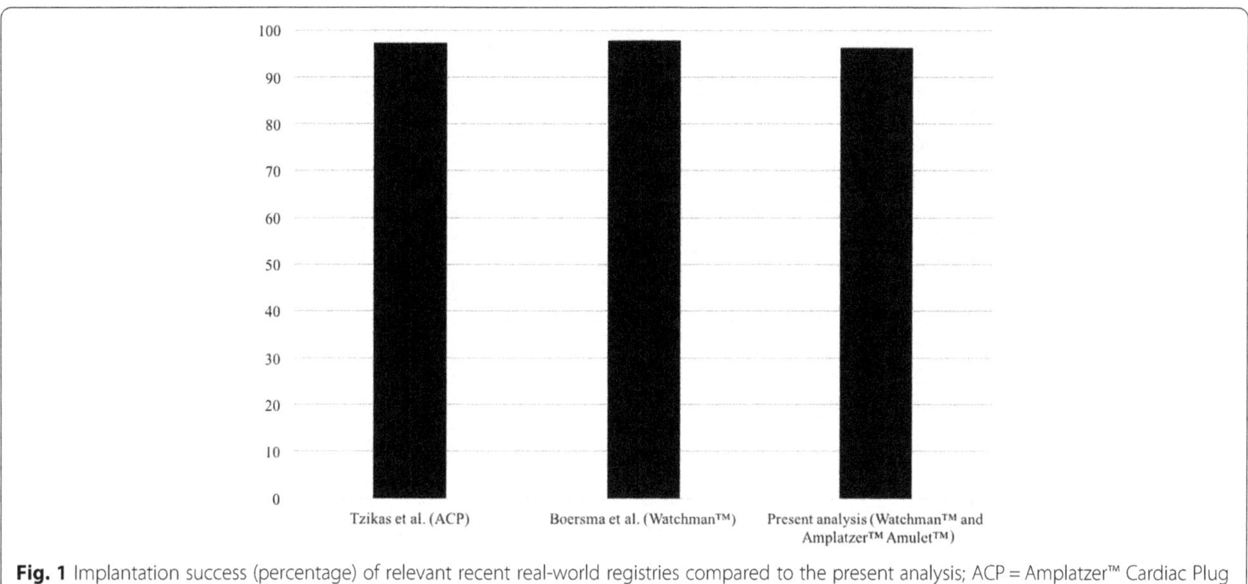

Fig. 1 Implantation success (percentage) of relevant recent real-world registries compared to the present analysis; ACP = Amplatzer™ Cardiac Plug

smaller peri-device leaks clinical irrelevance is assumed [23]. Any type of peri-device leak was infrequent in both groups ($p = 1.0$) and no device dislodgement was detected during follow-up. This was even though the Watchman™ device appeared significantly more compressed in follow-up TOE ($p = 0.015$). Limited to a 6 months post-intervention period, the LAAC technique's efficacy, i.e., the primary outcome measure, was demonstrated by only 1 thromboembolic event which occurred in a total of 142 clinically followed-up patients (0.7%; $p = 1.00$). As a deep vein thrombosis was detected being causal for a pulmonary embolism, this case was not to be registered as a cardioembolic event, but, nevertheless, it occurred based on OAC cessation after LAAC. More and more frequently, AF is characterized by a more comprehensive definition than being reduced to an atrial disorder with locoregional thrombogenic potential in the LAA. Indeed, AF seems to be associated with a general state of hypercoagulability [24] which could also be an explanation for the occurrence of the deep vein thrombosis.

By means of safety, the rate of major access site bleedings in the Amplatzer™ Amulet™ group (8.9 versus 1.4% of all implantations; $p = 0.046$) appears surprisingly high compared to 0.8% of major access site bleedings in the registry of Tzikas et al. with the first generation Amplatzer™ device [14]. The Amplatzer™ Amulet™ is not known to increase this rate [25]. It might be speculated, that the number of relevant access site bleedings may be overestimated by the small number of Amulet™ implantations and by the heterogeneous use of vascular closure techniques. However, this finding emphasis the fact that advantages of the interventional approach can only be achieved in the long run while the initial period is determined by complications of the complex procedure [20]. Of note, only one procedure-related death had to be registered, and no periprocedural thromboembolic event occurred.

Within follow-up, 5.6% of patients faced a major bleeding event ($p = 0.68$). All patients received more than one antithrombotic agent during the follow-up period, the majority a DAPT (95.6%; $p = 0.36$). Though being used as an alternative to OAC for ineligible patients in clinical practice, DAPT was shown not to be favourable to warfarin in lowering the bleeding risk [26]. Once again, the intervention's net benefit should be expected only after several years [11].

Study limitations

These analyses were based on retrospective observational registry data with the inherent limitations of this study type, e.g., a selection bias. Due to the retrospective character of this registry, conduction of the intervention was not influenced by the study investigators, and based on the operators' discretion. This individualized decision algorithm might have not insignificantly influenced the outcome measures but surely reflects the clinical practice. The operators could choose between two device types in only one centre, which created an imbalance in the total number of device implantations. Concerning the registration of bleeding events, the reservation must be made, that the grading of bleeding events unlike all other baseline characteristics was not objectively extractable out of the available patient data, but rather was based on the subjective assessment and documentation of the treating physician. Apparently, a bleeding event was more often considered relevant in centre 2. Since in centre 1 only the Watchman™ device was implanted, this circumstance impacted the proportional distribution of prior bleeding events. In addition, a HAS-BLED score > 3 was numerically more frequent in the Amplatzer™ Amulet™ group. Due to an imbalance in the total number of device implantations per group, this numerical variance might not be reflected by a statistical significant difference. That is also why we did not elaborate a regression analysis of outcome parameters on the factor "prior bleeding event". A follow-up TOE was available in only 69 and 62% of all successfully implanted patients, respectively, and the follow-up period was limited to 6 months, and, therefore, rates of thromboembolism and major bleedings could not be compared to the estimated annual rates from the CHA_2DS_2-VASc and the HAS-BLED score. Moreover, the limited sample size might not have insignificantly contributed to the non-detection of thromboembolic events during follow-up as these events are known to be infrequent after the LAAC procedure. However, despite the limitations of this observational registry, it is serving as a data source for a little studied topic.

Conclusions

Independent from the selected device type, technical success was high, and the interventional closure of the LAA presented with adequate efficacy and safety within 6 months follow-up in a real-world population. While this registry provides first insights into the comparison of different LAA closure devices in clinical practice, larger, whenever possible randomized studies or well-designed prospective registries will have to confirm these results.

Abbreviations

(N)OAC: (Non-Vitamin K antagonist) oral anticoagulation; AF: Atrial fibrillation; ASA: Acetylsalicylic acid; BARC: Bleeding Academic Research Consortium; CI: Conficence interval; DAPT: Dual antiplatelet therapy; IQR: Interquartile range; LA(A): Left atrial (appendage); LAAC: Left atrial appendage closure; LMWH: Low molecular weight heparin; LV: Left ventricular; n.s.: Not significant; OR: Odds ratio; RCT: Randomized controlled trial; SD: Standard deviation; TOE: Transoesophageal echocardiography

Funding

We acknowledge financial support by Deutsche Forschungsgemeinschaft and Ruprecht-Karls-Universität Heidelberg within the funding programme.

Authors' contributions

CF conceived the study, participated in its design and coordination, participated in data analysis and interpretation and helped to draft and revise the manuscript for important intellectual content. LH conceived the study, participated in its design and coordination, participated in data analysis and interpretation and helped to revise the manuscript for important intellectual content. MA participated in the study design and coordination, as well as data analysis and revised the manuscript. MB1 conceived the study, participated in its design and coordination, participated in data analysis and interpretation and helped to revise the manuscript for important intellectual content. SL conceived the study, participated in its design and coordination, participated in data analysis and interpretation and helped to revise the manuscript for important intellectual content. MB2 participated in the study design and coordination, as well as data acquisition and revised the manuscript for important intellectual content. IA conceived the study, participated in its design and coordination, participated in data analysis and interpretation and helped to draft and revise the manuscript for important intellectual content. CAN conceived the study, participated in its design and coordination, participated in data analysis and interpretation and helped to draft and revise the manuscript for important intellectual content. All authors read and approved the final manuscript.

Competing interests

Ibrahim Akin is a member of the Editorial Board of BMC Cardiovascular Disorders. The other authors declare that they have no competing interests concerning the content of this study.

Author details

[1]First Department of Medicine, University Medical Centre Mannheim (UMM), Faculty of Medicine Mannheim, University of Heidelberg, European Centre for AngioScience (ECAS), and DZHK (German Centre for Cardiovascular Research) partner site Heidelberg/Mannheim, Theodor-Kutzer-Ufer 1-3, 68167 Mannheim, Germany. [2]Department of Cardiology, University Hospital Rostock, Rostock, Germany. [3]Royal Brompton Hospital, London, United Kingdom and National Heart and Lung Institute, Imperial College London, London, UK.

References

1. Go AS, Hylek EM, Phillips KA, Chang Y, Henault LE, Selby JV, Singer DE. Prevalence of diagnosed atrial fibrillation in adults: national implications for rhythm management and stroke prevention: the AnTicoagulation and risk factors in atrial fibrillation (ATRIA) study. JAMA. 2001;285(18):2370–5.
2. Kannel WB, Benjamin EJ. Status of the epidemiology of atrial fibrillation. Med Clin North Am. 2008;92(1):17–40. ix
3. Kirchhof P, Benussi S, Kotecha D, Ahlsson A, Atar D, Casadei B, Castella M, Diener HC, Heidbuchel H, Hendriks J, et al. 2016 ESC guidelines for the management of atrial fibrillation developed in collaboration with EACTS. Eur Heart J. 2016;37(38):2893–962.
4. Waldo AL, Becker RC, Tapson VF, Colgan KJ, Committee NS. Hospitalized patients with atrial fibrillation and a high risk of stroke are not being provided with adequate anticoagulation. J Am Coll Cardiol. 2005;46(9):1729–36.
5. Vedovati MC, Verdecchia P, Giustozzi M, Molini G, Conti S, Pierpaoli L, Valecchi F, Aita A, Agnelli G, Becattini C. Permanent discontinuation of non vitamin K oral anticoagulants in real life patients with non-valvular atrial fibrillation. Int J Cardiol. 2017;236:363–9.
6. Kakkar AK, Mueller I, Bassand JP, Fitzmaurice DA, Goldhaber SZ, Goto S, Haas S, Hacke W, Lip GY, Mantovani LG, et al. Risk profiles and antithrombotic treatment of patients newly diagnosed with atrial fibrillation at risk of stroke: perspectives from the international, observational, prospective GARFIELD registry. PLoS One. 2013;8(5):e63479.
7. O'Brien EC, Holmes DN, Ansell JE, Allen LA, Hylek E, Kowey PR, Gersh BJ, Fonarow GC, Koller CR, Ezekowitz MD, et al. Physician practices regarding contraindications to oral anticoagulation in atrial fibrillation: findings from the outcomes registry for better informed treatment of atrial fibrillation (ORBIT-AF) registry. Am Heart J. 2014;167(4):601–9. e601
8. Okumura Y, Yokoyama K, Matsumoto N, Tachibana E, Kuronuma K, Oiwa K, Matsumoto M, Kojima T, Hanada S, Nomoto K, et al. Current use of direct oral anticoagulants for atrial fibrillation in Japan: findings from the SAKURA AF registry. J Arrhythm. 2017;33(4):289–96.
9. Blackshear JL, Odell JA. Appendage obliteration to reduce stroke in cardiac surgical patients with atrial fibrillation. Ann Thorac Surg. 1996;61(2):755–9.
10. Holmes DR, Reddy VY, Turi ZG, Doshi SK, Sievert H, Buchbinder M, Mullin CM, Sick P, Investigators PA. Percutaneous closure of the left atrial appendage versus warfarin therapy for prevention of stroke in patients with atrial fibrillation: a randomised non-inferiority trial. Lancet. 2009;374(9689): 534–42.
11. Reddy VY, Sievert H, Halperin J, Doshi SK, Buchbinder M, Neuzil P, Huber K, Whisenant B, Kar S, Swarup V, et al. Percutaneous left atrial appendage closure vs warfarin for atrial fibrillation: a randomized clinical trial. JAMA. 2014;312(19):1988–98.

12. Reddy VY, Mobius-Winkler S, Miller MA, Neuzil P, Schuler G, Wiebe J, Sick P, Sievert H. Left atrial appendage closure with the Watchman device in patients with a contraindication for oral anticoagulation: the ASAP study (ASA Plavix feasibility study with Watchman left atrial appendage closure technology). J Am Coll Cardiol. 2013;61(25):2551–6.
13. Urena M, Rodes-Cabau J, Freixa X, Saw J, Webb JG, Freeman M, Horlick E, Osten M, Chan A, Marquis JF, et al. Percutaneous left atrial appendage closure with the AMPLATZER cardiac plug device in patients with nonvalvular atrial fibrillation and contraindications to anticoagulation therapy. J Am Coll Cardiol. 2013;62(2):96–102.
14. Tzikas A, Shakir S, Gafoor S, Omran H, Berti S, Santoro G, Kefer J, Landmesser U, Nielsen-Kudsk JE, Cruz-Gonzalez I, et al. Left atrial appendage occlusion for stroke prevention in atrial fibrillation: multicentre experience with the AMPLATZER cardiac plug. EuroIntervention. 2016;11(10):1170–9.
15. Boersma LV, Ince H, Kische S, Pokushalov E, Schmitz T, Schmidt B, Gori T, Meincke F, Protopopov AV, Betts T, et al. Efficacy and safety of left atrial appendage closure with WATCHMAN in patients with or without contraindication to oral anticoagulation: 1-year follow-up outcome data of the EWOLUTION trial. Heart Rhythm. 2017;14(9):1302–8.
16. Boersma LV, Schmidt B, Betts TR, Sievert H, Tamburino C, Teiger E, Pokushalov E, Kische S, Schmitz T, Stein KM, et al. Implant success and safety of left atrial appendage closure with the WATCHMAN device: peri-procedural outcomes from the EWOLUTION registry. Eur Heart J. 2016; 37(31):2465–74.
17. Fastner C, Nienaber CA, Park JW, Brachmann J, Zeymer U, Goedde M, Sievert H, Geist V, Lewalter T, Krapivsky A, et al. Impact of left atrial appendage morphology on indication and procedural outcome after interventional occlusion - results from the prospective multicenter German LAARGE registry. EuroIntervention. 2018;14(2):151–7.
18. Figini F, Mazzone P, Regazzoli D, Porata G, Ruparelia N, Giannini F, Stella S, Ancona F, Agricola E, Sora N, et al. Left atrial appendage closure: a single center experience and comparison of two contemporary devices. Catheter Cardiovasc Interv. 2017;89(4):763–72.
19. Fastner C, Lehmann R, Behnes M, Sartorius B, Borggrefe M, Akin I. Veno-venous double lasso pull-and-push technique for transseptal retrieval of an embolized Watchman occluder. Cardiovasc Revasc Med. 2016;17(3):206–8.
20. Holmes DR Jr, Kar S, Price MJ, Whisenant B, Sievert H, Doshi SK, Huber K, Reddy VY. Prospective randomized evaluation of the Watchman left atrial appendage closure device in patients with atrial fibrillation versus long-term warfarin therapy: the PREVAIL trial. J Am Coll Cardiol. 2014;64(1):1–12.
21. Tzikas A, Bergmann MW. Left atrial appendage closure: patient, device and post-procedure drug selection. EuroIntervention. 2016;12(Suppl X):X48–54.
22. Shah M, Avgil Tsadok M, Jackevicius CA, Essebag V, Eisenberg MJ, Rahme E, Humphries KH, Tu JV, Behlouli H, Guo H, et al. Warfarin use and the risk for stroke and bleeding in patients with atrial fibrillation undergoing dialysis. Circulation. 2014;129(11):1196–203.
23. Viles-Gonzalez JF, Kar S, Douglas P, Dukkipati S, Feldman T, Horton R, Holmes D, Reddy VY. The clinical impact of incomplete left atrial appendage closure with the Watchman device in patients with atrial fibrillation: a PROTECT AF (percutaneous closure of the left atrial appendage versus warfarin therapy for prevention of stroke in patients with atrial fibrillation) substudy. J Am Coll Cardiol. 2012;59(10):923–9.
24. Watson T, Shantsila E, Lip GY. Mechanisms of thrombogenesis in atrial fibrillation: Virchow's triad revisited. Lancet. 2009;373(9658):155–66.
25. Gloekler S, Shakir S, Doblies J, Khattab AA, Praz F, Guerios E, Koermendy D, Stortecky S, Pilgrim T, Buellesfeld L, et al. Early results of first versus second generation Amplatzer occluders for left atrial appendage closure in patients with atrial fibrillation. Clin Res Cardiol. 2015;104(8):656–65.
26. Hohnloser SH, Pajitnev D, Pogue J, Healey JS, Pfeffer MA, Yusuf S, Connolly SJ, Investigators AW. Incidence of stroke in paroxysmal versus sustained atrial fibrillation in patients taking oral anticoagulation or combined antiplatelet therapy: an ACTIVE W substudy. J Am Coll Cardiol. 2007;50(22): 2156–61.

Telmisartan protects chronic intermittent hypoxic mice via modulating cardiac renin-angiotensin system activity

Wanyu Wang[1], Ailing Song[2], Yiming Zeng[3*], Xiaoyang Chen[3], Yixiang Zhang[3], Yonghong Shi[1], Yihua Lin[1] and Wen Luo[1]

Abstract

Background: To explore the effects of chronic intermittent hypoxia (CIH), which mimics sleep apnea syndrome, on the cardiac renin angiotensin system (RAS), and to investigate the cardiac protection of an angiotensin receptor blocker (ARB)telmisartan (TERT) against CIH.

Methods: 32 healthy male C57B6J mice were randomly divided into CIH, ARB, blank and air control groups. CIH lasted for 12 weeks. Cardiac angiotensin converting enzyme (ACE), angiotensin converting enzyme 2 (ACE 2) and angiotensin II (Ang II) were evaluated by immunohistochemistry. Myocardial apoptosis were assessed by TUNEL assay and myocardial cell ultrastructure were observed under transmission electron microscope.

Results: Cardiac ACE expression was higher in the CIH group than in blank and air control groups, which was decreased with TERT treatment. TERT treatment elevated the expression of cardiac ACE 2 and Ang II compared with CIH group. Myocardial cell and capillary endothelial cell apoptosis, mitochondrial injury were most severe in CIH groups, which were mitigated with TERT treatment.

Conclusions: CIH changes the expression of cardiac ACE, ACE2 and Ang II, which may cause myocardial damage. TERT protects mice from CIH-linked cardiac damage via modulating the activity of RAS in the hearts.

Keywords: Chronic intermittent hypoxia, Sleep apnea syndromes, Telmisartin, ACE, ACE 2, Ang II, Myocardial apoptosis; myocardial cell ultrastructure

Background

It has been well documented that the incidence of sleep apnea syndromes (SAS) is high in the general population and that SAS may lead to cardiovascular disease (CVDs) [1]. Chronic intermittent hypoxia (CIH) is one of the distinctive pathophysiological features of SAS, and is implicated in the development of SAS-associated CVDs. One of the mechanisms by which CIH promotes CVDs is the activation of the renin-angiotensin system (RAS) [2], a well-known contributor to the pathogenesis of CVDs. However, a key component of RAS, angiotensin converting enzyme 2 (ACE 2), inhibits RAS and exhibits vasodilatatory and anti-proliferative functions [3]. Currently, the effects of ACE 2 on the cardiovascular system have been investigated in diabetic animal models. However, the expression and function of ACE 2 in the hearts of CIH animals has not, to date, been explored. Previously, we reported that we successfully generated a CIH mouse model and studied the potential mechanisms by which CIH impaired cardiovascular function [4]. In our published work, we also investigated the protective effects of an angiotensin receptor blocker (ARB), telmisartan (TERT), that both has vasodilatory and anti-oxidative activity and is widely used clinically as an antihypertensive [5–7]. We found that CIH increased oxidative stress in the mouse hearts, as evidenced by increased levels of 8-hydroxy-2′-deoxyguanosine/8-hydroxyguanosine (8-OHdG/8-OHG), malondialdehyde (MDA), and NADPH oxydase p47, which were

* Correspondence: zeng_yi_ming@126.com; 13599513293@163.com
[3]Department of Pulmonary and Critical Care Medicine of the Second Affiliated Hospital of Fujian Medical University, Sleep and Breathing Disorders Research Institute of Fujian Medical University, No.34 Zhongshan North Road, Licheng District, Quanzhou 362000, Fujian, China
Full list of author information is available at the end of the article

suppressed by TERT treatment [4]. In the present study, we investigated the mechanisms by which CIH affects the RAS. Furthermore, we explored whether TERT could protect against CIH-induced cardiac damage via modulating the activity of the RAS. Our goal was to elucidate the mechanisms by which TERT, and more generally, ARB, may act in the treatment of SAS.

Methods

The experimental protocol was approved by Laboratory Animal Ethics Committee of the First Affiliated Hospital of Xiamen University. CIH, ARB treatment, blank control and air control groups, as described previously [4].

A total of 32 healthy male C57B6J mice, with a body weight between 20 and 25 g, were provided by the Laboratory Animals Center, Chinese Academy of Sciences, Shanghai (License number: SYXK (Fujian) 2008–0001). A self-made intermittent hypoxia box, an air control box, and a gas control system to control the gas cycle from oxygen and nitrogen gas to air were used in this study. The S-450 oxygen-detection alarm was purchased from American IST-AIM Company with a sensitivity of 0.1%. Medically compressed oxygen with a concentration higher than 99%, compressed nitrogen gas with a concentration higher than 99%, Atman-6500 air pump. The CIH profiles consisted of alternating room air (21% oxygen) and 5.5% oxygen every 120 s. Telmisartan (TERT) tablets (Micardis) were provided by the Shanghai Boehringer Ingelheim Company. Rabbit-anti-mouse antibodies against ACE, ACE 2 and Ang II were obtained from the Wuhan Boster Company. PV9001 kit and diaminobenzidine (DAB) coloring reagent kit were obtained from Beijing Zhong Shan Golden Bridge Inc. In Situ Cell Death Detection Kit (11684817910) was obtained from Roche. JEM-2100HC transmission electron microscope with a charge-coupled device camera (JEM-2100HC) operating at 120 Kv was purchased from Japan Electronics Co, Ltd.

CIH and ARB treatment model

The experimental mice were randomly divided into four groups (8 per group): CIH, ARB treatment, blank control and air control groups. An intermittent hypoxia system was used to generate the CIH model. Briefly, the self-made plexiglass box was constructed with an aperture closed by hyaline film and bilateral wells. The production well contained a one-way flap. The gas inside the box had a constant flow to avoid carbon dioxide retention. The gas control system contained a micro-computer chip, control procedures, relays, solenoid valves and monitors. Each gas supply had an individual air ventilation pipe, all of which were controlled by solenoid valve switches. The oxygen concentrations inside the box were tightly controlled. Each episodic hypoxia cycle time was 2 min (i.e. nitrogen 30 s, resting 30 s, oxygen 20 s and air 40 s). Each gas insufflation was shown on the control program monitor. The oxygen concentration in the box was monitored by the oxygen-detecting alarm.

Mice in CIH and ARB groups were placed in the intermittent hypoxia box. Intermittent hypoxia lasted for 12 weeks with 8 h per day. After eight weeks of intermittent hypoxia, the mice in ARB group were intragastrically administered TERT solution, which contained 0.2 mL normal saline with the TERT concentration 10 mg/kg/d [8], once per day for 4 weeks. In the air control group, the control system and plexiglass box used was the same as that of the CIH and ARB groups in order to reproduce the same environment. The cycle was similar to the one used in CIH and ARB groups in order to produce the same noise but only air was used. The blank control group had no any gaseous interference.

After 12 weeks, mice were sacrificed by heart dissection under anesthesia. Mice were fasted overnight followed by anesthesia with an intraperitoneal injection of 3% phenobarbital (30 mg/kg), all mice were weighted. Blood samples were collected through a direct cardiac puncture, and were centrifuged at 3000 g for 15 min at 4 °C while the supernatants (serum) were collected and stored at − 80 °C for further analysis. Mice were vascularly perfused through the heart with cold 100 mM phosphate buffer (pH 7.4). Tissues were immediately removed and the heart was dissected, and cut into small pieces within 1 mm cubes. The other part of the apex of the hearts was fixed in 10% neutral buffered formalin, stored in 70% ethanol, paraffin embedded and sectioned for subsequent histological analysis and TUNEL assay.

Determination of cardiac ACE, ACE 2 and Ang II, TUNEL assay, transmission electron microscope

Immunohistochemistry with the PV9001/DAB two stage method was used to detect the expression of ACE, ACE 2 and Ang II. The primary antibody was used at a concentration of 1:50. All positive staining was brown-yellow. The average optical density values were calculated by IPP 6.0 software. After dewaxing and rehydration, sections were incubating in proteinase K (400 μg/mL) for 10 min at 37 °C. TUNEL staining was then performed using In Situ Cell Death Detection Kit (Roche, 11,684,817,910) according to the instructions. After DAB substrate detection, sections were counterstaining with hematoxylin, mounted under glass coverslip and analyzed under light microscope. TUNEL-positive cardiomyocytes in each group were carefully evaluated under double-blinded conditions. Ten high-power fields (× 400) were randomly selected and scored, and the percentage of TUNEL-positive cells was determined by dividing the numbers of positive-staining nuclei by the numbers of total nuclei of the cells. The samples for transmission electron microscope were fixed with 2% glutaraldehyde in 0.1 m PBS overnight at 4 °C. After brief washing with PBS, the samples were post-fixed with 2% osmium tetroxide and 0.5% potassium ferricyanide in 25 mM cacodylate buffer at 22 °C, followed by dehydration, infiltration and embedding in Spurr's resin. Thin sections (70 nm) were made and post-stained with uranyl acetate and lead citrate. Samples were viewed under transmission electron microscope. Images were captured at magnifications of 15,000~ 40,000.

Statistical analysis

All of data are presented as the means ± standard error of the mean unless specified otherwise. One-way analysis of variance (ANOVA) followed by the Bonferroni post-hoc test was used to examine statistical comparisons of the mouse cardiac ACE2, and non-parametric Wilcoxon rank sum test was used to determine the statistical significance of cardiac ACE and Ang II data, the rate of apoptotic cells among these groups. The P values were calculated from two-tailed test. $P < 0.05$ was considered significant. Statistical analyses were performed using SPSS 20.0.

Results

TERT decreased the cardiac expression of ACE but increased the expression of ACE 2 and Ang II in CIH

Immunohistochemistry was used to determine the expression levels of ACE, ACE 2, and Ang II in the apex of mouse hearts obtained from different experimental groups, which are quantified and presented in Table 1. CIH and ARB groups showed stronger ACE staining (Fig. 1a-d) compared with the two control groups (Fig. 1e-h). Similarly, the expression level of cardiac ACE was significantly higher in the CIH group compared to that in the two control groups ($^{*}p < 0.001$, vs. two controls. Table 1). TERT treatment reduced the level of ACE, although this reduction did not reach statistical significance compared with the CIH group. No significant difference in ACE expression was found between blank control and air control groups. In the myocardium of the apex of the heart, Ang II staining was mainly localized in the cytoplasm (Fig. 2a-h), and its expression was higher in CIH group than in blank and air control groups ($^{\#}p < 0.05$ vs two control groups). However, TERT treatment significantly increased Ang II levels in the heart compared with other experimental groups. ($^{\&}p < 0.05$ vs. CIH). No significant difference in cardiac AngII expression was found between blank control and air control groups. ACE 2 positive cells showed a similar cytoplasmic staining pattern in cardiac samples obtained from each experimental group (Fig. 3a-h). The expression level of cardiac ACE 2 was higher in the CIH group than in blank and air control groups (+p < 0.05, Table 1), however, TERT treatment significantly increased ACE 2 expression in cardiac samples ($^{\$}P < 0.001$ vs. CIH). There were no significant differences between blank control and air control groups. Collectively, we conclude that TERT decreased the cardiac expression of ACE but increased the expression of ACE 2 and Ang II in CIH mouse hearts.

Pathological changes in myocardial cells under electron microscope

Next, we evaluated the pathological changes in myocardial cell and capillary endothelial cells in the four experimental groups under electron microscope. While in both the blank and air control groups the chromatin of myocardial nuclei was uniform and the nuclear membrane was intact, in CIH group the myocardial nuclei were pyknotic, the nucleolus dissolved and disappeared, and the heterochromatin clustered in the perinuclear region, which showed the apoptosis of myocardial cells in 8/8 CIH cases (Fig. 4a-d). Also, in CIH group, the number of mitochondria decreased, the size was abnormal, the mitochondrial membrane was incomplete, the number of cristae was reduced, and the arrangement was disordered, while in the blank and air control groups, the quantity and size of the mitochondrial are normal and the membrane is intact. The mitochondrial cristae filled

Table 1 TERT decreased the cardiac expression of ACE but increased the expression of ACE 2 and Ang II in CIH

Group	n	Cardiac ACE	Cardiac Ang II	Cardiac ACE 2	Apoptotic rate of myocardial cells by TUNEL assay (%)
CIH group	8	0.034900 ± 0.0130[a]	0.095922 ± 0.0328[d]	0.052200 ± 0.0192[b]	53.23 ± 5.292[f]
ARB treatment group	8	0.025100 ± 0.0061[a]	0.149025 ± 0.0217[d c]	0.072850 ± 0.0175[b c]	23.32 ± 2.827
Blank control group	8	0.004738 ± 0.0026	0.015019 ± 0.0070	0.017488 ± 0.0131	22.39 ± 3.715
Air control group	8	0.005238 ± 0.0026	0.020684 ± 0.0107	0.029313 ± 0.0136	23.72 ± 2.857

[a]$p < 0.001$ vs. blank and air control groups
[b]$p < 0.05$ vs. blank and air control groups
[c]$p < 0.001$ vs. CIH
[d]$p < 0.05$ vs. blank and air control groups
[e]$p < 0.05$ vs. CIH
[f]$p < 0.001$ vs. the other three experimental groups

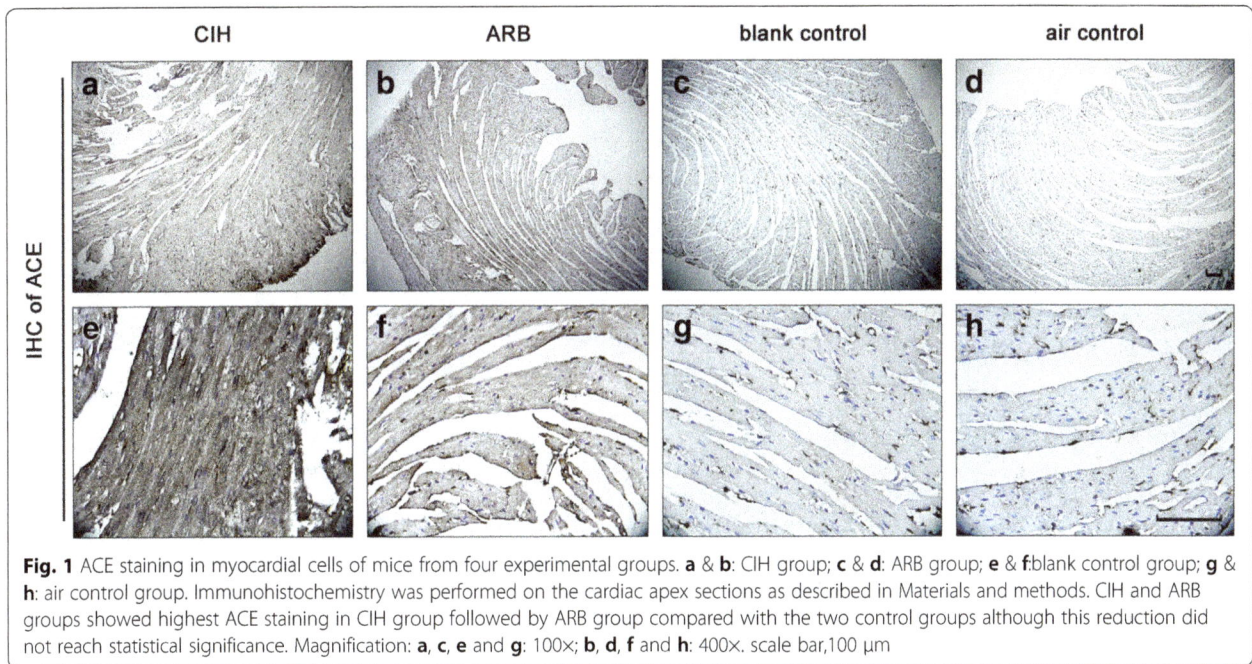

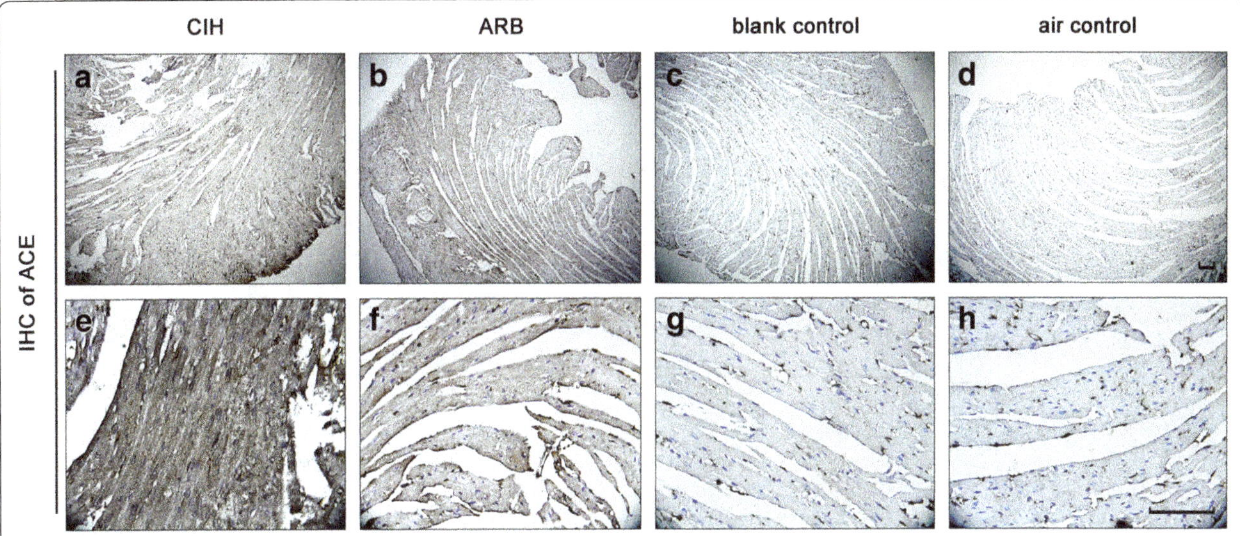

Fig. 1 ACE staining in myocardial cells of mice from four experimental groups. **a** & **b**: CIH group; **c** & **d**: ARB group; **e** & **f**:blank control group; **g** & **h**: air control group. Immunohistochemistry was performed on the cardiac apex sections as described in Materials and methods. CIH and ARB groups showed highest ACE staining in CIH group followed by ARB group compared with the two control groups although this reduction did not reach statistical significance. Magnification: **a**, **c**, **e** and **g**: 100×; **b**, **d**, **f** and **h**: 400×. scale bar,100 μm

the entire cavity of the mitochondrion and were arranged in parallel, regular and abundant in number (Fig. 5a-d). In addition, in CIH group, the cristae are broken, dissolved, destroyed, flocculent, as well as increased electron density of matrix increases in 7/8 CIH cases (Fig. 6a-d). The coarse and fine filaments were well arranged and each band was clearly visible in CIH group, blank and air control groups. Capillary endothelial cell nuclei were pyknotic, and the heterochromatin clustered in the perinuclear region which showed the apoptosis of capillary endothelial cell in 4/8 CIH cases (Fig. 7a-d) while no capillary endothelial cells were found apoptotic in the blank and air control groups.

The ultrastructural changes observed in the ARB group were in between those of the CIH group and the blank and air control groups. Visualization of cardiomyocyte and capillary endothelial cell apoptosis is rare under electron microscopy. The quantity and size of the mitochondria were normal with intact membranes. The electron density of the mitochondrial matrix increased similarly to that observed

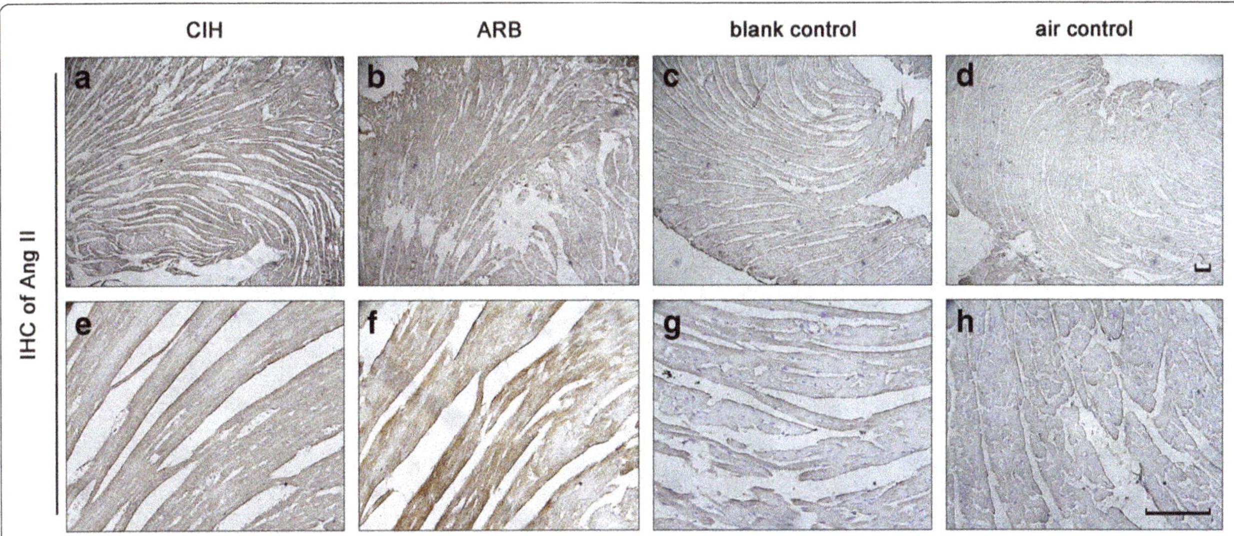

Fig. 2 Ang II staining in myocardial cells of mice from four experimental groups. **a** & **b**: CIH group; **c** & **d**:ARB group; **e** & **f**:blank control group; **g** & **h**: air control group. Immunohistochemistry was performed on the cardiac apex sections as described in Materials and methods. The expression level of cardiac AngII was highest in ARB group followed by CIH group compared with the two control groups. Magnification: **a**, **c**, **e** and **g**: 100×; **b**, **d**, **f** and **h**: 400×. scale bar, 100 μm

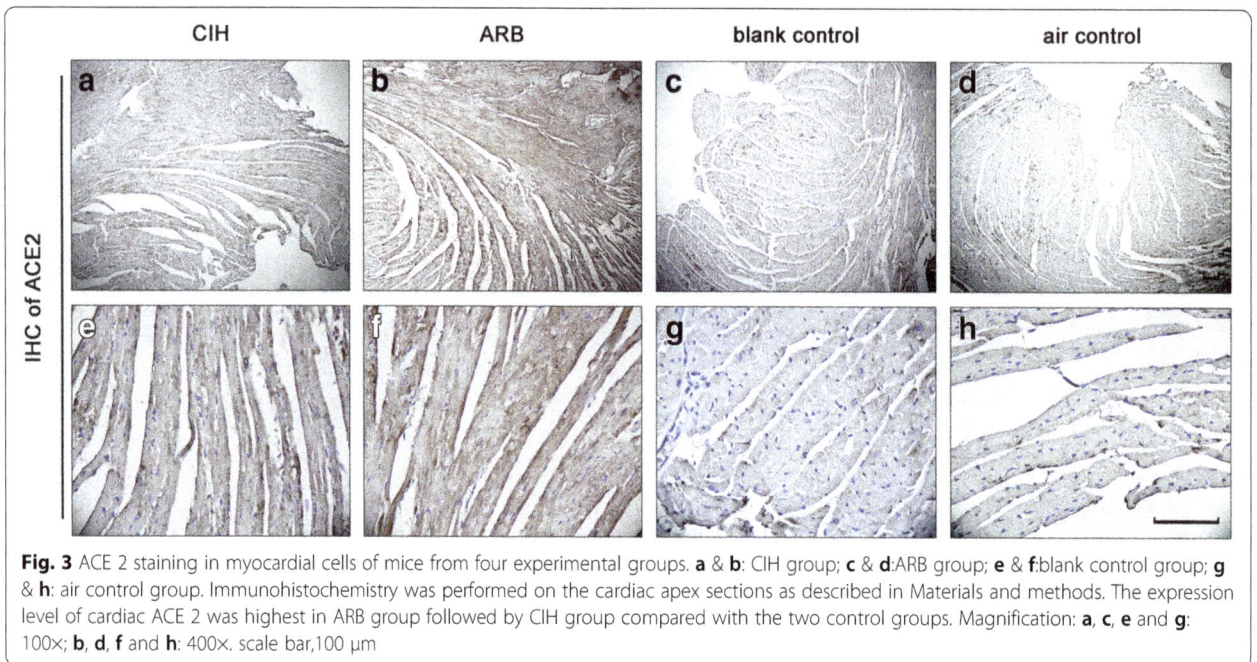

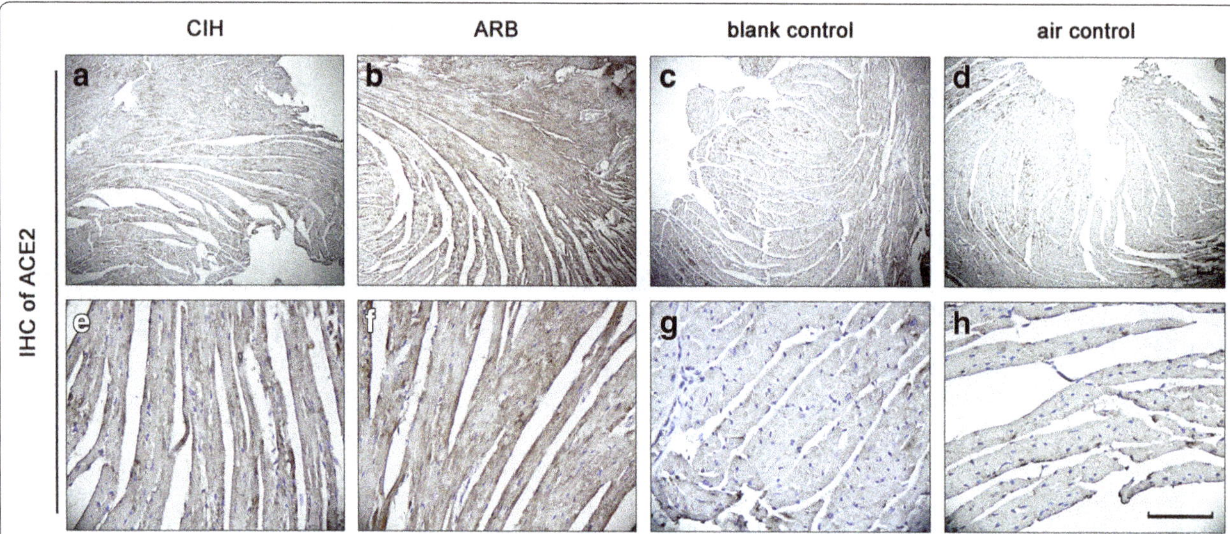

Fig. 3 ACE 2 staining in myocardial cells of mice from four experimental groups. **a** & **b**: CIH group; **c** & **d**:ARB group; **e** & **f**:blank control group; **g** & **h**: air control group. Immunohistochemistry was performed on the cardiac apex sections as described in Materials and methods. The expression level of cardiac ACE 2 was highest in ARB group followed by CIH group compared with the two control groups. Magnification: **a**, **c**, **e** and **g**: 100×; **b**, **d**, **f** and **h**: 400×. scale bar,100 μm

in the CIH group, however, the number of cristae was normal and well-arranged akin to that of the air and blank control groups. The changes under the electron microscope were closer to blank control and air control groups. Pathological changes were alleviated obviously in ARB group.

We also assessed apoptosis of myocardial cells of mice from these four groups with TUNEL assay. As shown in Fig. 8, while no significant difference in apoptotic rate of myocardial cells was observed between ARB group, blank control and air control groups, which are quantified and presented in Table 1. CIH had a significantly higher apoptotic rate compared with the other three experimental groups ($^{**}p < 0.001$). Thus, CIH impairs myocardial cells structure and increases myocardial cells and capillary endothelial cells apoptosis while these changes can be reversed with TERT treatment.

Discussion

SAS is closely linked to the development of cardiovascular disease, in which CIH plays an important role. In our experiment, each intermittent hypoxia cycle lasted approximately two minutes, mimicking 30 times intermittent hypoxia per hour, which was equivalent to severe SAS. Chen et al. [9] studied a CIH animal model and concluded that the lowest oxygen saturation was approximately 70%, equivalent to severe SAS. In another model, Song et al. [10] also demonstrated that, owing to the gas constant exchange in the box, there was no carbon dioxide accumulation. The partial pressure of carbon dioxide in the blood of mice had no correlation with the intermittent hypoxia cycle, which confirmed that the mice did not rebreathe. These findings eliminated the interference of carbon dioxide retention.

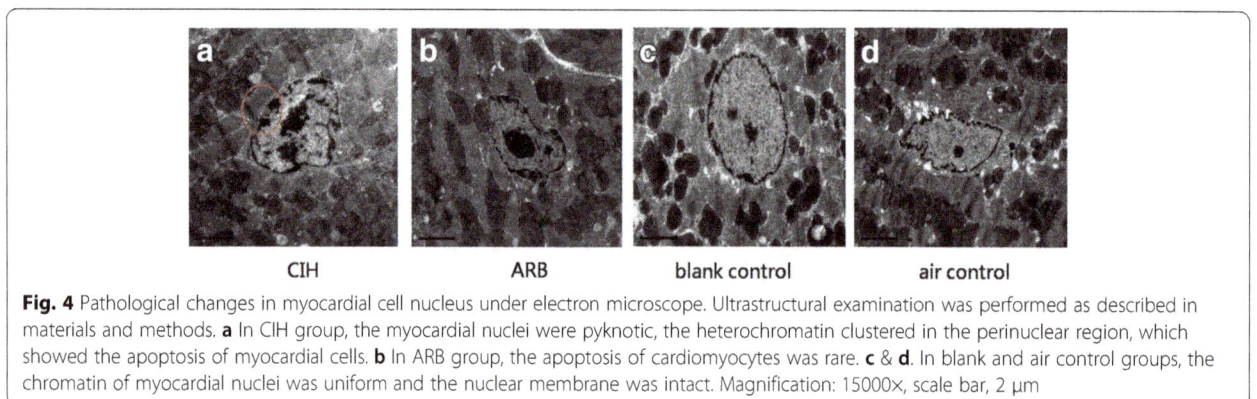

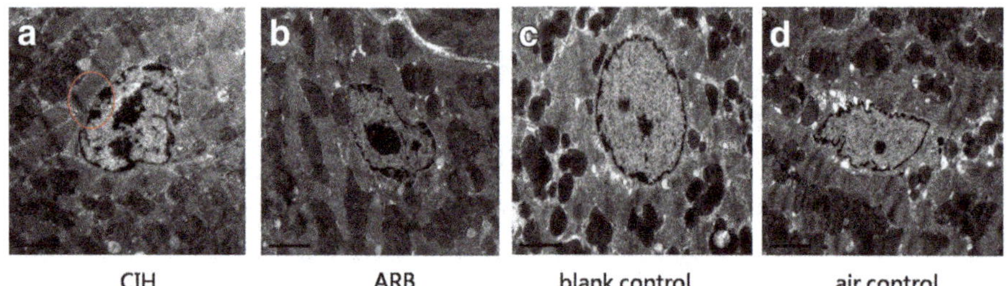

Fig. 4 Pathological changes in myocardial cell nucleus under electron microscope. Ultrastructural examination was performed as described in materials and methods. **a** In CIH group, the myocardial nuclei were pyknotic, the heterochromatin clustered in the perinuclear region, which showed the apoptosis of myocardial cells. **b** In ARB group, the apoptosis of cardiomyocytes was rare. **c** & **d**. In blank and air control groups, the chromatin of myocardial nuclei was uniform and the nuclear membrane was intact. Magnification: 15000×, scale bar, 2 μm

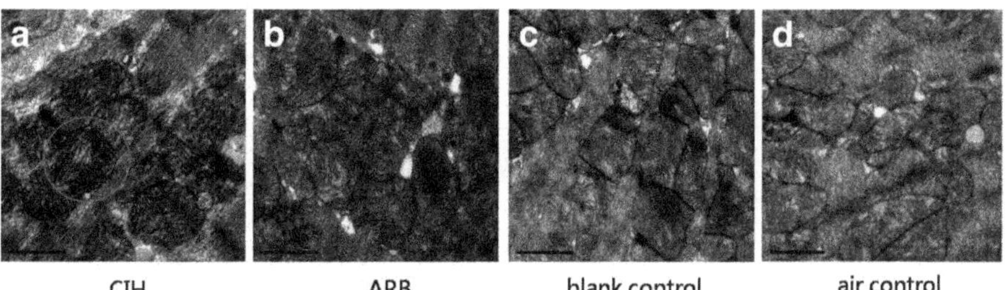

Fig. 5 Pathological changes in myocardial cell mitochondria under electron microscope. Ultrastructural examination was performed as described in materials and methods. **a** In CIH group the number of mitochondria decreased, the size was abnormal, the mitochondrial membrane was incomplete, the number of cristae was reduced, and the arrangement was disorder. The cristae were broken, dissolved, destroyed, flocculent, and the electron density of matrix increases. **b** In ARB group, the quantity and size of the mitochondrial are normal and the membrane is intact. The electron density of the mitochondrial matrix increased the same as CIH group while the number of cristae was normal and well arranged. **c** & **d** In blank and air control groups, the quantity and size of the mitochondrial are normal and the membrane is intact. The mitochondrial cristae were filled with the entire cavity of the mitochondrion and were arranged in parallel, regular and abundant in number. Magnification: 40000×, scale bar, 1 μm

CIH can stimulate hypoxic chemoreceptors in the carotid body, thus activating the systemic sympathetic nervous system and RAS [2], but how CIH affects local RAS and subsequently contributes to the development of CVD remains unknown. In our study, we found that ACE expression was highest in the CIH group (Fig. 1a, b), suggesting that CIH could facilitate the expression of ACE in mouse cardiac myocytes in vivo. ACE is the key enzyme of RAS and participates in the systemic and local effects of RAS through endocrine, autocrine and paracrine secretion. The most prominent physiological activity of ACE is to cleave Ang I to Ang II and inactivate bradykinin. Ang II is the product of ACE [11, 12], and ACE can damage the cardiovascular system through production of Ang II. Our study also demonstrated that Ang II expression was higher in the CIH group (Fig. 2a, b) than in the blank control and air control groups (Fig. 2e-h), indicating that CIH induced the expression of ACE and its product Ang II which is potentially implicated in CIH-linked CVD. AngII can act on the angiotensin type 1 receptor, and increase inflammation, oxidative stress, apoptosis, and cardiac remodeling, ultimately leading to heart failure. [13] As Ang II can up-regulate the expression of ACE [14], we believe that there was a positive feedback between Ang II and ACE.

ACE 2 is the homolog of ACE, which shares 42% sequence homology with ACE. The main function of ACE 2 is to cleave Ang I to Ang (1–9) and Ang II to Ang (1–7). The catalytic activity of cleaving Ang II to Ang (1–7) is 400 times higher than cleaving Ang I to Ang (1–9) [15]. Therefore, the main product of ACE 2 is Ang (1–7). Ang (1–7) exhibits anti-RAS activity, as well as functioning as a vasodilatation and anti-proliferative agent, suggesting that ACE 2 is the key enzyme in balancing the vasoconstrictive and proliferative effects of Ang II, as well as the anti-proliferative effect of Ang (1–7). In our study, we observed higher expression of ACE 2 in the myocardium of mice from CIH group (Fig. 3a, b) than that from blank and air control groups (Fig. 3e-h). Since increased ACE 2 levels offer benefits to cardiac structure and function, we speculate that CIH-induced expression of ACE 2 was an adaptive response. Indeed, Zhang R

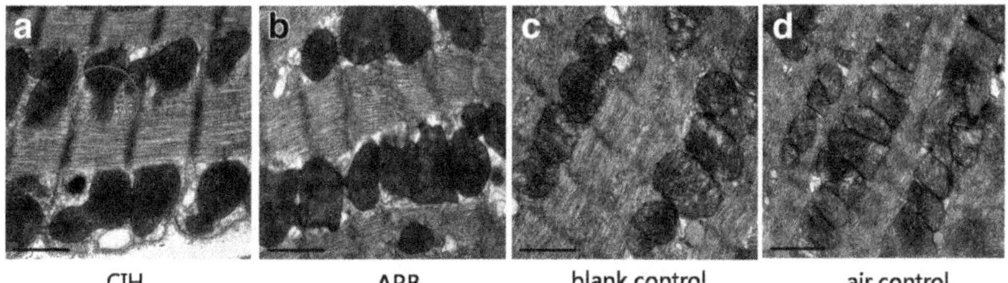

Fig. 6 Pathological changes in myocardial cell mitochondria and myoneme under electron microscope. Ultrastructural examination was performed as described in materials and methods. **a** In CIH group, the number of mitochondria decreased, the size was unequal and abnormal, the mitochondrial membrane was incomplete, and the electron density of matrix increased. **b** In ARB group, the electron density of the mitochondrial matrix increased the same as CIH group while the quantity and size of the mitochondria were normal and the membrane was intact. **c** & **d**. In blank and air control groups, the electron density of the mitochondrial matrix was nomal, the quantity and size of the mitochondria were normal and the membrane was intact. The coarse and fine filaments were well arranged and each band was clearly visible in four experimental groups (**a**-**d**). Magnification: 40000×, scale bar, 1 μm

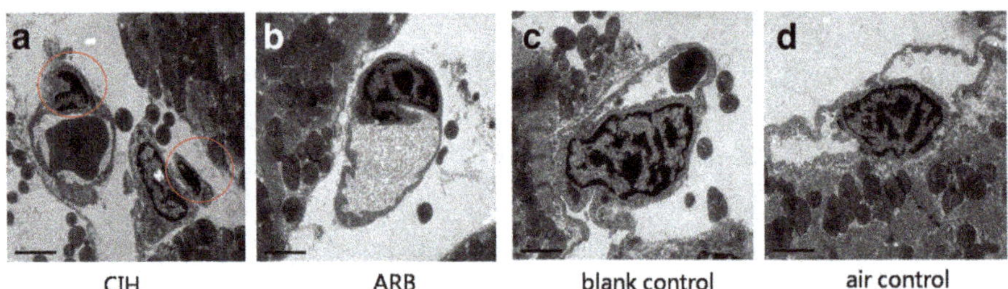

Fig. 7 Pathological changes in capillary endothelial cells under electron microscope. Ultrastructural examination was performed as described in materials and methods. Increased capillary endothelial cell apoptosis was observed in CIH group (**a**), which was rarely seen in ARB group (**b**), **c** & **d**. In blank and air control groups the chromatin of capillary endothelial cell was uniform and the nuclear membrane was intact. Magnification: 15000×, scale bar, 2 μm

[16] demonstrated that ACE 2 mRNA and protein expression increased in the early stages of hypoxia in pulmonary artery smooth muscle cells, but decreased at a later stage, which was accompanied by the accumulation of hypoxia inducible factor-1α (HIF-1α) and Ang II. Thus, it is possible that HIF-1α downregulates ACE 2 expression through Ang II. In our experiments, CIH lasted for 12 weeks, and ACE 2 expression remained higher in the CIH group than in blank and air control groups. Whether local accumulation of HIF-1α and Ang II at later hypoxic stages was responsible for the downregulation of ACE 2 remains unclear, and requires further study. This may include examining the correlation of the expression levels of myocardial ACE 2 with HIF1α and Ang II in hypoxic heart tissue for a prolonged CIH time more than 12 weeks.

In TUNEL assays, we also observed that myocardial cell apoptosis was the most severe in CIH group. Under

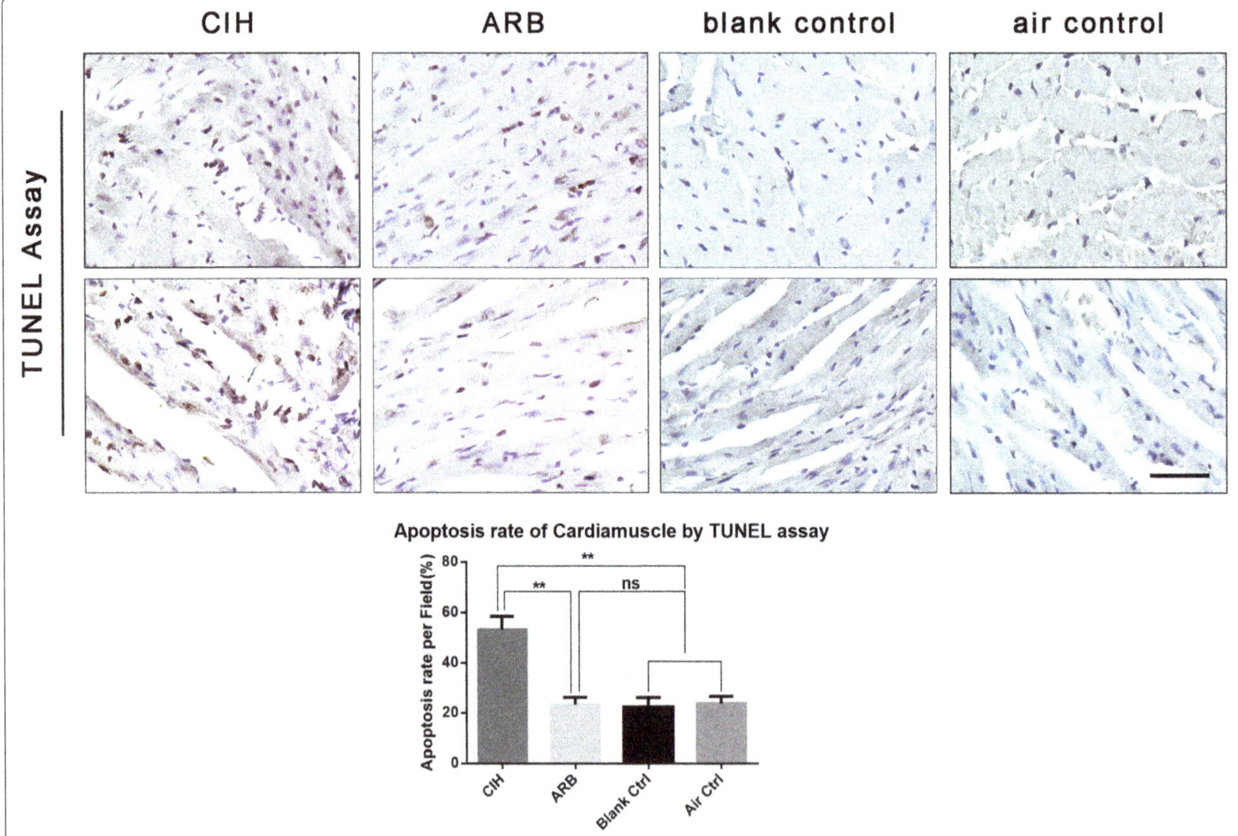

Fig. 8 Apoptotic rate of myocardial cells in four experimental groups. TUNEL staining was performed as described in materials and methods. CIH group exhibited the highest apoptotic rate compared with the other three experimental groups. **$p < 0.001$ vs. CIH group. Magnification: 400×, scale bar, 100 μm

electron microscopy, the apoptosis of cardiomyocyte and capillary endothelial cells were the most serious in CIH group. We also observed the ultrastructural changes of mitochondria and cristae, indicating that CIH can also cause mitochondrial damage. Chen et al. reported that the damage of CIH to mitochondria was related to myocardial apoptosis [17]. Mitochondrial damage is one of the primary mechanisms leading to apoptosis, and hyperactivity of RAS can produce apoptosis in early stages of cardiac disease [18]. Activated RAS can also exacerbate mitochondrial damage and increase apoptosis in endothelial cells, and mitochondria-ROS acts as a central regulator of RAS-mediated cell damage [19].We surmise that CIH can lead to myocardial damage by elevating the expression of ACE and Ang II, while the higher expression of ACE2 presents insufficiency of compensation.

Our study also showed that Ang II expression was highest in ARB group (Fig. 2c, d). ARBs can protect the cardiovascular system by blocking the activation of angiotensin type 1 receptor by Ang II, therefore, inhibit the negative feedback for the release of renin. Finally, ARBs increase renin, Ang I, Ang II and Ang (1–7) [20, 21]. Increased Ang II concentrations can interact with the angiotensin type 2 receptor. It is believed that this is mediated by bradykinin and nitric oxide (NO) [22], and the effect of this combination of mediators is both vasodilatory and anti-proliferative, which protects the cardiovascular system. Ang II has been shown to up-regulate the expression of ACE [14], which can be blocked by angiotensin type 1 receptor blocker (ARB) but not by angiotensin-2 receptor blockers, indicating that Ang II-induced expression of ACE was mainly achieved through angiotensin type 1 receptor- (AT-1) activation. In the present study, treatment with TERT, an ARB, reduced the level of ACE induced by CIH, which might alleviate the myocardial damage of CIH. Although this reduction did not reach statistical significance compared with the CIH group, maximal pharmacological effects of TERT were observed between four to eight treatment weeks, and we only treated mice with TERT for four weeks, which may account for this observation. Therefore, longer treatment with TERT is needed to further clarify if TERT could confer protection against CIH-induced cardiac injury via efficiently suppressing an increase in ACE.

In our study, we also observed that TERT treatment significantly elevated the expression of ACE 2 in the heart, suggesting that this may be one of the mechanisms by which TERT protects against hypoxia-induced heart injury. Previously, Koka et al. [14] showed that Ang II down-regulated ACE 2 expression in HK-2 cell line, which was blocked by the angiotensin type 1 receptor blocker losartan an extracellular signal-regulated kinase (ERK1/2) and p38 MAP kinase-specific antagonist, but not by the angiotensin type 2 receptor blocker PD123319, suggesting that Ang II suppressed ACE 2 expression through angiotensin type 1 receptor-ERK1/2 and p38 MAP kinase signaling. In the present study, Ang II expression in the hearts was increased in the CIH group, and this increase was further elevated by TERT treatment. These observations were in line with the TERT-induced increase in ACE 2. But increased Ang II expression did not suppress the expression of ACE 2 in mouse CIH hearts with TERT treatment, which was most likely due to the blockage of angiotensin type 1 receptor- by TERT.

Under electron microscopy and through TUNEL assay, we observed that the apoptosis of cardiomyocytes and capillary endothelial cells were rare in the ARB group. The ultrastructural changes of mitochondria and cristae induced by CIH were also alleviated by ARB treatment. We hypothesize that the blockade of the angiotensin type 1 receptor (AT1R) by ARB treatment can elevate the expression of ACE2, thus enhancing the protective effects of ACE 2 and alleviating the myocardial damage induced by ACE and AngII.

Furthermore, TERT, acting as an ARB, can block the effects of Ang II more thoroughly than ACEI, such as Ang II generated from chymotrypsin or other non-ACE pathways. Therefore, TERT may replace ACEI in long-term clinical use to avoid "AngII inhibition escape" phenomenon.

Conclusions

In conclusion, we demonstrate that CIH induces the expression of ACE and Ang II in mouse hearts which may impair cardiovascular function. CIH also increases the cardiac expression of ACE2, which may be a compensatory protection mechanism against CIH. TERT treatment further increased ACE 2 levels in myocardial cells but decreased ACE level, through blocking the interaction between Ang II and AT-1 receptor, impeding the effects of Ang II, thus conferring cardiac protection against CIH.

Abbreviations

ACE 2: angiotensin converting enzyme 2; ACE: angiotensin converting enzyme; Ang II: angiotensin II; ANOVA: analysis of variance; AT1R: Angiotensin type 1 receptor; CIH: Chronic intermittent hypoxia; CIH: chronic intermittent hypoxia; DAB: diaminobenzidine; MDA: malondialdehyde; RAS: renin-angiotensin system; SAS: sleep apnea syndromes; TERT': telmisartan; TUNEL: TdT-mediated dUTP nick end labeling

Authors' contribution

WW, AS, XC and YZ2 performed the research, WW, YS, YL, WL analyzed the data and wrote the manuscript, YZ1 designed the research study, contributed the animal model for the study and revised the manuscript. All authors Approval of the submitted and final versions.

Funding
2015 Innovative Project of Fujian Province supported by the Health and Family Planning Commission of Xiamen City, and Innovation Project of Medicine, Health, and Science & Technology (2015-CXB-36). The funder plays no role in the design of the study; the collection, analysis, and interpretation of data; or in writing the manuscript.

Competing interests
The authors declare that they have no competing interests.

Author details
[1]Pneumology Department of the First Affiliated Hospital of XiaMen University, The first clinical medical college of Fujian Medical University Teaching hospital of Fujian Medical University, Xiamen, China. [2]Pneumology Department of Wuxi Branch of Rijin Hospital affiliated to Shanghai jiaotong university medical college, Wuxi, China. [3]Department of Pulmonary and Critical Care Medicine of the Second Affiliated Hospital of Fujian Medical University, Sleep and Breathing Disorders Research Institute of Fujian Medical University, No.34 Zhongshan North Road, Licheng District, Quanzhou 362000, Fujian, China.

References

1. Somers VK, White DP, Amin R, Abraham WT, Costa F, Culebras A, Daniels S, Floras JS, Hunt CE, Olson LJ. Sleep apnea and cardiovascular disease: an American Heart Association/american college of cardiology foundation scientific statement from the American Heart Association Council for high blood pressure research professional education committee, council on clinical cardiology, stroke council, and council on cardiovascular nursing. In collaboration with the National Heart, Lung, and Blood Institute National Center on sleep disorders research (National Institutes of Health). Circulation. 2008;118:1080–111.
2. Rey S, Valdes G, Iturriaga R. Pathophysiology of obstructive sleep apnea-associated hypertension. Rev Med Chil. 2007;135:1333–42.
3. Patel SK, Velkoska E, Freeman M, Wai B, Lancefield TF, Burrell LM. From gene to protein-experimental and clinical studies of ACE2 in blood pressure control and arterial hypertension. Front Physiol. 2014;5:227.
4. Wang WY, Zeng YM, Chen XY, Zhang YX. Effect of Telmisartan on local cardiovascular oxidative stress in mouse under chronic intermittent hypoxia condition. Sleep Breath. 2013;17:181–7.
5. Yoo SM, Choi SH, Jung MD, Lim SC, Baek SH. Short-term use of telmisartan attenuates oxidation and improves Prdx2 expression more than antioxidant beta-blockers in the cardiovascular systems of spontaneously hypertensive rats. Hypertens Res. 2015;38:106–15.
6. Bakheit AH, Abd-Elgalil AA, Mustafa B, Haque A, Telmisartan WTA. Profiles of drug substances, excipients, and related methodology, vol. 40; 2015. p. 371–429.
7. Chen XP, Qian LR. The vasodilatory action of telmisartan on isolated mesenteric artery rings from rats. Iranian J Basic Med Sci. 2015;18:974–8.
8. Nagai N, Oike Y, Noda K, Urano T, Kubota Y, Ozawa Y, Shinoda H, Koto T, Shinoda K, Inoue M. Suppression of ocular inflammation in endotoxin-induced uveitis by blocking the angiotensin II type 1 receptor. Invest Ophthalmol Vis Sci. 2005;46:2925–31.
9. Chen XY, Zeng YM, Hunag ZY, Tao G, Zheng XZ, Li YJ. Effect of chronic intermittent hypoxia on hypoxia inducible factor-1alpha in mice. Zhonghua Jie He He Hu Xi Za Zhi. 2005;28(2):93–6.
10. Song AL, Zeng YM, CHEN XY. The chronic hypoxia / reoxygenation mice model. International journal of respiratory. Diseases. 2006;26:408–11.
11. Kramkowski K, Mogielnicki A, Buczko W. The physiological significance of the alternative pathways of angiotensin II production. J Physiol Pharmacol. 2006;57:529–39.
12. Igase M, Kohara K, Nagai T, Miki T, Ferrario CM. Increased expression of angiotensin converting enzyme 2 in conjunction with reduction of neointima by angiotensin II type 1 receptor blockade. Hypertens Res. 2008; 31:553–9.
13. Xu J, Carretero OA, Liao TD, Peng H, Shesely EG, Xu J, Liu TS, Yang JJ, Reudelhuber TL, Yang XP. Local angiotensin II aggravates cardiac remodeling in hypertension. Am J Physiol Heart Circ Physiol. 2010;299: H1328–38.
14. Koka V, Huang XR, Chung AC, Wang W, Truong LD, Lan HY. Angiotensin II up-regulates angiotensin I-converting enzyme (ACE), but down-regulates ACE2 via the AT1-ERK/p38 MAP kinase pathway. Am J Pathol. 2008;172: 1174–83.
15. Zhong Y, Li JF. ANG (1- 7) and its protective effects in hypertension. Chinese J Cardiovasc Dis Res. 2008;6:702–6.
16. Zhang R, Wu Y, Zhao M, Liu C, Zhou L, Shen S, Liao S, Yang K, Li Q, Wan H. Role of HIF-1alpha in the regulation ACE and ACE2 expression in hypoxic human pulmonary artery smooth muscle cells. Am J Physiol Lung Cell Mol Physiol. 2009;297:L631–40.
17. Zeng YM, Cheng XY, Huang ZY, Song AL. Effect of hypoxia/ reoxygenationon the ultrastructure of mice cardiomyocytes and kidney. Fudan University. J Med Sci. 2006;33:84–8.
18. Velez Rueda JO, Palomeque J, Mattiazzi A. Early apoptosis in different models of cardiac hypertrophy induced by high renin-angiotensin system activity involves CaMKII. Journal of Applied Physiol (Bethesda, Md : 1985). 2012;112:2110–20.
19. Chen F, Chen B, Xiao FQ, Wu YT, Wang RH, Sun ZW, Fu GS, Mou Y, Tao W, Hu XS. Autophagy protects against senescence and apoptosis via the RAS-mitochondria in high-glucose-induced endothelial cells. Cell Physiol Biochem. 2014;33:1058–74.
20. Ferrario CM, Trask AJ, Jessup JA. Advances in biochemical and functional roles of angiotensin-converting enzyme 2 and angiotensin-(1-7) in regulation of cardiovascular function. Am J Physiol Heart Circ Physiol. 2005; 289:H2281–90.
21. Ferrario CM, Jessup J, Chappell MC, Averill DB, Brosnihan KB, Tallant EA, Diz DI, Gallagher PE. Effect of angiotensin-converting enzyme inhibition and angiotensin II receptor blockers on cardiac angiotensin-converting enzyme 2. Circulation. 2005;111:2605–10.
22. Johren O, Dendorfer A, Dominiak P. Cardiovascular and renal function of angiotensin II type-2 receptors. Cardiovasc Res. 2004;62:460–7.

17

Value of the fT3/fT4 ratio and its combination with the GRACE risk score in predicting the prognosis in euthyroid patients with acute myocardial infarction undergoing percutaneous coronary intervention: a prospective cohort study

Tongtong Yu, Chunyang Tian, Jia Song, Dongxu He, Jiake Wu, Zongyu Wen, Zhijun Sun and Zhaoqing Sun*

Abstract

Background: Thyroid hormones deeply influence the cardiovascular system; however, the association between the fT3/fT4 ratio and the clinical outcome in euthyroid patients with acute myocardial infarction (AMI) undergoing percutaneous coronary intervention (PCI) is not well defined. Therefore, the present study aimed to assess the prognostic performance of the fT3/fT4 ratio in predicting the long-term prognosis in euthyroid patients with AMI undergoing PCI.

Methods: In a prospective cohort study with a 1-year follow-up, according to the clinical end point, 953 euthyroid individuals (61.0 ± 11.6; female, 25.8%) were divided into two groups: (1) the survival group ($n = 915$) and (2) the death group ($n = 38$).

Results: According to Cox regression multivariate analysis, fT4 (HR: 1.249, 95% CI: 1.053–1.480, $p = 0.010$) and the fT3/fT4 ratio (HR: 3.546, 95% CI: 1.705–7.377, $p = 0.001$) were associated with an increased risk of 1-year all-cause mortality. The prognostic performance of the fT3/fT4 ratio was similar to the Global Registry of Acute Coronary Events (GRACE) score in predicting 1-year all-cause mortality (C-statistic: $z = 0.261$, $p = 0.794$; IDI: -0.017, $p = 0.452$; NRI: -0.049, $p = 0.766$), but better than fT4 (C-statistic: $z = 2.438$, $p = 0.015$; IDI: 0.053, $p = 0.002$; NRI: 0.656, $p < 0.001$). The fT3/fT4 ratio also significantly improved the prognostic performance of the GRACE score (GRACE score vs GRACE score + fT3/fT4 ratio: C-statistic: $z = 2.116$, $p = 0.034$; IDI: 0.0415, $p = 0.007$; NRI: 0.614, $p < 0.001$).

Conclusions: In euthyroid patients with AMI undergoing PCI, the fT3/fT4 ratio was an independent predictor of 1-year all-cause mortality. Its prognostic performance was similar to the GRACE score, and also improved its prognostic performance (GRACE score vs GRACE score + fT3/fT4 ratio).

Keywords: fT3/fT4 ratio, GRACE risk score, Acute myocardial infarction, Percutaneous coronary intervention

* Correspondence: sunzhaoqing@vip.163.com
Department of Cardiology, Shengjing Hospital of China Medical University, Shenyang, Liaoning, People's Republic of China

Background

Despite the use of novel treatment strategies, patients with acute myocardial infarction (AMI) still suffer from an adverse prognosis [1]. Attention should still focus on revealing novel treatment targets and important risk factors. In AMI, serum triiodothyronine (T3) is decreased [2–5], while serum thyroxine (T4) remains almost unchanged [2–4] or declines [5]. In fact, the cardiovascular system is the foremost target of thyroid hormones, and is adversely affected even if these hormone levels only change slightly [6]. A decrease in serum T3 has been found to be a predictor of larger myocardial injury size [4, 5, 7], worse cardiac function [8, 9], greater thrombus burden [10], and a poorer prognosis [5, 11–14] in AMI. A recent study also confirmed the association between free T4 and adverse outcomes in acute coronary syndrome [15]. Serum T3, which is the most important bioactive thyroid hormone for cardiomyocytes, is mostly produced by the peripheral process of deiodination of T4 [6]. In AMI, the studies have suggested that the peripheral conversion of T4 into T3 was reduced [3, 4]. However, no previous study has focused on the clinical value of the disturbance of the conversion of T4 into T3 in patients with AMI. The fT3/fT4 ratio, a thyroid hormone index, could reflect deiodinase activity [16], and thus, represent the conversion of T4 to T3 [17]. The Global Registry of Acute Coronary Events (GRACE) score is widely recommended to calculate in-hospital and long-term mortality in acute coronary syndrome (ACS), which helps clinical decision-making and discriminates high-risk patients [18–22]. The GRACE score has passed rigorous validation since its conception in 2004; however, several changes has been approved in the diagnostic and management tools of ACS in the last 14 years. Moreover, the estimation of risk is a continuous process, and further refinement of current risk scores may help the decision-making process in real world practice. Furthermore, novel risk factors are not included in the GRACE score, such as thyroid hormone-related indicators including thyrotropin, fT3, fT4 and the fT3/fT4 ratio.

In the present study, we aimed to assess whether the fT3/fT4 ratio is a useful clinical parameter in predicting long-term prognosis in euthyroid patients with AMI undergoing PCI. In addition, we compared the prognostic performance of fT3, fT4, and the fT3/fT4 ratio using the GRACE score as the reference standard. Moreover, we confirmed whether fT3, fT4, and the fT3/fT4 ratio could improve the prognostic performance of the GRACE score.

Methods

Study design and setting

The present study was based on a prospective cohort. From January 1st 2015 to July 31st 2016, 1195 consecutive patients with AMI were hospitalized and underwent successful PCI at a large-scale hospital in Northeast China (Shengjing Hospital of China Medical University, Shenyang, China). AMI included non-ST-segment elevation myocardial infarction (NSTEMI) and ST-segment elevation myocardial infarction (STEMI). NSTEMI is defined as chest discomfort or anginal equivalent, ST-segment depression, transitory ST-segment elevation or prominent T-wave inversion, and positive cardiac biomarkers (CKMB, T/I troponin) [18–21]. STEMI is defined as chest pain and significant ST-segment elevation (≥ 0.1 mV in at least 2 standard leads or ≥ 0.2 mV in at least 2 contiguous precordial leads) or new left bundle branch block [18–21]. PCI was performed in accordance with current guidelines [18–21]. The duration of dual antiplatelet therapy was at least 12 months [18–21, 23]. Clinical and procedural data from all cases were collected by the investigators from electronic medical records. On admission, venous blood samples were drawn in standard tubes at room temperature, rapidly centrifuged, and the levels of thyrotropin (TSH), free T3 (fT3), and free T4 (fT4) were measured using a completely automated immunoassay analyzer (i2000, Abbott, USA) in the core laboratory of Shengjing Hospital. The reference intervals of our laboratory were as follows: TSH, 0.3–4.8 uIu/mL; fT3, 2.63–5.71 pmol/L; and fT4, 9.01–19.05 pmol/L. Patients with circulating levels of TSH, fT3, and fT4 all in the reference range were defined as euthyroid. Prospective clinical follow-up after discharge was performed regularly in all cases by direct hospital visits and telephone interviews with the patient's general practitioner/cardiologist, the patient, or the patient's family. All events were adjudicated and classified by two cardiologists. Exclusion criteria included: (1) no thyroid or GRACE score data (13 cases); (2) primary hypothyroidism or hyperthyroidism (27 cases); (3) subhypothyroidism or subhyperthyroidism or low T3 syndrome (132 cases); (4) any other abnormal thyroid status (43 cases); (5) concomitant treatment with synthetic thyroid hormones, antithyroid drugs, corticosteroids, dopamine, dobutamine, or amiodarone (7 cases); or (6) loss of follow-up (20 cases). Finally, the present study included 953 euthyroid patients with AMI undergoing PCI, all of whom underwent a 1-year follow-up. The clinical endpoint of the study was 1-year all-cause mortality. All patients were divided into two groups: (1) the survival group (n = 915, 96.0%) and (2) the death group (n = 38, 4.0%). The present study complies with the Declaration of Helsinki; and Shengjing Hospital of China Medical University Research Ethics Committee approved the research protocol. Written informed consent was formally obtained from all participants.

Statistical analysis

The cumulative event rate was estimated from Kaplan-Meier curves and compared using the log-rank test.

The Cox proportional-hazards regression model was used to analyze the effects of the variables on event-free survival. The variables that showed significance in univariate analysis (Table 1, $p < 0.1$) entered the final model. Results are reported as hazard ratios (HRs) with associated 95% confidence intervals (CIs). The predictive performance of fT3, fT4, the fT3/fT4 ratio, and the GRACE score was assessed by indices of discrimination (C-statistic). As continuous variables, the predictive performance of the GRACE score, the GRACE score + fT3, the GRACE score + fT4, and the GRACE score + the fT3/fT4 ratio was assessed by indices of discrimination (C-statistic), calibration (the Hosmer–Lemeshow (HL) test and Nagelkerke–R^2), and

Table 1 Baseline Characteristics of the study population, median (IQR), or N (%), or means±SD

Variable	All Patients (*n* = 953)	Survival Group (*n* = 915)	Death Group (*n* = 38)	*p* value
Demographics				
Age, yrs	61.0 ± 11.6	60.8 ± 11.6	67.6 ± 10.6	<0.001
Female	246 (25.8)	231 (25.2)	15 (39.5)	0.050
Medical history				
History of Diabetes Mellitus	281 (29.5)	269 (29.4)	12 (31.6)	0.773
History of Hypertension	533 (55.9)	502 (54.9)	31 (81.6)	0.001
History of MI	107 (11.2)	102 (11.1)	5 (13.2)	0.701
Prior PCI	90 (9.4)	89 (9.7)	1 (2.6)	0.143
Presentation				
Killip class III/IV on admission	19 (2.0)	11 (1.2)	8 (30.0)	<0.001
SBP on admission, mm Hg	134.4 ± 22.7	134.3 ± 22.6	138.5 ± 26.2	0.259
Heart rate on admission, bpm	76.6 ± 14.7	76.2 ± 14.3	86.4 ± 20.4	<0.001
GRACE score	127.7 ± 32.2	126.5 ± 31.6	158.0 ± 32.7	<0.001
Diagnosis on admission				0.573
STEMI	519 (54.5)	500 (54.6)	19 (50.0)	
NSTEMI	434 (45.5)	415 (45.4)	19 (50.0)	
Troponin-I on admission, ng/mL	4.06 (0.38, 31.77)	4.04 (0.37, 32.07)	5.31 (0.67, 25.01)	0.870
Creatinine on admission, umol/l	72 (61, 86)	72 (61, 86)	81 (62, 107)	0.090
Albumin on admission, g/L	39.4 ± 3.6	39.5 ± 3.5	37.5 ± 4.2	0.001
TSH, uIU/mL	1.546 ± 0.961	1.549 ± 0.965	1.485 ± 0.853	0.687
fT3, pmol/L	3.902 ± 0.588	3.913 ± 0.581	3.659 ± 0.694	0.009
fT4, pmol/L	13.11 ± 1.84	13.08 ± 1.82	14.02 ± 2.20	0.002
fT3/ fT4 ratio	0.302 ± 0.055	0.304 ± 0.054	0.262 ± 0.058	<0.001
Percutaneous coronary intervention details				
Left main disease	75 (7.9)	71 (7.8)	4 (10.5)	0.535
Three-vessel disease	242 (25.4)	232 (25.4)	10 (26.3)	0.894
TIMI flow grade 0/1 on arrival	741 (77.8)	714 (78.0)	27 (71.1)	0.311
TIMI flow grade 3 post PCI	947 (99.4)	910 (99.5)	37 (97.4)	0.111
Medical treatment at discharge				
Aspirin	950 (99.7)	912 (99.7)	38 (100)	0.724
Clopidogrel	865 (90.8)	830 (90.7)	35 (92.1)	0.771
Ticagrelor	75 (7.9)	72 (7.9)	3 (7.9)	0.995
Statin	943 (99.0)	905 (98.9)	38 (100)	0.517
ACEI/ARB	510 (53.5)	490 (53.6)	20 (52.6)	0.911
Beta-blockers	481 (50.5)	461 (50.4)	20 (52.6)	0.786

MI myocardial infarction, *PCI* percutaneous coronary intervention, *SBP* systolic blood pressure, *bpm* beats per minute, *STEMI* ST-segment elevation myocardial infarction, *NSTEMI* non-ST-segment elevation myocardial infarction, *TSH* thyrotropin, *fT3* free triiodothyronine, *fT4* free thyroxine, *ACEI/ARB* Angiotensin-converting enzyme inhibitors / Angiotensin receptor blockers

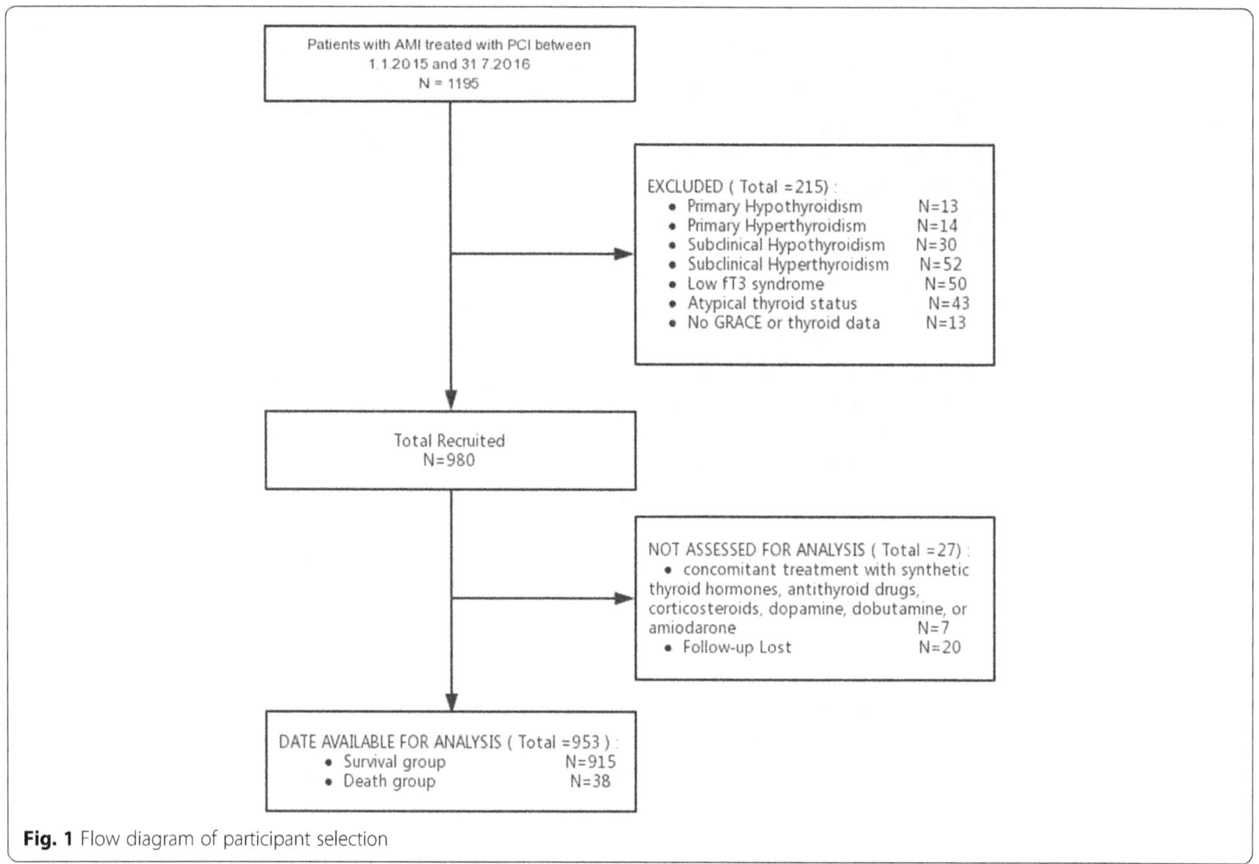

Fig. 1 Flow diagram of participant selection

precision (Brier scores). The C-statistic was compared using a nonparametric test developed by DeLong et al. [24]. Each model was entered into a logistic regression model to obtain the individual risk probability of all-cause death. The HL test and the Nagelkerke–R^2 from the regression model was used as an indicator of the goodness-of-fit of each risk model and to assess their calibration ability [25]. As continuous variables, Brier scores of the fT3 + GRACE, fT4 + GRACE, fT3/fT4 ratio + GRACE, and GRACE scores were also calculated [26]. Moreover, we used absolute integrated discrimination improvement (IDI) and category-free net reclassification improvement (NRI) to evaluate improvements in risk prediction quantitation of the fT3 + GRACE, fT4 + GRACE, fT3/fT4 ratio + GRACE, and GRACE scores as continuous variables [27]. All tests were two-sided, and the statistical significance is defined as $p < 0.05$. All statistical analyses were performed using the Statistical Analysis System version 9.4 (SAS, SAS Institute Inc., Cary, North Carolina, USA).

Results

Baseline characteristics

Figure 1 represents the flowchart of patient selection. The final study cohort consisted of 953 euthyroid patients with AMI undergoing PCI. The cohort was divided into two groups: (1) the survival group (915

Table 2 Effects of multiple variables on Clinical Outcomes in Univariate and Multivariate Analysis

	Univariate Analysis			Multivariate Analysis		
	HR	95% CI	*p* value	HR	95% CI	*p* value
TSH (per 1 uIU/mL increase)	0.930	0.660–1.311	0.680			
fT3 (per 1 pmol/L decrease)	2.154	1.207–3.842	0.009	0.887	0.463–1.700	0.718 [a]
fT4 (per 1 pmol/L increase)	1.282	1.095–1.499	0.002	1.249	1.053–1.480	0.010 [a]
fT3/fT4 ratio (per 0.1 unit decrease)	6.742	3.534–12.859	<0.001	3.546	1.705–7.377	0.001 [a]

[a]Adjusted for age, gender, history of hypertension, Killip class III/IV on admission, Heart rate on admission, creatinine on admission, albumin on admission

Table 3 C-statistic of different parameters for clinical outcomes prediction

	C-statistic	95% CI	*p* value
fT3	0.631	0.600–0.662	0.006
fT4	0.624	0.592–0.655	0.010
fT3/fT4 ratio	0.738	0.709–0.766	<0.001
GRACE	0.755	0.727–0.782	<0.001

patients (96.0%)) and (2) the death group (38 patients (4.0%)). The clinical characteristics of the two groups are shown in Table 1. Patients in the death group were older and had a significantly higher heart rate on admission, GRACE score, albumin on admission, and fT4; and a lower fT3 and fT3/fT4 ratio, as compared with those in the survival group (Table 1). The rates of hypertension and Killip class III/IV on admission were significantly higher in the death group (Table 1).

Prognostic performance of different thyroid hormone-related indicators in prognosis prediction

The univariate analysis revealed that fT3, fT4, and fT3/fT4 ratio, but not TSH, were associated with 1-year all-cause mortality (Table 2). In Cox regression multivariate analysis, fT4 and the fT3/fT4 ratio remained associated with 1-year all-cause mortality; 24.9% per pmol/L increase in fT4 concentration (HR: 1.249, 95% CI: 1.053–1.480, $p = 0.010$) and a 2.546-fold per 0.1 unit decrease in the fT3/fT4 ratio (HR: 3.546, 95% CI: 1.705–7.377, $p = 0.001$) (Table 2).

The C-statistic of fT3, fT4, the fT3/fT4 ratio, and the GRACE score in predicting all-cause mortality was 0.631 (95% CI: 0.600–0.662), 0.624 (95% CI: 0.592–0.655), 0.738 (95% CI: 0.709–0.766), and 0.755 (95% CI: 0.727–0.782), respectively (Table 3 and Fig. 2). The cut-off values for fT3, fT4, and the fT3/fT4 ratio were: 3.685 with a sensitivity of 0.605 and a specificity of 0.632; 14.21 with a sensitivity of 0.500 and a specificity of 0.748; and 0.255 with a sensitivity of 0.632 and a specificity of 0.820, respectively.

Based on the cut-off value for fT3, the cohort was divided into two groups: the high fT3 group (fT3 > 3.685 pmol/L, $n = 593$) and the low fT3 group (fT3 ≤ 3.685 pmol/L, $n = 360$. The unadjusted Kaplan-Meier estimate for all-cause mortality was significantly higher in the low fT3 group as compared with the high fT3 group (all-cause mortality: 6.4% vs 2.5%, $p = 0.003$) (Fig. 3a). Based on the cut-off value for fT4, the cohort was divided into two groups: the high fT4 group (fT4 ≥ 14.21 pmol/L, $n = 250$) and the low fT4 group (fT4 < 14.21 pmol/L, $n = 703$). The unadjusted Kaplan-Meier estimate for all-cause mortality was

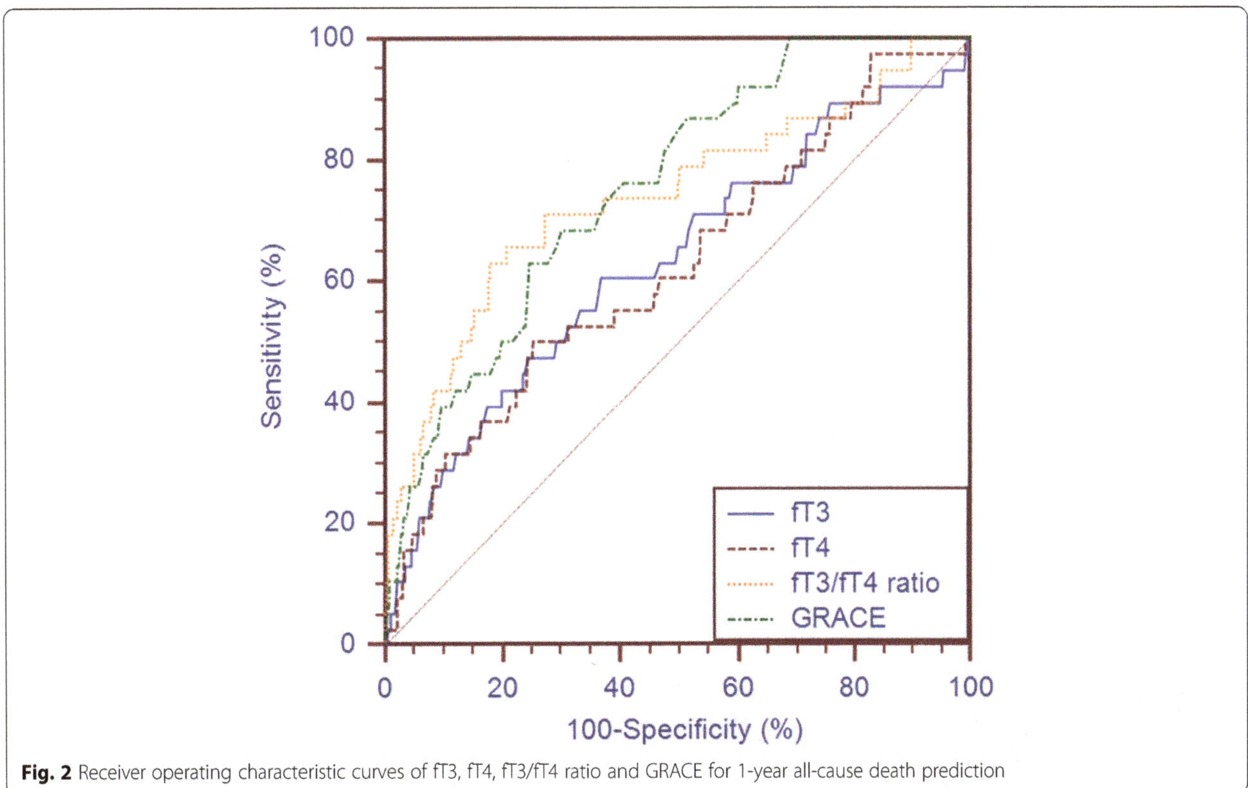

Fig. 2 Receiver operating characteristic curves of fT3, fT4, fT3/fT4 ratio and GRACE for 1-year all-cause death prediction

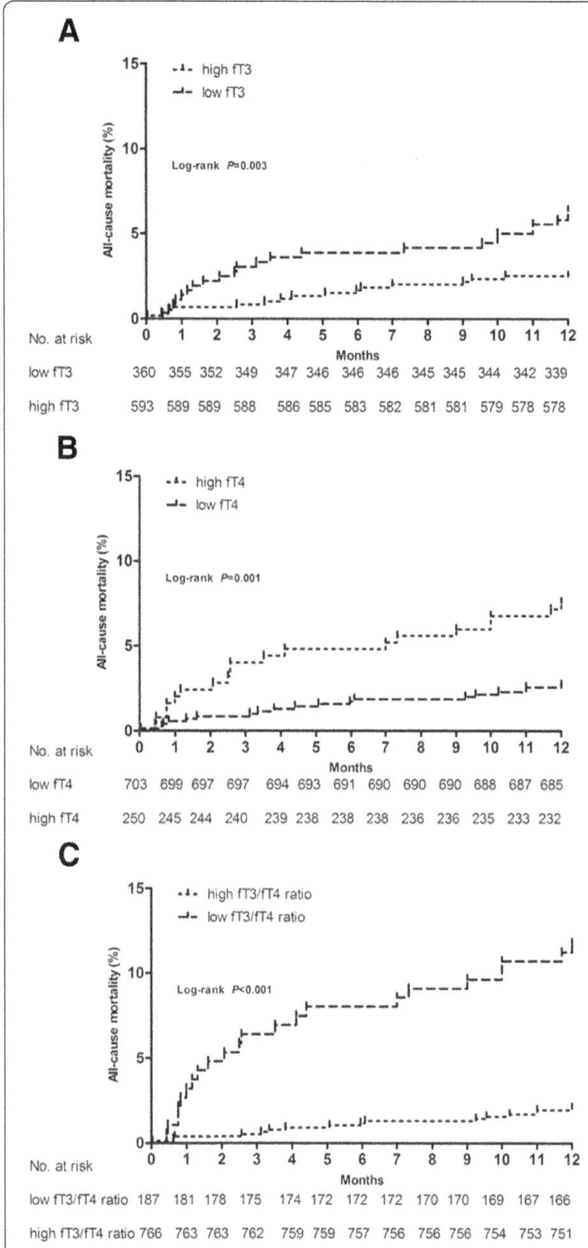

Fig. 3 Kaplan-Meier survival curves for 1-year all-cause death by the cut off values for (**a**) fT3, **b** fT4 and (**c**) fT3/fT4 ratio (high fT3 group: fT3>3.685 pmol/L and low fT3 group: fT3 ≤ 3.685 pmol/L; high fT4 group: fT4 ≥ 14.21 pmol/L and low fT4 group: fT4<14.21 pmol/L; high fT3/fT4 ratio group: fT3/fT4 ratio>0.255 and low fT3/fT4 ratio group: fT3/fT4 ratio ≤ 0.255)

significantly higher in the high fT4 group as compared with the low fT4 group (all-cause mortality: 7.6% vs 2.7%, $p = 0.001$) (Fig. 3b). Based on the cut-off value for the fT3/fT4 ratio, the cohort was divided into two groups: the high fT3/fT4 ratio group (fT3/fT4 ratio > 0.255, $n = 766$) and the low fT3/fT4 ratio group (fT3/fT4 ratio ≤ 0.255, $n = 187$). The unadjusted Kaplan-Meier estimate for all-cause mortality was significantly higher in the low fT3/fT4 ratio group as compared with the high fT3/fT4 ratio group (all-cause mortality: 11.8% vs 2.1%, $p < 0.001$) (Fig. 3c).

Comparison of the prognostic performance of fT3, fT4, the fT3/fT4 ratio, and the GRACE score in prognosis prediction

The prognostic performance of the fT3/fT4 ratio was similar to that of the GRACE score in predicting 1-year all-cause mortality (C-statistic: $z = 0.261$, $p = 0.794$; IDI: -0.017, $p = 0.452$; NRI: -0.049, $p = 0.766$), but better than that of fT3 (C-statistic: $z = 2.062$, $p = 0.039$; IDI: 0.056, $p = 0.001$; NRI: 0.625, $p < 0.001$) and fT4 (C-statistic: $z = 2.438$, $p = 0.015$; IDI: 0.053, $p = 0.002$; NRI: 0.656, $p < 0.001$) (Table 4).

Improvement in the prognostic performance of the GRACE score when combined with thyroid hormone-related indicators

The C-statistic of the GRACE score, the GRACE score + fT3, the GRACE score + fT4, and the GRACE score + the fT3/fT4 ratio in predicting all-cause mortality was 0.755 (95% CI: 0.727–0.782), 0.765 (95% CI: 0.736–0.791), 0.775 (95% CI: 0.747–0.801), and 0.836 (95% CI: 0.811–0.859), respectively (Table 5 and Fig. 4). Among the four models, the HL p-value of the GRACE score was the highest; the Nagelkerke-R^2 of the GRACE score + the fT3/fT4 ratio was the highest; and the Brier score of the GRACE score + the fT3/fT4 ratio was the lowest (Table 5). However, only the new model in which the GRACE score was combined with the fT3/fT4 ratio improved the prognostic performance, which was better than that of the GRACE score (C-statistic: $z = 2.116$, $p = 0.034$; IDI: 0.0415, $p = 0.007$; NRI: 0.614, $p < 0.001$). In contrast, the prognostic performance of the GRACE score + fT3 and the GRACE score + fT4 was similar to that of the GRACE score (C-statistic: $z = 0.608$, $p = 0.543$; IDI: 0.0047, $p = 0.277$; NRI: 0.198, $p = 0.231$; C-statistic: $z = 1.078$, $p = 0.281$; IDI: 0.0095, $p = 0.142$; NRI: 0.243, $p = 0.141$, respectively) (Table 6).

Discussion

The present study tested the association between the fT3/fT4 ratio and the long-term prognosis in euthyroid patients with AMI undergoing PCI. The main findings were as follows: (1) the fT3/fT4 ratio was an independent predictor of 1-year all-cause mortality; (2) the prognostic performance of the fT3/fT4 ratio was similar to that of the GRACE score, and better than that of fT3 and fT4; and (3) only the fT3/fT4 ratio could improve the prognostic performance of the original GRACE score model.

Table 4 Comparisons of the predictive performance of fT3, fT4, fT3/fT4 ratio and GRACE for the prognosis prediction

	z for C-statistic	*p* for C-statistic	NRI	*p* for NRI	IDI	*p* for IDI
fT3 vs. fT3/fT4 ratio	2.062	0.039	0.625	<0.001	0.056	0.001
fT4 vs. fT3/fT4 ratio	2.438	0.015	0.656	<0.001	0.053	0.002
GRACE vs. fT3/fT4 ratio	0.261	0.794	-0.049	0.766	-0.017	0.452
fT3 vs. GRACE	2.013	0.044	0.594	<0.001	0.039	0.005
fT4 vs. GRACE	2.202	0.028	0.531	0.001	0.036	0.011
fT3 vs. fT4	0.117	0.907	−0.075	0.649	−0.002	0.677

Thyroid hormones extensively affect the physiological and pathological processes of the cardiovascular system [6]. Previous studies have demonstrated that even mild thyroid dysfunction in cardiac patients results in an adverse prognosis: subclinical hypothyroidism is a strong indicator of atherosclerosis risk [28, 29]; subclinical hyperthyroidism is associated with an increased risk of atrial fibrillation [30]; a mildly altered thyroid status (including subclinical hypothyroidism, subclinical hyperthyroidism, and low T3 syndrome) is also associated with an increased risk of mortality in patients with cardiac disease [14, 31–33]. T3 and T4 are two main iodinated hormones secreted by the thyroid gland. Since the affinity of the thyroid hormone receptors is far higher for T3 than for T4, T3 is considered the biologically active hormone, and T4 must be converted to T3 to produce potent thyroid hormone receptormediated effects [6]. Less than 20% of circulating T3 is directly secreted by the thyroid gland, while more than 80% is produced by a peripheral process of deiodination of T4 [6]. Thus, the conversion of T4 to T3 is very important in the production of circulating T3 and the thyroid hormone action on the heart. In chronic and acute illness, this conversion has been reported to decline [3, 4, 34]. Furthermore, a disturbance in the conversion of T4 to T3 contributes to reduced T3 production in low T3 syndrome and its etiology [16, 34, 35]. Previous studies have demonstrated that the fT3/fT4 ratio could reflect deiodinase activity [16], and thus, represent the conversion of T4 to T3 [17]. A significant correlation between the fT3/fT4 ratio and infarct size has been observed [4]; however, no study has focused on the clinical value of a disturbance in the conversion of T4 to T3 in AMI patients. The present study demonstrates that in euthyroid patients with AMI undergoing PCI, the fT3/fT4 ratio was associated with 1-year all-cause mortality (all-cause mortality for low the fT3/fT4 ratio group vs the high fT3/fT4 ratio group: 11.8% vs 2.1%, *log-rank* test: $p < 0.001$). The results of Cox regression multivariate analysis further confirmed that a reduction in the fT3/fT4 ratio was associated with a 2.546-fold greater likelihood of 1-year all-cause death. The discriminative performance of the fT3/fT4 ratio was encouraging (C-statistic: 0.738; 95% CI: 0.709–0.766), far better than that of fT3 and fT4, and similar to that of the GRACE score in predicting 1-year all-cause mortality in euthyroid patients with AMI undergoing PCI. Taken together, the fT3/fT4 ratio is a very useful clinical parameter in predicting long-term prognosis in euthyroid patients with AMI undergoing PCI, can help risk stratification in AMI patients, and identify those patients at high risk of 1-year all-cause death. Therefore, the fT3/fT4 ratio may be taken as a better risk factor for AMI; however, further large cohort studies are needed in this regard.

The GRACE score, containing the main traditional risk factors for cardiovascular disease, was derived in the early twenty-first century. Since then, increasing amounts of novel risk factors have been studied; nevertheless, the GRACE score does not contain any of these new risk factors such as thyroid hormone-related indicators, including thyrotropin, fT3, fT4, and the fT3/fT4 ratio [6]. The present study found that the fT3/fT4 ratio was a valid adjunct to the GRACE score. The new model, the GRACE score + the fT3/fT4 ratio, showed good discrimination (C-statistic: 0.836), calibration (HL *p*-value: 0.180, R^2: 0.157), and precision (Brier score: 0.0348). The prognostic

Table 5 GRACE, GRACE+ fT3/fT4 ratio, GRACE+ fT3 and GRACE+ fT4 performance for the prognosis prediction

	Discrimination				Calibration		Precision
	C-statistic	Standard error	*p* value	95% CI	HL *p*-Value	R^2	Brier Score
GRACE	0.755	0.0364	<0.001	0.727–0.782	0.337	0.119	0.0366
GRACE+ fT3/fT4 ratio	0.836	0.0286	<0.001	0.811–0.859	0.180	0.157	0.0348
GRACE+ fT3	0.765	0.0359	<0.001	0.736–0.791	0.185	0.090	0.0364
GRACE+ fT4	0.775	0.0358	<0.001	0.747–0.801	0.029	0.101	0.0362

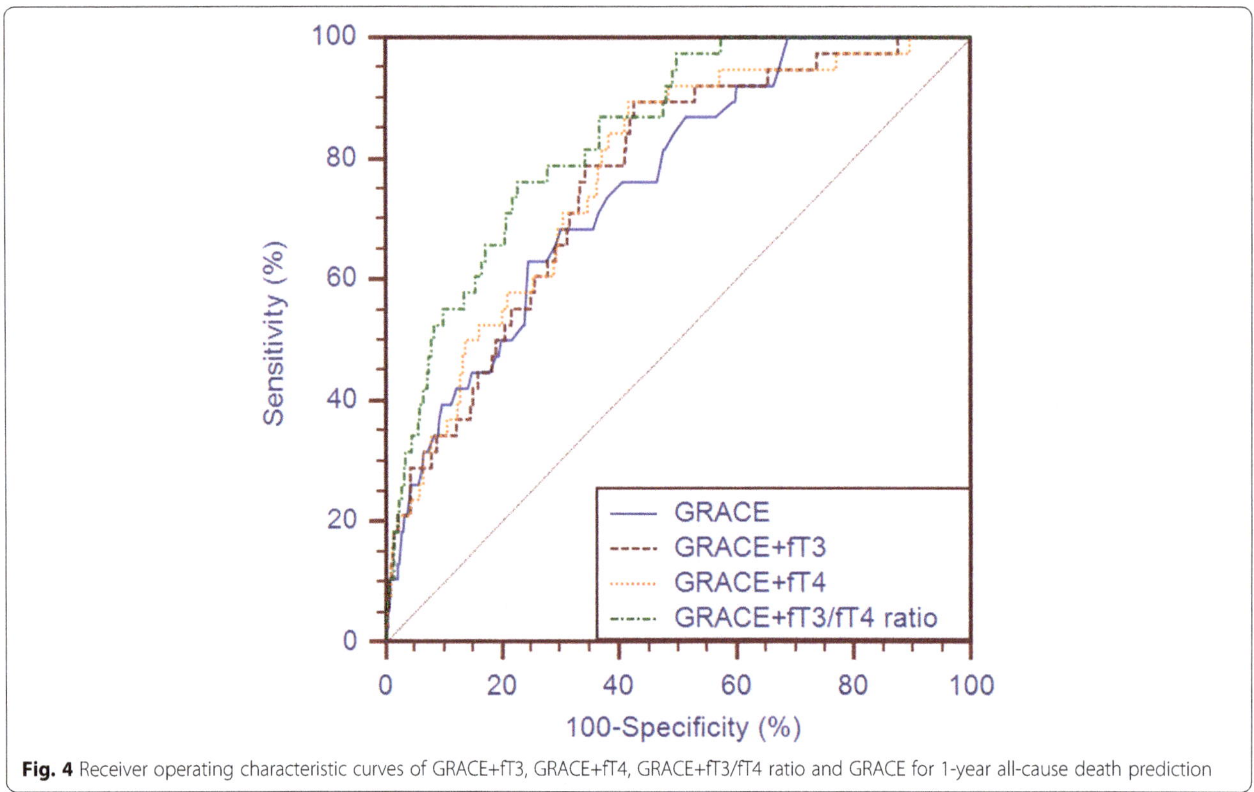

Fig. 4 Receiver operating characteristic curves of GRACE+fT3, GRACE+fT4, GRACE+fT3/fT4 ratio and GRACE for 1-year all-cause death prediction

performance of the new model was also better than that of the original model (only the GRACE score). In clinical practice, the new model, the GRACE score combined with the fT3/fT4 ratio, can also help make a more accurate assessment of the long-term mortality risk and more precise clinical decisions.

The present study has several limitations. Firstly, this was a single center, observational study; thus, potential confounders and selection bias could not be completely adjusted, since some important clinical data were collected from electronic medical records. However, it has the advantage of being a prospective study. Secondly, thyroid function tests were not repeated within 2–12 weeks to exclude transient forms of thyroid dysfunction as recommended by the guidelines [36], at euthyroid diagnosis. Thirdly, previous studies have indicated that iodinated contrast media may influence thyroid function [37, 38]; however, in the present study, the thyroid function of some patients was tested following the use of iodinated contrast media, since they needed emergency PCI. Fourthly, the present study did not test total T3 (TT3) and total T4 (TT4) levels, since only free T3 and free T4 can enter target cells and play a role, directly reflecting the state of thyroid function [6]. Fifthly, previous studies have found that reverse T3 increased in AMI [2–5], and that increased levels of reverse T3 were also independently associated with 1-year mortality [39]; however, the present study did not test reverse T3 (rT3). In the future, other studies should be performed to obtain the association between prognosis and more thyroid hormone-related indicators including TSH, TT3, TT4, fT3, fT4, rT3, and the fT3/fT4 ratio. Finally, the present study only included AMI patients in whom successful PCI was performed; thus, the results cannot be generalized to all ACS patients.

Conclusion

In euthyroid patients with AMI undergoing PCI, the fT3/fT4 ratio was an independent predictor of 1-year all-cause mortality, and could also significantly improve the prognostic performance of the GRACE score.

Table 6 Comparisons of the predictive performance of GRACE, GRACE+ fT3/fT4 ratio, GRACE+ fT3 and GRACE+ fT4 for the prognosis prediction

	z for C-statistic	*p* for C-statistic	NRI	*p* for NRI	IDI	*p* for IDI
GRACE vs. GRACE+ fT3/fT4 ratio	2.116	0.034	0.614	<0.001	0.0415	0.007
GRACE vs. GRACE+ fT3	0.608	0.543	0.198	0.231	0.0047	0.277
GRACE vs. GRACE+ fT4	1.078	0.281	0.243	0.141	0.0095	0.142

Abbreviations

ACEI/ARB: Angiotensin-converting enzyme inhibitors / Angiotensin receptor blockers; ACS: Acute coronary syndrome; AMI: Acute myocardial infarction; bpm: Beats per minute; CI: Confidence interval; fT3: Free serum triiodothyronine; fT4: Thyroxine; GRACE score: Global Registry of Acute Coronary Events score; HL: Hosmer-Lemeshow; HR: Hazard ratio; IDI: Integrated discrimination improvement; NRI: Net reclassification improvement; NSTEMI: Non-ST-segment elevation myocardial infarction; PCI: Percutaneous coronary intervention; SBP: Systolic blood pressure; STEMI: ST-segment elevation myocardial infarction; TSH: Thyrotropin

Acknowledgments

Thank Prof. Liqiang Zheng for his statistical assistance! He ensured that the statistical analyses in our manuscript were carried out correctly.

Funding

This research project was supported by grants from the Social Development Research Program of Liaoning Province (2011225020). It funded the collection of data and a revision of the written English.

Authors' contributions

ZS conceived and designed the experiments. TY, JS, DH, JW, ZW and CT performed the experiments. TY analyzed the data and wrote the paper. ZJS revised the paper. All authors have reviewed and agreed on the contents of this paper.

Competing interests

The authors declare that they have no competing interests.

References

1. Eapen ZJ, Tang WH, Felker GM, Hernandez AF, Mahaffey KW, Lincoff AM, et al. Defining heart failure end points in ST-segment elevation myocardial infarction trials: integrating past experiences to chart a path forward. Circ Cardiovasc Qual Outcomes. 2012;5(4):594–600.
2. Eber B, Schumacher M, Langsteger W, Zweiker R, Fruhwald FM, Pokan R, et al. Changes in thyroid hormone parameters after acute myocardial infarction. Cardiology. 1995;86(2):152–6.
3. Westgren U, Burger A, Levin K, Melander A, Nilsson G, Pettersson U. Divergent changes of serum 3,5,3'-triiodothyronine and 3,3',5'-triiodothyronine in patients with acute myocardial infarction. Acta Med Scand. 1977;201(4):269–72.
4. Smith SJ, Bos G, Gerbrandy J, Docter R, Visser TJ, Hennemann G. Lowering of serum 3,3',5-triiodothyronine thyroxine ratio in patients with myocardial infarction; relationship with extent of tissue injury. Eur J Clin Investig. 1978; 8(2):99–102.
5. Friberg L, Werner S, Eggertsen G, Ahnve S. Rapid down-regulation of thyroid hormones in acute myocardial infarction: is it cardioprotective in patients with angina? Arch Intern Med. 2002;162(12):1388–94.
6. Jabbar A, Pingitore A, Pearce SH, Zaman A, Iervasi G, Razvi S. Thyroid hormones and cardiovascular disease. Nat Rev Cardiol. 2017;14(1):39–55.
7. Kim DH, Choi DH, Kim HW, Choi SW, Kim BB, Chung JW, et al. Prediction of infarct severity from triiodothyronine levels in patients with ST-elevation myocardial infarction. Korean J Intern Med. 2014;29(4):454–65.
8. Lymvaios I, Mourouzis I, Cokkinos DV, Dimopoulos MA, Toumanidis ST, Pantos C. Thyroid hormone and recovery of cardiac function in patients with acute myocardial infarction: a strong association? Eur J Endocrinol. 2011;165(1):107–14.
9. Jankauskienė E, Orda P, Barauskienė G, Mickuvienė N, Brožaitienė J, Vaškelytė JJ, et al. Relationship between left ventricular mechanics and low free triiodothyronine levels after myocardial infarction: a prospective study. Intern Emerg Med. 2016;11(3):391–8.
10. Viswanathan G, Balasubramaniam K, Hardy R, Marshall S, Zaman A, Razvi S. Blood thrombogenicity is independently associated with serum TSH levels in post-non-ST elevation acute coronary syndrome. J Clin Endocrinol Metab. 2014;99(6):e1050–4.
11. Zhang B, Peng W, Wang C, Li W, Xu Y. A low fT3 level as a prognostic marker in patients with acute myocardial infarctions. Intern Med. 2012; 51(21):3009–15.
12. Özcan KS, Osmonov D, Toprak E, Güngör B, Tatlısu A, Ekmekçi A, et al. Sick euthyroid syndrome is associated with poor prognosis in patients with ST segment elevation myocardial infarction undergoing primary percutaneous intervention. Cardiol J. 2014;21(3):238–44.
13. Kang MG, Hahm JR, Kim KH, Park HW, Koh JS, Hwang SJ, et al. Prognostic value of total triiodothyronine and free thyroxine levels for the heart failure in patients with acute myocardial infarction. Korean J Intern Med. 2018; 33(3):512–21.
14. Wang B, Liu S, Li L, Yao Q, Song R, Shao X, et al. Non-thyroidal illness syndrome in patients with cardiovascular diseases: a systematic review and meta-analysis. Int J Cardiol. 2017;226:1–10.
15. Brozaitiene J, Mickuviene N, Podlipskyte A, Burkauskas J, Bunevicius R. Relationship and prognostic importance of thyroid hormone and N-terminal pro-B-type natriuretic peptide for patients after acute coronary syndromes: a longitudinal observational study. BMC Cardiovasc Disord. 2016;16:45.
16. Maia AL, Kim BW, Huang SA, Harney JW, Larsen PR. Type 2 iodothyronine deiodinase is the major source of plasma T3 in euthyroid humans. J Clin Invest. 2005;115(9):2524–33.
17. Itoh S, Yamaba Y, Oda T, Kawagoe K. Serum thyroid hormone, triiodothyronine, thyroxine, and triiodothyronine/thyroxine ratio in patients with fulminant, acute, and chronic hepatitis. Am J Gastroenterol. 1986;81(6):444–9.
18. Amsterdam EA, Wenger NK, Brindis RG, Casey DE Jr, Ganiats TG, Holmes DR Jr, et al. 2014 AHA/ACC guideline for the Management of Patients with non-ST-elevation acute coronary syndromes: a report of the American College of Cardiology/American Heart Association task force on practice guidelines. J Am Coll Cardiol. 2014;64(24):e139–228.
19. American College of Emergency Physicians; Society for Cardiovascular Angiography and Interventions, O'Gara PT, Kushner FG, Ascheim DD, Casey DE Jr, Chung MK, de Lemos JA, et al. 2013 ACCF/AHA guideline for the management of ST-elevation myocardial infarction: a report of the American College of Cardiology Foundation/American Heart Association task force on practice guidelines. J Am Coll Cardiol. 2013;61(4):e78–e140.
20. Roffi M, Patrono C, Collet JP, Mueller C, Valgimigli M, Andreotti F, et al. 2015 ESC guidelines for the management of acute coronary syndromes in patients presenting without persistent ST-segment elevation: task force for the Management of Acute Coronary Syndromes in patients presenting without persistent ST-segment elevation of the European Society of Cardiology (ESC). Eur Heart J. 2016;37(3):267–315.
21. Task Force on the management of ST-segment elevation acute myocardial infarction of the European Society of Cardiology (ESC), Steg PG, James SK, Atar D, Badano LP, Blömstrom-Lundqvist C, Borger MA, et al. ESC guidelines for the management of acute myocardial infarction in patients presenting with ST-segment elevation. Eur Heart J. 2012;33(20):2569–619.
22. Eagle KA, Lim MJ, Dabbous OH, Pieper KS, Goldberg RJ, Van de Werf F, et al. GRACE investigators. A validated prediction model for all forms of acute coronary syndrome: estimating the risk of 6-month postdischarge death in an international registry. JAMA. 2004;291(22):2727–33.
23. D'Ascenzo F, Moretti C, Bianco M, Bernardi A, Taha S, Cerrato E, et al. Meta-analysis of the duration of dual antiplatelet therapy in patients treated with second-generation drug-eluting stents. Am J Cardiol. 2016;117(11):1714–23.
24. DeLong ER, DeLong DM, Clarke-Pearson DL. Comparing the areas under two or more correlated receiver operating characteristic curves: a nonparametric approach. Biometrics. 1988;44(3):837–45.

25. Lemeshow S, Hosmer DW Jr. A review of goodness of fit statistics for use in the development of logistic regression models. Am J Epidemiol. 1982; 115(1):92–106.
26. Redelmeier DA, Bloch DA, Hickam DH. Assessing predictive accuracy: how to compare brier scores. J Clin Epidemiol. 1991;44(11):1141–6.
27. Pencina MJ, D'Agostino RB Sr, D'Agostino RB Jr, Vasan RS. Evaluating the added predictive ability of a new marker: from area under the ROC curve to reclassification and beyond. Stat Med. 2008;27(2):157–72. discussion 207–12
28. Hak AE, Pols HA, Visser TJ, Drexhage HA, Hofman A, Witteman JC. Subclinical hypothyroidism is an independent risk factor for atherosclerosis and myocardial infarction in elderly women: the Rotterdam study. Ann Intern Med. 2000;132(4):270–8.
29. Rodondi N, Aujesky D, Vittinghoff E, Cornuz J, Bauer DC. Subclinical hypothyroidism and the risk of coronary heart disease: a meta-analysis. Am J Med. 2006;119(7):541–51.
30. Cappola AR, Fried LP, Arnold AM, Danese MD, Kuller LH, Burke GL, et al. Thyroid status, cardiovascular risk, and mortality in older adults. JAMA. 2006; 295(9):1033–41.
31. Iervasi G, Pingitore A, Landi P, Raciti M, Ripoli A, Scarlattini M, et al. Low-T3 syndrome: a strong prognostic predictor of death in patients with heart disease. Circulation. 2003;107(5):708–13.
32. Iervasi G, Molinaro S, Landi P, Taddei MC, Galli E, Mariani F, et al. Association between increased mortality and mild thyroid dysfunction in cardiac patients. Arch Intern Med. 2007;167(14):1526–32.
33. Zhang M, Sara JD, Matsuzawa Y, Gharib H, Bell MR, Gulati R, et al. Clinical outcomes of patients with hypothyroidism undergoing percutaneous coronary intervention. Eur Heart J. 2016;37(26):2055–65.
34. Carter JN, Eastmen CJ, Corcoran JM, Lazarus L. Inhibition of conversion of thyroxine to triiodothyronine in patients with severe chronic illness. Clin Endocrinol. 1976;5(6):587–94.
35. Yu J, Koenig RJ. Regulation of hepatocyte thyroxine 5′-deiodinase by T3 and nuclear receptor coactivators as a model of the sick euthyroid syndrome. J Biol Chem. 2000;275(49):38296–301.
36. LeFevre ML. U.S. preventive services task force. Screening for thyroid dysfunction: U.S. preventive services task force recommendation statement. Ann Intern Med. 2015;162(9):641–50.
37. Gartner W, Weissel M. Do iodine-containing contrast media induce clinically relevant changes in thyroid function parameters of euthyroid patients within the first week? Thyroid. 2004;14(7):521–4.
38. van der Molen AJ, Thomsen HS, Morcos SK. Contrast media safety committee, European Society of Urogenital Radiology (ESUR). Effect of iodinated contrast media on thyroid function in adults. Eur Radiol. 2004; 14(5):902–7.
39. Friberg L, Drvota V, Bjelak AH, Eggertsen G, Ahnve S. Association between increased levels of reverse triiodothyronine and mortality after acute myocardial infarction. Am J Med. 2001;111(9):699–703.

18

Factors associated with door-in to door-out delays among ST-segment elevation myocardial infarction (STEMI) patients transferred for primary percutaneous coronary intervention: a population-based cohort study in Ontario, Canada

Oumin Shi[1,2*], Anam M. Khan[2], Mohammad R. Rezai[2], Cynthia A. Jackevicius[2,3,5], Jafna Cox[8], Clare L. Atzema[2,7], Dennis T. Ko[2,4,5], Thérèse A. Stukel[2,5], Laurie J. Lambert[9], Madhu K. Natarajan[6], Zhi-jie Zheng[1] and Jack V. Tu[2,4,5]

Abstract

Background: Compared to ST-segment elevation myocardial infarction (STEMI) patients who present at centres with catheterization facilities, those transferred for primary percutaneous coronary intervention (PCI) have substantially longer door-in to door-out (DIDO) times, where DIDO is defined as the time interval from arrival at a non-PCI hospital, to transfer to a PCI hospital. We aimed to identify potentially modifiable factors to improve DIDO times in Ontario, Canada and to assess the impact of DIDO times on 30-day mortality.

Methods: A population-based, retrospective cohort study of 966 STEMI patients transferred for primary PCI in Ontario in 2012 was conducted. Baseline factors were examined across timely DIDO status. Multivariate logistic regression was used to examine independent predictors of timely DIDO as well as the association between DIDO times and 30-day mortality.

Results: The median DIDO time was 55 min, with 20.1% of patients achieving the recommended DIDO benchmark of ≤30 min. Age ($OR_{>75 \text{ vs } 18-55}$ 0.30, 95% CI: 0.16–0.56), symptom-to-first medical contact (FMC) time ($OR_{61\text{-}120mins \text{ vs } <60mins}$ 0.60, 95% CI: 0.39–0.90; $OR_{>120mins \text{ vs } <60mins}$ 0.53, 95% CI:0.35–0.81) and emergency medical services transport with a pre-hospital electrocardiogram (ECG) ($OR_{EMS \text{ transport} + ECG \text{ vs self-transport}}$ 2.63, 95% CI:1.59–4.35) were the strongest predictors of timely DIDO. Patients with timely ECG were more likely to have recommended DIDO times (33.0% vs 12.3%; $P < 0.001$). A significantly higher proportion of those who met the DIDO benchmark had timely FMC-to-balloon times (78.7% vs 27.4%; $P < 0.001$). Compared to patients with DIDO time ≤ 30 min, those with DIDO times > 90 min had significantly higher adjusted 30-day mortality rates (OR 2.82, 95% CI:1.10–7.19).

(Continued on next page)

* Correspondence: somking214@alumni.sjtu.edu.cn
[1]School of Public Health, Shanghai Jiaotong University School of Medicine, South Chongqing Road No, Shanghai 227, China
[2]Institute for Clinical Evaluative Sciences, G1 06, 2075 Bayview Avenue, Toronto, ON, Canada
Full list of author information is available at the end of the article

(Continued from previous page)

Conclusions: While benchmark DIDO times were still rarely achieved in the province, we identified several potentially modifiable factors in the STEMI system that might be targeted to improve DIDO times. Our findings that patients who received a pre-hospital ECG were still being transferred to non-PCI capable centres suggest strategies addressing this gap may improve patient outcomes.

Keywords: ST-segment elevation myocardial infarction (STEMI), Primary percutaneous coronary intervention (PCI), Door-in to door-out (DIDO), Pre-hospital electrocardiogram (ECG), Mortality

Background

For patients with ST-Elevation myocardial infarction (STEMI), time-to-treatment is an important modifiable determinant of survival [1, 2]. Timely primary percutaneous coronary intervention (PCI) is considered the preferred method of reperfusion compared to fibrinolytic therapy, given its lower STEMI mortality rate [3]. However, about 25% of Canadian residents do not live within a one-hour drive of a PCI-capable centre and often have to be transferred from a non-PCI capable (referral) hospital [4]. Consequent lengthening in receipt of PCI therapy has a demonstrably negative impact on clinical outcomes [5, 6].

Delays in providing timely reperfusion therapy can occur at several points along the treatment pathway but take place frequently at the referral hospital [7, 8]. Guidelines for STEMI recommend that the time between arrival to, and transfer from a referral hospital to a PCI-capable hospital, also referred to as the door-in-door-out (DIDO) time, should be ≤30 min, and has been widely adopted as an important metric for quality of STEMI care [1, 9]. However, several studies have noted that this benchmark is rarely achieved [7, 8, 10–12].

In light of this, there is a clear need to develop new strategies or refine pre-existing ones that are responsible for prolonged DIDO times. One such suggestion is having emergency medical services (EMS) personnel administer a 12-lead electrocardiogram (ECG) prior to arrival at the hospital (pre-hospital ECG) for patients suspected of having a STEMI, although the impact on reducing DIDO times has not been well studied [13].

Utilizing a population-based cohort of STEMI patients in Ontario, Canada, we aimed to identify potentially modifiable factors to improve DIDO time. A secondary objective was to examine the impact of DIDO times on 30-day mortality rates adjusted for important confounders. Our findings could have important public health and policy implications, providing 'real world' evidence for areas in the STEMI system that should be targeted for improvement.

Methods

Data sources

The Ontario portion of the Canadian Institute for Health Information (CIHI) Discharge Abstract Database (DAD) and National Ambulatory Care Reporting System (NACRS) were used to identify all patients who were hospitalized or presented to an emergency department (ED) for a STEMI event in calendar year 2012. Detailed information on patients was obtained from their medical charts which were abstracted by trained cardiology nurses hired by the research team. Abstracted data included patient characteristics at baseline, key time variables, presenting information and information on the patient transport process. The data were securely transmitted electronically to a database housed at the Institute for Clinical Evaluative Sciences (ICES) in Toronto, Ontario. Given the low-risk nature of this study, Ontario privacy laws allow waivers of informed consent to abstract the data [14, 15].

Mortality information was obtained through linkage, utilizing encoded health card numbers, to the Registered Persons Database (RPDB). The RPDB contains socio-demographic and date of death information on all Ontario residents eligible for the Ontario Health Insurance Plan.

Study population

Figure 1 details the creation of the study cohort. International Classification of Diseases, tenth revision codes (Table S1 in the Data Supplement [see Additional file 1]) were used to identify 6631 patients who had a recorded STEMI event in administrative data. A random sample of ~ 50% of the patients in each health region, termed a Local Health Integration Network (LHIN), had their charts abstracted, affording us a representative sample of patients for use in the study. Based on chart reviews, individuals who did not meet the clinical criteria for a STEMI event or were determined to have had an in-hospital STEMI were further excluded. Among 3133 STEMI patients with abstracted charts, we focused on the 1616 patients (51.6%) who initially presented to a referral hospital and thus excluded those who were transported directly to a PCI-capable centre or who were discharged home or died in the first hospital. For the purpose of this study, in which timeliness of DIDO for primary PCI was examined, we further excluded those who received fibrinolytic therapy at the first hospital or were missing information on the variables required to

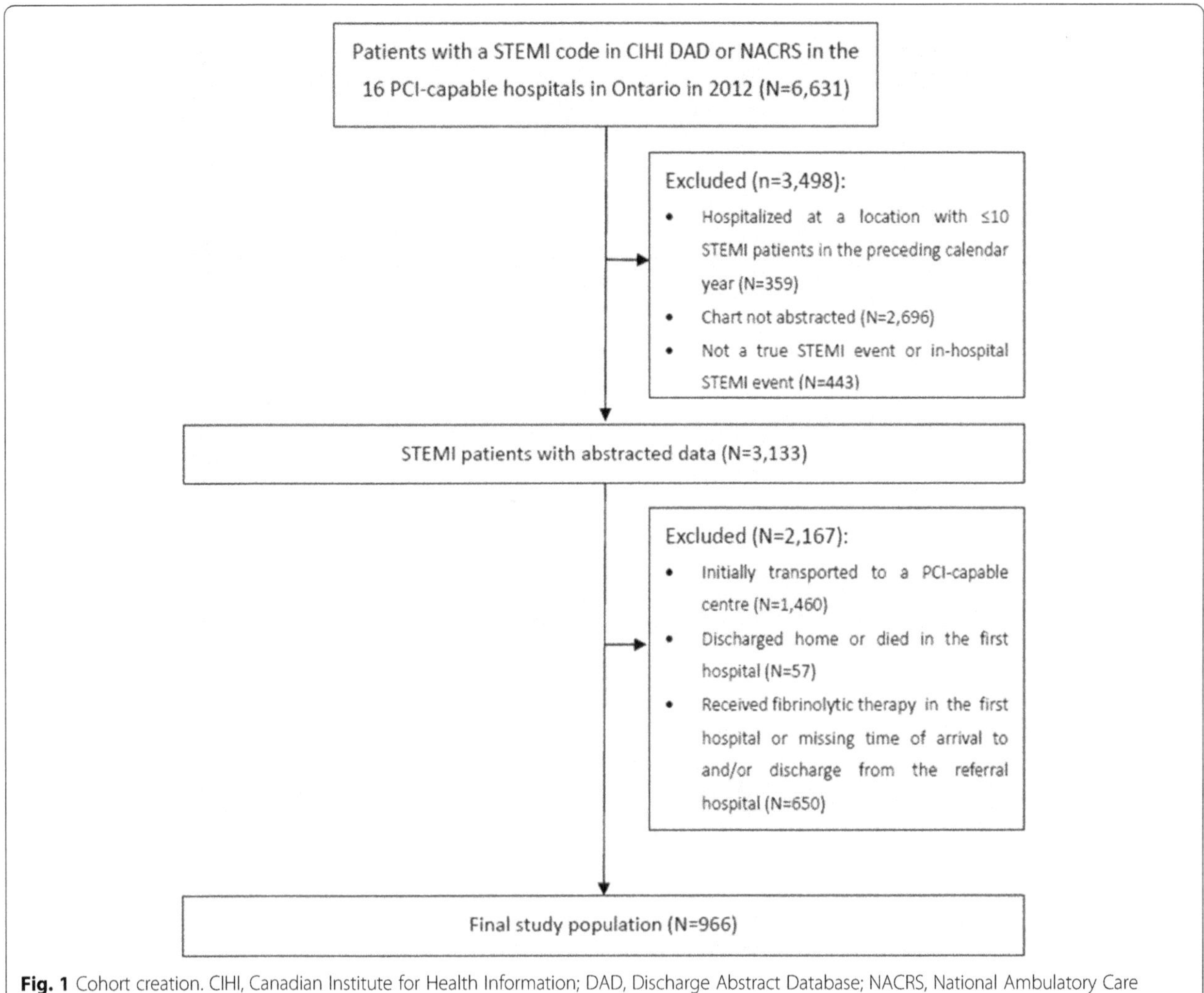

Fig. 1 Cohort creation. CIHI, Canadian Institute for Health Information; DAD, Discharge Abstract Database; NACRS, National Ambulatory Care Reporting System; PCI, percutaneous coronary intervention; STEMI, ST-segment elevation myocardial infarction

compute DIDO time, creating the final study population of 966 patients.

Process of care and clinical outcome definitions

We assessed several important process of care measures along the STEMI treatment pathway. Where appropriate, benchmarks were selected to be consistent with published Canadian and American guidelines for STEMI care [1, 9, 13, 16]. Details on the operationalization of the measures and their associated benchmarks can be found in Table S2 of the Data Supplement [see Additional file 1].

Our primary clinical outcome of interest was all-cause 30-day mortality, defined as death due to any cause within 30 days of the primary PCI procedure.

Statistical analyses

Baseline patient and process of care measures were examined across timely DIDO status. The proportion of those achieving timely DIDO who also met the benchmark first medical contact (FMC)-to-balloon time of ≤120 min was also examined.

The median durations of process of care indicators comprising the total symptom-to-reperfusion time were compared amongst those who were transported by EMS but did not receive a pre-hospital ECG, transported by EMS and received a pre-hospital ECG and those who transported themselves to hospital.

Generalized estimating equation (GEE) multivariate logistic regression was used to compute odds ratios and corresponding 95% confidence intervals (CI) to identify baseline characteristics independently associated with a DIDO time ≤ 30 min [17]. GEE models were used to account for clustering at the LHIN level given that patients residing in the same LHIN may be similarly affected by health system factors which effect STEMI care (e.g., regional STEMI networks) [13]. A similar regression model was used to assess the association between DIDO times and 30-day mortality adjusted for patient factors including demographics, traditional cardiac risk factors and co-morbidities, presenting features, symptom-to-FMC time, pre-hospital ECG status and the median durations of several process-of-care measures.

For comparative purposes, we also calculated the crude 30-day mortality rates amongst the 518 patients who received fibrinolytic therapy at the referral hospital and had data on the times of arrival to the hospital and administration of therapy. This group was not the major focus of this study and as noted earlier, was excluded in the cohort used for the main set of analyses.

Where there was missing data for a variable, it was < 1% of the sample size and was imputed to the most common value.

All analyses were conducted at ICES in Toronto, Canada using SAS version 9.3 (SAS Institute, Cary NC). This study was approved by the Research Ethics Boards at Sunnybrook Health Sciences Centre and each of the PCI centres in Ontario.

Results

Patient characteristics and timely DIDO

The distribution of DIDO times is shown in Figure S1 in the Data Supplement [see Additional file 1]. The median DIDO time was 55 min (interquartile range: 35–112 min). Only 194 patients (20.1%) achieved the DIDO benchmark, and ~ 1/3 of patients had DIDO times greater than 90 min.

Fewer patients with DIDO times ≤30 min, compared to patients with times > 30 min, were elderly, defined as older than 75 years of age (10.3% vs 19.9%; adjusted OR $[aOR]_{>75 \text{ vs } 18-55}$ 0.30, 95% CI: 0.16–0.56) (Table 1). Traditional cardiovascular risk factors, co-morbidities and presenting information were not found to be significantly associated with DIDO timeliness.

Approximately 43% of patients with timely DIDO had acceptable symptom-to- FMC contact times of between 0 and 60 min, in contrast to only 27.5% of those with untimely DIDO (Table 1). We observed a strong gradient for timeliness of DIDO, such that those who had the longest symptom-to-FMC times had an almost 2-fold decrease in timely DIDO rates compared to those with the shortest time ($aOR_{61\text{-}120mins \text{ vs. } 0-60 \text{ min}}$ 0.60, 95% CI: 0.39–0.90; $aOR_{>120mins \text{ vs. } 0-60 \text{ min}}$ 0.53, 95% CI: 0.35–0.81) (Table 1).

Process of care measures

As depicted in Fig. 2a, receipt of a timely ECG (time to first ECG was less than 10 min) was significantly associated with timely DIDO ($P < 0.0001$). Amongst process of care measures, EMS transport with receipt of a pre-hospital ECG was the strongest independent predictor of timely DIDO ($aOR_{EMS + \text{pre-hospital ECG vs self-transport}}$ 2.63, 95% CI: 1.59–4.35) (Table 1; Fig. 2b).

Table 1 Baseline characteristics of the study cohort across Door-in to door-out (DIDO) status, Ontario, Canada, 2012

	DIDO time (mins)		aOR (95% CI)[a] (timely DIDO vs. untimely)[b]
	≤30 min (*N* = 194)	> 30 min (*N* = 772)	
	Frequency (column %)		
Age group, years			
18–55	87 (44.8)	230 (29.8)	Ref.
56–65	51 (26.3)	234 (30.3)	0.57 (0.39–0.87)
66–75	36 (18.6)	154 (19.9)	0.61 (0.37–0.99)
> 75	20 (10.3)	154 (19.9)	0.30 (0.16–0.56)
Sex, females	33 (17.0)	194 (25.1)	0.72 (0.46–1.15)
Cardiovascular risk factors			
Diabetes mellitus	39 (20.1)	167 (21.6)	0.95 (0.62–1.45)
Current smoker	88 (45.4)	302 (39.1)	0.96 (0.67–1.39)
Hypertension	93 (47.9)	390 (50.5)	0.98 (0.68–1.41)
Previous cardiovascular clinical events			
Myocardial infarction	21 (10.8)	99 (12.8)	0.68 (0.70–3.03)
Angina	8 (4.1)	41 (5.3)	0.93 (0.39–2.22)
COPD	7 (3.6)	38 (4.9)	0.94 (0.38–2.33)
Stroke	7 (3.6)	30 (3.9)	1.43 (0.58–3.57)
Presenting characteristics			
Cardiac arrest at scene	13 (6.7)	51 (6.6)	0.69 (0.71–2.04)
Elevated cardiac enzymes[c]	171 (88.1)	675 (87.4)	1.22 (0.71–2.04)
Off-hours presentation[d]	122 (62.9)	508 (65.8)	0.91 (0.64–1.28)
Symptom to FMC time, mins			
0–60	84 (43.3)	212 (27.5)	Ref.
61–120	56 (28.9)	268 (34.7)	0.60 (0.39–0.90)
> 120	54 (27.8)	292 (37.8)	0.53 (0.35–0.81)
Transport to first hospital			
Self-transport	103 (53.1)	510 (66.1)	Ref.
EMS transport with ECG	36 (18.6)	71 (9.2)	2.63 (1.59–4.35)
EMS transport without ECG	55 (28.4)	191 (24.7)	1.45 (0.95–2.22)

Abbreviations: *aOR* adjusted odds ratio, *CI* confidence interval, *COPD* chronic obstructive pulmonary disease, *DIDO* door-in to door-out, *ECG* electrocardiogram, *EMS* emergency medical services, *FMC* first medical contact, *mins* minutes, *Ref* reference

[a]Logistic regression model fully adjusted for all the variables in the table

[b]Door-in to door-out times were considered timely if they were ≤ 30 min

[c]Elevated cardiac enzyme levels were defined as having at least one of the following occur within the first 24 h of the first medical contact: 1) a rise in troponin levels above the upper reference limit or the level indicative of acute myocardial infarction, or 2) a rise in creatine kinase MB or creatine kinase more than twice the upper limit of normal as defined on the lab report

[d]Defined as presentation to a hospital before 9 am or after 5 pm on weekdays and anytime on weekends

Timely reperfusion

A significantly ($P < 0.0001$) higher proportion of those who met the DIDO benchmark also had timely FMC-to-balloon times, with rates almost three times higher in the former group (78.7% vs 27.4%) (Fig. 2c).

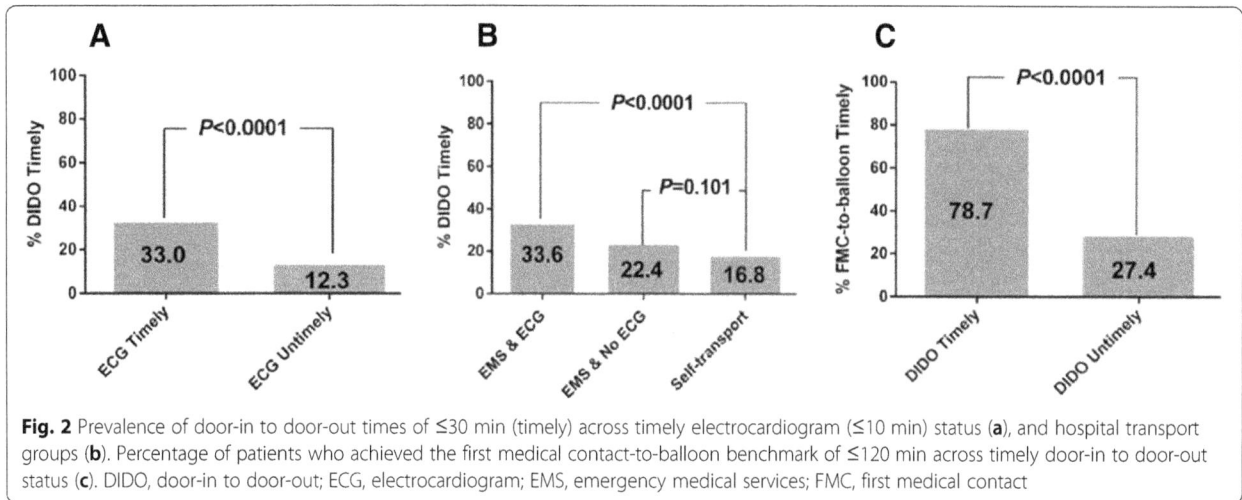

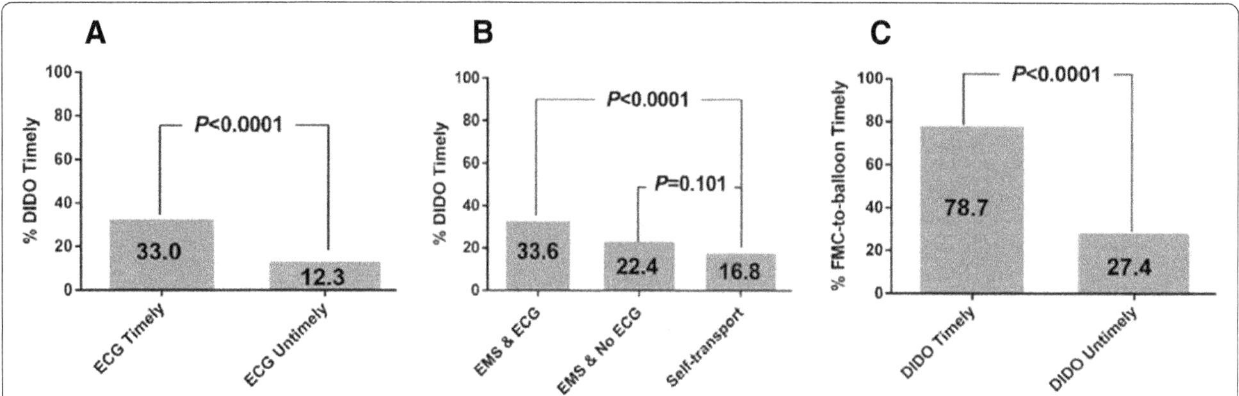

Fig. 2 Prevalence of door-in to door-out times of ≤30 min (timely) across timely electrocardiogram (≤10 min) status (**a**), and hospital transport groups (**b**). Percentage of patients who achieved the first medical contact-to-balloon benchmark of ≤120 min across timely door-in to door-out status (**c**). DIDO, door-in to door-out; ECG, electrocardiogram; EMS, emergency medical services; FMC, first medical contact

Overall, 47.4% of the transferred patients in our study met the FMC-to-balloon time benchmark.

The breakdown of the components of median reperfusion time across those who self-transported to hospital, were transported by EMS but did not receive a pre-hospital ECG, and those who were transported by EMS and had a pre-hospital ECG are shown in Fig. 3. The median times were 225, 216 and 199 min, respectively. Symptom-to-door time accounted for the greatest duration of median reperfusion time, followed by DIDO times, which were significantly shorter amongst those who were transported by EMS and received pre-hospital ECG compared to the self-transport group (Symptom-to-door time: 85 min vs 106 min, DIDO: 47 min vs 56 min; $P < 0.05$). 33.6% of those in the former group had timely DIDO compared to only 22.4% and 16.8% in the EMS and no pre-hospital ECG group and self-transport groups, respectively (Fig. 2B).

30-day mortality

Table 2 shows 30-day mortality rates across DIDO times. Crude 30-day mortality rates ranged from 4.1% amongst those with DIDO times of ≤30 min to 11.6% in those with DIDO times in excess of 90 min. While only patients with DIDO times > 90 min had significantly higher mortality rates (aOR 2.82, 95% CI: 1.10–7.19) a mortality gradient was evident.

Patients who received fibrinolytic therapy in the first hospital were excluded from the main analyses, but their crude 30-day mortality rate (6.6%) did not differ

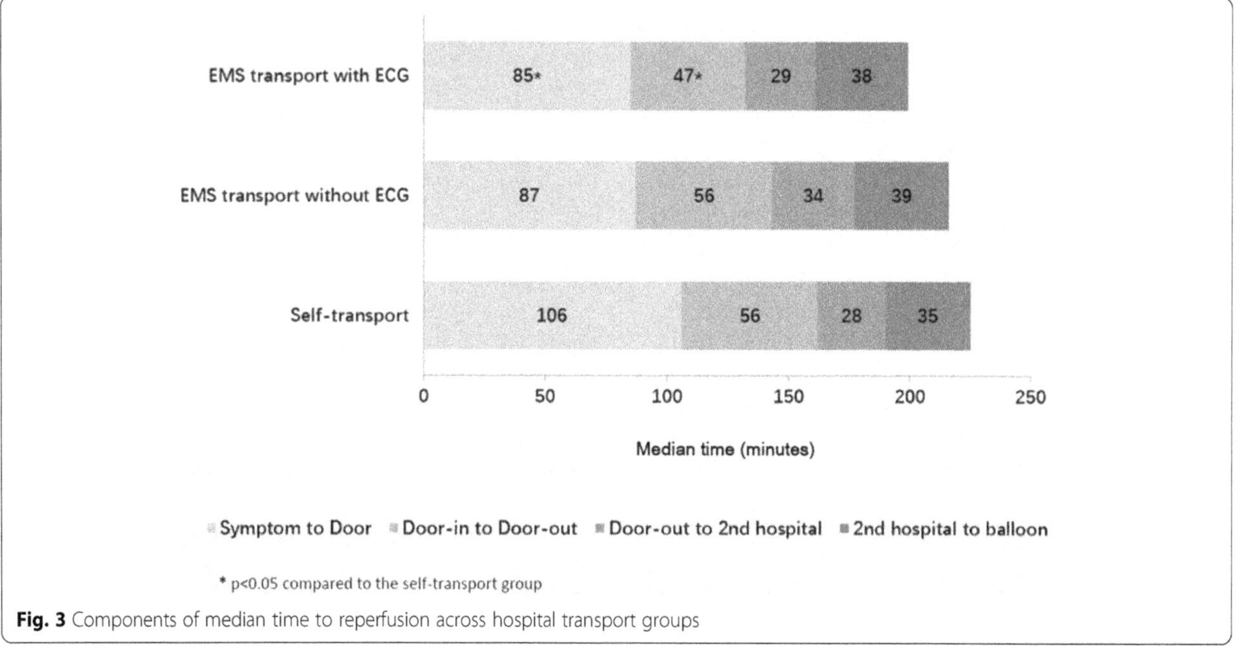

Fig. 3 Components of median time to reperfusion across hospital transport groups

Table 2 Association between door-in to door-out times and 30-day all-cause mortality amongst patients transferred for primary percutaneous coronary intervention, Ontario, Canada, 2012

	Number of events / Patient population	Crude 30-day mortality rate (%)	aOR (95% CI)[a]
DIDO time (mins)			
≤ 30 (timely)	8/194	4.1	Ref.
31–60	17/ 333	5.1	1.05 (0.38–2.89)
61–90	12/145	8.3	1.73 (0.58–5.09)
> 90	34/294	11.6	2.82 (1.10–7.19)
Overall	71/966	7.3	N/A

Abbreviations: *aOR* adjusted odds ratios, *CI* confidence intervals, *DIDO* door-in to door-out, *mins* minutes, *N/A* not applicable, *Ref* reference

[a]Logistic regression model was adjusted for patient demographics, traditional cardiac risk factors and co-morbidities, presenting features, symptom-to-FMC time, pre-hospital ECG status and times for process-of-care measures

significantly from patients transferred for primary PCI (7.3%; $P = 0.676$). Crude mortality rates for those administered fibrinolytic therapy can be found in Table S3 in the Data Supplement [see Additional file 1]. Patients with DIDO times >90 min had significantly higher crude mortality rates than those who got timely fibrinolytic therapy (11.6% vs. 5.5%; $P = 0.012$).

Discussion

In the present study, we utilized a population-based cohort of STEMI patients in Ontario, Canada to identify potentially modifiable factors that can improve DIDO times and the impact of DIDO times on long-term mortality. Only 20% of STEMI patients who were transferred from a referral hospital to a PCI-capable centre for primary PCI met the DIDO time of ≤30 min. Age was the strongest patient-level predictor of DIDO times. Transport to hospital by EMS in combination with receiving a pre-hospital ECG was the strongest process of care measure associated with DIDO times. In particular, this group had substantively shorter symptom to reperfusion times compared to those who transported themselves to hospital, driven largely by significantly shorter symptom to door and DIDO times. The mortality gradient for DIDO times observed in our study is important as it demonstrates poor long-term outcomes for those who experienced longer DIDO times. The crude 30-day mortality rates in patients transferred for primary PCI was higher than those who got fibrinolytic therapy, in particular for those with DIDO times over 90 min.

Our finding that achievement of benchmark DIDO time was low (20%) is consistent with previous studies [7, 8, 10–12]. A study using national registry data from the United States reported that only 11% of patients achieved DIDO benchmarks, and other studies reported rates of ~10% [8, 10, 11]. Canadian studies have reported higher rates than American-based studies, one reported 14% in Quebec [7, 10]. Several factors could account for the disparities in rates including varying characteristics of the study population, regional differences in policies and design of the STEMI system and/or changes in trends over time [7, 8, 10–12]. The latter may be especially pertinent in this case given that our work is more recent than other cited studies.

The guidelines indicate that 90% of patients transferred from a referring hospital should meet the 120-min time-to-treatment standard [1]. Less than 50% of transferred patients in our study met the FMC-to-balloon time benchmark. We observed stark differences in achievement of FMC-to-balloon time benchmark across DIDO status. Most transferred patients with DIDO time > 30 min do not have absolute contraindications for fibrinolytic therapy [18, 19]. In our and previous studies, about half of transferred patients had a DIDO time > 60 min, with few of these individuals receiving timely PCI [7, 8, 10–12]. Delayed transfer of STEMI patients with DIDO time > 60 min may not be a superior strategy to the timely use of fibrinolytic therapy [1, 3, 20]. One potential option to address prolonged DIDO times might be to increase the use of fibrinolytic therapy at referral hospitals, followed by transfer for catheterization post-lytic therapy [21].

Elderly age was found to be one of the strongest predictors of DIDO time in our study which is in light with previous studies [7, 10]. Elderly individuals may be less likely to present with classic STEMI symptoms (e.g., retrosternal chest pain) and/or more likely to have ECGs which are complex to interpret, that may delay diagnosis and recognition of a STEMI. Our findings highlight there is a need to bring awareness to the complexity and non-traditional nature of the symptoms with which these elderly patients sometimes present in order to improve DIDO times for this group. Prior studies have shown the disparities in time to reperfusion for STEMI patients in the elderly [22, 23]. Better software that can accurately read difficult ECGs, enhanced training for medical personnel and public awareness campaigns might improve DIDO times.

We observed that patients transported by EMS personnel, whether in association with a pre-hospital ECG or not, resulted in shorter symptom-to-door times compared to those self-transported patients. However,

DIDO times were found to be significantly shorter compared to patients who self-transported only amongst those who received a pre-hospital ECG, suggesting that while EMS transport, irrespective of pre-hospital ECG status affects symptom-to-door time, for DIDO times it is the receipt of pre-hospital ECG that makes a difference. Provision of a pre-hospital ECG was not a universally adopted or mandated practice in Ontario in 2012 [9]. However, the findings of the present study suggest that policies which mandate and fund equipping ambulances with this technology and training EMS personnel to administer these ECG's might have a significant impact on reduction of DIDO times and mortality.

Ideally, provision of a pre-hospital ECG should allow for a quicker diagnosis, thus facilitating the activation of STEMI protocols, result in more direct transfers to PCI-capable centres or mitigate delays in the referral ED [24]. Notably, our study found that a fair proportion (11.1%) of individuals received a pre-hospital ECG and were still initially transferred to a non-PCI capable hospital. Contributing factors may include diagnostic uncertainty, incorrect interpretation of the ECG and/or a clinically unstable patient. It is also plausible that some ambulances continue to bring patients to the nearest community hospital, regardless of ECG findings because the PCI-capable centre is further away, which would identify an area to target for improvement. Increased clarity in the guidelines around when EMS personnel should bypass the closest centre in favor of a more distant PCI-capable hospital, which is integrated within a STEMI protocol, may in part help alleviate this problem. In 2015, a STEMI bypass protocol in Ontario enables paramedics to bypass local hospitals and transport patients with STEMI directly to PCI-capable centres if arrival at the PCI centre will be ≤60 min from the first medical contact [9]. These guidelines came into effect in the province in 2017 and future studies should examine whether new guidelines have reduced the number of patients with STEMI-positive ECG's being transferred to non-PCI capable hospitals. Our findings show that the major delay in reperfusion times occurs at the referral hospital, in line with previous studies' findings [10, 25]. However, it should also be recognized that it may be difficult in EDs to provide care within guideline recommendations for every patient, especially for those with atypical presentations.

The present study aids in generalizability of findings to other populations. The fact that we examined important process of care measures including receipt of pre-hospital ECG's, which have not been extensively studied enabled us to assess the impact of current STEMI management recommendations and guidelines on DIDO times so that we can ascertain a more complete picture of the STEMI care system and identify areas for improvement. Additionally, the present study found DIDO times to be an independent predictor of 30-day mortality, with the observed gradient strengthening the conclusion, and suggests the adverse impact of long DIDO times extends beyond the hospital visit itself. Previous studies have observed similar gradients for in-hospital mortality only or have been underpowered to make inferences regarding longer-term mortality outcomes adjusted for important confounders [10].

However, the present study presents with some important limitations. First, information on key time intervals was ascertained through retrospective chart review and recorded times could not be independently validated. Secondly, we were unable to collect information on the distance to the referral hospital or between the referral hospital and the PCI-capable centre or the details of patient symptoms as they were not available or well documented. Lastly, the administrative STEMI codes we used have not been validated. However, they were applied consistently across all records and those who were identified as STEMI cases from administrative data had their diagnosis verified via chart review by a trained cardiology research nurse, making it unlikely that non-STEMI cases were included in the study.

Conclusions

In conclusion, our findings suggest that benchmark DIDO times were not achieved for a majority of transferred STEMI patients in the province. Patient age and process of care measures, namely symptom-to-FMC time and receipt of a pre-hospital ECG, were identified to be strong independent predictors of DIDO time. Despite provision of pre-hospital ECGs, a fair proportion of patients were still transferred to non-PCI capable hospitals, suggesting that policies and system-level changes aimed at bypassing non-PCI capable hospitals in favor of PCI-capable hospitals for those with STEMI positive ECGs could have an important impact on outcomes.

Abbreviations

AOR: Adjusted odds ratio; CI: Confidence interval; CIHI: Canadian Institute for Health Information; COPD: Chronic obstructive pulmonary disease; D2B: Door-to-balloon time; DAD: Discharge Abstract Database; DIDO: Door-in to door-out; ECG: Electrocardiogram; EMS: Emergency medical services; FMC: First medical contact; mins: Minutes; NACRS: National Ambulatory Care Reporting System; PCI: Percutaneous coronary intervention; Ref: Reference; STEMI: ST-segment elevation myocardial infarction; TRANSFER-AMI: Trial of Routine Angioplasty and Stenting after Fibrinolysis to Enhance Reperfusion in Acute Myocardial Infarction

Acknowledgements

Parts of this material are based on data and/or information compiled and provided by the Canadian Institute for Health Information (CIHI). The analyses, conclusions, opinions, and statements expressed in the material are those of the authors and not necessarily those of CIHI. This study was supported by the Institute for Clinical Evaluative Sciences (ICES), which is funded by an annual grant from the Ontario Ministry of Health and Long-Term Care (MOHLTC). The opinions, results and conclusions reported in this paper are those of the authors and are independent from the funding sources. No endorsement by ICES or the Ontario MOHLTC is intended or should be inferred.

Funding

Supported by operating grants from the Institute of Circulatory and Respiratory Health (ICRH)- Canadian Institutes of Health Research (CIHR) Chronic Diseases Team (grant no. TCA 118349 and grant no. FRN 111035). Dr. Tu is supported by a Tier 1 Canada Research Chair in Health Services Research and an Eaton Scholar award from the Department of Medicine, University of Toronto.

Authors' contributions

JVT was involved in obtaining data used for this study. JVT, CAJ, JC, CLA and DTK designed the study. OS and MRR analyzed the data. OS, AMK, CAJ, JC, CLA, DTK, TAS, LJL, MKN, ZZ and JVT interpreted the study findings. OS, JVT and AMK drafted the manuscript. All authors read and approved the final manuscript.

Competing interests

The authors declare that they have no competing interests.

Author details

[1]School of Public Health, Shanghai Jiaotong University School of Medicine, South Chongqing Road No, Shanghai 227, China. [2]Institute for Clinical Evaluative Sciences, G1 06, 2075 Bayview Avenue, Toronto, ON, Canada. [3]Western University of Health Sciences, 309 E 2nd St, Pomona, California, USA. [4]Schulich Heart Centre, Sunnybrook Health Sciences Centre, 2075 Bayview Avenue, Toronto, ON, Canada. [5]University of Toronto, 27 King's College Circle, Toronto, ON, Canada. [6]Department of Medicine, Hamilton Health Sciences, McMaster University, 1200 Main St W, Hamilton, ON, Canada. [7]Sunnybrook Health Sciences Centre, 2075 Bayview Avenue, Toronto, ON, Canada. [8]Dalhousie University, 6299 South St, Halifax, NS, Canada. [9]Cardiology Evaluation Unit, Institut national d'excellence en santé et en services sociaux (INESSS), 2021, Avenue Union, Bureau 10.083, Montréal, Québec, Canada.

References

1. O'Gara PT, Kushner FG, Ascheim DD, Casey DE, Chung MK, de Lemos JA, et al. 2013 ACCF/AHA guideline for the management of ST-elevation myocardial infarction: a report of the American College of Cardiology Foundation/American Heart Association task force on practice guidelines. Circulation. 2013;127(4):e362–425.
2. Rathore SS, Curtis JP, Chen J, Wang Y, Nallamothu BK, Epstein AJ, et al. Association of door-to-balloon time and mortality in patients admitted to hospital with ST elevation myocardial infarction: national cohort study. BMJ. 2009;338:b1807.
3. Keeley EC, Boura JA, Grines CL. Primary angioplasty versus intravenous thrombolytic therapy for acute myocardial infarction: a quantitative review of 23 randomised trials. Lancet. 2003;361(9351):13–20.
4. Hameed SM, Schuurman N, Razek T, Boone D, Van Heest R, Taulu T, et al. Access to trauma Systems in Canada. J Trauma. 2010;69(6):1350–61.
5. Jollis JG, Roettig ML, Aluko AO, Anstrom KJ, Applegate RJ, Babb JD, et al. Implementation of a statewide system for coronary reperfusion for ST-segment elevation myocardial infarction. JAMA. 2007;298(20):2371–80.
6. Lambert L, Brown K, Segal E, Brophy J, Rodes-Cabau J, Bogaty P. Association between timeliness of reperfusion therapy and clinical outcomes in ST-elevation myocardial infarction. JAMA. 2010;303(21):2148 –55.
7. Lambert LJ, Brown KA, Boothroyd LJ, Segal E, Maire S, Kouz S, et al. Transfer of patients with ST-elevation myocardial infarction for primary percutaneous coronary intervention: a province-wide evaluation of "door-in to door-out" delays at the first hospital. Circulation. 2014;129(25):2653–60.
8. Miedema MD, Newell MC, Duval S, Garberich RF, Handran CB, Larson DM, et al. Causes of delay and associated mortality in patients transferred with ST-segment-elevation myocardial infarction. Circulation. 2011;124(15):1636–44.
9. CCN. Recommendations for Best Practice STEMI Management in Ontario. 2013.
10. Wang TY, Nallamothu BK, Krumholz HM, Li S, Roe MT, Jollis JG, et al. Association of door-in to door-out time with reperfusion delays and outcomes among patients transferred for primary percutaneous coronary intervention. JAMA. 2011;305(24):2540–7.
11. Herrin J, Miller LE, Turkmani DF, Nsa W, Drye EE, Bernheim SM, et al. National performance on door-in to door-out time among patients transferred for primary percutaneous coronary intervention. Arch Intern Med. 2011;171(21):1879–86.
12. Glickman SW, Lytle BL, Ou FS, Mears G, O'Brien S, Cairns CB, et al. Care processes associated with quicker door-in-door-out times for patients with ST-elevation-myocardial infarction requiring transfer: results from a statewide regionalization program. Circ Cardiovasc Qual Outcomes. 2011;4(4):382–8.
13. CCN. Cardiac Care Network of Ontario Ontario STEMI Bypass Protocol. 2015.
14. Kulynych J, Korn D. The effect of the new federal medical-privacy rule on research. N Engl J Med. 2002;346(3):201–4.
15. Tu JV, Willison DJ, Silver FL, Fang J, Richards JA, Laupacis A, et al. Impracticability of informed consent in the registry of the Canadian stroke network. N Engl J Med. 2004;350(14):1414–21.
16. Roffi M, Patrono C, Collet J, Mueller C, Valgimigli M, Andreotti F, et al. 2015 ESC guidelines for the management of acute coronary syndromes in patients presenting without persistent ST-segment elevation. Eur Heart J. 2016;37(3):267–315.
17. Chin CT, Chen AY, Wang TY, Alexander KP, Mathews R, Rumsfeld JS, et al. Risk adjustment for in-hospital mortality of contemporary patients with acute myocardial infarction: the acute coronary treatment and intervention outcomes network (ACTION) registry®–get with the guidelines (GWTG)™ acute myocardial infarction mortality model and risk score. Am Heart J. 2011;161(1):113–22.
18. Cantor WJ, Fitchett D, Borgundvaag B, Ducas J, Heffernan M, Cohen EA, et al. Routine early angioplasty after fibrinolysis for acute myocardial infarction. N Engl J Med. 2009;360(26):2705–18.
19. Bøhmer E, Hoffmann P, Abdelnoor M, Arnesen H, Halvorsen S. Efficacy and safety of immediate angioplasty versus ischemia-guided management after thrombolysis in acute myocardial infarction in areas with very long transfer distances. J Am Coll Cardiol. 2010;55(2):102–10.
20. Andersen HR, Nielsen TT, Vesterlund T, Grande P, Abildgaard U, Thayssen P, et al. Danish multicenter randomized study on fibrinolytic therapy versus acute coronary angioplasty in acute myocardial infarction: rationale and design of the danish trial in acute myocardial infarction-2 (DANAMI-2). Am Heart J. 2003;146(2):234–41.
21. Bhan V, Cantor WJ, Yan RT, Mehta SR, Morrison LJ, Heffernan M, et al. Efficacy of early invasive management post-fibrinolysis in men versus women with ST-elevation myocardial infarction: a subgroup analysis from trial of routine angioplasty and stenting after fibrinolysis to enhance reperfusion in acute myocardial infarction (TRANSFER-AMI). Am Heart J. 2012;164(3):343–50.
22. Avezum A, Makdisse M, Spencer F, Gore JM, Fox KA, Montalescot G, et al. Impact of age on management and outcome of acute coronary syndrome: observations from the global registry of acute coronary events (GRACE). Am Heart J. 2005;149(1):67–73.
23. Glickman SW, Granger CB, Ou FS, O'Brien S, Lytle BL, Cairns CB, et al. Impact of a statewide ST-segment-elevation myocardial infarction regionalization program on treatment times for women, minorities, and the elderly. Circ Cardiovasc Qual Outcomes. 2010;3(5):514–21.
24. Davis MT, Dukelow A, McLeod S, Rodriguez S, Lewell M. The utility of the prehospital electrocardiogram. CJEM. 2011;13(06):372–7.
25. Bradley EH, Herrin J, Wang Y, Barton BA, Webster TR, Mattera JA, et al. Strategies for reducing the door-to-balloon time in acute myocardial infarction. N Engl J Med. 2006;355(22):2308–20.

19

The value of shock index in prediction of cardiogenic shock developed during primary percutaneous coronary intervention

Zhonghai Wei*†, Jian Bai†, Qing Dai†, Han Wu, Shuaihua Qiao, Biao Xu and Lian Wang*

Abstract

Background: Shock index(SI) is a conventional predictive marker for haemodynamic state. Its breakpoint varies by different conditions according to previous studies. The current study was performed to evaluate the capability of SI in prediction of cardiogenic shock(CS) developed during primary percutaneous coronary intervention (pPCI).

Methods: Total 870 patients of ST segment elevation myocardial infarction(STEMI) who were haemodynamic stable before pPCI were involved in the study. In this cohort, 625 consecutive patients composed analysis series and 245 consecutive patients composed validation series. Multivariate regression analysis was used to evaluate whether SI was a significant predictor of developed CS and Hosmer-Lemeshow test was used to assess the goodness of model fitness. Receiver-operating characteristics (ROC) analysis was used to compare the predictive capability of SI with other predictors. The sensitivity, specificity, accuracy, positive and negative predictive values of SI at different cutoff values was compared to identify a best breakpoint.

Results: In the analysis series, SI and Killips classification were identified as independent predictors. ROC analysis demonstrated the diagnostic capability of SI was superior to pre-procedural systolic blood pressure(SBP) or heart rate(HR) alone (0.8113 vs 0.7582, $P = 0.04$ and 0.8113 vs 0.7111, $P < 0.001$). The diagnostic capability of SI was equivalent to that of combination of SBP, HR and Killips claasification(0.8133 vs 0.8137, $P = 0.97$). SI had a high specificity and low sensitivity. When the cutoff value was set at 0.93, the positive predictive value, negative predictive value and diagnostic accuracy was 42.6%, 95.1% and 87.4% respectively. In validation series, the area under ROC curve was 0.8245, which was similar to that in the analysis series. The positive predictive value, negative predictive value and diagnostic accuracy at the cutoff value of 0.93 was 53.8%, 93.2% and 88.9% respectively.

Conclusions: SI has a high predictive accuracy for developing CS during pPCI in STEMI patients. It is an excellent exclusion diagnosis index rather than confirmative diagnosis index.

Keywords: Shock index, Myocardial infarction, Cardiogenic shock, Reperfusion

* Correspondence: weizhnjjs@yeah.net; wanglianglyy@163.com
†Zhonghai Wei, Jian Bai and Qing Dai contributed equally to this work.
Department of Cardiology, Drum Tower Hospital, Medical School of Nanjing University, 321 Zhongshan Road, Nanjing 210008, Jiangsu Province, China

Background

In the past three decades, the in-hospital and 1-year mortality of ST segment elevation myocardial infarction (STEMI) have been remarkably decreased due to timely revascularization [1]. However, the worsening of cardiac function after STEMI is still rising despite of optimal reperfusion and pharmacological therapy. The infarct-related heart failure will no doubt increase the long-term comorbidity and mortality, which may counterbalance the benefits from the timely reperfusion. Previous studies have revealed that approximate 50% of final infarct myocardium caused by reperfusion injury (RI) [2, 3]. RI is therefore regarded as the leading cause of infarct size extension after blood flow recovery of infarct-related artery (IRA), which could possibly lead to cardiogenic shock (CS) during primary percutaneous coronary intervention (pPCI). It has been reported that patients of STEMI complicated with CS have 30-day or in-hospital mortality as high as nearly 50% [4–7]. Hence, those stable patients of STEMI but probably developing to CS during pPCI should be identified in advance and it may provide the target patients to doctors to take measures for ease of RI.

Shock index (SI) is a marker assessing the haemodynamic state, which is calculated as heart rate (HR) divided by systolic blood pressure (SBP) [8]. Patients with elevated SI, even with normal blood pressure and heart rate, should be paid more attention for the high risk of shock. In the acute coronary syndrome (ACS) or STEMI patients cohort, SI has been proven the independent predictor of long-term major adverse cardiac events (MACE) or mortality [9–11]. Nevertheless, there are few studies on the efficacy of this marker in prediction of developing CS during emergency reperfusion. The current study was aimed to evaluate the predictive capability of CS developed during pPCI in the cohort of STEMI.

Methods

Study population

The study cohort was retrieved from the database of our center. The including criteria was as follows: (1) the patients were diagnosed STEMI; (2)there was no cardiogenic shock when admitted in emergency room; (3) the patients accepted PCI after emergency angiography. The exclusion criteria was as follows: (1)the patients presented cardiogenic shock when arrived emergency room;(2) the patients rejected emergency angiography; (3) the patients did not need emergency revascularization or need emergency coronary artery bypass graft (CABG) surgery; (4)the patients were deployed prophylactic IABP before revascularization.

From January 2010 to May 2017, total 1250 STEMI patients were admitted in our hospital. 250 patients were excluded because they did not accepted emergency PCI due to over the time window of emergency revascularization. 59 patients were excluded due to cardiogenic shock when admitted in emergency room. 37 patients were excluded for sake of prophylactic use of IABP. 23 patients were excluded because of referral to emergency CABG or referral to elected procedure. 11 patients were excluded due to refusal of emergency angiography. Therefore, the remaining 870 patients were eligible for the study cohort. The study population consisted of 2 series: 1 analysis series (625 consecutive patients for analysis and identification of predictive capability) and 1 validation series (245 consecutive patients for validation the predictive capability).

Procedure details

All the patients with acute chest pain in emergency room accepted ECG within 10 min. STEMI was defined as new onset of ST segment elevation at the J point in at least 2 contiguous leads of more than 2 mm in men or more than 1.5 mm in women in V2 and V3 lead and/or of more than 1 mm in other leads. The presentation of new left bundle branch block was considered equivalent to STEMI [12]. Cardiogenic shock was defined that the systolic blood pressure of the patients is below 90 mmHg more than 30 min or the inotropic agents are needed to maintain the systolic blood pressure above 90 mmHg accompanied with pulmonary congestion and/or peripheral perfusion impairment [13].

The patients ready to accept primary PCI were administered a loading dose of aspirin 300 mg and ticagrelor 180 mg before the procedure. Clopidogrel 600 mg was given if ticagrelor was contraindicated or unavailable. After a radial or femoral artery puncture, a 6F sheath was inserted. Heparin was administered at a dose of 70–100 IU/kg, while tirofiban, urokinase or argatroban were used if necessary. Thrombus aspiration catheter was used if it was considered high burden of thrombus under angiography. After blood flow recovery of IRA, the stent was deployed immediately or delayed according to the discretion of coronary lesions and interventionists' experience. If CS occurred after the reperfusion of IRA, rescue IABP support was transfemorally placed preferentially. If the patients were not suitable for IABP, inotropic agents were alternative. All of the procedures were accomplished by experienced and qualified interventionists.

Statistics

Continuous normally distributed variables were shown as mean ± standard deviation (mean ± SD) and were compared using T-test between two groups. While those that were not normally distributed were presented as median (M) and interquartile range (IQR)

Table 1 Characteristic of patients cohort

	Non-Shock (*n* = 769)	Developed Shock (*n* = 101)	*P* value
Age,year[M(IQR)]	64(55–74)	63(55–73)	0.52
Male sex,n(%)	610(79.3)	76(75.6)	0.35
Anterior myocardial infarction,n(%)	389(50.6)	58(57.6)	0.2
Hypertension,n(%)	505(65.7)	69(68.8)	0.60
Diabetes,n(%)	215(28.0)	34(33.3)	0.23
Prior Stroke,n(%)	101(13.1)	30(30.3)	< 0.001
Hyperlipidemia,n(%)	64(9.7)	9(9.1)	0.84
Smoke,n(%)	450(58.5)	53(52.1)	0.25
Prior myocardial infarction, n(%)	73(9.53)	8(7.98)	0.61
Creatinine,μmol/L[M(IQR)]	72(62–87)	69(60–81)	0.22
EF,%[M(IQR)]	47(41–50)	44(40–48)	0.03
Triglyceride, mmol/L[M(IQR)]	1.38(1.00–2.05)	1.39(0.90–2.10)	0.72
Cholesterol, mmol/L[M(IQR)]	4.28(3.63–4.98)	4.49(3.83–4.88)	0.46
LDL-C, mmol/L[M(IQR)]	2.31(1.84–2.80)	2.29(1.91–2.79)	0.93
HDL-C, mmol/L[M(IQR)]	0.93(0.76–1.14)	0.91(0.77–1.11)	0.79
Pre-procedure SBP, mmHg[M(IQR)]	123(112–138)	104(96–108)	< 0.001
Pre-procedure HR, bpm[M(IQR)]	79(69–89)	91(82–100)	0.008
Total ischemic time,min[M(IQR)]	342(234–610)	360(267–713)	0.26
Killips class II/III, n(%)	185(24.0)	30(28.7)	0.50
Double vessel disease, n(%)	310(40.3)	34(33.3)	0.20
Triple vessel disease, n(%)	235(30.6)	40(39.4)	0.07
IRA			
LAD, n(%)	389(50.6)	58(57.6)	0.20
LCX/OM, n(%)	123(16)	1(0.99)	< 0.001
RCA, n(%)	195(25.4)	43(42.4)	< 0.001
PDA/PL, n(%)	65(8.5)	0	–
PTCA, n(%)	12(1.51)	0	–
Stents			
Sirolimus, n(%)	481(62.6)	58(57.6)	0.32
Everolimus, n(%)	231(30.1)	30(30.3)	0.95
Zotarolimus, n(%)	155(20.1)	24(24.2)	0.40
Paclitaxel, n(%)	6(0.76)	0	–
Mediction			
Aspirin, n(%)	769(100)	101(100%)	1.00
Clopidogrel, n(%)	516(67.1)	64(63.4)	0.45
Ticagrelor, n(%)	253(32.9)	37(36.6)	0.45
ACEI/ARB, n(%)	511(66.5)	64(63.6)	0.54
β-blocker, n(%)	606(78.8)	70(69.4)	< 0.001
Spironolactone, n(%)	442(57.5)	63(62.7)	0.35
Diuretics, n(%)	359(46.7)	55(54.5)	0.14
Statin, n(%)	767(99.8)	100(99.6)	0.31

EF ejection fraction, *LDL-C* low density lipoprotein cholesterol, *HDL-C* high density lipoprotein cholesterol, *SBP* systolic blood pressure, *HR* heart rate, *IRA* infarct related artery, *LAD* left anterior descending branch, *LCX* left circumflex branch, *OM* obtuse marginal branch, *RCA* right coronary artery, *PDA* posterior descending artery, *PL* posterior branch of left venticule, *ACEI* angiotensin converting enzyme inhibitor, *ARB* angiotensin receptor blocker

Table 2 Univariate regression analysis for the risk factors

Variables	OR	SE	*P* value	95% CI
Age	1.00	0.01	0.57	[0.99 1.03]
Female sex	1.14	0.34	0.65	[0.64 2.04]
Pre-Procedural SBP	0.94	0.01	< 0.01	[0.92 0.96]
Pre-Procedural HR	1.05	0.01	< 0.01	[1.03 1.06]
Total ischemic duration (per 1 h change)	1.01	0.01	0.51	[0.98 1.02]
Killips classification				
Killips = 2 vs =1	2.45	0.67	0.001	[1.43 4.19]
Killips = 3 vs =1	6.20	3.44	0.001	[2.09 18.4]
Multiple vessel disease	1.44	0.39	0.18	[0.85 2.43]
Extensive anterior MI	0.89	0.26	0.69	[0.50 1.58]
Prior MI	0.96	0.73	0.95	[0.22 4.25]
Prior hypertension	0.61	0.15	0.05	[0.37 1.00]
Prior diabetes	0.72	0.22	0.28	[0.40 1.30]
Prior stroke	1.64	0.53	0.13	[0.87 3.10]
Prior dyslipidemia	1.06	0.45	0.89	[0.46 2.44]
Smoking	0.96	0.24	0.88	[0.59 1.58]
Serum creatinine	1.00	0.01	0.58	[0.99 1.01]

SBP systolic blood pressure, *HR* heart rate, *MI* myocardial infarction

and compared using Wilcoxon rank-sum test between two groups. Categorical variables were shown as frequencies and percentages and were compared with χ^2 test or Fisher exact test. In the regression analysis, the following variables in the analysis series were set in the univariate regression analysis initially: age, gender, pre-procedural systolic blood pressure(SBP), pre-procedural heart rate(HR), Killips classification, total ischemic duration, multiple vessel disease, extensive anterior myocardial infarction(MI), infarct related artery(IRA), hypertension, diabetes, dyslipidemia, prior MI, prior stroke, smoking hobby, serum creatinine. The variables significant in univariate analysis were subsequently set in the multivariate analysis. The variables were selected using backwards method. The regression models were calibrated with Hosmer-Lemeshow χ^2 test for the goodness of fit. Thereafter, the significant covariates were tested for the accuracy with receiver-operating characteristics (ROC) analysis. The area under curve (AUC) was calculated to compare the diagnostic capability of the predictors. Specificity, sensitivity and Youden index (specificity+sensitivity-1) were calculated for identification of a reasonable cutoff value. In the validation series, the predictors were analyzed with ROC in order to identify the predictive value. The statistical analysis was performed by Stata version 12.0 (StataCop., College Station, Texus, USA). All the tests were 2 sided. Values of $P < 0.05$ were considered statistically significant.

Results

Characteristics of study population

Total 870 patients were valid for the current study. The median age was 65y with interquartile range of 55y-74y. There were 686 male patients (78.9%) and 184 female patients(21.1%). 769 patients were hemodynamic stable during pPCI(Non Shock Group), whereas 101 patients had developed CS during the procedure(Developed Shock Group). Compared with Developed Shock Group, Non Shock Group had lower proportion patients with prior stroke ($P < 0.001$), higher EF value ($P = 0.03$), higher pre-procedural SBP($P < 0.001$) and lower pre-procedural HR($P = 0.008$). Furthermore, more patients had left circumflex branch(LCX) or obtuse marginal branch(OM) as IRA and less patients had right coronary artery(RCA) as IRA in the Non Shock Group(P < 0.001). As regard to pharmacological therapy, there were more patients taking β-blocker in Non Shock Group in comparison with that in

Table 3 Multivariate regression analysis for risk factors

Variables	OR	SE	*P* value	95% CI
Pre-Procedural SBP	0.95	0.01	< 0.01	[0.93 0.96]
Pre-Procedural HR	1.05	0.01	< 0.01	[1.03 1.07]
Killips classification				
Killips = 2 vs =1	2.34	0.76	0.01	[1.24 4.44]
Killips = 3 vs =1	5.30	2.86	0.02	[1.27 22.1]

SBP systolic blood pressure, *HR* heart rate

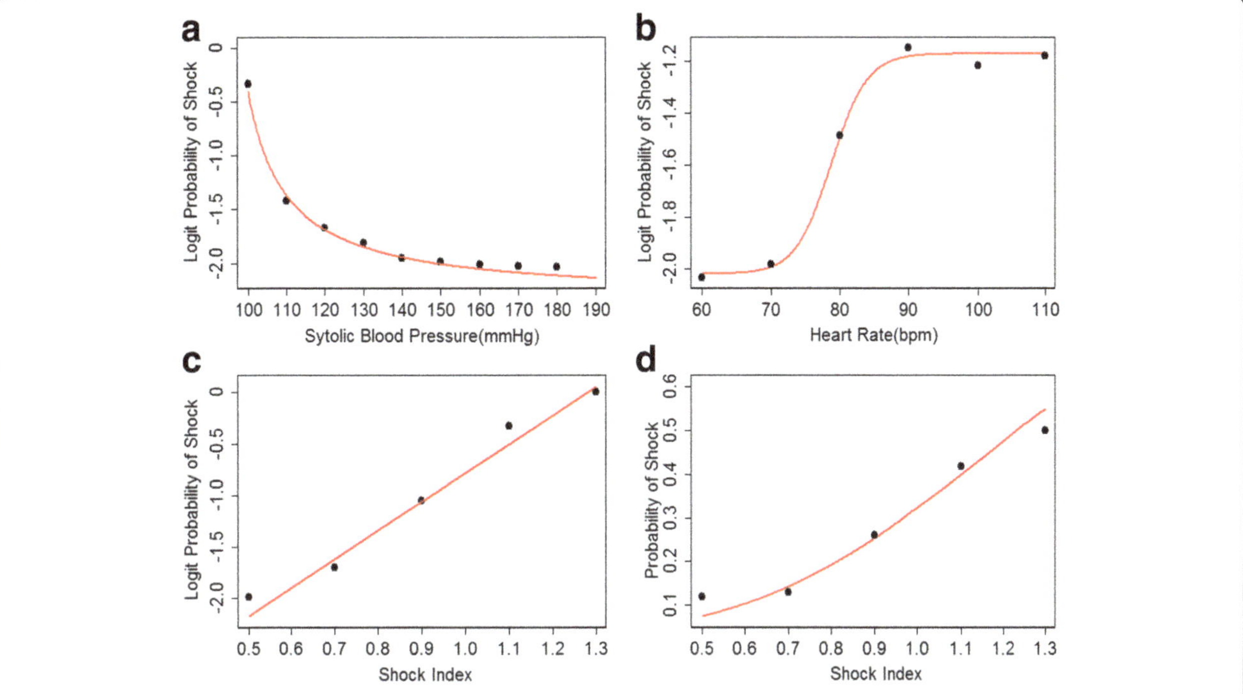

Fig. 1 (**a**) The logit probability of developing CS showed inverse proportional to the pre-procedural SBP. (**b**) The relationship between pre-procedural HR and logit probability of developing CS formed a sigmoid curve. (**c**) The logit probability of developing CS was positive linear correlated to the SI. (**d**) The relationship between probability of developing CS and SI was fitted into a logistic function. The curve shown in the graph was just at the rapid descending part of the logistic curve, which was very close to a line. SBP: systolic blood pressure; HR: heart rate; SI: shock index; CS: cardiogenic shock

Developed Shock Group(P < 0.001), while other medication was no different between two groups (Table 1).

Identification of relevant risk factors

In the analysis series, 72 patients were subjected to the CS during primary PCI. We took CS as dependent variable, the following factors as independent variables: age, sex category, pre-procedural SBP and pre-procedural HR, Killips classification, total ischemic duration, multiple vessel disease, extensive anterior MI, IRA, renal function, prior related history including hypertension, diabetes, dyslipidemia, MI, stroke and smoking habit. On univariate analysis, pre-procedural SBP and pre-procedural HR, Killips classification were the significant variables. Prior history of hypertension had a trend toward to statistical significance (Table 2).

In multivariate analysis, the above statistical significant variables together with some clinical significant variables including age, total ischemic duration, multiple vessel disease were set in the multivariate regression analysis. Table 3 showed the pre-procedural SBP, pre-procedural HR and Killips classification were the independent predictors. Hosmer-Lemeshow test demonstrated the model was well fitted ($\chi^2 = 6.43$, $P = 0.599$).

Model fit of SI

The regression model revealed the risk of developing CS was positively correlated with pre-procedural HR and negatively correlated with pre-procedural SBP. Furthermore, the scatter plot showed the relationship between logit probability of shock and pre-procedural SBP was nonlinear and a inverse proportional function was well fitted ($P < 0.001$,adjust R square = 0.9904)(Fig. 1a). The relationship between logit probability of shock and pre-procedural HR was also nonlinear and a logistic function was fitted ($P < 0.001$, adjust R square = 0.9973)(Fig. 1b). SI was formulated as the ratio of pre-procedural HR to pre-procedural SBP. The logit probability of shock was positively linear correlated with SI (P < 0.001, adjust R square = 0.9549). The

Table 4 Multivariate regression analysis for shock index

Variables	OR	SE	*P* value	95% CI
Shock index (per 0.1 change)	1.93	0.16	< 0.01	[1.64 2.28]
Killips classification				
Killips = 2 vs =1	2.21	0.69	0.01	[1.21 4.06]
Killips = 3 vs =1	5.94	3.92	0.01	[1.63 21.7]
Shock index * Killips			> 0.05#	

P > 0.05 indicated there was no significant interaction between shock index and Killips classification in the multivariate regression analysis

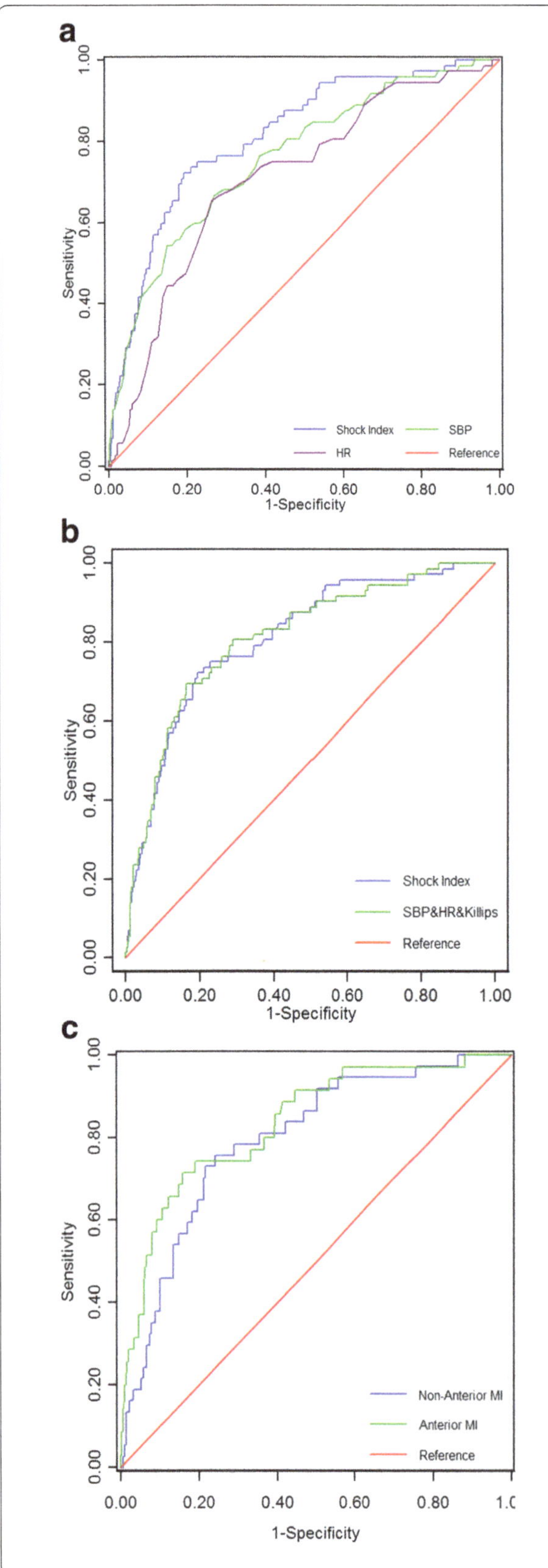

Fig. 2 (**a**) SI had a better diagnostic capability than pre-procedural SBP or pre-procedural HR alone. (**b**) The diagnostic capability of SI was similar to that of the combination of pre-procedural SBP and pre-procedural HR and Killips classification. (**c**) The diagnostic capability of SI had no difference between non-anterior MI subgroup and anterior MI subgroup. SI: shock index; SBP: systolic blood pressure; HR: heart rate; MI: myocardial infarction

relationship between probability of shock and SI was located at the rapid rise part of a sigmoid curve and the logistic function was well fitted (P < 0.001, adjust R square = 0.9898) (Fig. 1c and d). Regression analysis demonstrated that SI was a significant independent predictor (Hosmer--Lemeshow $\chi^2 = 8.12$, $P = 0.42$)(Table 4). However, there was no interplay between SI and Killips classification no matter in CS cohort, non-CS cohort or global cohort. That meant Killips classification was not able to further promote the discriminability of SI.

Diagnostic capability assessment

With the calibration of ROC analysis, the AUC of SI was significantly higher than that of pre-procedural SBP(0.8113 vs 0.7582, $P = 0.04$) and pre-procedural HR(0.8113 vs 0.7111, $P < 0.001$) respectively(Fig. 2a). The AUC of SI was similar to the AUC of combination of SBP, HR and Killips classification(0.8133 vs 0.8137, $P = 0.97$) (Fig. 2b). Moreover, the AUC of SI in anterior MI patients was not significantly different from that in non-anterior MI patients(0.8332 vs 0.7944, $P = 0.46$)(Fig. 2c).

The diagnostic parameters were calculated at different cutoff of SI (Table 5). Of note, SI had a high specificity and low sensitivity because of the relatively low incidence of developing CS during pPCI. In other words, it was suitable for exclusion diagnosis. When the cutoff was between 0.90~ 0.95, the accuracy were all above 85% and the negative predictive value were higher than 90%. If the cutoff was set at 0.93, the negative predictive value was as high as 95%.

Predictive capability validation of SI

In the validation series, total 29 patients had undergone CS during primary PCI. Logistic regression analysis demonstrated that the odd ratio of SI (per 0.1 changes) for predicting this event was 1.94(95% CI: 1.54–2.46). Hosmer-Lemeshow test revealed a excellent model fit($\chi^2 = 8.57$, $P = 0.38$). The ROC curve of SI was depicted in Fig. 3. The AUC of this curve was 0.8245(95% CI: 0.7441–0.9048). The incidence of developing CS at different breakpoints was shown in Fig. 4. If the cutoff value was set at 0.93, the sensitivity, specificity, positive predictive value and negative predictive value was 48.3%, 94.4%, 53.8% and 93.2% respectively. The accuracy and Youden index was 88.9% and 42.7% respectively.

Table 5 The diagnostic capability assessment of shock index

Cutoff	Sensitivity(%)	Specificity(%)	Youden index(%)	Accuracy(%)	Positive predictive value(%)	Negative predictive value(%)
0.90	31.9	93.7	25.6	86.6	39.7	91.4
0.91	30.6	94.0	24.6	86.7	40.0	91.2
0.92	29.2	94.9	24.1	87.4	42.9	91.2
0.93	27.8	95.1	22.9	87.4	42.6	95.1
0.94	26.4	95.3	21.7	87.4	42.2	90.9
0.95	22.2	96.2	18.4	87.7	43.2	90.5

Discussion

SI is a reliable predictor for early shock in different situation, such as trauma, infection, pulmonary embolism, which is usually set 0.9 as the threshold of elevation [14–18]. However, there are several other cutoff values in different studies [17, 19, 20], which means the diagnostic capability of SI varies over different conditions. Theoretically, SI should be more sensitive in reflexing the pre-shock state because heart rate usually elevates before the systolic blood pressure goes down as a compensatory response. Surprisingly, the consequence in our data was beyond our expectation.

Pre-procedural SBP, pre-procedural HR and Killips classification have been identified independent predictors of developing CS during emergency reperfusion in the current study, which is consistent with the previous findings [21, 22]. Further analysis showed the relationship of logit probability of CS with pre-procedural SBP and pre-procedural HR were both not linear. The scatter dots were fitted into an inverse proportional function in the former relationship and a logistic function in the latter relationship. Despite the monotone change could make SBP and HR predictors, there were flat parts in the both curves, which probably caused the makers less sensitive. On the contrary, SI had much better feature in this regard. The logit probability of shock was positive linear related to SI, which was an ideal relationship for the binary variables model. A recent study performed by Laust Obling et al. demonstrated that the odd ratio was 1.26 for per 10% change in the patients developing CS after leaving catheter laboratory [22]. In our data, the odd ratio was 1.93 for per 10% change. Of note, SI was not an independent predictor in Laust Obling's study, while it did in our study. The leading cause may be the ejection fraction (EF) was set in the regression analysis in the previous study. EF was highly associated with CS and probably masked the effect of SI. But EF was not available before pPCI in our setting.

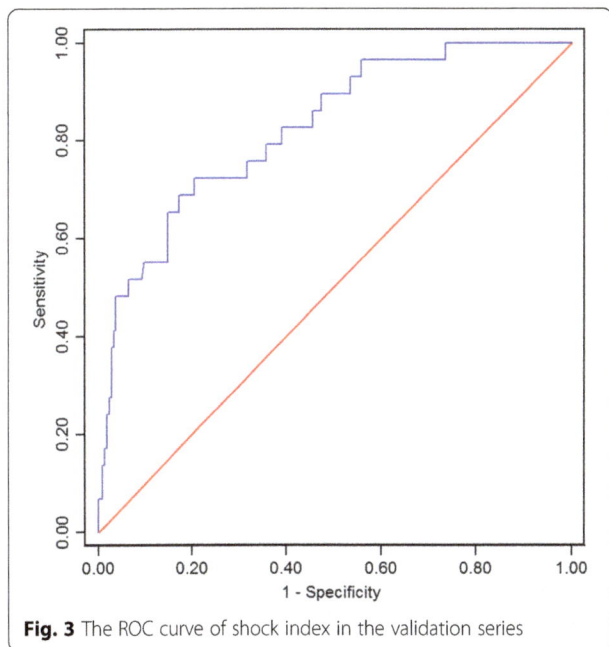

Fig. 3 The ROC curve of shock index in the validation series

ROC analysis proved that SI had a better diagnostic capability than either SBP or HR alone, while it had an equivalent diagnostic capability with the combination of SBP, HR and Killips classification. Killips classification could not further improve the diagnostic capability due to no interaction between SI and Killips classification. Therefore, we had reason using SI instead of the other independent predictors. The AUC of SI in the analysis series was highly close to that in the validation series, which implied SI was a reliable predictor. Nonetheless,

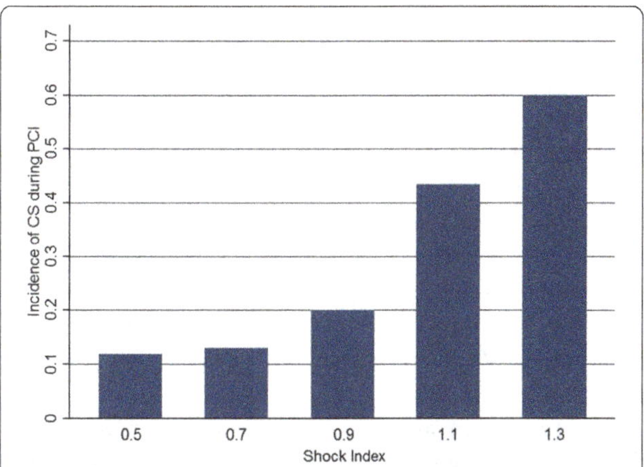

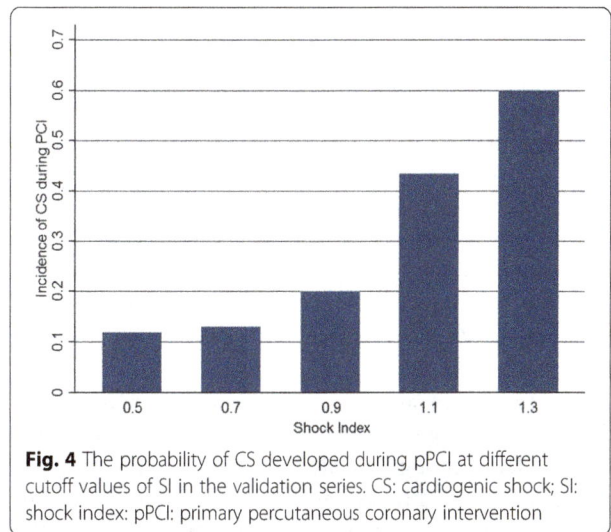

Fig. 4 The probability of CS developed during pPCI at different cutoff values of SI in the validation series. CS: cardiogenic shock; SI: shock index: pPCI: primary percutaneous coronary intervention

SI had a high specificity and low sensitivity despite the predictive accuracy was above 85%. The sensitivity and positive predictive value varied markedly, while the specificity and negative predictive value remained as high as about 95%. The incidence of CS developed during pPCI in the study cohort influenced the sensitivity and positive predictive value. Generally speaking, the incidence of developing CS was not very high however. It meant SI was not a good index for confirmative diagnosis but a good index for exclusion of developing CS.

In the previous studies, the cutoff values were arbitrary and also varied over different settings. Nevertheless, SI norms change by age and gender just because the blood pressure and heart rate varies by age and gender [18, 23]. SI declines about 0.01~ 0.02 per every 5 years in male population and about 0.02~ 0.03 per every 5 years in female population [18], which forms a slow declined curve. In other words, the same threshold might not be sensitive as to the aged population. Several studies have used age modified SI (age×SI) as a better predictor to offset the disadvantage of SI [24–26]. In our data, the breakpoint of SI was set at 0.93 as an ideal threshold for exclusion of developing CS. We did not use age modified SI just because age was not significant predictors. Moreover, we also attempted to modified SI using Killips classification to create a novel and better index, but failed in the end, which was mainly due to no interaction between SI and Killips classification.

Conclusions

According to the current study, SI had advantage in prediction of developing CS during pPCI for STEMI patients. It had an excellent negative predictive capability, but the positive predictive capability was not as so good.

Limitations

Firstly, the negative predictive value of SI had been proven approximate 95% by analysis and validation series. However, the difference of positive predictive value between analysis series and validation series was markedly due to a bit small sample size of validation series. Secondly, left main artery(LM) as IRA is a strong predictor of developing CS, which has been reported in previous study [22]. In our center, all the patients with LM as IRA had accepted prophylactic IABP support, which exclude these patients from current study. Therefore, we could not investigate the possible interaction of LM with SI. Thirdly, SI norms changes by age as aforementioned. We did not analyze the predictive value by age stratification due to age not being significant covariate by regression analysis. Maybe the age range in the data was not large enough or the analysis series sample was not large enough for SI to discriminate the diagnostic capability in different age groups. The last but not least, diabetes usually worsens the prognosis of the patients with acute myocardial infarction accompanied with multivessel disease [27, 28]. It may affect the anti-apoptotic properties of atherosclerotic plaques and reduce the mobilization of stem cells to repair the damaged myocardial tissue [29, 30]. However, in the current study, diabetes did not play an important role in developing CS during primary PCI. It may be considered that diabetes influences the long-term prognosis rather than instant consequence of acute myocardial infarction. Moreover, incretin, a novel antidiabetic drug, has been identified a protective effect on the cardiovascular events. It could improve the cardiovascular prognosis of diabetic patients by pleiotropic effect [27, 28]. In our patient cohort, we did not have the detail percentage of the patients who had accepted incretin therapy, which preclude us to evaluate whether incretin therapy could protect the patients against developing CS during primary PCI.

Abbreviations

ACEI: Angiotensin converting enzyme inhibitor; ACS: Acute coronary syndrome; ARB: Angiotensin receptor blocker; AUC: Area under curve; CABG: Coronary artery bypass graft; CS: Cardiogenic shock; HR: Heart rate; IABP: Intra-aortic balloon counterpulsation; IRA: Infarct-related artery; LAD: Left anterior descending branch; LCX: Left circumflex branchor; MACE: Major adverse cardiac events; MI: Myocardial infarction; OM: Obtuse marginal branchas; PDA: Posterior descending artery; PL: Posterior branch of left venticule; pPCI: Primary percutaneous coronary intervention; RCA: Right coronary artery; ROC: Receiver-operating characteristics; SBP: Systolic blood pressure; SI: shock index; STEMI: ST segment elevation myocardial infarction

Fundings

This study was supported by the National Natural Science Foundation of China (No. 81700392) and the Municipal Medical Science Technology Development Foundation of Nanjing(No. YKK17085).

Authors' contributions

ZHW: Conception and design, manuscript writing, data analysis and interpretation. JB: manuscript writing, accountable for all aspects of the work in ensuring that questions related to the accuracy or integrity of any part of the work are appropriately investigated and resolved. QD: data analysis and interpretation. HW: data acquisition and graph making. SHQ: data acquisition and management. BX: manuscript revising for important intellectual content. LW: manuscript and data revising, approval of the version to be published. All the authors have read and approved the manuscript and ensure that this is the case.

Competing interests

The authors of this article have no competing interest.

References

1. O'Gara PT, Kushner FG, Ascheim DD, Casey DE Jr, Chung MK, de Lemos JA, et al. 2013 ACCF/AHA guideline for the management of ST-elevation myocardial infarction: a report of the American College of Cardiology Foundation/American Heart Association task force on practice guidelines. Circulation. 2013;127:e362–425.
2. Yellon DM, Hausenloy DJ. Myocardial reperfusion injury. N Engl J Med. 2007; 357:1121–35.
3. Frohlich GM, Meier P, White SK, Yellon DM, Hausenloy DJ. Myocardial reperfusion injury: looking beyond primary PCI. Eur Heart J. 2013;34:1714–22.
4. Goldberg RJ, Spencer FA, Gore JM, Lessard D, Yarzebski J. Thirty-year trends (1975 to 2005) in the magnitude of, management of, and hospital death rates associated with cardiogenic shock in patients with acute myocardial infarction: a population-based perspective. Circulation. 2009;119:1211–9.
5. De Luca L, Olivari Z, Farina A, Gonzini L, Lucci D, Di Chiara A, et al. Temporal trends in the epidemiology, management, and outcome of patients with cardiogenic shock complicating acute coronary syndromes. Eur J Heart Fail. 2015;17:1124–32.
6. Harjola VP, Lassus J, Sionis A, Kober L, Tarvasmaki T, Spinar J, et al. Clinical picture and risk prediction of short-term mortality in cardiogenic shock. Eur J Heart Fail. 2015;17:501–9.
7. Babaev A, Frederick PD, Pasta DJ, Every N, Sichrovsky T, Hochman JS. Trends in management and outcomes of patients with acute myocardial infarction complicated by cardiogenic shock. JAMA. 2005;294:448–54.
8. Spyridopoulos I, Noman A, Ahmed JM, Das R, Edwards R, Purcell I, et al. Shock-index as a novel predictor of long-term outcome following primary percutaneous coronary intervention. Eur Heart J Acute Cardiovasc Care. 2015;4:270–7.
9. Hemradj VV, Ottervanger JP, de Boer MJ, Suryapranata H. Shock index more sensitive than cardiogenic shock in ST-elevation myocardial infarction treated by primary percutaneous coronary intervention. Circ J. 2017;81:199–205.
10. Abe N, Miura T, Miyashita Y, Hashizume N, Ebisawa S, Motoki H, et al. Long-term prognostic implications of the admission shock index in patients with acute myocardial infarction who received percutaneous coronary intervention. Angiology. 2017;68:339–45.
11. Yu T, Tian C, Song J, He D, Sun Z. Derivation and validation of shock index as a parameter for predicting long-term prognosis in patients with acute coronary syndrome. Sci Rep. 2017;7:11929.
12. Thygesen K, Alpert JS, Jaffe AS, Simoons ML, Chaitman BR, White HD, et al. Third universal definition of myocardial infarction. Circulation. 2012;126: 2020–35.
13. Thiele H, Zeymer U, Neumann FJ, Ferenc M, Olbrich HG, Hausleiter J, et al. Intraaortic balloon support for myocardial infarction with cardiogenic shock. N Engl J Med. 2012;367:1287–96.
14. McMahon CG, Kenny R, Bennett K, Little R, Kirkman E. The effect of acute traumatic brain injury on the performance of shock index. J Trauma. 2010; 69:1169–75.
15. Bircan A, Karadeniz N, Ozden A, Cakir M, Varol E, Oyar O, et al. A simple clinical model composed of ECG, shock index, and arterial blood gas analysis for predicting severe pulmonary embolism. Clin Appl Thromb Hemost. 2011;17:188–96.
16. Birkhahn RH, Gaeta TJ, Terry D, Bove JJ, Tloczkowski J. Shock index in diagnosing early acute hypovolemia. Am J Emerg Med. 2005;23:323–6.
17. Sankaran P, Kamath AV, Tariq SM, Ruffell H, Smith AC, Prentice P, et al. Are shock index and adjusted shock index useful in predicting mortality and length of stay in community-acquired pneumonia? Eur J Intern Med. 2011; 22:282–5.
18. Rappaport LD, Deakyne S, Carcillo JA, McFann K, Sills MR. Age- and sex-specific normal values for shock index in National Health and nutrition examination survey 1999-2008 for ages 8 years and older. Am J Emerg Med. 2013;31:838–42.
19. Keller AS, Kirkland LL, Rajasekaran SY, Cha S, Rady MY, Huddleston JM. Unplanned transfers to the intensive care unit: the role of the shock index. J Hosp Med. 2010;5:460–5.
20. Guyette F, Suffoletto B, Castillo JL, Quintero J, Callaway C, Puyana JC. Prehospital serum lactate as a predictor of outcomes in trauma patients: a retrospective observational study. J Trauma. 2011;70:782–6.
21. De Luca G, Savonitto S, Greco C, Parodi G, Dajelli Ermolli NC, Silva C, et al. Cardiogenic shock developing in the coronary care unit in patients with ST-elevation myocardial infarction. J Cardiovasc Med (Hagerstown). 2008;9:1023–9.
22. Obling L, Frydland M, Hansen R, Moller-Helgestad OK, Lindholm MG, Holmvang L, et al. Risk factors of late cardiogenic shock and mortality in ST-segment elevation myocardial infarction patients. Eur Heart J Acute Cardiovasc Care. 2018;7:7–15.
23. Park MK. Blood pressure tables. Pediatrics. 2005;115:826–7 author reply 7.
24. Yu T, Tian C, Song J, He D, Sun Z. Age shock index is superior to shock index and modified shock index for predicting long-term prognosis in acute myocardial infarction. Shock. 2017;48:545–50.
25. Zarzaur BL, Croce MA, Fischer PE, Magnotti LJ, Fabian TC. New vitals after injury: shock index for the young and age x shock index for the old. J Surg Res. 2008;147:229–36.
26. Torabi M, Moeinaddini S, Mirafzal A, Rastegari A, Sadeghkhani N. Shock index, modified shock index, and age shock index for prediction of mortality in emergency severity index level 3. Am J Emerg Med. 2016;34:2079–83.
27. Marfella R, Sardu C, Balestrieri ML, Siniscalchi M, Minicucci F, Signoriello G, et al. Effects of incretin treatment on cardiovascular outcomes in diabetic STEMI-patients with culprit obstructive and multivessel non obstructive-coronary-stenosis. Diabetol Metab Syndr. 2018;10:1.
28. Marfella R, Sardu C, Calabro P, Siniscalchi M, Minicucci F, Signoriello G, et al. Non-ST-elevation myocardial infarction outcomes in patients with type 2 diabetes with non-obstructive coronary artery stenosis: effects of incretin treatment. Diabetes Obes Metab. 2018;20:723–9.
29. Balestrieri ML, Rizzo MR, Barbieri M, Paolisso P, D'Onofrio N, Giovane A, et al. Sirtuin 6 expression and inflammatory activity in diabetic atherosclerotic plaques: effects of incretin treatment. Diabetes. 2015;64:1395–406.
30. Marfella R, Rizzo MR, Siniscalchi M, Paolisso P, Barbieri M, Sardu C, et al. Peri-procedural tight glycemic control during early percutaneous coronary intervention up-regulates endothelial progenitor cell level and differentiation during acute ST-elevation myocardial infarction: effects on myocardial salvage. Int J Cardiol. 2013;168:3954–62.

Serum matrix metalloproteinase-9 is a valuable biomarker for identification of abdominal and thoracic aortic aneurysm: a case-control study

Tan Li[1], Bo Jiang[2], Xuan Li[2], Hai-yang Sun[1], Xin-tong Li[2], Jing-jing Jing[3] and Jun Yang[1*]

Abstract

Background: Matrix metalloproteinase-9 (MMP9) has been reported to play a key role in the pathogenesis of aortic aneurysm. However, few studies have assessed serum MMP9 levels in both abdominal aortic aneurysm (AAA) and thoracic aortic aneurysm (TAA). In this study, we investigated the serum levels of MMP9 in aortic aneurysm to evaluate its predictive and diagnostic efficacy for AAA and TAA, and explored the association of MMP9 with circulating laboratory markers.

Methods: A total of 296 subjects were enrolled, including 105 AAA patients, 79 TAA patients and 112 healthy controls. The levels of serum MMP9 were detected by enzyme-linked immunosorbent assay (ELISA).

Results: Compared to control group, both AAA and TAA patients had higher serum MMP9 levels in the overall comparison and subgroup analysis based on subjects aged<65 years, either male or female, hypertension, non-diabetes and non-hyperlipidemia (all $P<0.05$). Moreover, MMP9 levels were significantly higher in TAA group than those in AAA group in the total comparison, and this discrepancy was also found in the non-diabetes, non-hyperlipidemia and aortic diameter ≥ 5.5 cm subgroup analysis. Serum MMP9 levels were influenced by age and hypertension. There was a positive association of serum MMP9 with CRP ($r = 0.33$, $P < 0.001$) and Hcy ($r = 0.199$, $P = 0.033$). Multiple logistic analyses showed that serum MMP9 was an independent risk factor for AAA and TAA. Based on receiver operating characteristic (ROC) analysis, the area under the curve (AUC) of MMP9 for predicting TAA was 0.83 with 70% sensitivity and 91% specificity, while the AUC of MMP9 to detect AAA was 0.69 and the sensitivity and specificity were 50% and 88%.

Conclusions: Serum MMP9 was closely related to the existence of aortic aneurysms and could be a valuable marker for the discrimination of aortic aneurysm, especially for TAA.

Keywords: Matrix metalloproteinase-9, Abdominal aortic aneurysm, Thoracic aortic aneurysm, C- reactive protein

Background

Aortic aneurysm is a complex and dangerous vascular disease that results from the multifactorial interaction of genetic and environmental factors [1]. According to anatomical locations, aortic aneurysm is generally divided into abdominal aortic aneurysm (AAA) and thoracic aortic aneurysm (TAA). They may share some similarities in pathogenesis and histological phenotypes that both involve the metabolic imbalance and progressive weakening of aortic wall [2, 3], but not for syndrome and bicuspid valve associated TAA. Matrix metalloproteinase-9 (MMP9) is a gelatinase with proteolytic activity on extracellular matrix degradation in aortic wall and its excessive production can lead to progressive aortic remodeling and dilatation [2]. Any cause increasing the activity of aortic endothelial cells, smooth muscle cells and infiltrating

* Correspondence: yangjun@cmu1h.com
[1]Department of Cardiovascular Ultrasound, the First Hospital of China Medical University, No.155 Nanjing Bei Street, Heping District, Shenyang 110001, China
Full list of author information is available at the end of the article

inflammatory cells can produce a large amount of MMP9 released into blood circulation [4].

Evidence has demonstrated higher circulating MMP9 levels in AAA patients [5, 6]. As for TAA, studies often focused on the gene variation and tissue expression of MMP9 [7, 8], but much less is known about the association between serum MMP9 and TAA. A study by Meffert et al. suggested no different expression of serum MMP9 between TAA with hyperlipidemia and without hyperlipidemia [9]. Based on small sample sizes, Tsarouhas et al. revealed that there were increased MMP9 levels in TAA serum and tissue [10], however, Karapanagiotidis et al. showed that TAA patients had lower serum MMP9 levels [11]. To our knowledge, there were no studies available on detailed comparison of serum MMP9 levels in AAA and TAA, and the performance of serum MMP9 for identification of aortic aneurysm is still unknown. To date, circulating biomarkers, such as C-reactive protein (CRP), homocysteine (Hcy) and Cystatin C (Cys-c), have been analyzed in aortic aneurysmal diseases, but it remains unclear whether the studied biomarkers are correlated with serum MMP9.

In the present study, we attempted to explore the overall and stratified comparative differences in serum MMP9 levels and evaluate its potential clinical applicability for predicting AAA and TAA. Meanwhile, we intended to determine the relationship between serum MMP9 and other laboratory markers to discuss their possible interaction relevant for aortic aneurysm.

Methods

Subjects

This was a single center, case-control study. A total of 105 AAA patients, 79 TAA patients and 112 controls were recruited from the First Hospital of China Medical University between October 2016 and October 2017. Thoracoabdominal aortic aneurysms and AAA cases with extension to the iliac artery were not included in this study. The diagnosis of all patients was based on the computed tomography angiography (CTA). Exclusion criteria included the subjects accompanied by congenital genetic disorders, severe cardiovascular diseases, autoimmune diseases, severe organ failure, infectious diseases, malignant tumors, hematological system diseases, previous aortic surgery or received non-steroidal anti-inflammatory drugs or steroids. Demographic data, risk factors and laboratory parameters were obtained from clinical records. Hypertension was defined as having a systolic blood pressure (SBP) ≥ 140 mmHg and/or having a diastolic blood pressure (DBP) ≥90 mmHg and/or being under antihypertensive treatment. Diabetes was defined as fasting serum glucose (FPG) ≥7 mmol/L (126 mg/dL) and (or) being on treatment for diabetes [12]. Hyperlipidemia was defined as serum total cholesterol (TC) ≥6.22 mmol/L (240 mg/dL), or serum triglyceride (TG) ≥2.26 mmol/L (200 mg/dL), or serum low-density lipoprotein cholesterol (LDL-C) ≥4.14 mmol/L (160 mg/dL) [13]. For subjects with AAA or TAA, the maximal aortic diameter was assessed via CTA using the average of three measurements. This study was approved by the Ethics Committee of the First Hospital of China Medical University (Shenyang, China). Written informed consent was obtained from each subject.

Detection of serum MMP9

Blood samples were collected using standardized sterile tubes and centrifuged at 3500 r/min for 10 min at 4 °C, and the serum was separated, and stored at – 80 °C until being assayed. Serum MMP9 levels were measured by enzyme-linked immunosorbent assay (ELISA) using MMP9 ELISA kits (Wuhan Boster Biotechnology Company, Wuhan, Hubei, China), according to the manufacturer's protocol.

Statistical analysis

All statistical analyses were performed using SPSS version 17.0 software. Continuous variables were reported as mean values and standard deviations, and categorical variables were represented as numbers and percentages. Differences among categories were evaluated using ANOVA, independent-sample t-test or χ^2 test as appropriate. Spearman's rank correlation test was used to examine the associations of serum MMP9 levels with laboratory markers and maximal aortic diameter. Multiple logistic regression models were performed to determine the predictive value of serum MMP9 in AAA or TAA risk with the adjustment for the potential confounding factors. Receiver operating characteristic (ROC) curves and the area under the curve (AUC) were used to evaluate the diagnostic effects of serum MMP9 and to determine appropriate cut-off points. A two-sided $P<0.05$ was considered statistically significant.

Results

Characteristics of the study subjects

The detailed clinical characteristics of the cases and controls were described and compared in Table 1. Male members made up a larger proportion in three groups. AAA and TAA patients tended to have higher heart rate, leucocyte count and blood pressure compared with control subjects.

Serum MMP9 levels between different groups in the total and stratified comparisons

Serum MMP9 levels in control, AAA and TAA groups were 258.79 ± 133.00, 333.45 ± 138.57 and 385.17 ± 109.23 ng/ml, respectively. In the total comparison, there were significantly higher serum MMP9 levels in AAA and TAA groups than those in control

Table 1 Clinical characteristics of the study subjects

Variables	Control $N = 112$	AAA $N = 105$	TAA $N = 79$
Age, years	62.32 ± 11.23	66.75 ± 10.28$^{\#}$	59.04 ± 11.55*†
Males, n (%)	83(74.1%)	78(74.2%)	57(72.2%)
Height, cm	167.70 ± 7.20	169.49 ± 7.06	169.61 ± 7.10
Weight, kg	70.12 ± 10.13	66.40 ± 12.36$^{\#}$	73.38 ± 11.80†
Heart rate, bmp	73.58 ± 9.67	79.70 ± 13.58$^{\#}$	79.92 ± 15.65*
Leucocyte, $\times 10^9$/L	5.82 ± 1.77	7.94 ± 3.53$^{\#}$	11.16 ± 4.87*†
Thrombocyte, $\times 10^9$/L	221.51 ± 56.72	218.65 ± 81.38	207.88 ± 64.66
SBP, mmHg	134.48 ± 17.19	141.79 ± 19.56$^{\#}$	152.69 ± 28.98*†
DBP, mmHg	77.70 ± 11.67	80.65 ± 12.22	86.44 ± 18.33*
TC, mmol/L	4.90 ± 0.87	4.75 ± 1.01	4.41 ± 0.91*†
TG, mmol/L	1.53 ± 0.88	1.40 ± 1.06	1.35 ± 0.90
LDL-C, mmol/L	3.13 ± 0.77	3.15 ± 0.91	2.68 ± 0.74*†
HDL-C, mmol/L	1.32 ± 0.34	1.04 ± 0.31$^{\#}$	1.13 ± 0.37*
FPG, mmol/L	5.55 ± 1.63	5.74 ± 1.56	6.43 ± 1.84*†
CRP, mg/L	–	32.97 ± 51.71	64.95 ± 47.47†
Hcy, umol/L	–	18.60 ± 11.60	18.52 ± 12.77
Cys-c, mg/L	–	1.14 ± 0.44	1.40 ± 0.76†
Max. aortic diameter, cm	–	5.64 ± 1.61	5.28 ± 0.95

AAA abdominal aortic aneurysm, *TAA* thoracic aortic aneurysm
$P^{\#}$: AAA vs. Control, P^{*}: TAA vs. Control, $P^{\dagger}$: TAA vs. AAA

group, while TAA subjects had higher serum MMP9 levels when compared with AAA patients(all $P<0.05$).

Furthermore, we compared serum MMP9 levels between different groups stratified by age, gender, hypertension, diabetes or hyperlipidemia status and maximal aortic diameter, as shown in Table 2. The results showed that MMP9 levels were significantly increased from control to AAA to TAA group in the subjects aged<65 years. Compared to control group, AAA and TAA patients had increased MMP9 levels in either male or female, and this discrepancy was also found in hypertension status. Meanwhile, serum MMP9 levels in TAA patients were significantly higher than those in AAA subjects in male subgroup comparison. However, in the non-diabetes and non-hyperlipidemia status, MMP9 levels were obviously higher from control to AAA to TAA group (all $P < 0.05$). When stratified by maximal aortic diameter, TAA patients tended to have higher MMP9 levels than AAA cases only in the subgroup with max. Aortic diameter ≥ 5.5 cm.

Influence of age, gender, risk factors and maximal aortic diameter on serum MMP9

Table 2 also showed the comparison results in the individual group. We found that the≥65 years group had much higher serum MMP9 levels compared with the <65 years group in the control and AAA group. Serum MMP9 levels were significantly higher in subjects with hypertension than those without hypertension in each group (all $P<0.05$). However, there were no significant differences in the serum MMP9 levels between male and female, diabetes and non-diabetes, hyperlipidemia and non- hyperlipidemia, max. Aortic diameter ≥ 5.5 cm and <5.5 cm groups.

Correlation of serum MMP9 with laboratory biomarkers and maximal size of aneurysm

We evaluated a possible correlation between MMP9 levels and CRP, Cys-c, Hcy and maximal aortic diameter. Serum MMP9 levels had a positive association with the concentration of CRP($r = 0.330$, $P < 0.001$) and Hcy($r = 0.199$, $P = 0.033$) (Fig. 1). However, there was no significant relationship of MMP9 levels with Cys-c($r = 0.097$, $P = 0.272$) and maximal aortic diameter($r = 0.008$, $P = 0.918$).

Predictive and diagnostic value of serum MMP9 for aortic aneurysm

We further performed multiple logistic regressions to evaluate the risk prediction value of serum MMP9 for AAA and TAA under different adjustment models, as shown in Table 3. When all potential confounding factors were adjusted, serum MMP9 was still significantly associated with AAA risk (OR = 1.004 per unit increase, 95% CI

Table 2 Serum MMP9 levels in age, gender, risk factors and maximal aortic diameter

		Control			AAA			TAA		$P^{\#}$	P^{*}	$P^{\dagger}$
		MMP9(ng/ml)	*P*		MMP9(ng/ml)	*P*		MMP9(ng/ml)	*P*			
Total		258.79 ± 133.00			333.45 ± 138.57			385.17 ± 109.23		<0.001	<0.001	0.015
Age	<65y(60)	200.78 ± 139.20	<0.001	<65y(47)	299.44 ± 160.84	0.029	<65y(52)	378.63 ± 96.80	0.464	0.004	<0.001	0.013
	≥65y(52)	325.73 ± 86.94		≥65y(58)	361.01 ± 111.50		≥65y(27)	397.77 ± 131.00		0.087	0.005	0.143
Gender	male(83)	260.57 ± 135.13	0.812	male(78)	328.11 ± 144.39	0.505	male(55)	390.09 ± 110.19	0.548	0.008	<0.001	0.017
	female(29)	253.69 ± 128.88		female(27)	348.88 ± 121.38		female(24)	373.90 ± 108.47		0.004	0.001	0.462
Hypertension	Yes(46)	291.13 ± 114.98	0.026	Yes(64)	362.45 ± 140.89	0.007	Yes(53)	405.44 ± 91.35	0.038	0.013	<0.001	0.141
	No(66)	236.25 ± 140.71		No(41)	288.17 ± 123.34		No(26)	343.87 ± 131.23		0.053	0.001	0.099
Diabetes	Yes(14)	308.00 ± 110.55	0.11	Yes(23)	316.37 ± 153.51	0.506	Yes(33)	379.07 ± 124.77	0.677	0.997	0.177	0.301
	No(98)	251.76 ± 134.93		No(82)	338.24 ± 134.72		No(46)	389.55 ± 97.79		<0.001	<0.001	0.043
Hyperlipidemia	Yes(26)	273.10 ± 128.94	0.494	Yes(23)	359.34 ± 151.80	0.313	Yes(16)	402.51 ± 100.01	0.481	0.099	0.002	0.644
	No(86)	253.56 ± 134.85		No(82)	326.19 ± 134.73		No(63)	380.77 ± 111.77		0.002	<0.001	0.026
Max. aortic diameter	NA	–	–	<5.5(60)	334.62 ± 131.26	0.923	<5.5(55)	371.19 ± 112.91	0.085	–	–	0.114
	NA	–		≥5.5(45)	331.89 ± 149.26		≥5.5(24)	417.22 ± 94.82		–	–	0.005

AAA abdominal aortic aneurysm, *TAA* thoracic aortic aneurysm

$P^{\#}$: AAA vs. Control, P^{*}: TAA vs. Control, $P^{\dagger}$: TAA vs. AAA

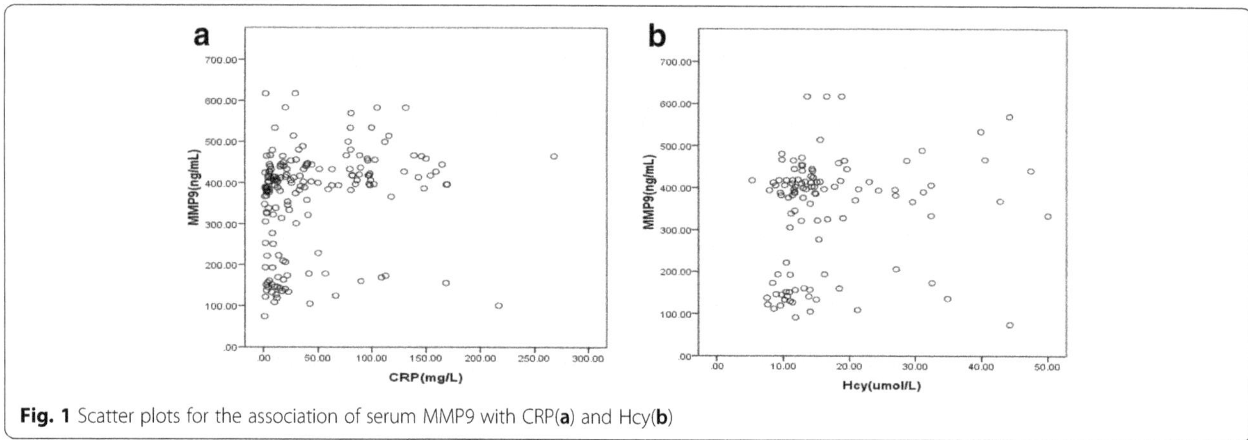

Fig. 1 Scatter plots for the association of serum MMP9 with CRP(**a**) and Hcy(**b**)

= 1.001–1.007, P = 0.018) and TAA risk (OR = 1.014 per unit increase, 95% CI = 1.006–1.022, $P < 0.001$).

In addition, the ROC curves of MMP9 levels for predicting AAA and TAA (Fig. 2). The ROC curve analysis illustrated that MMP9 levels had strong diagnostic value for TAA with the AUC of 0.83(95% CI: 0.77–0.90; $P < 0.001$) and an optimal cut-off point of 393.00 ng/ml associated with corresponding validity parameters of 70% sensitivity and 91% specificity. However, the AUC of MMP9 for predicting AAA was 0.69(95% CI: 0.62–0.76; $P < 0.001$) and MMP9 ≥ 385.32 ng/ml had a sensitivity of 50% and a specificity of 88%.

Discussion

Serum MMP9 levels represent the leakage of enzyme into the bloodstream during periods of matrix catabolism and its elevation may reflect a more active state of degeneration of the aortic wall. In the current study, our results suggested higher MMP9 levels in either AAA or TAA group than those in control group. Interestingly, we also found that TAA patients tended to have higher MMP9 levels than AAA subjects in the overall comparison, which might depend on their different embryological feature, wall mechanics and arterial hemodynamics [2]. Compared to the abdominal aorta, thoracic aorta has thicker aortic media [14, 15] and a higher degree of wall shear stress [16, 17], which were possibly linked to higher MMP9 production for aneurysm formation.

In the subgroup comparisons stratified by age, gender, hypertension, diabetes and hyperlipidemia, we found that both AAA and TAA patients had higher MMP9 levels in the subjects aged <65 years, either male or female, and hypertensive status compared with controls. In addition, MMP9 levels showed to increase from control to AAA to TAA group in the non-diabetes and non-hyperlipidemia status. Hypertension is a well-known risk factor associated with aortic aneurysm. However, although diabetes and hyperlipidemia are recognized cardiovascular risk factors strongly associated with most acquired cardiovascular pathologies, they seem to be relatively weak risk factors for aortic aneurysm. Some studies indicated that the presence of diabetes had a reduced risk for aortic aneurysm, resulting from decreased MMPs production and activation in the aortic wall [18, 19]. Recent research also found that diabetes inhibited experimental aortic aneurysm progression through reducing macrophage infiltration and medial elastolysis, and lowering serum glucose could diminish its protective effects [20, 21]. Hyperlipidemia and its associated effect on extracellular matrix have also

Table 3 Multiple logistic regression analysis of serum MMP9 levels for AAA and TAA risk

Variables	AAA		TAA	
	OR(95%CI)	P	OR(95%CI)	P
Model 1				
MMP9, ng/mL	1.004(1.002–1.006)	<0.001	1.010(1.007–1.013)	<0.001
Model 2				
MMP9, ng/mL	1.004(1.001–1.007)	0.006	1.012(1.007–1.018)	<0.001
Model 3				
MMP9, ng/mL	1.004(1.001–1.007)	0.018	1.014(1.006–1.022)	<0.001

Model 1: age and gender were adjusted
Model 2: Model 1 plus height, weight, heart rate, leucocyte and thrombocyte
Model 3: Model 2 plus hypertension, diabetes and hyperlipidemia

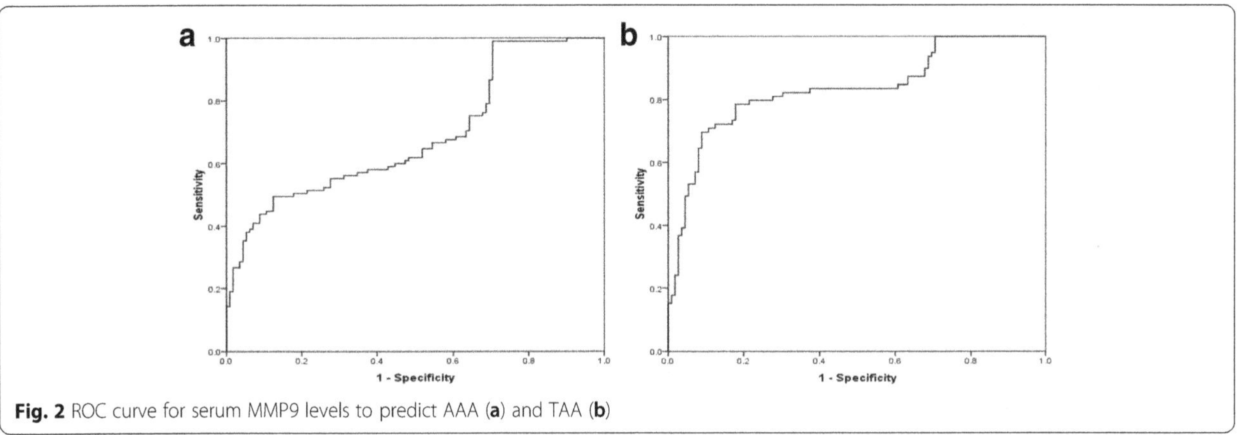

Fig. 2 ROC curve for serum MMP9 levels to predict AAA (**a**) and TAA (**b**)

been demonstrated to limit AAA formation in mice [21], and showed a negative association with AAA risk [22, 23]. These observations identified the protective role of diabetes and hyperlipidemia in aneurysm formation, which might partly account for our findings that the different MMP9 levels were obviously reflected in non-diabetic and non-hyperlipidemia subgroup analysis. Furthermore, we analyzed the effects of traditional cardiovascular risk factors on serum MMP9 levels. We found that subjects aged ≥65 years had higher MMP9 levels than those aged <65 years. Additionally, hypertensive participants exhibited much higher serum MMP9 levels than non-hypertensive ones in each group.

Maximal aortic diameter, as a surrogate clinical marker of the growth rate, has been used to discuss its potential correlation with MMP9 levels [16]. MMP9 activity varied with aortic diameter in AAA, and its expression was reported to be elevated in aneurysms with a diameter of 5.0 to 6.9 cm [24]. Freestone et al. [25] indicated an increased activity of MMP9 in aneurysms with a diameter ≥ 5.5 cm. On the contrary, neither Hovsepian nor Eugster had observed a significant correlation between serum MMP9 and aneurysm size of AAA [26, 27]. A recent study also suggested no relationship between serum MMP9 and TAA diameter [9]. In our study, serum MMP9 levels were not influenced by maximal aortic diameter in either AAA or TAA group, however, TAA patients were prone to have higher MMP9 levels than AAA subjects in aortic diameter ≥ 5.5 cm subgroup comparison.

Various systemic laboratory diagnostic biomarkers have been investigated and linked to the risk for aortic aneurysm or its outcomes, such as CRP, Hcy and Cys-c. CRP, a sensitive and non-specific inflammatory marker, has been recognized as an independent risk factor in the detection of vascular inflammation [4]. It has been considered to be associated with aortic aneurysm presence and progression [28, 29]. Moreover, CRP can induce MMP9 production in human mononuclear cells in a concentration-dependent manner [30, 31]. Hcy, a sulfur containing amino acid, has been suggested to play a key role in aortic aneurysm [32, 33]. Moreover, Hcy can produce marked vascular remodeling and elastolysis of the aortic wall by excessive MMPs production and activation [10, 34]. Above evidence might explain our findings that serum MMP9 levels were positively correlated with circulating CRP and Hcy, which could partly reflect the fact that multiple biomarkers responded to aortic aneurysm related events. Although circulating Cys-c has been proved to be related to AAA and may favor proteolysis in the pathogenesis of AAA [35], we found no association of serum MMP9 with Cys-c.

To further assess the clinical application value of serum MMP9 in aortic aneurysm, we explored its predictive and diagnostic efficacy for identifying AAA or TAA. In multiple logistic analyses after adjusting the possible confounders, we demonstrated that serum MMP9 was an independent risk factor for the existence of AAA or TAA. With a low expected incidence, the focus for a biomarker should primarily be on specificity. Based on ROC curves, elevated MMP9 levels suggested a higher specificity than sensitivity in recognizing either AAA or TAA, which represented that serum MMP9 conferred a crucial role in safely ruling out aortic aneurysm. Moreover, AUCs, cut-off points for serum MMP9, and the sensitivity and specificity were much better with its use for predicting TAA than AAA. Therefore, serum MMP9 may be a valuable diagnostic biomarker for aortic aneurysm, especially for TAA.

Our study has some limitations. First, our sample size was small, and a more precise localization and detailed classification for TAA cases were lacking. Second, the serial measurements of MMP9 levels for evaluating dynamic changes were not investigated. Third, there were no complete records of potential confounders relevant to aortic aneurysm and MMP9 levels, such as the history of smoking and drinking. In addition, histological samples and MMP9 tissue expression were not investigated in this study. Further prospective studies based on larger scale cohorts will be needed to validate the clinical applicability of serum MMP9 on the identification of aortic aneurysm initiation and progression in the future practice.

Conclusions

Our results suggested that MMP9 levels were significantly increased in AAA and TAA group. Furthermore, we also found TAA patients tended to have higher levels of MMP9 than AAA subjects in the overall comparison, and in the non-diabetes, non-hyperlipidemia and aortic diameter ≥ 5.5 cm subgroup analysis. Moreover, MMP9 levels were affected by age and hypertension, and were positively associated with circulating CRP and Hcy. Multiple logistic analyses further suggested that serum MMP9 was an independent risk factor for aortic aneurysm. Serum MMP9 showed a high specificity for the diagnosis of either AAA or TAA. Therefore, MMP9 might be a useful biomarker with clinical predictive and diagnostic value for aortic aneurysm, especially for TAA.

Abbreviations

AAA: Abdominal aortic aneurysm; AUC: Area under the curve; CRP: C-reactive protein; CTA: Computed tomography angiography; Cys-c: Cystatin C; DBP: Diastolic blood pressure; ELISA: Enzyme-linked immunosorbent assay; FPG: Fasting serum glucose; Hcy: Homocysteine; HDL-C: High-density lipoprotein cholesterol; LDL-C: Low-density lipoprotein cholesterol; MMP9: Matrix metalloproteinase-9; ROC: Receiver operating characteristic; SBP: Systolic blood pressure; TAA: Thoracic aortic aneurysm; TC: Total cholesterol; TG: Triglyceride

Acknowledgments

The authors would like to thank Professor Yuan Yuan and Shi-jie Xin for their assistance for the coordination of this study.

Funding

This work is supported by grants from the Natural Science Foundation of Liaoning Province (Ref No. 2015020506).

Authors' contributions

TL performed the experiments, analyzed the data and drafted the manuscript. BJ and XL contributed to the clinical data and blood sample collection. HYS, XTL and JJJ participated in the experiments. JY was involved in supervisory role in study design. All authors have read and approved the final manuscript.

Competing interests

All authors declare that they have no competing interests.

Author details

[1]Department of Cardiovascular Ultrasound, the First Hospital of China Medical University, No.155 Nanjing Bei Street, Heping District, Shenyang 110001, China. [2]Department of Vascular and Thyroid Surgery, the First Hospital of China Medical University, Shenyang 110001, China. [3]Tumor Etiology and Screening Department of Cancer Institute and General Surgery, the First Hospital of China Medical University, Shenyang 110001, China.

References

1. Baumann F, Makaloski V, Diehm N. Aortic aneurysms and aortic dissection: epidemiology pathophysiology and diagnostics. Der Internist. 2013;54(5): 535–42.
2. Guo DC, Papke CL, He R, Milewicz DM. Pathogenesis of thoracic and abdominal aortic aneurysms. Ann N Y Acad Sci. 2006;1085:339–52.
3. Matsumoto KI, Satoh K, Maniwa T, Tanaka T, Okunishi H, Oda T. Proteomic comparison between abdominal and thoracic aortic aneurysms. Int J Mol Med. 2014;33(4):1035–47.
4. Wen D, Zhou XL, Li JJ, Hui RT. Biomarkers in aortic dissection. Clin Chim Acta. 2011;412(9–10):688–95.
5. Grodin JL, Powell-Wiley TM, Ayers CR, Kumar DS, Rohatgi A, Khera A, McGuire DK, de Lemos JA, Das SR. Circulating levels of matrix metalloproteinase-9 and abdominal aortic pathology: from the Dallas heart study. Vasc Med. 2011;16(5):339–45.
6. Takagi H, Manabe H, Kawai N, Goto SN, Umemoto T. Circulating matrix metalloproteinase-9 concentrations and abdominal aortic aneurysm presence: a meta-analysis. Interact Cardiovasc Thorac Surg. 2009;9(3):437–40.
7. Rabkin SW. Differential expression of MMP-2, MMP-9 and TIMP proteins in thoracic aortic aneurysm - comparison with and without bicuspid aortic valve: a meta-analysis. Vasa. 2014;43(6):433–42.
8. Zhang X, Wu D, Choi JC, Minard CG, Hou X, Coselli JS, Shen YH, LeMaire SA. Matrix metalloproteinase levels in chronic thoracic aortic dissection. J Surg Res. 2014;189(2):348–58.
9. Meffert P, Tscheuschler A, Beyersdorf F, Heilmann C, Kocher N, Uffelmann X, Discher P, Rylski B, Siepe M, Kari FA. Characterization of serum matrix metalloproteinase 2/9 levels in patients with ascending aortic aneurysms. Interact Cardiovasc Thorac Surg. 2017;24(1):20–6.
10. Tsarouhas K, Tsitsimpikou C, Apostolakis S, Haliassos A, Tzardi M, Panagiotou M, Tsatsakis A, Spandidos DA. Homocysteine and metalloprotease-3 and -9 in patients with ascending aorta aneurysms. Thromb Res. 2011;128(5):e95–9.
11. Karapanagiotidis GT, Antonitsis P, Charokopos N, Foroulis CN, Anastasiadis K, Rouska E, Argiriadou H, Rammos K, Papakonstantinou C. Serum levels of matrix metalloproteinases −1,-2,-3 and −9 in thoracic aortic diseases and acute myocardial ischemia. J Cardiothorac Surg. 2009;4:59.
12. Li T, Chen S, Guo X, Yang J, Sun Y. Impact of hypertension with or without diabetes on left ventricular remodeling in rural Chinese population: a cross-sectional study. BMC Cardiovasc Disord. 2017;17(1):206.
13. Expert Panel on Detection E, Treatment of High Blood Cholesterol in A. Executive summary of the third report of the National Cholesterol Education Program (NCEP) expert panel on detection, evaluation, and treatment of high blood cholesterol in adults (adult treatment panel III). Jama. 2001;285(19):2486–97.
14. Davis FM, Rateri DL, Daugherty A. Mechanisms of aortic aneurysm formation: translating preclinical studies into clinical therapies. Heart. 2014; 100(19):1498–505.
15. Ito S, Akutsu K, Tamori Y, Sakamoto S, Yoshimuta T, Hashimoto H, Takeshita S. Differences in atherosclerotic profiles between patients with thoracic and abdominal aortic aneurysms. Am J Cardiol. 2008;101(5):696–9.
16. Astrand H, Ryden-Ahlgren A, Sundkvist G, Sandgren T, Lanne T. Reduced aortic wall stress in diabetes mellitus. Eur J Vasc Endovasc Surg. 2007;33(5): 592–8.
17. Castier Y, Brandes RP, Leseche G, Tedgui A, Lehoux S. p47phox-dependent NADPH oxidase regulates flow-induced vascular remodeling. Circ Res. 2005; 97(6):533–40.
18. Gertz SD, Gavish L, Mintz Y, Beeri R, Rubinstein C, Gavish LY, Berlatzky Y, Appelbaum L, Gilon D. Contradictory effects of hypercholesterolemia and diabetes mellitus on the progression of abdominal aortic aneurysm. Am J Cardiol. 2015;115(3):399–401.

19. Golledge J, Karan M, Moran CS, Muller J, Clancy P, Dear AE, Norman PE. Reduced expansion rate of abdominal aortic aneurysms in patients with diabetes may be related to aberrant monocyte-matrix interactions. Eur Heart J. 2008;29(5):665–72.
20. Dua MM, Miyama N, Azuma J, Schultz GM, Sho M, Morser J, Dalman RL. Hyperglycemia modulates plasminogen activator inhibitor-1 expression and aortic diameter in experimental aortic aneurysm disease. Surgery. 2010; 148(2):429–35.
21. Miyama N, Dua MM, Yeung JJ, Schultz GM, Asagami T, Sho E, Sho M, Dalman RL. Hyperglycemia limits experimental aortic aneurysm progression. J Vasc Surg. 2010;52(4):975–83.
22. Chun KC, Teng KY, Chavez LA, Van Spyk EN, Samadzadeh KM, Carson JG, Lee ES. Risk factors associated with the diagnosis of abdominal aortic aneurysm in patients screened at a regional veterans affairs health care system. Ann Vasc Surg. 2014;28(1):87–92.
23. Golledge J, van Bockxmeer F, Jamrozik K, McCann M, Norman PE. Association between serum lipoproteins and abdominal aortic aneurysm. Am J Cardiol. 2010;105(10):1480–4.
24. McMillan WD, Tamarina NA, Cipollone M, Johnson DA, Parker MA, Pearce WH. Size matters: the relationship between MMP-9 expression and aortic diameter. Circulation. 1997;96(7):2228–32.
25. Freestone T, Turner RJ, Coady A, Higman DJ, Greenhalgh RM, Powell JT. Inflammation and matrix metalloproteinases in the enlarging abdominal aortic aneurysm. Arterioscler Thromb Vasc Biol. 1995;15(8):1145–51.
26. Eugster T, Huber A, Obeid T, Schwegler I, Gurke L, Stierli P. Aminoterminal propeptide of type III procollagen and matrix metalloproteinases-2 and -9 failed to serve as serum markers for abdominal aortic aneurysm. Eur J Vasc Endovasc Surg. 2005;29(4):378–82.
27. Hovsepian DM, Ziporin SJ, Sakurai MK, Lee JK, Curci JA, Thompson RW. Elevated plasma levels of matrix metalloproteinase-9 in patients with abdominal aortic aneurysms: a circulating marker of degenerative aneurysm disease. J Vasc Interv Radiol. 2000;11(10):1345–52.
28. Golledge J, Tsao PS, Dalman RL, Norman PE. Circulating markers of abdominal aortic aneurysm presence and progression. Circulation. 2008; 118(23):2382–92.
29. Hellenthal FA, Buurman WA, Wodzig WK, Schurink GW. Biomarkers of abdominal aortic aneurysm progression. Part 2: inflammation. Nat Rev Cardiol. 2009;6(8):543–52.
30. Nabata A, Kuroki M, Ueba H, Hashimoto S, Umemoto T, Wada H, Yasu T, Saito M, Momomura S, Kawakami M. C-reactive protein induces endothelial cell apoptosis and matrix metalloproteinase-9 production in human mononuclear cells: implications for the destabilization of atherosclerotic plaque. Atherosclerosis. 2008;196(1):129–35.
31. Singh U, Dasu MR, Yancey PG, Afify A, Devaraj S, Jialal I. Human C-reactive protein promotes oxidized low density lipoprotein uptake and matrix metalloproteinase-9 release in Wistar rats. J Lipid Res. 2008;49(5):1015–23.
32. Moroz P, Le MT, Norman PE. Homocysteine and abdominal aortic aneurysms. ANZ J Surg. 2007;77(5):329–32.
33. Narayanan N, Tyagi N, Shah A, Pagni S, Tyagi SC. Hyperhomocysteinemia during aortic aneurysm a plausible role of epigenetics. Int J Physiol Pathophysiol Pharmacol. 2013;5(1):32–42.
34. Giusti B, Marcucci R, Lapini I, Sestini I, Lenti M, Yacoub M, Pepe G. Role of hyperhomocysteinemia in aortic disease. Cell Mol Biol. 2004;50(8):945–52.
35. Schulte S, Sun J, Libby P, Macfarlane L, Sun C, Lopez-Ilasaca M, Shi GP, Sukhova GK. Cystatin C deficiency promotes inflammation in angiotensin II-induced abdominal aortic aneurisms in atherosclerotic mice. Am J Pathol. 2010;177(1):456–63.

Association between the intima-media thickness of the extracranial carotid arteries and metabolic syndrome in ethnic Kyrgyzs

Alina S. Kerimkulova[1*], Olga S. Lunegova[1], Aibek E. Mirrakhimov[2], Saamay S. Abilova[1], Malik P. Nabiev[1], Ksenia V. Neronova[1], Erkaiym E. Bektasheva[1], Ulan M. Toktomamatov[1], Jyldyz E. Esenbekova[1] and Erkin M. Mirrakhimov[1,3]

Abstract

Background: It is known that atherosclerosis is the leading cause of cardiovascular disease. We aimed to study the correlation between components of metabolic syndrome (MS) and subclinical carotid atherosclerosis in a group of ethnic Kyrgyzs.

Methods: In a descriptive study we assessed 144 ethnic Kyrgyzs (69 males, 75 females) aged 36–73 years (average age 51.03 ± 8.2). All participants underwent a clinical investigation and an anthropometric evaluation (weight, height, waist circumference (WC)). Abdominal obesity (AO) was confirmed at WC ≥ 94 cm in males and ≥ 88 cm in females. Fasting plasma glucose and lipid spectrum tests were performed. An ultrasound assessment of carotid intima-media thickness (IMT) was performed using a 7.5 MHz transducer (Phillips-SD 800).

Results: MS was revealed in 61 (42.4%; 47.8% in men and 37.3% in women) of the investigated patients. IMT was significantly increased with the presence of MS components in males (no components vs 2 components of MS: 0. 67 ± 0.007 and 0.81 ± 0.009 respectively; $p < 0.05$) and females (no components vs 3 components of MS: 0.63 ± 0.007 and 0.76 ± 0.01 respectively; $p < 0.01$). IMT trended towards an increase in the presence of a greater number of MS components in patients with and without AO ($p < 0.01$). In order to identify independent factors affecting IMT we carried out a multifactorial logistic regression analysis. Arterial hypertension was found to have the greatest influence on the development of MS (OR = 3.81, $p < 0.0001$).

Conclusion: In the group of ethnic Kyrgyzs, a greater number of MS components, with AO or without AO, is associated with higher carotid IMT.

Keywords: Carotid atherosclerosis, Intima-media, Carotid arteries, Metabolic syndrome, Kyrgyz

Background

It is known that atherosclerosis is the leading cause of cardiovascular disease (CVD), accompanied by increased mortality and disability [1]. Therefore, it is important to identify people at high risk of CVD at the earliest stage. Indeed, the presence of more than one atherosclerosis risk factors significantly aggravates the overall CVD risk. Based on this concept, metabolic syndrome (MS) has been highlighted as a cluster of risk factors for atherosclerosis.

An accessible method for estimating pre-clinical atherosclerosis is thickness of the carotid intima-media complex (CIMT), which is measured using non-invasive ultrasound scanning [2]. At the same time, CIMT is an important predictor of coronary atherosclerosis [3, 4]. Along with coronary atherosclerosis, studies demonstrated a gender correlation between IMT and metabolic syndrome [5]. However, as has been shown in epidemiological studies, the correlation between CIMT and MS was identified based on the Western population, or by using the MS criteria for Adult Treatment Panel (ATP) III [6, 7].

* Correspondence: alinakg@gmail.com
[1]Kyrgyz State Medical Academy named after I.K. Akhunbaev, T.Moldo street 3, Bishkek 720040, Kyrgyz Republic
Full list of author information is available at the end of the article

It should be emphasized that there have been no studies carried out on the relationship between CIMT and MS in ethnic Kyrgyz. Moreover, it is interesting to know whether each component of MS equally contributes to an increase in CIMT, and which MS components have the strongest association with the increase in CIMT [6, 8, 9].

The purpose of this research is to study the correlation between MS components and sub-clinical carotid atherosclerosis in a group of ethnic Kyrgyz.

Methods

The research included the ethnic Kyrgyz over 35 years of age, who are residents of the Kyrgyz Republic, and who responded to an announcement of the forthcoming study. This study excluded patients with severe chronic liver, kidney or thyroid dysfunction, as well as people who received corticosteroids or insulin, and pregnant and lactating women. The flowchart of the study is presented in Fig. 1.

The patients underwent a clinical examination including an assessment of complaints and anamnesis, as well as an objective examination with the measurement of anthropometric parameters including height, weight, waist circumference (WC), and systolic (SBP) and diastolic (DBP) blood pressure (BP). The average BP was calculated as the arithmetic mean of SBP and DBP. The body mass index (BMI) was calculated using the formula: BMI = weight (kg)/height (m)2. Obesity was established at BMI ≥30 kg/m2.

The laboratory tests included the blood plasma analysis of glucose (fasting), the lipid spectrum (total cholesterol (TC), triglycerides (TG) and high-density lipoprotein cholesterol (HDL-C). The blood samples were collected and centrifuged, then the serum was separated and frozen at − 20 °C. All the biochemical analyses were conducted at the Dir Adjoint du Département

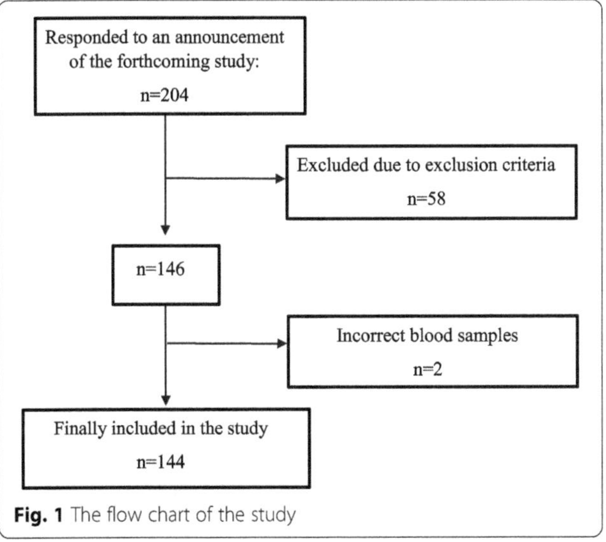

Fig. 1 The flow chart of the study

Hommes, Natures, Musée de l'Homme (Paris, France). Low-density lipoprotein cholesterol (LDL-C) was calculated according to Friedwald's formula [10].

The measurement of CIMT

The sub-clinical and structural changes in the extracranial section of the right and left common carotid arteries were evaluated using a 7.5 MHz linear vascular sensor (echocardiograph Phillips-SD 800). The measurement of CIMT was performed in the middle third of the common carotid artery, along with the back wall of the vessel, and in the areas free of atherosclerotic plaques. CIMT was evaluated based on systole and diastole, then the obtained data were averaged. For calculations, the arithmetic mean of the left and right carotid arteries were used. The measurements of carotid parameters were evaluated in accordance with the criteria of the European Carotid Surgery Trialists 1991 [11].

The definition of MS

MS was diagnosed using the modified criteria that include the presence of abdominal obesity (AO) and two or more of the following conditions: arterial hypertension (AH), dyslipidemia and hyperglycemia [12]. For AO, the following values were taken from the Kyrgyz average WC of ≥94 cm in men and ≥ 88 cm in women [13]. AH was established at SBP ≥130 mmHg or at DPB ≥ 85 mmHg, or in patients taking antihypertensive drugs. Dyslipidemia was established at a TG level of 1.7 mmol/L and/or HDL-C < 1.03 in men and < 1.29 mmol/L in women, or in patients using lipid-lowering drugs. Hyperglycemia was determined at a fasting glucose level > 5.6 mmol/L, or in patients receiving treatment for type 2 diabetes mellitus (DM) [14].

The statistical analysis was carried out with the aid of STATISTICA 7.0 (StatSoft Inc., USA). The variable distribution was analyzed using the Kolmogorov-Smirnov test. The variables with normal and non-parametric distributions are presented as a mean ± standard deviation and median (25th–75th percentiles), respectively. The differences in the characteristics of patients with MS and without MS were analyzed using the Student's t-test for parametric variables and the Mann-Whitney test for non-parametric variables. Furthermore, a comparison of the groups by their binary features was carried out by the $\chi 2$ test. The effect of MS and the increase in the number of MS components in CIMT was assessed by the single-factor parametric variance analysis (ANOVA). The a posteriori group comparison was performed by post-hoc analysis with the Bonferroni amendment. In order to identify independent factors impacting on CIMT, we carried out a multifactorial logistic regression analysis to find out which MS component is significantly associated with an elevated level of IMT. In particular, values from 75 percentiles of IMT and higher were considered as the elevated level of IMT. The independent variables included gender, age, arterial hypertension, level of glycemia and triglycerides. Were conducted by a post-hoc sample size calculation was performed to estimate the sampling size (by using the calculator available at http://clincalc.com/stats/SampleSize.aspx).

The criterion for statistical significance was set at $p < 0.05$.

Results

One hundred and forty-four (144) ethnic Kyrgyzs (69 men and 75 women) aged 36 to 73 years were examined; the average age of the patients was 51.03 ± 8.2 years (for men: 51.9 ± 8.7 years, for women: 50.2 ± 7.7 years).

We conducted the post-hoc sample size calculation. According to the results of the sample size calculation, 120 patients (60 in both groups) are required to have an 80% chance of detecting, as significant at the 5% level. The sample size required per group – 60. The total sample size required – 120 (Alpha – 0.05; Beta – 0.2; Power – 0.8). The subgroups (men and women, with and without metabolic syndrome): men: the sample size required per group – 34. The total sample size required – 68 (Alpha – 0.05; Beta – 0.2; Power – 0.8). Women: the sample size required per group – 25. The total sample size required – 50 (Alpha – 0.05; Beta – 0.2; Power – 0.8).

MS was detected in 61 (42.4%) of the examined patients (47.8% of men and 37.3% of women). Table 1 presents the clinical and biochemical characteristics of patients depending upon whether they had MS or not. In patients with MS, there were large values of BMI, WC, SBP, DBP, TG, blood glucose and a lower level of HDL-C. Besides, the women with MS were older than those without MS, whilst the men were of a comparable in age (Table 1).

We analyzed the pharmacological agents taken by patients (see Table 2). In men, there were no statistically significant differences in the medication use in the groups with and without MS. Among women, those with MS in comparison to women without MS were more likely to take ACE inhibitors (28.6% and 8.5% respectively, $p < 0, 05$). There were no statistically significant differences in other groups by use of medications (Table 2). All patients with diabetes mellitus were managed with glibenclamide, but none was on metformin. There were no statistically significant differences between the subgroups with and without MS (Table 2). The patients in both groups did not take statins. After obtaining the results of the lipid spectrum, the patients were recommended to take statins, as well as the recommendations were provided for correcting cardiometabolic risk factors.

A comparison of the CIMT values depending on the presence or absence of MS and the number of MS components is shown in Table 3. Taking into account that

Table 1 Characteristics of the examined patients, depending on the presence of metabolic syndrome

	Men		Women	
	MS not present ($n = 36$)	MS present ($n = 33$)	MS not present ($n = 47$)	MS present ($n = 28$)
Age	52.3 ± 9.5	51.6 ± 8.0	48.6 ± 7.2	52.9 ± 7.9*
BMI, kg/m^2	26.4 ± 3.1	29.8 ± 3.7$	26 ± 4.5	31.3 ± 4.5^
WC, cm	93.8 ± 8.5	103.5 ± 8.3$	83.4 ± 9.5	96.8 ± 6.5^
SBP#, mmHg.	135 (128–152)	146 (135–157)*	128 (119–136)	140 (134–160)&
DBP#, mmHg.	89 (81–96)	93 (89–102)**	83 (77–91)	91 (80–96)
TC, mmol/L	5.1 ± 0.9	5.5 ± 0.9	5.02 ± 0.9	4.97 ± 1.3
TG#, mmol/L	1.2 (0.9–1.4)	2.2 (1.7–3.5)^	1.0 (0.8–1.2)	1.5 (1.1–2.0)$
HDL-C#, mmol/L	1.15 (1.02–1.4)	0.83 (0.7–1.0)^	1.4 (1.3–1.6)	1.03 (0.8–1.2)^
LDL-C, mmol/L	3.2 ± 0.8	3.4 ± 0.9	3.1 ± 0.8	3.2 ± 1.03
Glucose#, mmol/L	5.2 (5.04–5.4)	6.2 (5.7–6.6)^	5.2 (4.9–5.5)	5.8 (5.5–6.3)^
Smoking, n (%)	15 (41.7)	11 (33.3)	0 (0)	0 (0)
AH, n (%)	18 (50)	27 (81.8)*	12 (25.5)	18 (64.3)**
Dyslipidemia, n (%)	12 (33.3)	32 (96.7)^	14 (29.8)	27 (96.4)^
Hyperglycemia, n (%)	5 (13.9)	25 (75.8)^	7 (14.9)	20 (71.4)^
IMT#, mm	0.72 ± 0.01	0.78 ± 0.01	0.66 ± 0.009	0.72 ± 0.01*

BMI body mass index, *WC* waist circumference, *SBP* systolic blood pressure, *DBP* diastolic blood pressure, *TC* total cholesterol, *TG* triglycerides, *HDL-C* cholesterol of high-density lipoproteins, *LDL-C* low-density lipoprotein cholesterol. Hereinafter in Tables 2 and 3: *AH* arterial hypertension, *MS* metabolic syndrome, *IMT* the average thickness of the intima-media complex; # = the data are represented as median (25–75%), * - $p < 0.05$; ** - $p < 0.01$; & - $p < 0.001$; $ - $p < 0.0001$; ^ - $p < 0.00001$

Table 2 Characteristics of medications use depending on the presence or the absence of metabolic syndrome

Parameters	Men		Women	
	MS + (n = 36)	MS - (n = 33)	MS + (n = 47)	MS - (n = 28)
ACEI, n (%)	5 (15,2)	3 (8,3)	8 (28,6)	4 (8,5)*
Amlodipine, n (%)	0 (0)	1 (2,8)	1 (3,6)	1 (2,1)
Other Ca antagonists (Verapamil, Nifedipine), n (%)	1 (3,03)	0 (0)	1 (3,6)	0 (0)
Beta blockers (atenolol), n (%)	3 (9,1)	2 (5,6)	1 (3,6)	3 (6,4)
Indapamide, n (%)	1 (3,03)	0 (0)	0 (0)	0 (0)
Oral glucose lowering drug (glibenclamide), n (%)	2 (6,1)	0 (0)	1 (3,6)	0 (0)

ACEI angiotensin converter enzyme inhibitors, *MS* metabolic syndrome; * - $p < 0.05$ in women

the studies have shown that carotid IMT in men differs from IMT in women [15], we analysed IMT separately for each gender.

In both sexes, there was a tendency for an increase in CIMT in persons with MS compared to those without MS. Moreover, in women, this trend was statistically significant ($p < 0.05$). All patients were divided up into four groups based on the number of MS components: group 1 in which the patients did not have any component of MS; groups 2–4 included patients with the presence of one to three components of MS: AH, dyslipidemia and hyperglycemia, respectively. In both men ($p < 0.05$) and in women ($p < 0.01$), a gradual increase was observed as the number of MS components increased. In addition, CIMT in men with two components of MS was significantly greater than in patients without a single component of MS. The women with three MS components had greater CIMT than the patients with two and without a single MS component (Table 3).

The effect of the increase in the number of MS components in IMT was analyzed depending on the presence or absence of AO (Fig. 2). In patients with or without AO, there was a tendency for an increase in IMT as the number of MS components increased. At the same time, in the cases where persons did not have AO, this tendency was statistically significant ($p < 0.01$) (Fig. 2).

Table 3 IMT depending on the presence or absence of metabolic syndrome and the number of components

	Men		Women	
	n	IMT. mm	n	IMT. mm
MS not present	36	0.72 ± 0.01	47	0.66 ± 0.009
MS present	33	0.78 ± 0.01	28	0.72 ± 0.01
		$p = 0.07$		$p < 0.05$
Number of MS components				
0	10	0.67 ± 0.007	18	0.63 ± 0.007
1	20	0.72 ± 0.01	28	0.68 ± 0.009
2	18	0.81 ± 0.009*	17	0.69 ± 0.01
3	21	0.76 ± 0.01	12	0.76 ± 0.01*#
		$p < 0.05$		$p < 0.01$

* - $p < 0.01$ - in comparison with patients without a single MS component; # - $p < 0.05$ in comparison with patients with two components of MS

To determine the independent association of MS components with carotid IMT, a multiple regression analysis was performed (Table 4). In men age ($\beta = 0.523$, $p <$ 0.00001), and in women age ($\beta = 0.354$, $p < 0.001$) and the mean BP ($\beta = 0.369$, $p < 0.001$) were significantly associated with carotid IMT.

Discussion

After having analyzed the results of the 144 ethnic Kyrgyzs, we found that the combination of MS components affects CIMT. Amongst the components of MS, the factors that had the strongest associations with CIMT were arterial hypertension and AO.

The effect of an increase in the number of the MS components on carotid atherosclerosis has been shown in some epidemiological studies [6, 16, 17]. In our work, we also found an increase in IMT as the number of MS components increased in patients of both sexes.

Nevertheless, in the analysis of IMT depending on the number of components of MS and AO, the association between IMT and MS was not statistically significant. In this case, we showed that IMT in patients with AO and without AO was similar with the same number of MS components. In other studies [18], a more frequent occurrence of carotid atherosclerosis was observed in persons with a large number of MS components, regardless of the presence of AO. Moreover, Lee et al. [19] showed the similar risk of developing coronary heart disease in patients with both AO and without AO. These results suggest that the central type of obesity is not always indicative of an increased risk of CVD.

It is known that AO is a significant predictor of insulin resistance, which, in turn, leads to impaired glucose tolerance, hypertension and dyslipidemia [20]. The results obtained by us suggest that AO may not be the immediate cause of atherosclerosis. However, AO is included in a cluster of risk factors, including AH, dyslipidemia, and hyperglycemia. The research has shown that AO has a key position in the set of risk factors associated with the development of atherosclerosis [21].

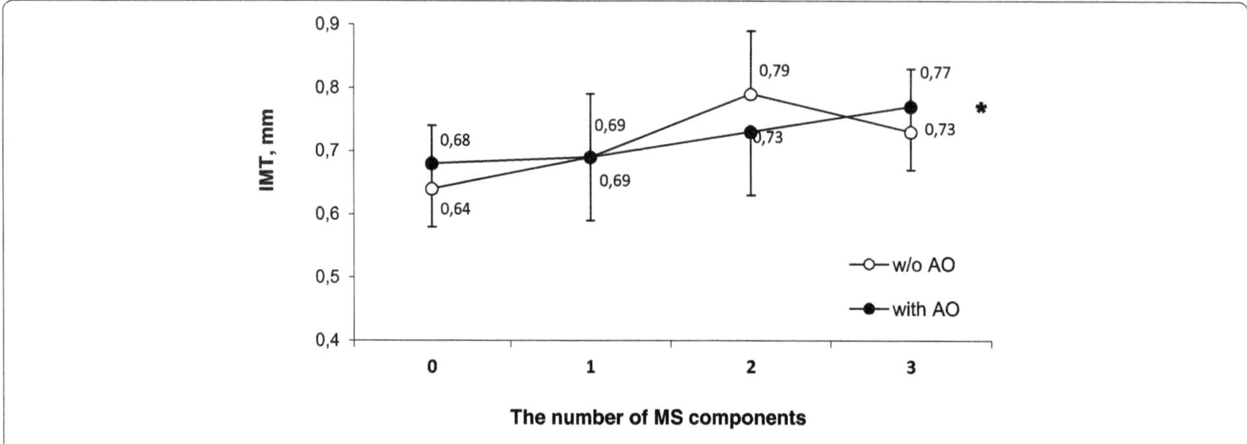

Fig. 2 IMT in the carotid artery depending on the presence or absence of abdominal obesity. Notes: IMT - intima-media complex thickness; AO - abdominal obesity; MS - metabolic syndrome; the data are presented as mean ± standard deviation; * $p < 0.01$

In our study, CIMT was associated with MS, but a relationship with AO could not be identified. However, it is not prudent to ignore patients with normal WC, but with a combination of other components of MS, since such patients still, have a risk of further worsening IMT.

In the present work, it was initially planned to determine whether the MS components were equally associated with IMT. We examined the effect of each component of MS on IMT and found that, in patients with AO, in contrast to those with dyslipidemia and hyperglycemia, there were significantly higher rates of IMT than in patients without a single MS component. These results suggest that not all components of MS have a similar atherosclerotic risk. The most important determinants contributing to the development of thickening of IMT appear to be AH and age.

AH is recognized as an important risk factor for the development of atherosclerosis, CVD, and strokes. In a study by Ishizaka et al. [22], it was shown that among the five components of MS according to the ATP III criteria, carotid atherosclerosis was strongly associated with AH. Furthermore, Su et al. [23], studied risk factors such as hypertension, hypercholesterolemia, hypertriglyceridemia and type II diabetes, and recognized AH as the most significant risk factor for increased IMT and the development of carotid stenosis.

Table 4 Logistic regression analysis with the dependent variable – increased IMT value

	Controlling for age, sex, AH, serum glucose, TG		
	OR	95 CI	p<
Male sex	0.42	0.44–0.60	0.0001
Age	1.13	49.67–52.38	0.0001
AH	3.81	0.44–0.60	0.0001
Glucose, mmol/l	1.21	5.56–6.17	0.0001
TG, mmol/l	1.23	1.38–1.73	0.0001

AH arterial hypertension, *TG* triglycerides

In the present study, we found that arterial hypertension has the highest association with CIMT. At the same time, some population-based studies have confirmed an association between CIMT and AH as well as other traditional risk factors for atherosclerosis such as smoking, dyslipidemia and hyperglycemia [24, 25]. Furthermore, the studies have shown that the risk of MS is not always determined by the number of its components in an individual. Thus, we have shown significant influence on IMT clusters by different components of MS, whilst the composition of clusters consistently included elevated blood pressure [26, 27]. Although hypertension is a significant risk factor for increasing CIMT, we should not ignore individuals with other risk factors.

We believe that every component of MS including AH, dyslipidemia, and hyperglycemia is a risk factor for increasing CIMT. At the same time, the effect of MS components on CIMT can be uneven. This study shows that patients with AH probably have a higher risk of carotid arteriosclerosis than patients without AH. The presence of hypertension amongst MS components in an individual suggests that additional preventative approaches are used in such patients.

It ought to be mentioned that there are some limitations to interpreting the results of this study. Firstly, the examined patients may not meet strict criteria for the representativeness of the Kyrgyz population as a whole. We included patients who responded to the announcement of the forthcoming study, so there could be the possibility (or there was room for) of a systematic error in the selection process. In this study, the incidence of MS was slightly higher than in previous studies of ethnic Kyrgyzs [28], and, the prevalence of MS was higher than in the studies of Europeans [7]. Secondly, the present results were obtained in a cross-sectional study, which does not allow us to conclude the temporal sequence of the observed association. In this regard, prospective studies are needed to assess the long-term effects of MS on CIMT. Thirdly, it is necessary to note that, a relatively small number of patients was included in the study. However, the post-hoc sample size calculation showed that the included number of patients was sufficient. Fourthly, the ultrasound of carotid arteries was conducted once by a single provider blinded to the study. We did not study endothelial function, because it did not fall within the primary study objective. Nonetheless, the determination of endothelial function is also crucial for the early diagnosis of atherosclerosis [29, 30].

Conclusion

This study shows that an increase in the number of components of MS, with or without AO, is associated with greater CIMT. We also found that the risk of CIMT differs among MS components. The most important determinants of CIMT were age and AH. Our results support the view that simply diagnosing MS is not sufficient to establish risk factors for atherosclerosis in an individual and recommend a qualitative and quantitative assessment of multiple components of MS.

Abbreviations

AH: Arterial hypertension; AO: abdominal obesity; ATP: Adult Treatment Panel; BMI: Body mass index; BP: Blood pressure; CIMT: Thickness of the carotid intima-media complex; CVD: Cardiovascular disease; DBP: Diastolic blood pressure; DM: Diabetes mellitus; HDL-C: High-density lipoprotein cholesterol; IMT: Intima-media thickness; LDL-C: Low-density lipoprotein cholesterol; MS: metabolic syndrome; SBP: systolic blood pressure; TC: total cholesterol; TG: triglycerides; WC: waist circumference

Acknowledgements

The authors express their gratitude to E. Heyer, Dir Adjoint du Département Hommes, Natures, Musée de l'Homme (Paris, France) for conducting the laboratory analysis.

Authors' contributions

KAS, MEM conceived the study. MEM supervised the study and endorsed the submission of the article. KAS, LOS, MAE, ASS, NMP, NKV, BEE, TUM, EJE analyzed and interpreted the data. KAS, MAE, MEM drafted the manuscript. All authors revised the manuscript critically for important intellectual content. All authors read and approved the final manuscript. All authors take responsibility for all aspects of the reliability and freedom from bias of the data presented and their discussed interpretation. There are no conflicts of interest.

Competing interests

The authors declare that they have no competing interests.

Author details

[1]Kyrgyz State Medical Academy named after I.K. Akhunbaev, T.Moldo street 3, Bishkek 720040, Kyrgyz Republic. [2]Kyrgyz Society of Cardiology, Bishkek, Kyrgyz Republic. [3]National Center of Cardiology and Internal Medicine named after academician M.M. Mirrakhimov, Bishkek, Kyrgyz Republic.

References

1. GBD 2013 Mortality and Causes of Death Collaborators. Global, regional, and national age-sex specific all-cause and cause-specific mortality for 240 causes of death, 1990–2013: a systematic analysis for the Global Burden of Disease Study 2013. Lancet. 2015;385(9963):117–71.
2. Randrianarisoa E, Rietig R, Jacob S, Blumenstock G, Haering HU, Rittig K, et al. Normal values for intima-media thickness of the common carotid artery-- an update following a novel risk factor profiling. Vasa. 2015;44(6):444–50.
3. Ciccone MM, Scicchitano P, Zito A, Agati L, Gesualdo M, Mandolesi S, Carbonara R, Ciciarello F, Fedele F. Correlation between coronary artery disease severity, left ventricular mass index and carotid intima media thickness, assessed by radio-frequency. Cardiovasc Ultrasound. 2011;9:32.
4. Ciccone MM, Niccoli-Asabella A, Scicchitano P, Gesualdo M, Notaristefano A, Chieppa D, Carbonara S, Ricci G, Sassara M, Altini C, Quistelli G, Lepera ME, Favale S, Rubini G. Cardiovascular risk evaluation and prevalence of silent myocardial ischemia in subjects with asymptomatic carotid artery disease. Vasc Health Risk Manag. 2011;7:129–34.
5. A S, Orru' M, Morrell CH, Tarasov K, Schlessinger D, Uda M, Lakatta EG. Associations of large artery structure and function with adiposity: effects of age, gender, and hypertension. The SardiNIA study. Atherosclerosis. 2012; 221(1):189–97.
6. Pietri P, Vlachopoulos C, Vyssoulis G, Ioakeimidis N, Stefanadis C. Macro- and microvascular alterations in patients with metabolic syndrome: sugar makes the difference. Hypertens Res. 2014;37:452–6.
7. Scuteri A, Laurent S, Cucca F, Cockcroft J, Cunha PG, Mañas LR, Mattace Raso FU, Muiesan ML, Ryliškytė L, Rietzschel E, Strait J, Vlachopoulos C, Völzke H, Lakatta EG, Nilsson PM. Metabolic syndrome and arteries research (MARE) consortium. Metabolic syndrome across Europe: different clusters of risk factors. Eur J Prev Cardiol. 2015;22(4):486–91.
8. Iglseder B, Cip P, Malaimare L, Ladurner G, Paulweber B. The metabolic syndrome is a stronger risk factor for early carotid atherosclerosis in women than in men. Stroke. 2005;36:1212–7.
9. Kawamoto R, Tomita H, Oka Y, Kodama A, Kamitani A. Metabolic syndrome amplifies the LDL-cholesterol associated increases in carotid atherosclerosis. Intern Med. 2005;44:1232–8.
10. Friedewald WT, Levy RI, Fredrickson DS. Estimation of the concentration of low density lipoprotein cholesterol in plasma, without use of the preparative ultracentrifuge. Clin Chem. 1972;18:499–502.
11. European Carotid Surgery Trialists' Collaborative Group. MRC - European carotid surgery trial: interim results for symptomatic patients with severe (70 - 99%) or with mild (0 - 29%) carotid stenosis. Lancet. 1991;337:1235–43.
12. Ford ES. Prevalence of the metabolic syndrome defined by the international diabetes federation among adults in the U.S. Diabetes Care. 2005;28:2745–9.
13. Mirrakhimov AE, Lunegova OS, Kerimkulova AS, Moldokeeva CB, Nabiev MP, Mirrakhimov EM. Cut off values for abdominal obesity as a criterion of metabolic syndrome in an ethnic Kyrgyz population (central Asian region). Cardiovasc Diabetol. 2012;22(11):16.
14. Alberti KGMM, Zimmet P, Shaw J. The metabolic syndrome—a new worldwide definition. Lancet. 2005;366(9491):1059–62.
15. Ciccone MM, Bilianou E, Balbarini A, Gesualdo M, Ghiadoni L, Metra M, Palmiero P, Pedrinelli R, Salvetti M, Scicchitano P, Zito A, Novo S, Mattioli AV. Task force on: 'Early markers of atherosclerosis: influence of age and sex'. J Cardiovasc Med (Hagerstown). 2013;14(10):757–66.
16. Pollex RL, Al-Shali KZ, House AA, Spence JD, Fenster A, Mamakeesick M, et al. Relationship of the metabolic syndrome to carotid ultrasound traits. Cardiovasc Ultrasound. 2006;4:28–35.
17. Roberson LL, Aneni EC, Maziak W, Agatston A, Feldman T, Rouseff M, Tran T, Blaha MJ, Santos RD, Sposito A, Al-Mallah MH, Blankstein R, Budoff MJ, Nasir

K. Beyond BMI: the "metabolically healthy obese" phenotype & its association with clinical/subclinical cardiovascular disease and all-cause mortality -- a systematic review. BMC Public Health. 2014;14:14.

18. Noda H, Iso H, Yamashita S, Ueno H, Yokode M, Yamada N, et al. Defining vascular disease (DVD) research group. Risk stratification based on metabolic syndrome as well as non-metabolic risk factors in the assessment of carotid atherosclerosis. J Atheroscler Thromb. 2011;18:504–12.
19. Lee J, Ma S, Heng D, Tan CE, Chew SK, Hughes K, et al. Should central obesity be an optional or essential component of the metabolic syndrome? Ischemic heart disease risk in the Singapore cardiovascular cohort study. Diabetes Care. 2007;30:343–7.
20. Matsuzawa Y, Funahashi T, Nakamura T. The concept of metabolic syndrome: contribution of visceral fat accumulation and its molecular mechanism. J Atheroscler Thromb. 2011;18:629–39.
21. Yasuda T, Matsuhisa M, Fujiki N, Sakamoto F, Tsuji M, Fujisawa N, et al. Is central obesity a good predictor of carotid atherosclerosis in Japanese type 2 diabetes with metabolic syndrome? Endocr J. 2007;54:695–702.
22. Ishizaka N, Ishizaka Y, Toda E, Hashimoto H, Nagai R, Yamakado M. Hypertension is the most common component of metabolic syndrome and the greatest contributor to carotid arteriosclerosis in apparently healthy Japanese individuals. Hypertens Res. 2005;28:27–34.
23. Su TC, Jeng JS, Chien KL, Sung FC, Hsu HC, Lee YT. Hypertension status is the major determinant of carotid atherosclerosis: a community -based study in Taiwan. Stroke. 2001;32:2265–71.
24. Johnson HM, Douglas PS, Srinivasan SR, Bond MG, Tang R, Li S, et al. Predictors of carotid intima-media thickness progression in young adults: the Bogalusa heart study. Stroke. 2007;38:900–5.
25. Hong EG, Ohn JH, Lee SJ, Kwon HS, Kim SG, Kim DJ, Kim DS. Clinical implications of carotid artery intima media thickness assessment on cardiovascular risk stratification in hyperlipidemic Korean adults with diabetes: the ALTO study. BMC Cardiovasc Disord. 2015;15:114.
26. Scuteri A, Franco OH, Majiid A, Jolita B, Sergey B, Cheng HM, Chen CH, Choi SW, Francesco C, De Buyzere ML, Alessandro D, Marcus D, Gunnar E, Albert H, Seul-Ki J, Kweon SS, Michel L, Lee YH, Mattace Raso F, Olle M, Morrell CH, Park KS, Rietzschel ER, Kristina R, Ryliskyte L, Ulf S, David S, Shin MH, Irina S, Shih-Hsien S, Olga T, Völzke H, Lakatta EG, Nilsson P, Consortium MARE. The relationship between the metabolic syndrome and arterial wall thickness: a mosaic still to be interpreted. Atherosclerosis. 2016;255:11–6.
27. Scuteri A, Najjar SS, Orru' M, Usala G, Piras MG, Ferrucci L, Cao A, Schlessinger D, Uda M, Lakatta EG. The central arterial burden of the metabolic syndrome is similar in men and women: the SardiNIA study. Eur Heart J. 2010;31(5):602–13.
28. Mirrakhimov EM, Kerimkulova AS, Lunegova OS, Mirrakhimov AE, Nabiev MP, Neronova KV, et al. The association of leptin with dyslipidemia, arterial hypertension and obesity in Kyrgyz (central Asian nation) population. BMC Res Notes. 2014;7:411.
29. Scuteri A, Stuehlinger MC, Cooke JP, Wright JG, Lakatta EG, Anderson DE, Fleg JL. Nitric oxide inhibition as a mechanism for blood pressure increase during salt loading in normotensive postmenopausal women. J Hypertens. 2003;21(7):1339–46.
30. Scuteri A, Tesauro M, Rizza S, Iantorno M, Federici M, Lauro D, Campia U, Turriziani M, Fusco A, Cocciolillo G, Lauro R. Endothelial function and arterial stiffness in normotensive normoglycemic first-degree relatives of diabetic patients are independent of the metabolic syndrome. Nutr Metab Cardiovasc Dis. 2008;18(5):349–56.

Comparative evaluation of cannabinoid receptors, apelin and S100A6 protein in the heart of women of different age groups

Irena Kasacka[1*], Żaneta Piotrowska[1], Anna Filipek[2] and Wojciech Lebkowski[3]

Abstract

Background: Recent studies have shown a significant role of the endocannabinoid system, apelin and S100A6 protein in the regulation of cardiovascular system functioning. The aim of the study was to compare and evaluate the distribution of cannabinoid receptors (CB1 and CB2), apelin and S100A6 protein in the heart of healthy women in different age groups.

Methods: The study was conducted on the hearts of 10 women (organ donors) without a history of cardiovascular disease, who were divided into two age groups: women older than 50 years and women under 50 years of age. Paraffin heart sections were processed by immunohistochemistry for detection of cannabinoids receptors (CB1 and CB2), apelin and S100A6 protein.

Results: CB1 and CB2 immunoreactivity in the cytoplasm of cardiomyocytes in the heart of women over 50 was weaker than in younger individuals. There was also strong immunoreactivity of CB1 in intercalated discs (ICDs) of the heart, only in women over 50. The presence of this receptor in this location was not found in women under 50. Apelin- and S100A6-immunoreactivity in the cardiomyocytes was stronger in older women compared to women under 50.The CB1, apelin and S100A6 immunostaining in the endothelium of myocardial vessels was weaker in women over 50 than in younger women, while intensity of CB2- immunoreaction in coronary endothelium was similar in both groups of women.
The results of the study indicate the important role of endocannabinoids, apelin, and S100A6 protein in cardiac muscle function.

Conclusion: This report might contribute to a better understanding of the role of endocannabinoid system, apelin and S100 proteins in heart function as well as shed new light on processes involved in age-related cardiomyopathy.

Keywords: CB1, CB2, Apelin, S100A6, Women, Heart

Background

Since the discovery of the endocannabinoid system in the 1990's, evidence indicating its key importance in various physiological and pathological processes within the body has been emerging [1]. The endocannabinoid system contributes to the control of mental health, eating behaviour, reproductive function, pain sensation and immune response [1]. Latest reports have also revealed a substantial role of the endocannabinoid system in cardiovascular system performance [1]. The cannabinoid receptors CB1 and CB2 and their endogenous ligands, called endocannabinoids, have been identified in cardiovascular tissues of human and several mammal species [1]. It has been proved that the endocannabinoid system participates in the regulation of blood pressure, heart rate and myocardial contractility [1, 2]. The endocannabinoid system also determines cardiomyocytes survivability and is involved in histopathological changes in the heart [3–8]. CB1 receptor axis promotes cardiomyocytes injury, augments collagen deposition and cardiomyocyte overgrowth in experimental models of cardiovascular diseases [3–5]. By contrast, treatment with CB2 receptor agonist limits cardiomyocytes apoptosis and prevents heart hypertrophy and fibrosis in

* Correspondence: kasacka@umb.edu.pl
[1]Department of Histology and Cytophysiology, Medical University of Bialystok, Mickiewicza 2C street, 15-222 Białystok, Poland
Full list of author information is available at the end of the article

rodents subjected to myocardial infarction (MI) and ischemia–reperfusion (I/R) heart injury [6–8].

Recent studies have shown the relevance of apelin in cardiovascular homeostasis [9]. Both the apelin receptor (APJ) and the apelin peptide have been detected in human and rat heart [9]. Clinical, experimental and in vitro studies have revealed that apelin lowers blood pressure, increases heart rate, evokes positive inotropic effect, and modulates cardiac loading [9, 10]. Literature data have also indicated the cardioprotective action of apelin. Treatment with apelin reduces myocardial injury, limits hypertrophy and fibrosis of cardiac tissue in rodents with MI, I/R heart injury and heart pressure overload [11–16]. Several reports have indicate the existence of a functional interaction between endocannabinoid system and apelin [17–19]. It was found that cannabinoid signalling modulates the expression of the apelin gene in the adipocyte and skeletal muscle cells [17–19]. In this way, it can be concluded that the endocannabinoid system influences the biological function of apelin, including its cardiovascular action.

It is known that the contractility of myocardial cells is strictly dependent on the fluctuation of intracellular calcium content. Cannabinoids and apelin modulate the calcium flow in cardiomyocytes by affecting calcium channels (L - type Ca^{2+} channels, T-type Ca^{2+} channels, $Na+/Ca^{2+}$ exchanger) and calcium circulation between the sarcoplasmic reticulum and cytosol [1, 9, 10].

The calcium signalling in myocardial cells is regulated by various calcium-binding proteins. They also include proteins belonging to the S100 family that have two EF-hand type calcium-binding domains [20].

Recent studies on the S100 proteins family have revealed that its members, S100A6, fulfils an important role in maintaining heart functionality [21]. It has been demonstrated that S100A6 regulates calcium transition between the sarcoplasmic reticulum and the cytosol in cardiomyocytes [21]. This finding indicates the involvement of S100A6 in intracellular calcium cycling during cardiac muscle cells contraction. Moreover, it has been stated that S100A6 regulates cardiomyocytes differentiation and exerts a beneficial effect on cardiomyocytes viability [21, 22]. Studies on mice and cultured neonatal rat cardiomyocytes proved protective role of S100A6, limiting apoptosis of cardiac muscle cells [21, 22]. By contrast, in vitro studies on carcinoma cells lines have demonstrated that S100A6 might participate in programmed cell death pathways [23, 24].

Aging is a major risk factor for cardiovascular morbidity and mortality [25]. Clinical and experimental data have demonstrated that aging is accompanied by histopathological changes in the heart such as cardiomyocyte apoptosis, cardiac muscle cell hypertrophy and heart fibrosis [26]. Age-associated heart remodelling is followed by cardiac dysfunction. Haemodynamic studies have revealed that elderly patients have a slower heart rate, decreased cardiac output, impaired cardiac systolic and diastolic function compared to younger individuals [26].

Considering the above-mentioned unfavourable impact of aging on the cardiovascular system and the involvement of the cannabinoid system, apelin and S100A6 protein in control of cardiac function, we decided to perform immunohistochemical detection and comparative evaluation of the distribution of cannabinoid receptors (CB1 and CB2), apelin and S100A6 in the heart of healthy women in different age groups.

Methods

Sample collection

Ten adult women (organ donors) without history of cardiovascular disease were used in the study. The women were in age range from 19 to 64 yrs., mean body weight 63,2 kg and mean BMI (body mass index) 23,3 kg/m^2.

The women were divided into two groups: subjects older than 50 years (over 50) and subjects under 50 years old (under 50).

Each study participant presented with clinical symptoms of brain death, was considered to be an organ donor. Irreversible brain damage was confirmed by special clinical examination and angiography (no blood flow within the brain arteries). After brain death was diagnosed and confirmed, heart samples were collected from each body after other organs (kidneys, liver) for transplantation were harvested.

Heart samples were immediately fixed in Bouin's solution and routinely embedded in paraffin. Sections (4 µm) were stained with haematoxylin-eosin for general histological examination and processed by immunohistochemistry for detection of cannabinoids receptors (CB1 and CB2), apelin and S100A6 protein.

Ethical issues

The study protocol was approved by the Ethics Committee, Medical University of Białystok (R-I-002/345/2007), and a written informed consent had previously been obtained from each woman or from her family member(s).

Immunohistochemistry

Paraffin blocks were cut into 4-µm sections (3 sections from each subject for each antibody) and attached to positively charged glass slides. Immunohistochemistry was performed, using an EnVision Plus-HRP Rabbit Detection Kit K4011 (Dako Denmark) [27]. Immunostaining was performed by the following protocol: paraffin-embedded sections were deparaffinized and hydrated in pure alcohols. For antigen retrieval, the sections were subjected to pre-treatment in a pressure chamber heated for 1 min at 21 psi at 125 °C (one pound force per square inch (1 psi) equates to 6.895 kPa, the conversion factor has been provided by the United Kingdom National Physical Laboratory). During antigen retrieval sections were incubated with Target Retrieval Solution Citrate pH = 6.0 S 2369 (Dako Denmark) for CB2 and S100A6, or Target Retrieval Solution with pH 9.0 (S 2367, Dako Denmark) for CB1 and apelin. After cooling down to room temperature, the sections were incubated with Peroxidase Blocking Reagent S 2001 (Dako, Denmark) for 10 min to block endogenous peroxidase activity. Subsequently, the sections were incubated overnight with the primary antibodies against CB1 (No ab23703 purchased from Abcam, UK), CB2 (No ab3561 purchased from Abcam, UK) S100A6 (purchased from Nencki Institute of Experimental Biology, produced in-house) and apelin (No. bs-2425R purchased from Bioss Antibodies) at 4 °C in a humidified chamber. The antisera were previously diluted in Antibody Diluent (S 0809, Dako Denmark), in proportion 1:1000 for CB1, 1:200 for CB2 and apelin, 1:5000 for S100A6. The procedure was followed by incubation with secondary antibody (conjugated to horseradish peroxidase-labelled polymer). The bound antibodies were visualized by 1 min incubation with liquid 3,3′-diaminobenzidine (DAB) substrate chromogen. The sections were finally counterstained in QS haematoxylin (H-3404, Vector Laboratories, Burlingame, CA, USA), mounted and evaluated under light microscope. Appropriate washing with S 3006 Wash Buffer (Dako Denmark) was performed between each step. Specificity tests, performed for the CB1, CB2, apelin and S100A6 antibody included: negative control, where the antibodies were replaced by normal rabbit serum (Vector Laboratories, Burlingame, CA, USA) at respective dilution. For negative control, no immunostaining was observed in heart tissues under the omission of the primary antibodies.

Histological preparations were subjected to a visual analysis using an Olympus BX41 light microscope with Olympus DP12 digital camera and a PC computer and documented.

Quantitative analysis

Images from five randomly selected microscopic fields, each field of 0.785 mm^2, in magnification of 200× (20× the lens and 10× the eyepiece) from all heart sections were submitted for morphometric evaluation by using NIS Elements AR 3.10 Nikon software for microscopic image analysis.

The intensity of immunohistochemical reaction was measured, using a 0 to 256 grey scale level, where the completely **white or bright pixels** were scored **0** and completely **black** pixels were scored **256**.

Statistical analysis

All data were analysed for statistical significance using software computer package Statistica Version 12.0. The mean values were computed automatically; significant differences were determined by Student's t-test; $p < 0.05$ was accepted as significant.

Results

Routine tests (H + E staining) showed no microscopic pathological changes in the hearts of women.

The mean values of age, body weight and body mass index (BMI) in the two groups of women are presented in Table 1. The average body weight and BMI of women in our study was similar.

The performed immunohistochemical tests revealed a positive reaction of CB1, CB2 receptors, apelin and S100A6 in the heart of all studied women, although the density and intensity of reactions varied between age groups (Figs. 1, 2, 3 and 4). There was no immunoreactivity when the primary antibodies were omitted from the staining procedure.

Immunolabelling of CB1 in the hearts of women under 50 gave a moderate to strong reaction in the cytoplasm of cardiomyocytes (Fig. 1a). In women over 50, the intensity of CB1 immunoreactivity in the cytoplasm of myocardial cells was significantly weaker, but in the hearts of these women strong reactivity of the CB1 receptors in the intercalated discs was observed (ICDs) (Fig. 1b). In the heart of women under 50 was noted also weak CB1-immunostaining in endothelium of coronary vasculature (Fig. 1a), in vessels supplying the heart of older women the CB1-immunoreaction was residual or not detected (Fig. 1b).

The same perinuclear CB2 receptor in cardiomyocytes was found in the hearts of women in both groups (Fig. 2a and b). The intensity of CB2-immunoreaction in cardiac muscle cells was weaker in the hearts of older women compared to those under 50 (Fig. 2b). In all studied women was observed similar, very weak CB2-staining in endothelium of myocardial vessels (Fig. 2a and b).

Antisera against apelin strongly immunostained vascular endothelial cells and gave a very weak reaction in the cardiomyocytes in the hearts of younger women (Fig. 3a). In the hearts of women older than 50 years, the apelin immunosignal in endothelial cells was very weak or negative (Fig. 3b), whereas the density and intensity of the reaction showing apelin in the cardiomyocytes of

Table 1 Age (year), weight (kg) and BMI (body mass index - kg/m^2) of women expressed as mean ± SE

Group of women	age (years)	weight (kg)	BMI (kg/m^2)
women under 50 years old			
$n = 5$	31.4 ± 4.36	61.9 ± 2.21	22.6 ± 0.93
women over 50 years old			
$n = 5$	57.0 ± 2.04 *	66.6 ± 4.44	24.5 ± 2.17

*$p < 0.05$ women over 50 vs women under 50

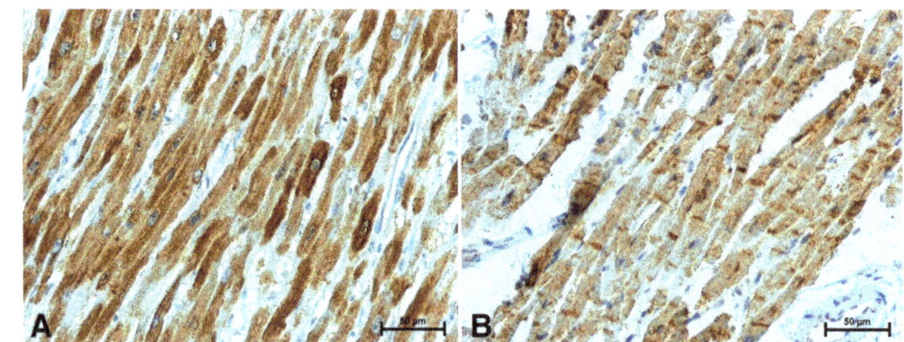

Fig. 1 Immunolocalization of CB1 receptor in the heart of woman (**a**) under 50 years old; strong CB1-immunosignal in cardiomyocytes (**b**) over 50 years old; weak CB1 immunoreactivity in the cytoplasm of cardiomyocytes and very strong CB1-immunolabelling in ICDs

women over the age of 50 was far stronger than in younger women (Fig. 3a and b).

In the hearts of younger women a weak S100A6-immunoreactivity in the cytoplasm of cardiac muscle cells was noted. The S100A6-immunosignal was observed in the form of brown-stained granules in the vicinity of cardiomyocyte nuclei (Fig. 4a). The S100A6-immunoreaction in the cardiomyocytes of older women was considerably stronger compared to subjects under 50 (Fig. 4b). The S100A6 was identified also in endothelial cells of coronary vasculature. In the hearts of women under 50, the S100A6-immunostaining in endothelial cells was moderate (Fig. 4a), while in the hearts of women over 50 weakened S100A6-immunoreaction in vascular endothelium was noted (Fig. 4b).

Computer image analysis confirmed the visually perceived changes in the intensity of the immunohistochemical reaction against CB1, CB2, apelin and S100A6 in the hearts of women over 50 and under 50 years of age (Table 2).

Discussion

The cardiovascular system is subject to precise regulation in order to ensure appropriate blood supply to different body tissues under a wide range of circumstances. The results of the latest research demonstrate that the endocannabinoid system, apelin and S100A6 participate in the complex process controlling the cardiovascular system function since they exert a significant influence on blood pressure, heart rate and myocardial contractility [1, 9, 21].

To the best of our knowledge, the current report is the first comparison of CB1, CB2, apelin and S100A6 distribution in the hearts of healthy women of different age groups. Our study demonstrated decreased immunoreactivity for both cannabinoid receptors, while increased immunohistochemical reaction for apelin and S100A6 in the cardiomyocyte cytoplasm in the hearts of older women. Noteworthy is the fact that in women over 50 the presence of CB1 receptor was detected also in ICDs, which was not the case in younger women. Presented research indicate also on decrease of CB1, apelin and S100A6 immunoreactivity, but no significant changes in intensity of CB2 immunostaining in the endothelium of coronary vessels in women over 50.

Aging is associated with substantial alterations in cardiovascular structure and function. Aging-related vascular stiffness and blood pressure elevation leads to considerable cardiac workload. The increasing pressure acting on the heart's wall results in myocardial hypertrophy and fibrotic remodelling of the cardiac wall in older individuals [26, 28].

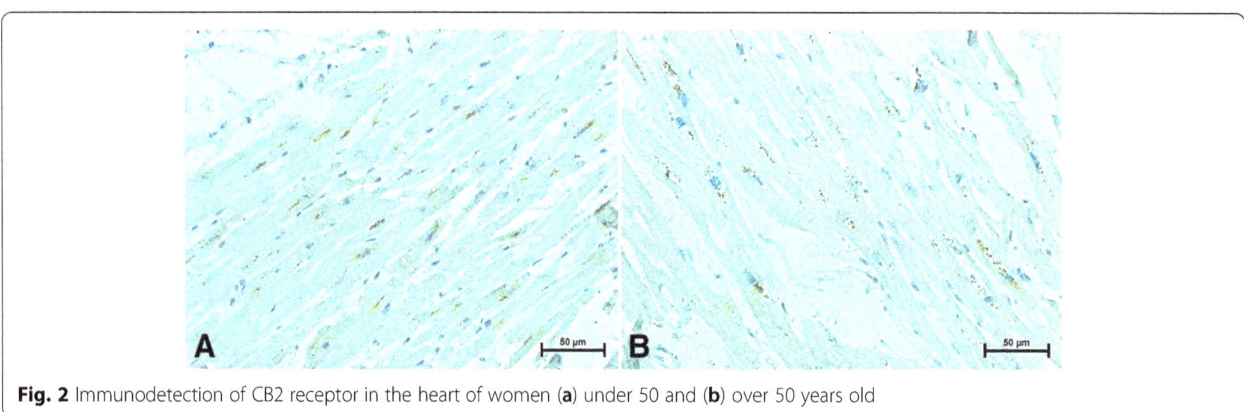

Fig. 2 Immunodetection of CB2 receptor in the heart of women (**a**) under 50 and (**b**) over 50 years old

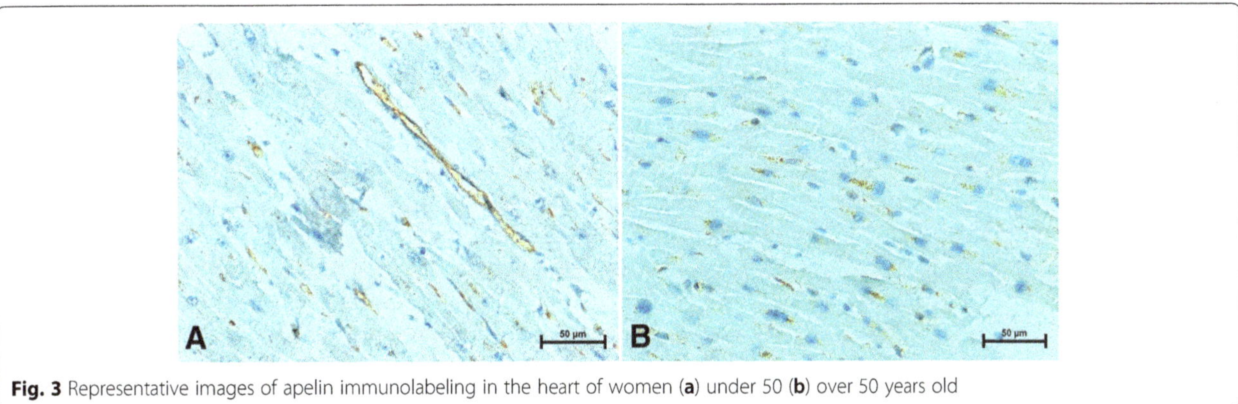

Fig. 3 Representative images of apelin immunolabeling in the heart of women (**a**) under 50 (**b**) over 50 years old

Moreover, aging leads to the activation of multiple molecular mechanisms resulting in cardiomyocyte damage. These include a decrease in the efficiency of somatic mutations repair, the accumulation of defective proteins as well as increased oxidative stress due to the impairment of mitochondrial bioenergetics [28].

The growing body of evidence points to the involvement of the endocannabinoid system, apelin-APJ system and S100A6 protein in histopathological changes in the heart [1, 9, 21]. The activation of CB1 and CB2 receptors exerts a significant impact on cardiomyocyte survival. Recent investigations on mice models of cardiomyopathy have demonstrated that CB1-signalling contributes to programmed cell death while the CB2-axis produces a cardioprotective effect [3–8]. In vivo and in vitro studies have revealed that cardiac muscle cell viability is also dependent on apelin. Apelin prevented cardiomyocyte death in cases of I/R heart injury or glucose deprivation [11–13]. A few previous studies have demonstrated the importance of S100A6 in cardiomyocyte survival. Mofid et al. [21] and Tsoporis et al. [22] demonstrated that S100A6 markedly reduced the apoptosis of cardiomyocytes exposed to TNF-α and hypoxia/reoxygenation conditions. By contrast, other researchers have stated that S100A6 promotes apoptosis in different cultured cell types [23, 24].

Experimental data indicate that the endocannabinoid system participates in the process of cardiac fibrosis. It has been noted that the CB1 receptor-axis determines collagen deposition in the heart of rodents subjected to MI, doxorubicin-induced myocardial injury and diabetic cardiomyopathy [3–5]. In turn, the stimulation of CB2 receptor decreased fibrotic remodelling of the heart's wall in mice undergoing an I/R episode and MI [7, 8]. Some recent evidence highlights the antifibrotic action of apelin in cardiovascular disease. Apelin has been found to restrict cardiac fibrosis in rodents subjected to heart pressure overload, Dahl-salt hypertension, pulmonary hypertension or MI [14, 15, 29]. Recent investigations indicate that S100A6 protein attenuates the pathological fibrotic remodelling of the cardiac wall. It has been demonstrated that mice overexpressing S100A6 have less collagen-rich scar content in the heart post I/R injury compared to animals in which S100A6 gene was not influenced [21].

The endocannabinoid system performs a relevant role in the progression of heart hypertrophy. Studies on mice with experimental MI and diabetes have demonstrated that the CB1-pathway is implicated in cardiomyocyte overgrowth, whereas CB2-signalling is associated with protection against cardiac hypertrophy [4, 5, 8]. Several recent reports have demonstrated that apelin limits the development of heart hypertrophy. Apelin treatment

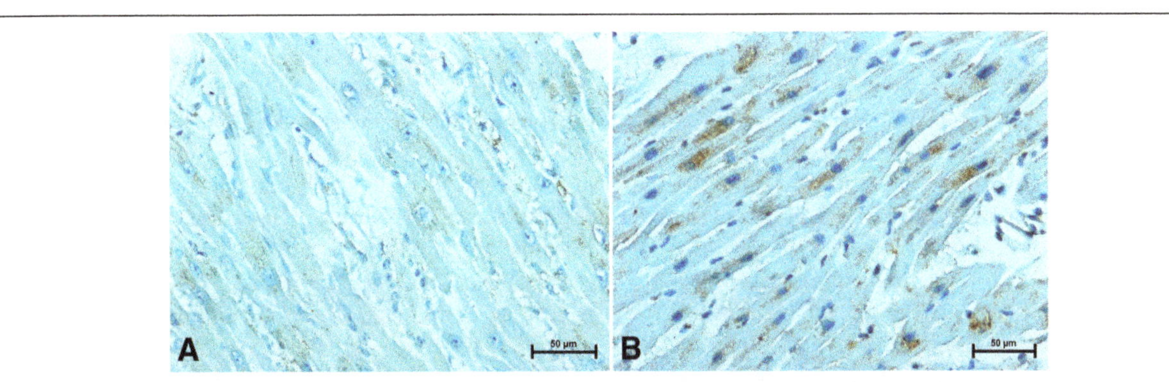

Fig. 4 Positive S100A6-immunostaining in heart of women (**a**) under 50 years old and (**b**) women over 50

Table 2 Intensity of immunoreaction against CB1, CB2, apelin and S100A6 in women heart (mean ± SE). (Scale from 0 (white pixel) to 256 (black pixel))

Intensity of immunohistochemical reaction in women heart	women under 50 years old	women over 50 years old	
CB1			
cardiomyocyte cytoplasm	146.7 ± 2.99	108.2 ± 2.45*	↓*
intercalated discs	ND	180.7 ± 4.63*	↑*
endothelium of coronary vessels	61.6 ± 2.16	45.7 ± 2.43*	↓*
CB2			
cardiomyocyte cytoplasm	110.7 ± 2.57	91.1 ± 3.57*	↓*
endothelium of coronary vessels	49.9 ± 2.15	48.1 ± 1.98	
apelin			
cardiomyocyte cytoplasm	73.6 ± 2.26	95.0 ± 2.72*	↑*
endothelium of coronary vessels	135.9 ± 3.65	73.9 ± 2.43*	↓*
S100A6			
cardiomyocyte cytoplasm	81.0 ± 1.85	125.9 ± 3.30*	↑*
endothelium of coronary vessels	97.4 ± 3.84	79.1 ± 2.48*	↓*

*$p < 0.05$ women over 50 vs women under 50
↓ weakening of immunohistochemical reaction
↑ intensification of immunohistochemical reaction
ND not detected

substantially reduced cardiac hypertrophy in rodents with heart pressure overload and various models of hypertension [14, 15, 30]. In the past decade researches have confirmed the involvement of S100A6 protein in cardiac hypertrophy. It has been stated that S100A6 abolishes cardiomyocyte overgrowth induced by various hypertrophic factors and reduces cardiac hypertrophy in mice exposed to I/R heart injury [21, 31].

In view of the aforementioned, the changes in CB1, CB2, apelin and S100A6 levels in the hearts of women over 50 observed in our study might suggest the involvement of the endocannabinoid system, apelin and S100A6 protein in age-related heart remodelling. However, as the current study provides novel findings, further research should be performed to thoroughly understand the importance of CB1, CB2, apelin and S100A6 in age-induced cardiovascular changes.

It is known that in patients above the age of 50–60, dysfunction of the mechanical action of the heart occurs [26]. There are overwhelming literature data proving the impact of the endocannabinoid system on the frequency and strength of cardiac contraction. The activation of CB1 receptors evokes bradycardia and negative inotropic effect [1, 2]. In contrast to CB1 receptor, the stimulation of CB2-receptor triggers a positive contractile response in cardiac muscle cells [1, 2]. The systolic and diastolic heart function is also regulated by the apelin-APJ system [10]. Apelin treatment has significantly increased cardiomyocyte contractility in physiological and pathological conditions [10, 14, 15, 29]. A few reports have indicated that S100A6 might influence cardiac contractility. It has been demonstrated that S100A6 regulates calcium cycling between the sarcoplasmic reticulum and the cytosol in cardiomyocytes, which is necessary for the occurrence of the contraction cycle [21].

On the basis of this, a possible link might be suspected between impaired cardiac performance in older individuals and the alterations in the cannabinoid system, apelin and S100A6 in the hearts of women over 50 demonstrated in the present study.

Clinical and experimental studies have demonstrated abnormal activity of the endocannabinoid system in cardiovascular diseases including myocardial infarction, I/R heart injury, obesity-related circulatory dysfunction, diabetic cardiomyopathy and doxorubicin-induced heart failure [1, 3, 6, 8]. Numerous literature reports have indicated that cardiovascular diseases progress together with the impairment of apelin expression. Reduced circulating apelin levels have been observed in patients with heart failure, coronary artery disease and lone atrial fibrillation as well as in experimental models of isoproterenol-induced cardiomyopathy, I/R heart injury and heart failure [11, 32–36]. Cardiovascular events have also been linked with S100A6 upregulation. Increased S100A6 serum levels have been found in patients with acute coronary syndrome and in the rat model of MI [37].

Considering the above, the alterations in CB1, CB2, apelin and S100A6 distribution in the hearts of older women might be related with the development of cardiovascular complications in older individuals.

Conducted immunohistochemical identification of cannabinoid receptors in heart of women gave positive reaction for CB1 and CB2 receptors in cytoplasm of cardiac cells. The presented observation is consistent with results of Weis et al. [38], who similarly stated immunoreactivity for cannabinoid receptors in cardiomyocytes cytoplasm in human heart. Cannabinoid receptors belong to G-protein coupled membrane receptor family [1].

The G-protein coupled receptors are localized not only on cell membrane, they have been identified also on intracellular organelles including mitochondria [39]. Mendizabal-Zubiaga et al. [40] investigated distribution of cannabinoid receptors in cardiac muscle cells using immunogold staining method and electron microscope. Authors revealed that cannabinoid receptors are disposed on cardiomyocytes sarcolemma and also on the membrane of intracellular organelles. The greatest density of immunoparticles showing cannabinoid receptors was observed on mitochondrial membrane [40]. Described in our report cytoplasmic immunostaining for cannabinoid receptors in cardiomyocytes might be explained by the attachment of antibodies against CB1 and CB2 to receptors located on organelles membrane.

In the current study we observed the appearance of a strong CB1-immunosignal in ICDs in the hearts of women over 50, while in younger women CB1 was not detectable in this location. Intercalated discs ensure communication between cardiomyocytes in order to coordinate their function. ICDs construction contains adherens junctions, desmosomes and gap junctions and also a number of ion channels enabling the simultaneous spread of electrical potential across cardiac muscle cells. Voltage-dependent Ca^{2+} and Na^{+} channels are also among ion channels identified in ICDs [41]. Experimental studies have demonstrated that CB1 signalling modulates the activity of calcium and sodium voltage-gated channels [1]. Perhaps, the observed displacement of CB1 receptor to intercalated discs in the hearts of women over 50 is associated with the role of CB1 receptors in the regulation of ion current through channels occurring in ICDs.

Aging proceeds with progressive endothelial dysfunction, involving impaired secretion of vasoactive, proinflammatory and prothrombotic factors by endothelial cells as well as endothelial cell injury induced by intensified production of reactive oxygen species [42].

Enlarging literature data indicate on significant effect of cannabinoids, apelin and S100A6 on endothelial cell functioning. CB1-signaling impairs endothelium-dependent vascular dilatation and promotes endothelial cells apoptosis via inducing oxidative stress in those cells [43]. Whereas the CB2-pathway evokes endothelial-protective effect by attenuating endothelial cell response to proinflammatory molecules and limiting adhesion of monocytes to vascular endothelium [43]. Apelin triggers the endothelial release of vasodilator substances such as nitric oxide, therefore is involved in endothelial-dependent regulation of vascular tone [44]. The S100A6 protein regulates proliferative potential of endothelial cells and increases viability of those cells [45].

In the presented study we observed decrease of CB1 immunoreaction while unaltered immunoreactivity for CB2 in endothelium of coronary vasculature in older women. Having regard to above-mentioned, our findings might suggest inhibition of CB1-pathway in favour of CB2-signaling as adaptive process limiting endothelial dysfunction during ageing. However, this aspect should be subjected to further detailed investigation.

The current research revealed also weakened apelin and S100A6 immunostaining in endothelium of myocardial vessels in women over 50, which might indicate on participation of apelin and S100A6 in age-related deterioration of endothelial functioning.

Conclusion

The presented results of immunohistochemical study demonstrate alterations in the cannabinoid system, apelin and S100A6 in the hearts of women over 50.

The observed changes in CB1, CB2, apelin and S100A6 in heart of older women might be the result of ageing induced dysregulation of heart homeostasis or an adaptive mechanism attenuating the development of cardiac complications in older individuals.

The role of endocannabinoid system, apelin and S100 protein in regulating the heart's function during ageing and their importance in age-related cardiomyopathy require further investigation.

Abbreviations

APJ: The apelin receptor; CB1: The cannabinoid receptor type 1; CB2: The cannabinoid receptor type 2; I/R: Ischemia/reperfusion; ICDs: Intercalated discs; MI: Myocardial infarction; TNF-α: Tumour necrosis factor-alpha

Funding

This work was supported by statutory funds from the Medical University of Bialystok N/ST/ZB/17/001/2232.

Authors' contributions

IK, WL and AF conceived of and designed the experiments. IK, and ZP analyzed the data. IK, AF, and WL contributed reagents/materials/analysis tools. Writing – original draft preparation: ZP. Writing – review and editing: IK. Approval of final manuscript: all authors.

Competing interests

The authors declare that they have no competing interests.

Author details

[1]Department of Histology and Cytophysiology, Medical University of Bialystok, Mickiewicza 2C street, 15-222 Białystok, Poland. [2]Nencki Institute of Experimental Biology, Laboratory of Calcium Binding Proteins, Ludwika Pasteura 3 street, 02-093 Warszawa, Poland. [3]Department of Neurosurgery, Medical University of Bialystok, Marii Skłodowskiej-Curie 24A street, 15-276 Białystok, Poland.

References

1. Kaschina E. Cannabinoid CB1/CB2 receptors in the heart: expression, regulation, and function. In: Meccariello R, editor. Cannabinoids in health and disease. IntechOpen; 2016. p. 169–86.
2. Sterin-Borda L, Del Zar CF, Borda E. Differential CB1 and CB2 cannabinoid receptor-inotropic response of rat isolated atria: endogenous signal transduction pathways. Biochem Pharmacol. 2005;69:1705–13.
3. Mukhopadhyay P, Rajesh M, Bátkai S, Patel V, Kashiwaya Y, Liaudet L, Evgenov OV, Mackie K, Haskó G, Pacher P. CB1 cannabinoid receptors promote oxidative stress and cell death in murine models of doxorubicin-induced cardiomyopathy and in human cardiomyocytes. Cardiovasc Res. 2010;85:773–84.

4. Slavic S, Lauer D, Sommerfeld M, Kemnitz UR, Grzesiak A, Trappiel M, Thöne-Reineke C, Baulmann J, Paulis L, Kappert K, Kintscher U, Unger T, Kaschina E. Cannabinoid receptor 1 inhibition improves cardiac function and remodelling after myocardial infarction and in experimental metabolic syndrome. J Mol Med (Berl). 2013;91:811–23.
5. Rajesh M, Bátkai S, Kechrid M, Mukhopadhyay P, Lee WS, Horváth B, Holovac E, Cinar R, Liaudet L, Mackie K, Haskó G, Pacher P. Cannabinoid 1 receptor promotes cardiac dysfunction, oxidative stress, inflammation, and fibrosis in diabetic cardiomyopathy. Diabetes. 2012;61:716–27.
6. Wang PF, Jiang LS, Bu J, Huang XJ, Song W, Du YP, He B. Cannabinoid-2 receptor activation protects against infarct and ischemia-reperfusion heart injury. J Cardiovasc Pharmacol. 2012;59:301–7.
7. Li X, Han D, Tian Z, Gao B, Fan M, Li C, Li X, Wang Y, Ma S, Cao F. Activation of cannabinoid receptor type II by AM1241 ameliorates myocardial fibrosis via Nrf2-mediated inhibition of TGF-β1/Smad3 pathway in myocardial infarction mice. Cell Physiol Biochem. 2016;39:1521–36.
8. Duerr GD, Heinemann JC, Suchan G, Kolobara E, Wenzel D, Geisen C, Matthey M, Passe-Tietjen K, Mahmud W, Ghanem A, Tiemann K, Alferink J, Burgdorf S, Buchalla R, Zimmer A, Lutz B, Welz A, Fleischmann BK, Dewald O. The endocannabinoid-CB2 receptor axis protects the ischemic heart at the early stage of cardiomyopathy. Basic Res Cardiol. 2014;109:425.
9. Chandrasekaran B, Dar O, McDonagh T. The role of apelin in cardiovascular function and heart failure. Eur J Heart Fail. 2008;10:725–32.
10. Szokodi I, Tavi P, Földes G, Voutilainen-Myllylä S, Ilves M, Tokola H, Pikkarainen S, Piuhola J, Rysä J, Tóth M, Ruskoaho H. Apelin, the novel endogenous ligand of the orphan receptor APJ, regulates cardiac contractility. Circ Res. 2002;91:434–40.
11. Wang W, McKinnie SM, Patel VB, Haddad G, Wang Z, Zhabyeyev P, Das SK, Basu R, McLean B, Kandalam V, Penninger JM, Kassiri Z, Vederas JC, Murray AG, Oudit GY. Loss of Apelin exacerbates myocardial infarction adverse remodeling and ischemia-reperfusion injury: therapeutic potential of synthetic Apelin analogues. J Am Heart Assoc. 2013;2:000249.
12. Tao J, Zhu W, Li Y, Xin P, Li J, Liu M, Li J, Redington AN, Wei M. Apelin-13 protects the heart against ischemia-reperfusion injury through inhibition of ER-dependent apoptotic pathways in a time-dependent fashion. Am J Physiol Heart Circ Physiol. 2011;301:1471–86.
13. Zhang Z, Yu B, Tao GZ. Apelin protects against cardiomyocyte apoptosis induced by glucose deprivation. Chin Med J. 2009;122:2360–5.
14. Falcão-Pires I, Gonçalves N, Henriques-Coelho T, Moreira-Gonçalves D, Roncon-Albuquerque R Jr, Leite-Moreira AF. Apelin decreases myocardial injury and improves right ventricular function in monocrotaline-induced pulmonary hypertension. Am J Physiol Heart Circ Physiol. 2009;296:2007–14.
15. Koguchi W, Kobayashi N, Takeshima H, Ishikawa M, Sugiyama F, Ishimitsu T. Cardioprotective effect of apelin-13 on cardiac performance and remodeling in end-stage heart failure. Circ J. 2012;76:137–44.
16. Pchejetski D, Foussal C, Alfarano C, Lairez O, Calise D, Guilbeau-Frugier C, Schaak S, Seguelas MH, Wanecq E, Valet P, Parini A, Kunduzova O. Apelin prevents cardiac fibroblast activation and collagen production through inhibition of sphingosine kinase 1. Eur Heart J. 2012;33:2360–9.
17. Bellocchio L, Cervino C, Vicennati V, Pasquali R, Pagotto U. Cannabinoid type 1 receptor: another arrow in the adipocytes' bow. J Neuroendocrinol. 2008;20:130–8.
18. Haddad M. What does Rimonabant do in rat primary skeletal muscle cells? Biomed Pharmacol J. 2014;7:81–92.
19. Geurts L, Lazarevic V, Derrien M, Everard A, Van Roye M, Knauf C, Valet P, Girard M, Muccioli GG, François P, de Vos WM, Schrenzel J, Delzenne NM, Cani PD. Altered gut microbiota and endocannabinoid system tone in obese and diabetic leptin-resistant mice: impact on apelin regulation in adipose tissue. Front Microbiol. 2011;2:149.
20. Donato R. Functional roles of S100 proteins, calcium-binding proteins of the EF-hand type. Biochim Biophys Acta. 1999;1450:191–231.
21. Mofid A, Newman NS, Lee PJ, Abbasi C, Matkar PN, Rudenko D, Kuliszewski MA, Chen HH, Afrasiabi K, Tsoporis JN, Gramolini AO, Connelly KA, Parker TG, Leong-Poi H. Cardiac overexpression of S100A6 attenuates cardiomyocyte apoptosis and reduces infarct size after myocardial ischemia-reperfusion. J Am Heart Assoc. 2017;6:004738.
22. Tsoporis JN, Izhar S, Parker TG. Expression of S100A6 in cardiac myocytes limits apoptosis induced by tumor necrosis factor-alpha. J Biol Chem. 2008; 283:30174–83.
23. Joo JH, Yoon SY, Kim JH, Paik SG, Min SR, Lim JS, Choe IS, Choi I, Kim JW. S100A6 (calcyclin) enhances the sensitivity to apoptosis via the upregulation of caspase-3 activity in Hep3B cells. J Cell Biochem. 2008;103:1183–97.
24. Slomnicki LP, Nawrot B, Leśniak W. S100A6 binds p53 and affects its activity. Int J Biochem Cell Biol. 2008;41:784–90.
25. Finegold JA, Asaria P, Francis DP. Mortality from ischaemic heart disease by country, region, and age: statistics from World Health Organisation and United Nations. Int J Cardiol. 2013;168:934–45.
26. Strait JB, Lakatta EG. Aging-associated cardiovascular changes and their relationship to heart failure. Heart Fail Clin. 2012;8:143–64.
27. Herman GE, Elfont EA. The taming of immunohistochemistry: the new era of quality control. Biotech Histochem. 1991;66:194–9.
28. Földes G, Horkay F, Szokodi I, Vuolteenaho O, Ilves M, Lindstedt KA, Mäyränpää M, Sármán B, Seres L, Skoumal R, Lakó-Futó Z, deChâtel R, Ruskoaho H, Tóth M. Circulating and cardiac levels of apelin, the novel ligand of the orphan receptor APJ, in patients with heart failure. Biochem Biophys Res Commun. 2003;308:480–5.
29. Tycinska AM, Sobkowicz B, Mroczko B, Sawicki R, Musial WJ, Dobrzycki S, Waszkiewicz E, Knapp MA, Szmitkowski M. The value of apelin-36 and brain natriuretic peptide measurements in patients with first ST-elevation myocardial infarction. Clin Chim Acta. 2010;411:2014–8.
30. Ellinor PT, Low AF, Macrae CA. Reduced apelin levels in lone atrial fibrillation. Eur Heart J. 2006;27:222–6.
31. Jia YX, Pan CS, Zhang J, Geng B, Zhao J, Gerns H, Yang J, Chang JK, Tang CS, Qi YF. Apelin protects myocardial injury induced by isoproterenol in rats. Regul Pept. 2006;133:147–54.
32. Iwanaga Y, Kihara Y, Takenaka H, Kita T. Down-regulation of cardiac apelin system in hypertrophied and failing hearts: possible role of angiotensin II-angiotensin type 1 receptor system. J Mol Cell Cardiol. 2006;41:798–806.
33. Cai XY, Lu L, Wang YN, Jin C, Zhang RY, Zhang Q, Chen QJ, Shen WF. Association of increased S100B, S100A6 and S100P in serum levels with acute coronary syndrome and also with the severity of myocardial infarction in cardiac tissue of rat models with ischemia-reperfusion injury. Atherosclerosis. 2011;217:536–42.
34. Marín-García J. Signaling in the aging heart. In: Marín-García J. Signaling in the heart. Boston: Springer; 2011. p. 221–43.
35. Kuba K, Zhang L, Imai Y, Arab S, Chen M, Maekawa Y, Leschnik M, Leibbrandt A, Markovic M, Schwaighofer J, Beetz N, Musialek R, Neely GG, Komnenovic V, Kolm U, Metzler B, Ricci R, Hara H, Meixner A, Nghiem M, Chen X, Dawood F, Wong KM, Sarao R, Cukerman E, Kimura A, Hein L, Thalhammer J, Liu PP, Penninger JM. Impaired heart contractility in Apelin gene-deficient mice associated with aging and pressure overload. Circ Res. 2007;101:32–42.
36. Foussal C, Lairez O, Calise D, Pathak A, Guilbeau-Frugier C, Valet P, Parini A, Kunduzova O. Activation of catalase by apelin prevents oxidative stress-linked cardiac hypertrophy. FEBS Lett. 2010;584:2363–70.
37. Tsoporis JN, Marks A, Haddad A, O'Hanlon D, Jolly S, Parker TG. S100A6 is a negative regulator of the induction of cardiac genes by trophic stimuli in cultured rat myocytes. Exp Cell Res. 2005;303:471–81.
38. Weis F, Beiras-Fernandez A, Sodian R, Kaczmarek I, Reichart B, Beiras A, Schelling G, Kreth S. Substantially altered expression pattern of cannabinoid receptor 2 and activated endocannabinoid system in patients with severe heart failure. J Mol Cell Cardiol. 2010;48:1187–93.
39. Lyssand JS, Bajjalieh SM. The heterotrimeric G protein subunit G alpha i is present on mitochondria. FEBS Lett. 2007;581:5765–8.
40. Mendizabal-Zubiaga J, Melser S, Bénard G, Ramos A, Reguero L, Arrabal S, Elezgarai I, Gerrikagoitia I, Suarez J, Rodríguez De Fonseca F, Puente N, Marsicano G, Grandes P. Cannabinoid CB1 receptors are localized in striated muscle mitochondria and regulate mitochondrial respiration. Front Physiol. 2016;7:476.
41. Estigoy CB, Pontén F, Odeberg J, Herbert B, Guilhaus M, Charleston M, Ho JWK Cameron D, Dos Remedios CG. Intercalated discs: multiple proteins perform multiple functions in non-failing and failing human hearts. Biophys Rev. 2009;1:43.
42. Donato AJ, Morgan RG, Walker AE, Lesniewski LA. Cellular and molecular biology of aging endothelial cells. J Mol Cell Cardiol. 2015;89:122–35.
43. Singla S, Sachdeva R, Mehta JL. Cannabinoids and atherosclerotic coronary heart disease. Clin Cardiol. 2012;35:329–35.
44. Tatemoto K, Takayama K, Zou MX, Kumaki I, Zhang W, Kumano K, Fujimiya M. The novel peptide apelin lowers blood pressure via a nitric oxide-dependent mechanism. Regul Pept. 2001;99:87–92.
45. Bao L, Odell AF, Stephen SL, Wheatcroft SB, Walker JH, Ponnambalam S. The S100A6 calcium-binding protein regulates endothelial cell-cycle progression and senescence. FEBS J. 2012;279:4576–88.

Time trends in statin use and incidence of recurrent cardiovascular events in secondary prevention between 1999 and 2013: a registry-based study

Nele Laleman[1], Séverine Henrard[1,2], Marjan van den Akker[1,3], Geert Goderis[1], Frank Buntinx[1,3], Gijs Van Pottelbergh[1] and Bert Vaes[1,2*]

Abstract

Background: The current study evaluated time trends of statin use and incidence of recurrent CVD in secondary prevention from 1999 to 2013 and investigated which factors were associated with statin use in secondary prevention.

Methods: Intego is a primary care registration network with 111 general practitioners working in 48 practices in Flanders, Belgium. This retrospective registry-based study included patients aged 50 years or older with a history of CVD. The time trends of statin use and incidence of recurrent CVD in secondary prevention were determined by using a joinpoint regression analysis. Multivariable mixed-effect logistic regression analysis was used to assess factors associated with statin use in patients in secondary prevention in 2013.

Results: The overall prevalence of statin use increased and showed two trends: a sharp increase from 1999 to 2005 (annual percentage change (APC) 25.4%) and a weaker increase from 2005 to 2013 (APC 3.7%). The average increase in statin use was the highest in patients aged 80 and older. Patients aged 70–79 years received the most statins. Men used more statins than women did, but both genders showed similar time trends. The incidence of CVD decreased by an average APC of 3.9%. There were no differences between men and women and between different age groups. A significant decrease was only observed in older patients without statins prescribed. In 2013, 61% of the patients in secondary prevention did not receive a statin. The absence of other secondary preventive medication was strongly associated with less statin use. Gender, age and comorbidity were associated with statin use to a lesser degree.

Conclusions: The prevalence of statin use in secondary prevention increased strongly from 1999 to 2013. Less than 50% of patients with a history of CVD received a statin in 2013. Especially patients who did not receive other secondary preventive medication were more likely to not receive a statin. Despite the strong increase in statin use, there was only a small decrease in the incidence of recurrent CVD, and this occurred mainly in older patients without statins prescribed.

Keywords: Statins, Secondary prevention, Cardiovascular diseases, Trends

* Correspondence: bert.vaes@kuleuven.be
[1]Department of Public Health and Primary Care, Universiteit Leuven (KU Leuven), Kapucijnenvoer 33, Blok J, 3000 Leuven, Belgium
[2]Institute of Health and Society, Université catholique de Louvain (UCL), Brussels, Belgium
Full list of author information is available at the end of the article

Introduction

Cardiovascular diseases (CVD) are still the leading cause of death in Europe: in 2012 they were responsible for 47% of all deaths [1, 2]. In the last few decades survival rates after CVD have increased and cardiovascular mortality has decreased [1, 2]. However, individuals with established CVD have a high risk of a recurrent event [2]. The currently recommended pharmacological intervention in secondary prevention is a combination of antithrombotic therapy, statins and, in some cases, antihypertensive agents, independent of age and gender [3–5].

Statins have proven to reduce the risk of recurrent CVD and of cardiovascular and total mortality in secondary prevention [3, 4, 6–8]. Nevertheless, there remains a large gap between current recommendations and clinical practice: previous studies reported that only a minority of patients with a history of CVD receives statins [9–31]. However, to date, no study described time trends of statin use in secondary prevention in combination with the evolution of recurrent CVD in the general population. Although statin non-use is very prevalent, the current study hypothesized that the use of statins in secondary prevention has increased substantially and that this possibly coincides with a lower incidence of recurrent CVD. Furthermore, factors associated with less statin use such as female gender, older age, comorbidity (diabetes, heart failure), smoking, low cholesterol level, longer time after diagnosis and type of CVD have been described [9, 10, 12, 15, 23, 26, 32–36]. However, a recent evaluation of statin use in secondary prevention and a description of factors related to statin use in a real world population are still lacking.

Therefore, the first aim of this retrospective registry-based study was to evaluate time trends of statin use and incidence of recurrent CVD in secondary prevention from 1999 to 2013. The second aim was to investigate which factors are associated with statin use in secondary prevention.

Methods

Study design and study population

Data were obtained from Intego, a general-practice-based morbidity registration network at the Department of Public Health and Primary Care of the University of Leuven, Belgium [37]. The Intego procedures were approved by the ethical review board of the Medical School of the University of Leuven (N° ML 1723) and by the Belgian Privacy Commission (no SCSZG/13/079). In 2013, 111 general practitioners (GPs), all using the medical software Medidoc®, collaborated in the Intego project. They worked in 48 practices evenly spread over Flanders, the Northern part of Belgium. GPs applied for inclusion in the registry. Before acceptance of their data, registration performance was audited using a number of algorithms that compared their results with those of all other applicants. Only the data of the practices with an optimal registration performance were included in the database. The Intego GPs prospectively and routinely registered all new diagnoses together with new drug prescriptions, laboratory test results and some background information (including gender and year of birth), using computer-generated keywords internally linked to codes. New data were coded and collected from the GPs' personal computers with specially framed extraction software and entered into a central database. Registered data were continuously updated and historically accumulated for each patient. New diagnoses were classified according to a very detailed thesaurus automatically linked to the International Classification of Primary Care (ICPC-2). Drugs were classified according to the WHO's Anatomical Therapeutic Chemical (ATC) classification system.

The current study is a retrospective cohort study that used Intego data from January 1st 1999 to December 31st 2013. In every yearly contact group (patients in contact with their GP for either reason during a year) between 1999 and 2013, we selected all patients aged 50 years or older with a history of CVD (myocardial infarction (MI) (K75), stroke (K90), transient ischemic attack (TIA) (K89), ischemic heart disease (IHD) with and without angina (K74 and K76, respectively) and peripheral arterial disease (PAD) (K92)). Recurrent CVD was defined as an incident case of MI, stroke or TIA in all selected patients, or an incident diagnosis of IHD or PAD in patients without a previous diagnosis of IHD or PAD. MI and stroke were considered as major events. TIA, IHD and PAD were considered as minor events. The prevalence of statin (ATC code C10AA) use (at least 2 prescriptions in the selected year) was registered for each year.

Clinical characteristics

Comorbidity

The medical history of all patients in secondary prevention in 1999 and in 2013 was registered. Besides the history of CVD as defined above, other relevant comorbidities were registered, such as atrial fibrillation, hypercholesterolemia, hypertension and mental disorders (anxiety, depression or overstrain). Furthermore, comorbidities were registered in order to construct the modified Charlson Comorbidity Index (mCCI) [38, 39]. For the presence of renal insufficiency, the glomerular filtration rate (GFR) was estimated (MDRD equation) based on the last creatinine measurement in the 2 years before 1999 or 2013. Whether or not LDL (low-density lipoprotein) had been measured in the 3 years before 1999 or 2013 was registered for all patients included.

Pharmacotherapy

The prescription of cardiovascular medication was registered for all patients in secondary prevention in 1999 and in 2013. Data were collected on the prescription of aspirin (ATC code B01AC06), agents acting on the renin-angiotensin system (RAS) (ATC code C09), non-RAS antihypertensive agents (ATC codes C03, C07 and C08) and other lipid lowering medication (LLM) (ATC code C10 except C10AA). Medication use in a specific year was considered positive when at least two prescriptions had been made in that year.

Statistical analysis

To analyse time trends in age-standardized rates between 1999 and 2013, a joinpoint regression analysis was performed [40]. A joinpoint is a point in the trend curve where a statistically significant change in trend over time is observed. A minimum number of 3 observations from a joinpoint to either end of the data, and a minimum number of 4 observations between two joinpoints were required. The age-standardized rates were computed taken the Flemish population in Belgium as the standard population, using 10-year age groups until 79 years, and 80 years and older as the last age group for standardization. The reference year for the standard population was 1999. From the joinpoint regression model, the annual percentage change (APC) and the average annual percentage change (AAPC) were extracted. APC is calculated for each significant trend from a piecewise log-linear model on the logarithm of the age-standardised rate versus the year. AAPC represents the average of APC estimates per significant trend weighted by the corresponding trend length (number of years in the trend). The trend analysis using the joinpoint regression model was performed using the SEER*-Stat software (Joinpoint Trend Analysis software from the Surveillance Research Program of the US National Cancer Institute (available at http://surveillance.cancer.-gov/joinpoint)).

Continuous data were summarized using median [P_{25}; P_{75}], and categorical data using proportions. Factors associated with statin use in patients in secondary prevention in 2013 were assessed using mixed effects logistic regression, which belongs to generalized linear mixed models (GLMM). Each GP practice was treated as a random effect to explore the variability between GP practices in addition to individual patient observations themselves, by age group (50–59 years, 60–79 years, 80+ years). The log-likelihood was estimated using the Laplace approximation. All variables in univariate analysis were candidate for the multivariable model. A stepwise approach was then used to select the best multivariable model. The goodness of fit of the model was assessed using the Akaike information criteria (AIC), Hosmer-Lemeshow test, c-index of the receiver operating characteristic (ROC) curve and the Somers' D_{xy} rank correlation. The c-index assesses the predictive performance of the model and the Somers' D_{xy} is an estimate of the rank correlation of the observed binary outcome and the predicted probabilities. In addition, at each step, the maximum variance inflation factor value associated with each parameter in the model was required to be less than 10 for the model to be chosen. A two-sided p-value < 0.05 was considered statistically significant. Statistical analyses of the factors associated with statin use in patients in secondary prevention were performed using R Software Version 3.0.3 (Free Software Foundation Inc., Boston, MA, USA) (lme4, pgirmess, gof and ROCR packages) [41].

Results

The age-standardized prevalence rate of statin prescription in secondary prevention increased from 8.4% in 1999 to 39.3% in 2013. Table 1 shows the trends in the prevalence of statin use between 1999 and 2013. Two trends were apparent: there was a sharp increase from 1999 to 2005 and a weaker, but also significant increase from 2005 to 2013 (APC 25.4% (95% CI 21.8–29.0) and 3.7% (95% CI 1.7–5.6), respectively). Figure 1 shows the age-standardized prevalence rate of statin prescription in secondary prevention according to age groups. The average increase in statin prescription was the highest in the oldest age group (AAPC 23.2% and 28.0% in women and men, respectively) and differed significantly with other age groups. In 2013, people aged 70–79 years most often received statins (51%). While patients aged 69 years or younger reached a plateau after 2005, the statin use of patients aged 70 years or older increased further, but less strongly than before. Men used more statins in secondary prevention than women did, but the time trends were similar in both genders (AAPC 12.3% and 12.6%, respectively, AAPC difference – 0.3% (95% CI -2.6; 2.0)).

Figure 2 and Table 2 show the time trends for the age-standardized incidence rate of recurrent CVD. The incidence was 52/1000 patient years in 1999, it did not show a significant trend until 2001, after which a significant decrease was observed (APC -2.2% (95% CI -3.8; – 0.6)). There were no significant differences in AAPC between men and women and between different age groups. Figure 3 shows the age-standardized incidence rate of recurrent CVD in patients receiving statins and in those without. The incidence rate of recurrent CVD in 1999 was higher in patients without statin prescription (57/1000 patient years vs 27/1000 patient years). A significant decrease of recurrent CVD was seen in patients without statin prescription (AAPC -3.9% (95% CI -5.6; – 2.2) and – 2.5% (95% CI -4.8; – 0.1), in patients with a major or minor first event, respectively). In

Table 1 Age-standardized prevalence rate of statin use in secondary prevention

Group	ASPR of statin use in 1999	Summary	Trend 1		Trend2		Trend3	
		AAPC	Years	APC	Years	APC	Years	APC
Total	8.4%	12.5 [10.9; 14.1]*	1999–2005	25.4 [21.8; 29.0]*	2005–2013	3.7 [1.7; 5.6]*		
Women	6.5%	12.6 [10.9; 14.3]*	1999–2005	25.0 [21.3; 28.8]*	2005–2013	4.1 [2.1; 6.2]*		
50–59	7.6%	8.3 [5.7; 10.8]*	1999–2005	21.0 [15.5; 26.9]*	2005–2013	−0.4 [− 3.4; 2.6]		
60–69	13.6%	7.3 [5.1; 9.6]*	1999–2006	15.2 [11.4; 19.2]*	2006–2013	−0.1 [− 3.4; 3.3]		
70–79	6.6%	14.0 [12.1; 16.0]*	1999–2004	31.0 [27.7; 34.4]*	2004–2008	11.2 [5.0; 17.8]*	2008–2013	1.3 [− 1.3; 3.9]
80+	1.2%	23.2 [17.3; 29.4]*	1999–2005	40.0 [26.8; 54.5]*	2005–2013	11.9 [5.0; 19.3]*		
Men	10.0%	12.3 [10.7; 13.9]*	1999–2005	25.4 [21.8; 29.0]*	2005–2013	3.4 [1.5; 5.3]*		
50–59	18.3%	6.5 [4.7; 8.4]*	1999–2005	17.2 [13.2; 21.4]*	2005–2013	−0.8 [− 3.0; 1.5]		
60–69	12.7%	10.7 [9.0; 12.4]*	1999–2005	24.9 [21.2; 28.8]*	2005–2013	1.0 [− 0.9; 3.1]		
70–79	7.6%	15.5 [13.7; 17.4]*	1999–2005	29.2 [25.1; 33.3]*	2005–2013	6.2 [4.1; 8.4]*		
80+	0.8%	28.0 [22.8; 33.3]*	1999–2005	59.1 [46.5; 72.9]*	2005–2013	8.7 [3.0; 14.6]*		

*$p < 0.05$; *ASPR* age-standardized prevalence rate, *AAPC* average annual percentage change, *APC* annual percentage change

patients receiving statins no significant trend was observed (AAPC 0.9% (95% CI -3.4; 5.4) and - 0.3% (95% CI -2.9; 2.4) in patients with a major or minor first event, respectively). The decrease in recurrent CVD was mainly seen in older patients (≥60 years) without statin prescription (Table 3).

The first part of Table 4 shows the main characteristics of patients in secondary prevention in 1999 and in 2013. Mean age, gender distribution and prevalence of different CVD were similar. The crude prevalence of statin use in secondary prevention increased sharply from 7.4% in 1999 to 39.3% in 2013. In 2013, more people received other secondary preventive medications (aspirin, RAS- and non-RAS-antihypertensive agents) than in 1999. In terms of comorbidity, there was an increase of hypercholesterolemia, hypertension, COPD, diabetes and cancer between 1999 and 2013.

In the second part of Table 4, the 2013 study population was split in different age groups (50–59 years, 60–79 years and 80+ years), because important differences in prevalence of statin use were observed (32.8%, 50.3% and 25.7%, respectively). Age groups 60–69 years and 70–79 years were combined because the prevalence of statin use was similar. In every age group, the prevalence of statin use was compared in subjects with and without specific clinical characteristics. In all age groups, women, subjects with an LDL-measurement in the past 3 years, subjects with no registered history of hypercholesterolemia, MI or IHD with angina, and subjects with no GFR estimated or not receiving any other preventive medication, showed a lower prevalence of statin use. People in the oldest age groups with a history of stroke, TIA or dementia were less often prescribed statins than people without these conditions. At younger age (50–79 years),

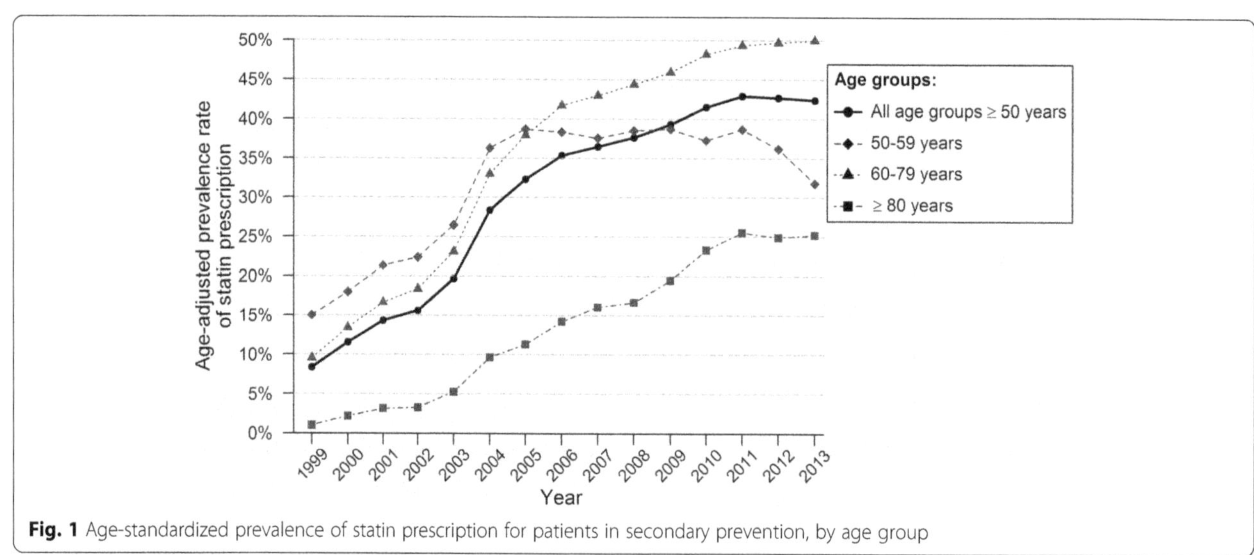

Fig. 1 Age-standardized prevalence of statin prescription for patients in secondary prevention, by age group

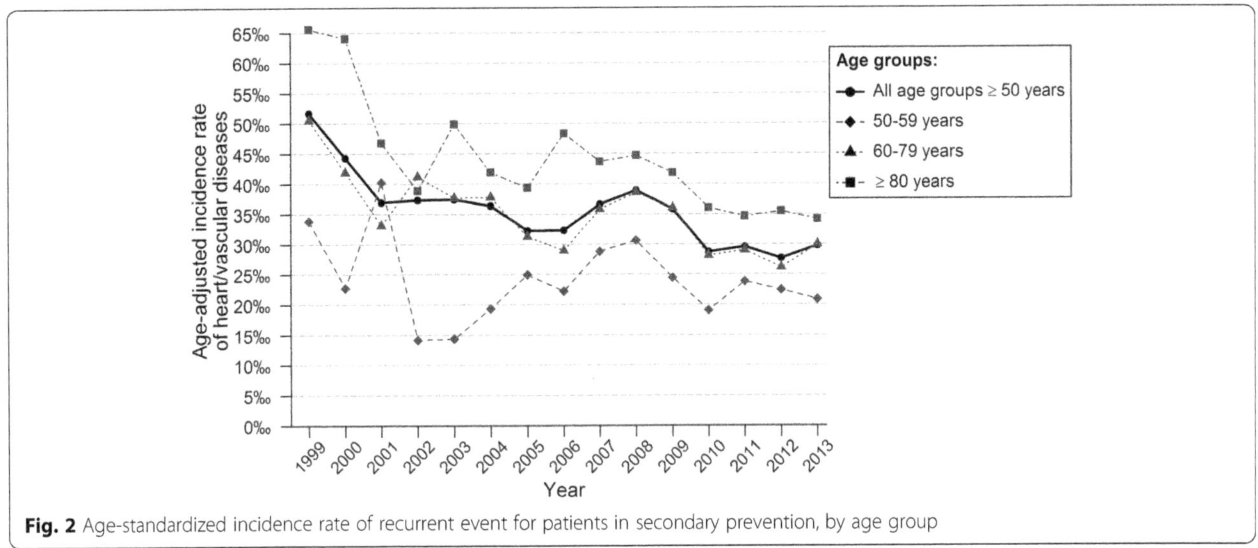

Fig. 2 Age-standardized incidence rate of recurrent event for patients in secondary prevention, by age group

individuals with cancer or PAD were less likely to receive a statin than peers without these conditions, whereas the opposite was observed for patients with diabetes.

Table 5 shows the results of the multivariable mixed-effect logistic regression analysis. In all age groups, the absence of other preventive medication was strongly associated with less statin use: patients who did not receive aspirin, RAS- or non-RAS-antihypertensive agents showed an OR of 0.03 (95% CI 0.01–0.06), 0.04 (95% CI 0.03–0.05) and 0.02 (95% CI 0.01–0.03), in age groups 50–59 years, 60–79 years and 80+, respectively. The prescription of other LLM than statins decreased the odds of having a statin prescribed. Women were less likely to receive statins in secondary prevention than men. In subjects aged 60–79 older age predicted greater statin use (OR 1.25 (95% CI 1.02–1.52)). On the other hand, older age predicted lower statin use in the oldest age group (OR 0.87 (95% CI 0.84–0.90)). In all age groups, hypertension was associated with less statin use, whereas hypercholesterolemia predicted greater statin use. Diabetes was associated with a higher statin use in subjects aged 60–79 years (OR 1.52 (95% CI 1.22–1.88)).

The c-index of the full model was 0.86, 0.84 and 0.90 in the respective age groups (50–59 years, 60–79 years and 80+ years), demonstrating a good total discriminant ability to identify patients with statin use. The c-index of the model that included only co-medication was 0.83, 0.80 and 0.86, respectively. The c-index of the model without co-medication was 0.76, 0.73 and 0.80, respectively. The Somers' D_{xy} rank correlation of the full model between the predicted probabilities and the observed outcome was 0.72, 0.68 and 0.80, respectively. Finally, the p-values associated with the Hosmer and Lemeshow

Table 2 Age-standardized incidence rate of CV/heart diseases in secondary prevention

Group	ASIR of CV/heart disease in 1999	Summary	Trend 1		Trend2	
		AAPC	Years	APC	Years	APC
Total	51.7‰	−3.9 [− 7.4; −0.4]*	1999–2001	−13.7 [− 34.4; 13.5]	2001–2013	−2.2 [− 3.8; − 0.6]*
Women	50.3‰	−2.8 [− 4.5; − 1.1]*	1999–2013	−2.8 [− 4.5; − 1.1]*		
50–59	34.5‰	−1.2 [− 6.5; 4.4]	1999–2013[a]	−1.2 [− 6.5; 4.4]		
60–69	33.2‰	− 0.7 [− 3.8; 2.5]	1999–2013	− 0.7 [− 3.8; 2.5]		
70–79	50.5‰	−3.3 [− 6.7; 0.1]	1999–2013	−3.3 [− 6.7; 0.1]		
80+	66.6‰	−3.7 [−5.4; − 2.1]*	1999–2013	−3.7 [− 5.4; − 2.1]*		
Men	52.8‰	−3.3 [− 5.1; − 1.5]*	1999–2013	−3.3 [− 5.1; − 1.5]*		
50–59	33.5‰	−1.1 [− 4.9; 2.9]	1999–2013	− 1.1 [− 4.9; 2.9]		
60–69	51.4‰	− 3.3 [− 5.4; − 1.1]*	1999–2013	− 3.3 [− 5.4; − 1.1]*		
70–79	58.0‰	−3.7 [− 6.3; − 1.1]*	1999–2013	−3.7 [− 6.3; − 1.1]*		
80+	64.1‰	−3.2 [− 5.5; − 0.8]*	1999–2013	−3.2 [− 5.5; − 0.8]*		

*$p < 0.05$; [a]without 2002 because it was 0, *ASIR* age-standardized incidence rate, *AAPC* average annual percentage change, *APC* annual percentage change

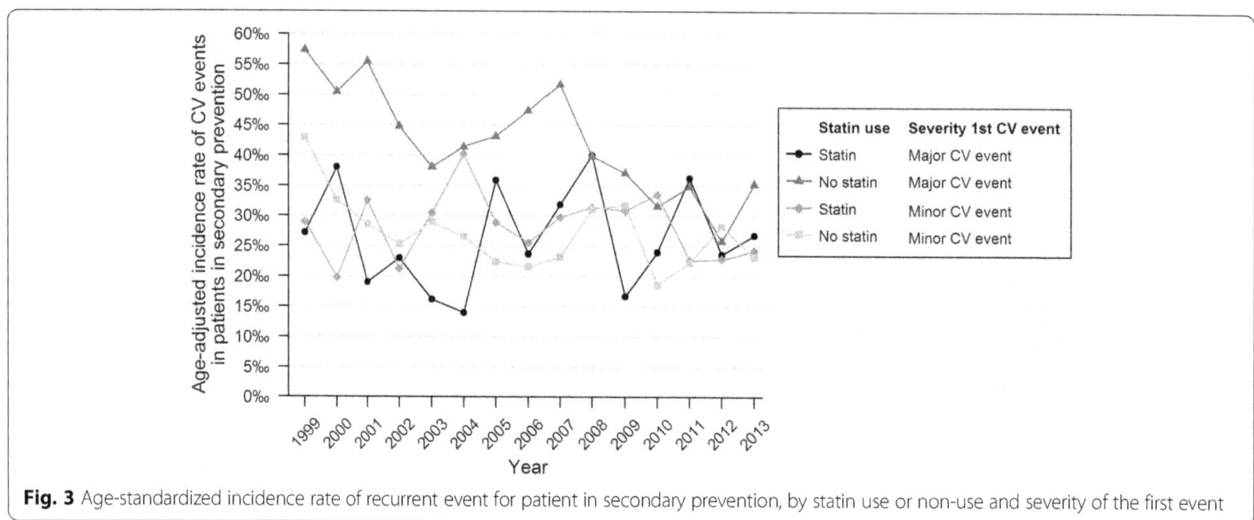

Fig. 3 Age-standardized incidence rate of recurrent event for patient in secondary prevention, by statin use or non-use and severity of the first event

test of the full model were 0.62, 0.10 and 0.73, respectively, demonstrating that the predicted values from the model fit the observed values.

Discussion

Major findings

This large registry-based study showed that the prevalence of statin use in secondary prevention increased strongly from 1999 to 2005, and more slightly from 2005 to 2013. Despite the strong increase in statin use in secondary prevention, there was rather a modest decline in the incidence of CVD, and this occurred mainly in older patients without statins prescribed. In 2013, less than 50% of the patients with a history of CVD received a statin. The absence of other secondary preventive medication was strongly associated with less statin use. Gender, age and comorbidity were associated with statin use to a lesser degree.

Time trends in age-standardized prevalence rate of statin use

Analogous to previous studies, we found that the prevalence of statin use in secondary prevention has increased over the last few decades [9–18, 20, 21, 23–36, 42–44]. The rise in statin use has been linked to guideline changes, promotions by the pharmaceutical industry, media reports, reimbursement conditions, entrance of generic medication and reductions of the price [10, 12, 15, 17, 18, 21, 24, 25, 28, 32, 33, 42, 43, 45].

This study computed AAPC of the prevalence of statin use in secondary prevention, which showed two trends: there was a sharp increase from 1999 to 2005 and a weaker, but also statistical significant increase from 2005 to 2013. This suggests that the steep increase in statin use in secondary prevention in the first time period was mainly linked to the growing literature in support of statins and to guideline changes. After 2005, when statins became less expensive for Belgian patients, the

Table 3 Age-standardized incidence rate of CV/heart diseases in secondary prevention among statin users and statin non-users

Group	ASIR of CV/heart disease in 1999	Summary	Trend 1		Trend2	
		AAPC	Years	APC	Years	APC
Total	51.7‰	−3.9 [− 7.4; − 0.4]*	1999–2001	− 13.7 [− 34.4; 13.5]	2001–2013	−2.2 [− 3.8; − 0.6]*
Statin users	69.5‰	−3.4 [− 6.7; 0.1]	1999–2001	− 34.5 [− 62.6; 14.7]	2001–2013	−0.4 [− 3.7; 2.9]
50–59[a]	28.3‰[a]	2.6 [−4.3; 9.9]	2001–2013	2.6 [− 4.3; 9.9]		
60–79	37.3‰	−0.5 [− 2.8; 1.9]	1999–2013	−0.5 [− 2.8; 1.9]		
80 + [b]	55.9‰[b]	−7.2 [− 29.0; 21.3]	2004–2013	−7.2 [− 29.0; 21.3]		
Statin non-users	52.6‰	−3.2 [−4.4; − 2.0]*	1999–2001	− 14.1 [− 33.8; 11.6]	2001–2013	− 2.3 [− 3.8; − 0.8]*
50–59	37.3‰	−1.8 [−6.7; 3.3]	1999–2013	− 1.8 [− 6.7; 3.3]		
60–79	51.7‰	−3.2 [− 4.6; − 1.7]*	1999–2013	−3.2 [− 4.6; − 1.7]*		
80+	64.2‰	−3.4 [− 5.0; − 1.8]*	1999–2013	−3.4 [− 5.0; − 1.8]*		

*$p < 0.05$, [a]data for years 1999 to 2000 were excluded because of the small sample size ($N < 100$), [b]data for years 1999 to 2003 were excluded because of the small sample size ($N < 100$), *ASIR* age-standardized incidence rate, *AAPC* average annual percentage change, *APC* annual percentage change

Table 4 Characteristics of patients on secondary prevention

Variables	1999	2013	Age group in 2013								
	Total (n = 4007)	Total (n = 6295)	50–59 years (n = 1077)			60–79 years (n = 3211)			80+ years (n = 2077)		
	n (%) or Median [P25; P75]	n (%) or Median [P25; P75]	n (%) or Median [P25; P75]	Statin use cat.[a] %	Statin use ref. cat.[b] %	*n* (%) or Median [P25; P75]	Statin use cat.[a] %	Statin use ref. cat.[b] %	n (%) or Median [P25; P75]	Statin use cat.[a] %	Statin use ref. cat.[b] %
Statin use, *n* (%)	295 (7.4)	2477 (39.3)	330 (32.8)			1614 (50.3)			533 (25.7)		
Baseline characteristics											
Age (years), median [IQR]	73 [66; 79]	74 [64; 82]	55 [52; 57]			70 [65; 75]			85 [82; 89]		
Women, *n* (%)	1839 (45.9)	2871 (45.6)	448 (44.5)	24.1***	39.7	1280 (39.9)	41.6***	56.0	1143 (55)	20.4***	32.1
LDL measurement, *n* (%)	1559 (38.9)	2405 (38.2)	421 (42.0)	23.3***	39.6	1040 (32.4)	38.8***	55.8	944 (45.5)	14.6***	34.9
Type of CVD history											
MI, *n* (%)	848 (21.2)	1507 (23.9)	331 (32.9)	36.3*	31.1	786 (24.5)	59.0***	47.4	390 (18.8)	31.0**	24.4
Stroke, *n* (%)	831 (20.7)	1496 (23.8)	248 (24.6)	29.8	33.7	672 (20.9)	46.3**	51.3	576 (27.7)	20.5***	27.6
TIA, *n* (%)	631 (15.7)	963 (15.3)	67 (6.7)	41.8	32.1	414 (12.9)	49.3	50.4	482 (23.2)	21.8**	26.8
IHD without angina, *n* (%)	754 (18.8)	1147 (18.2)	144 (14.3)	42.4**	31.2	648 (20.2)	61.3***	47.5	355 (17.1)	33.2***	24.1
IHD with angina, *n* (%)	1582 (39.5)	1809 (28.7)	173 (17.2)	46.8***	29.9	938 (29.2)	54.1**	48.7	698 (33.6)	27.5	24.7
PAD, *n* (%)	1011 (25.2)	1669 (26.5)	242 (24.0)	27.3**	34.5	873 (27.2)	45.9**	51.9	554 (26.7)	27.4	25.0
Comorbidities											
Atrial fibrillation, *n* (%)	430 (10.7)	870 (13.8)	24 (2.4)	45.8	32.5	359 (11.2)	53.8	49.8	487 (23.4)	21.1**	27.0
Hypercholesterolemia, *n* (%)	1040 (26.0)	2075 (33.0)	292 (29.0)	50.7***	25.5	1134 (35.3)	60.6***	44.6	649 (31.2)	34.2***	21.8
Hypertension, *n* (%)	1396 (34.8)	2772 (44.0)	344 (34.2)	36.6*	30.8	1422 (44.3)	51.7	49.1	1006 (48.4)	24.8	26.5
Mental disorder, *n* (%)	625 (15.6)	1310 (20.8)	289 (28.7)	32.5	32.9	627 (19.5)	45.1**	51.5	394 (19.0)	17.5***	27.6
Co-medications											
Aspirin and antihypertensive agents											
Aspirin + RAS and Non-RAS	75 (1.9)	707 (11.2)	88 (8.7)	Ref cat		458 (14.3)	Ref cat		161 (7.8)	Ref cat	
Aspirin + RAS or Non-RAS, *n* (%)	295 (7.4)	1464 (23.3)	171 (17.0)	73.5	80.7	959 (29.9)	73.7**	81.0	334 (16.1)	63.0**	70.8
Aspirin alone, *n* (%)	68 (1.7)	226 (3.6)	45 (4.5)	68.9	80.7	147 (4.6)	58.5***	81.0	34 (1.6)	44.1***	70.8
RAS or Non-RAS and no aspirin, *n* (%)	702 (17.5)	1808 (28.7)	256 (25.4)	38.7***	80.7	1014 (31.6)	60.4***	81.0	538 (25.9)	44.8***	70.8
None of these 3 categories, *n* (%)	2942 (73.4)	2797 (44.4)	535 (53.1)	12.7***	80.7	1091 (34.0)	16.1***	81.0	1171 (56.4)	4.6***	70.8
Other lipid-lowering medication	73 (4.3)	237 (3.8)	37 (3.7)	48.6**	32.2	164 (5.1)	43.3*	50.6	36 (1.7)	30.6	25.6
Charlson comorbidity index											
mCCI index[c], median [IQR]	5 [3; 6]	5 [4; 7]	3 [2; 4]			5 [4; 6]			7 [6; 8]		
MI/ IHD w/o angina, *n* (%)	1395 (34.8)	2364 (37.6)	442 (43.9)	36.4**	29.9	1269 (39.5)	59.3***	44.3	653 (31.4)	32.3***	22.6

Table 4 Characteristics of patients on secondary prevention *(Continued)*

Variables	1999	2013	Age group in 2013								
	Total (n = 4007)	Total (n = 6295)	50–59 years (n = 1077)			60–79 years (n = 3211)			80+ years (n = 2077)		
	n (%) or Median [P25; P75]	n (%) or Median [P25; P75]	*n* (%) or Median [P25; P75]	Statin use cat.[a] %	Statin use ref. cat.[b] %	*n* (%) or Median [P25; P75]	Statin use cat.[a] %	Statin use ref. cat.[b] %	n (%) or Median [P25; P75]	Statin use cat.[a] %	Statin use ref. cat.[b] %
Heart failure, *n* (%)	364 (9.1)	500 (7.9)	20 (2.0)	55.0**	32.3	156 (4.9)	59.6**	49.8	324 (15.6)	19.1**	26.9
PAD, *n* (%)	1011 (25.2)	1669 (26.5)	242 (24.0)	27.3**	34.5	873 (27.2)	45.9**	51.9	554 (26.7)	27.4	25.0
TIA/stroke, *n* (%)	1333 (33.3)	2283 (36.3)	305 (30.3)	31.8	33.2	1014 (31.6)	46.6**	51.9	964 (46.4)	21.1***	29.6
Dementia, *n* (%)	94 (2.3)	301 (4.8)	17 (1.7)	23.5	32.9	87 (2.7)	40.2*	50.5	197 (9.5)	14.7***	26.8
COPD/asthma, *n* (%)	579 (14.4)	1580 (25.1)	276 (27.4)	31.9	33.1	862 (26.8)	48.4	51.0	442 (21.3)	24.7	25.9
GI ulcer, *n* (%)	471 (11.8)	647 (10.3)	65 (6.5)	30.8	32.9	331 (10.3)	49.5	50.3	251 (12.1)	21.9	26.2
Liver disease, *n* (%)	110 (2.7)	361 (5.7)	52 (5.2)	40.4	32.4	200 (6.2)	48.0	50.4	109 (5.2)	20.2	26.0
Diabetes mellitus, *n* (%)	644 (16.1)	1587 (25.2)	235 (23.3)	38.7**	31.0	855 (26.6)	58.9***	47.1	497 (23.9)	27.4	25.1
Paralysis, *n* (%)	122 (3.0)	141 (2.2)	18 (1.8)	55.6**	32.4	65 (2.0)	43.1	50.4	58 (2.8)	15.5*	26.0
Cancer, *n* (%)	382 (9.5)	1207 (19.2)	191 (19.0)	20.9***	35.5	631 (19.7)	43.3***	52.0	385 (18.5)	23.4	26.2
Leukaemia, *n* (%)	9 (0.2)	40 (0.6)	10 (1.0)	20.0	32.9	15 (0.5)	46.7	50.3	15 (0.7)	33.3	25.6
Hodgkin's lymphoma, *n* (%)	12 (0.3)	44 (0.7)	6 (0.6)	16.7	32.9	27 (0.8)	40.7	50.3	11 (0.5)	36.4	25.6
HIV-infection/ AIDS, *n* (%)	NA	NA	NA								
Renal insufficiency[d], *n* (%)											
Yes vs no	468 (11.7)	665 (10.6)	14 (1.4)	50.0	37.7	192 (6.0)	49.5	54.6	459 (22.1)	25.3**	31.9
Not measured vs measured	755 (18.8)	970 (15.4)	214 (21.3)	13.6***	38.0	372 (11.6)	19.6***	54.3	384 (18.5)	6.0***	30.1

IQR inter-quartile range, *LDL* low-density lipoprotein, *CVD* cardiovascular disease, *MI* myocardial infarction, *TIA* transient ischemic attack, *IHD* ischemic heart disease, *PAD* peripheral arterial disease, *RAS* renin-angiotensin system, *mCCI* modified Charlson comorbidity index, *COPD* chronic obstructive pulmonary disease, *GI* gastro-intestinal (duodenal or gastric)

***$p < 0.001$, **$p < 0.05$, *$p < 0.10$ (p-values are derived from a simple logistic regression model)

[a]Statin use cat.: statin use in the category of interest; [b]Statin use ref. cat.: statin use in the category of reference; [c]Missing kidney function is treated as a score of 0; [d]the last value of the creatinine was taken if it was measured in the last 3 years. The eGFR was computed using the MDRD formula and if eGFR< 45 = > renal insufficiency

Table 5 Determinants of statin use in secondary prevention (mixed-effect logistic regression)

Variables	Multivariable analysis (50–59 years)		Multivariable analysis (60–79 years)		Multivariable analysis (80+ years)	
	OR [95%CI]	*p*-value	OR [95% CI]	*p*-value	OR [95% CI]	*p*-value
Baseline characteristics						
Age, per year increase			1.25 [1.02; 1.52]	0.030	0.87 [0.84; 0.90]	< 0.001
Women	0.59 [0.42; 0.84]	0.003	0.64 [0.54; 0.77]	< 0.001	0.68 [0.51; 0.89]	0.005
LDL measurement			0.64 [0.49; 0.83]	0.001	0.50 [0.37; 0.68]	< 0.001
Type of CVD history						
MI			1.42 [1.15; 1.75]	0.001		
IHD without angina			1.40 [1.12; 1.75]	0.003	1.48 [1.06; 2.09]	0.022
IHD with angina	1.60 [1.04; 2.45]	0.030			1.36 [1.03; 1.80]	0.033
Comorbidities						
Atrial fibrillation					0.66 [0.48; 0.92]	0.013
Hypercholesterolemia	3.59 [2.45; 5.30]	< 0.001	2.40 [1.98; 2.92]	< 0.001	2.93 [2.18; 3.97]	< 0.001
Hypertension	0.65 [0.44; 0.96]	0.030	0.58 [0.48; 0.70]	< 0.001	0.65 [2.18; 3.97]	0.002
Mental disorder					0.63 [0.43; 0.91]	0.015
Co-medications						
Aspirin and antihypertensive agents						
Reference: Aspirin + RAS and Non-RAS	1.00		1.00		1.00	
Aspirin + RAS or Non-RAS	0.63 [0.28; 1.35]	0.236	0.61 [0.44; 0.85]	0.004	0.67 [0.40; 1.12]	0.126
Aspirin alone	0.48 [0.19; 1.19]	0.110	0.23 [0.15; 0.36]	< 0.001	0.30 [0.13; 0.71]	0.006
RAS or Non-RAS	0.15 [0.08; 0.28]	< 0.001	0.36 [0.27; 0.47]	< 0.001	0.37 [0.24; 0.57]	< 0.001
None of these 3 categories	0.03 [0.01; 0.06]	< 0.001	0.04 [0.03; 0.05]	< 0.001	0.02 [0.01; 0.03]	< 0.001
Other lipid lowering medication	0.39 [0.17; 0.88]	0.024	0.24 [0.17; 0.35]	< 0.001	0.19 [0.08; 0.42]	< 0.001
Charlson comorbidity index						
mCCI index[a]			0.89 [0.83; 0.95]	< 0.001		
Liver disease					0.54 [0.28; 1.00]	0.054
Diabetes, mellitus			1.52 [1.22; 1.88]	< 0.001		
Paralysis	5.12 [1.51; 17.60]	0.009				
Cancer	0.63 [0.39; 1.01]	0.059				
Renal insufficiency						
Yes	1.88 [0.53; 6.60]	0.318	0.98 [0.65; 1.46]	0.904		
Not measured	0.34 [0.20; 0.55]	< 0.001	0.39 [0.27; 0.55]	< 0.001		

OR odds ratio, *CI* confidence interval, *LDL* low-density lipoprotein, *CVD* cardiovascular disease, *MI* myocardial infarction, *IHD* ischemic heart disease, *RAS* renin-angiotensin system, *mCCI* modified Charlson comorbidity index
[a]Missing kidney function is treated as a score of 0

prevalence of statin use in secondary prevention rather seemed to reach a plateau. This finding is in line with previous studies [14, 15, 21, 24, 26, 27, 33, 36].

Incidence of recurrent CVD

The current study showed that the incidence of recurrent CVD did not decrease much compared to the strong increase in the prevalence of statin use. Possible explanations are a higher prevalence of other cardiovascular risk factors and an inadequate control of other risk factors and perhaps the benefits of statins in most clinical trials do not translate to real world populations, which differ in ways that may adversely affect the risk-benefit balance (more comorbidities, polypharmacy, disability, etc). The current study also showed an increase in prevalence of diabetes, hypertension and hypercholesterolemia between 1999 and 2013. Unfortunately, insufficient data on the body mass index (BMI) and smoking status are available in the Intego registry. However, the Intego registry is representative for the Flemish population and the Belgian Health Interview Survey showed that the prevalence of overweight and smoking status in the age group 55+ years in Flanders did not change considerably from 1997 to 2013 (from 56.3 to 59% and from 17.6 to 16.9%, respectively) [46]. Moreover, the Euroaspire surveys described time trends in lifestyle, risk factor control and use of evidence-based medications in patients with coronary heart disease in Europe [14]. These surveys concluded that there was an increase of obesity and diabetes and that the proportion of smokers and the level of physical activity had remained stable from 1999 to 2013. Other studies showed similar results of cardiovascular risk factor control in secondary prevention [22, 28, 47–49].

The minor decrease of the incidence of recurrent CVD was only observed in patients without statins prescribed. The incidence in this group was higher in 1999 and evolved towards the lower incidence of recurrent CVD in patients with statins prescribed in the 15 years thereafter, to be around 25 per 1000 patient years. However, since this study was only an observational study, both groups cannot be considered identical. Therefore, no conclusions could be drawn about the possible effect of statins on the incidence of recurrent CVD. This study was only designed to observe trends and generate hypotheses. Furthermore, no data were available on other factors that might have led to improved CVD outcomes in the same time period, like a reduction in trans fat consumption or attention to the treatment of sleep apnea.

Factors associated with statin use

Despite the strong increase in statin use in secondary prevention, the current study confirmed, in line with the results of previous studies, that less than 50% of patients in secondary prevention received a statin in 2013 [9–18, 20, 21, 23–36, 42–44].

The absence of other secondary preventive medications (aspirin, RAS and non-RAS antihypertensive agents) was strongly associated with less statin use in secondary prevention. Possible explanations of these findings could be doctor-related factors such as poor knowledge and application of the guidelines, preference against polypharmacy or the doctor's reading of the evidence that may be at variance with the guidelines, and patient-related factors such as poor adherence to therapy. Previous studies also found an association between the use of statins, aspirin and antihypertensive agents [11, 23].

Women were less likely to receive statins in secondary prevention than men. This finding is also in line with previous studies [9, 12, 15, 19, 23, 29, 31–34]. Some of these studies showed that women also received less intensive statin therapy [9, 27, 34]. A possible reason for this observation might be the fact that women have a higher risk of statin adverse effects [50]. Furthermore, although statin therapy was shown to be an effective intervention in the secondary prevention of cardiovascular events in women, there was no benefit on stroke and all-cause mortality in women [51].

In the age group 60–79 years, higher age was associated with more statin use, whereas it was associated with less statin use in the oldest age group. This pattern of age-related statin use was also seen in other studies [12, 15, 21, 32, 33]. Although the most recent guidelines do not recommend age limitations for the use of statins in secondary prevention, current evidence does not support a favorable risk-benefit balance for statins in older persons [32]. Statins have shown to reduce the risk of coronary disease in older persons (70–82 years), but failed to reduce the risk for all-cause mortality and showed a statistically significant 25% increase in incident cancer [52]. Moreover, in the oldest old no trials have been performed and higher cholesterol concentrations have even been associated with longevity in this age group [53]. Furthermore, older age has also been linked to a greater risk of statin adverse effects [50].

The current study showed several comorbidities or cardiovascular risk factors were associated to statin use to a lesser degree. First, hypercholesterolemia was associated with more statin use in secondary prevention. This suggests that physicians prescribe statins as a function of cholesterol levels, despite the fact that statins are recommended in secondary prevention independently of cholesterol level [19, 20, 25, 32]. Second, diabetes predicted greater statin use in the age group 60–79 years. A possible explanation for this is the entrance of a diabetes care program in Belgium, with improved follow-up of these patients and increased awareness of recurrent CVD among patients with diabetes. Furthermore, diabetes has been classified as a coronary heart disease risk equivalent and as a stroke risk equivalent [54]. On the other hand, statin therapy has also been shown to be associated with a slightly increased risk of development of diabetes [55]. Moreover, statins have shown to raise glucose preferentially in patients at risk for diabetes, and to have increased occurrence of adverse effects in patients with diabetes [56]. Third, hypertension was associated with less statin use, possibly because patients and doctors are reluctant to polypharmacy. It has also been shown that geriatric patients of physicians who on average prescribed more medications like cholesterol lowering dugs, had an increased risk of mortality [57]. On the other hand, Xi et al. found that patients with hypertension after stroke are more likely to receive a statin [25]. Furthermore, the ALLHAT-LLT trial showed that pravastatin did not reduce either all-cause mortality or coronary heart disease in older persons with well-controlled hypertension [58]. Fourth, the observed associations between comorbidities like stroke, TIA, dementia and PAD and less statin use could possibly be explained by the higher risk of adverse effects [50, 59–61], the limited effect of statins in people with these conditions [62, 63] and possibly the greater risk of drug errors in people with cognitive problems. Other interesting associations between less statin use and cancer and more statin use and paralysis should be confirmed by further research.

Based on the current findings future research should be organized. First, the effect of a statin treatment in secondary prevention could be estimated in this real world population by using propensity score matching, although this approach is not able to capture key issues of healthy user effects. Second, qualitative research could focus on the reason behind the finding that less than 50% of patients in secondary prevention receive a statin prescription. Although guidelines recommend statins in all age groups, clinicians might be aware of the failure of evidence to support net benefit in key patient groups, including elderly (age > 70 years), or might be reluctant to prescribe statins because of the risk for adverse effects. Furthermore, the impact of patient-related factors and patient preferences should be explored. Third, the current study suggests investigating what factors may be leading to declining CVD risk in older non-statin users.

Strengths and limitations

The major strengths of the current study are the inclusion of a large real-world study population, representative of the general Flemish population, and the long follow-up period. This study was the first to compute AAPC of the prevalence of statin use in secondary prevention and to examine the prevalence of statin use parallel with the incidence of recurrent CVD in the same population. Furthermore, we were able to examine multivariable models to explain statin use in different age groups and have included a broad range of factors that may be associated with statin use.

However, this study also has limitations. First, this study was an observational study and statin users and non-users could not be considered identical. Therefore, no conclusions could be drawn about the causal effect of statins on the incidence of recurrent CVD. Second, no data were available on mortality. Third, only electronic GP prescriptions were taken into account. Manual prescriptions made during a house visit or prescriptions made by specialists were not included, which might underestimate the real prevalence of statin use. Fourth, we did not investigate the dosage and types of statin patients used and had insufficient data on actual cholesterol levels. Last, no information on smoking status, BMI, race, socio-economic status and time after diagnosis of the first CVD was available. Furthermore, secular trends that may alter CVD risk, like trans fat consumption or treatment of sleep apnea, were not examined.

Conclusion

The prevalence of statin use in secondary prevention increased strongly from 1999 to 2013, with the increase principally affecting elderly patients. Still, fewer than 50% of the patients with a history of CVD received a statin in 2013. Greater statin use was associated with male sex, medium-older age (increasing up to age 79 years, decreasing thereafter) and diabetes. Persons with cancer, stroke and hypertension were less likely to receive statins. But, the absence of other preventive medications was most strongly correlated with less statin use. The sizable increase in statin use was attended by only a small decline in recurrent cardiovascular events. Moreover, this decline was focused in elderly who were not on statins.

Abbreviations

AAPC: Average annual percentage change; AIC: AKAIKE information criteria; APC: Annual percentage change; ATC: Anatomical therapeutic chemical; BMI: Body mass index; CI: Confidence interval; COPD: Chronic obstructive pulmonary disease; CVD: Cardiovascular disease; GFR: Glomerular filtration rate; GLMM: Generalized linear mixed models; GP: General practitioner; IHD: Ischaemic heart disease; LDL: Low-density lipoprotein; LLM: Lipid lowering medication; mCCI: Modified Charlson comorbidity index; MDRD: Modification of diet in renal disease; MI: Myocardial infarction; OR: Odds ratio; PAD: Peripheral arterial disease; RAS: Renin-angiotensin system; ROC: Receiver operating characteristic; TIA: Transient ischaemic attack

Acknowledgements

The authors would like to thank all the participating general practitioners.

Funding

Intego is funded on a regular basis by the Flemish Government (Ministry of Health and Welfare). This work would not have been possible without the collaboration of all general practitioners of the Intego network. We hereby state the independence of the researchers from the funders.

Authors' contributions

SH and BV performed the analyses and NL and BV wrote the manuscript. FB and GG are responsible for the study concept and design and the recruitment of subjects and acquisition of data. All authors participated in the interpretation of the data. All authors approved the final version of the manuscript.

Competing interests

The authors declare that they have no competing interests.

Author details
[1]Department of Public Health and Primary Care, Universiteit Leuven (KU Leuven), Kapucijnenvoer 33, Blok J, 3000 Leuven, Belgium. [2]Institute of Health and Society, Université catholique de Louvain (UCL), Brussels, Belgium. [3]Department of Family Medicine, Maastricht University, Maastricht, The Netherlands.

References

1. European Cardiovascular Diseaese Statistics, 2012, https://www.escardio.org/static_file/Escardio/Press-media/press-releases/2013/EU-cardiovascular-disease-statistics-2012.pdf (Accessed 25 Feb 2017).
2. Bansilal S, Castellano JM, Fuster V. Global burden of CVD: focus on secondary prevention of cardiovascular disease. Int J Cardiol. 2015;201 Suppl 1:S1–7.
3. De Backer G, Ambrosioni E, Borch-Johnsen K, Brotons C, Cifkova R, Dallongeville J, et al. European guidelines on cardiovascular disease prevention in clinical practice: third joint task force of European and other societies on cardiovascular disease prevention in clinical practice (constituted by representatives of eight societies and by invited experts). Eur J Cardiovasc Prev Rehabil. 2003;10:S1–S10.
4. Stone NJ, Robinson JG, Lichtenstein AH, Bairey Merz CN, Blum CB, Eckel RH, et al. 2013 ACC/AHA guideline on the treatment of blood cholesterol to reduce atherosclerotic cardiovascular risk in adults: a report of the American College of Cardiology/American Heart Association task force on practice guidelines. J Am Coll Cardiol. 2014;63:2889–934.
5. Graham I, Atar D, Borch-Johnsen K, Boysen G, Burell G, Cifkova R, et al. European guidelines on cardiovascular disease prevention in clinical practice: executive summary. Fourth Joint Task Force of the European Society of Cardiology and other societies on cardiovascular disease prevention in clinical practice (constituted by representatives of nine societies and by invited experts). Eur J Cardiovasc Prev Rehabil. 2007;14 Suppl 2:E1–40.
6. Ong HT. The statin studies: from targeting hypercholesterolaemia to targeting the high-risk patient. QJM. 2005;98:599–614.
7. Scandinavian Simvastatin Study Group. Randomised trial of cholesterol lowering in 4444 patients with coronary heart disease: the Scandinavian Simvastatin Survival Study (4S). Lancet. 1994;344:1383–9.
8. Descamps OS, De Backer G, Annemans L, Muls E, Scheen AJ. New European guidelines for the management of dyslipidaemia in cardiovascular prevention. Rev Med Liege. 2012;67:118–27.
9. Dodhia H, Kun L, Logan Ellis H, Crompton J, Wierzbicki AS, Williams H, et al. Evaluating quality and its determinants in lipid control for secondary prevention of heart disease and stroke in primary care: a study in an inner London borough. BMJ Open. 2015;5:e008678.
10. Wallach Kildemoes H, Vass M, Hendriksen C, Andersen M. Statin utilization according to indication and age: a Danish cohort study on changing prescribing and purchasing behaviour. Health Policy. 2012;108:216–27.
11. Bejot Y, Zeller M, Lorgis L, Troisgros O, Aboa-Eboule C, Osseby GV, et al. Secondary prevention in patients with vascular disease. A population based study on the underuse of recommended medications. J Neurol Neurosurg Psychiatry. 2013;84:348–53.
12. Jorgensen CH, Gislason GH, Ahlehoff O, Andersson C, Torp-Pedersen C, Hansen PR. Use of secondary prevention pharmacotherapy after first myocardial infarction in patients with diabetes mellitus. BMC Cardiovasc Disord. 2014;14:4.
13. Park JH, Ruiz MC, Shields D, Orr DJ. Socioeconomic deprivation does not affect prescribing of secondary prevention in patients with peripheral arterial disease. Int Angiol. 2013;32:593–8.
14. Kotseva K, De Bacquer D, Jennings C, Gyberg V, De Backer G, Ryden L, et al. Time trends in lifestyle, risk factor control, and use of evidence-based medications in patients with coronary heart disease in Europe: results from 3 EUROASPIRE surveys, 1999-2013. Glob Heart. 2016. https://doi.org/10.1016/j.gheart.2015.11.003.
15. DeWilde S, Carey IM, Bremner SA, Richards N, Hilton SR, Cook DG. Evolution of statin prescribing 1994-2001: a case of agism but not of sexism? Heart. 2003;89:417–21.
16. Subherwal S, Patel MR, Kober L, Peterson ED, Jones WS, Gislason GH, et al. Missed opportunities: despite improvement in use of cardioprotective medications among patients with lower-extremity peripheral artery disease, underuse remains. Circulation. 2012;126:1345–54.
17. Fitzgerald TN, Popp C, Dardik A, Federman DG. Lipid goal achievement and trends in lipid-lowering therapy in veterans undergoing carotid endarterectomy. Vasc Med. 2009;14:21–7.
18. Tu JV, Gong Y. Trends in treatment and outcomes for acute stroke patients in Ontario, 1992-1998. Arch Intern Med. 2003;163:293–7.
19. Ovbiagele B, Schwamm LH, Smith EE, Hernandez AF, Olson DM, Pan W, et al. Recent nationwide trends in discharge statin treatment of hospitalized patients with stroke. Stroke. 2010;41:1508–13.
20. Lemaitre RN, Furberg CD, Newman AB, Hulley SB, Gordon DJ, Gottdiener JS, et al. Time trends in the use of cholesterol-lowering agents in older adults: the cardiovascular health study. Arch Intern Med. 1998;158:1761–8.
21. Whincup PH, Emberson JR, Lennon L, Walker M, Papacosta O, Thomson A. Low prevalence of lipid lowering drug use in older men with established coronary heart disease. Heart. 2002;88:25–9.
22. Young F, Capewell S, Ford ES, Critchley JA. Coronary mortality declines in the U.S. between 1980 and 2000 quantifying the contributions from primary and secondary prevention. Am J Prev Med. 2010;39:228–34.
23. Tonstad S, Rosvold EO, Furu K, Skurtveit S. Undertreatment and overtreatment with statins: the Oslo health study 2000-2001. J Intern Med. 2004;255:494–502.
24. Deambrosis P, Saramin C, Terrazzani G, Scaldaferri L, Debetto P, Giusti P, et al. Evaluation of the prescription and utilization patterns of statins in an Italian local health unit during the period 1994-2003. Eur J Clin Pharmacol. 2007;63:197–203.
25. Li X, Gao Y, Li J, Feng F, Liu JM, Zhang HB, et al. Underuse of statins in patients with atherosclerotic ischemic stroke in China. Chin Med J (Engl). 2012;125:1703–7.
26. Di Martino M, Degli Esposti L, Ruffo P, Bustacchini S, Catte A, Sturani A, et al. Underuse of lipid-lowering drugs and factors associated with poor adherence: a real practice analysis in Italy. Eur J Clin Pharmacol. 2005;61:225–30.
27. Shalev V, Weil C, Raz R, Goldshtein I, Weitzman D, Chodick G. Trends in statin therapy initiation during the period 2000-2010 in Israel. Eur J Clin Pharmacol. 2014;70:557–64.
28. Girot M, Mackowiak-Cordoliani MA, Deplanque D, Henon H, Lucas C, Leys D. Secondary prevention after ischemic stroke. Evolution over time in practice. J Neurol. 2005;252:14–20.
29. Balder JW, Scholtens S, de Vries JK, van Schie LM, Boekholdt SM, Hovingh GK, et al. Adherence to guidelines to prevent cardiovascular diseases: the LifeLines cohort study. Neth J Med. 2015;73:316–23.
30. Sheppard JP, Fletcher K, McManus RJ, Mant J. Missed opportunities in prevention of cardiovascular disease in primary care: a cross-sectional study. Br J Gen Pract. 2014;64:e38–46.
31. Shah NS, Huffman MD, Ning H, Lloyd-Jones DM. Trends in myocardial infarction secondary prevention: the National Health and nutrition examination surveys (NHANES), 1999-2012. J Am Heart Assoc. 2015;4. https://doi.org/10.1161/JAHA.114.001709.
32. Wallach-Kildemoes H, Stovring H, Holme Hansen E, Howse K, Petursson H. Statin prescribing according to gender, age and indication: what about the benefit-risk balance? J Eval Clin Pract. 2016;22:235–46.
33. Rasmussen JN, Gislason GH, Abildstrom SZ, Rasmussen S, Gustafsson I, Buch P, et al. Statin use after acute myocardial infarction: a nationwide study in Denmark. Br J Clin Pharmacol. 2005;60:150–8.
34. Cho L, Hoogwerf B, Huang J, Brennan DM, Hazen SL. Gender differences in utilization of effective cardiovascular secondary prevention: a Cleveland clinic prevention database study. J Women's Health (Larchmt). 2008;17:515–21.
35. Mohammed MA, El Sayed C, Marshall T. Patient and other factors influencing the prescribing of cardiovascular prevention therapy in the general practice setting with and without nurse assessment. Med Decis Mak. 2012;32:498–506.
36. Kildemoes HW, Stovring H, Andersen M. Driving forces behind increasing cardiovascular drug utilization: a dynamic pharmacoepidemiological model. Br J Clin Pharmacol. 2008;66:885–95.

37. Truyers C, Goderis G, Dewitte H, Akker M, Buntinx F. The Intego database: background, methods and basic results of a Flemish general practice-based continuous morbidity registration project. BMC Med Inform Decis Mak. 2014;14:48.
38. Vaes B, Beke E, Truyers C, Elli S, Buntinx F, Verbakel JY, et al. The correlation between blood pressure and kidney function decline in older people: a registry-based cohort study. BMJ Open. 2015;5:e007571.
39. Charlson ME, Pompei P, Ales KL, MacKenzie CR. A new method of classifying prognostic comorbidity in longitudinal studies: development and validation. J Chronic Dis. 1987;40:373–83.
40. Kim HJ, Fay MP, Feuer EJ, Midthune DN. Permutation tests for joinpoint regression with applications to cancer rates. Stat Med. 2000;19:335–51.
41. Dean CB, Nielsen JD. Generalized linear mixed models: a review and some extensions. Lifetime Data Anal. 2007;13:497–512.
42. de Ruijter W, de Waal MW, Gussekloo J, Assendelft WJ, Blom JW. Time trends in preventive drug treatment after myocardial infarction in older patients. Br J Gen Pract. 2010;60:47–9.
43. Appelros P, Jonsson F, Asberg S, Asplund K, Glader EL, Asberg KH, et al. Trends in stroke treatment and outcome between 1995 and 2010: observations from Riks-stroke, the Swedish stroke register. Cerebrovasc Dis. 2014;37:22–9.
44. Ko DT, Mamdani M, Alter DA. Lipid-lowering therapy with statins in high-risk elderly patients: the treatment-risk paradox. JAMA. 2004;291:1864–70.
45. Fraeyman J, Van Hal G, De Loof H, Remmen R, De Meyer GR, Beutels P. Potential impact of policy regulation and generic competition on sales of cholesterol lowering medication, antidepressants and acid blocking agents in Belgium. Acta Clin Belg. 2012;67:160–71.
46. Health Interview Survey, Belgium, 2013, https://his.wiv-isp.be/nl/SitePages/Rapporten.aspx (Accessed 25 Feb 2017).
47. Steinberg BA, Bhatt DL, Mehta S, Poole-Wilson PA, O'Hagan P, Montalescot G, et al. Nine-year trends in achievement of risk factor goals in the US and European outpatients with cardiovascular disease. Am Heart J. 2008;156:719–27.
48. Wong ND, Patao C, Wong K, Malik S, Franklin SS, Iloeje U. Trends in control of cardiovascular risk factors among US adults with type 2 diabetes from 1999 to 2010: comparison by prevalent cardiovascular disease status. Diab Vasc Dis Res. 2013;10:505–13.
49. Tang L, Patao C, Chuang J, Wong ND. Cardiovascular risk factor control and adherence to recommended lifestyle and medical therapies in persons with coronary heart disease (from the National Health and nutrition examination survey 2007-2010). Am J Cardiol. 2013;112:1126–32.
50. Golomb BA, Evans MA. Statin adverse effects: a review of the literature and evidence for a mitochondrial mechanism. Am J Cardiovasc Drugs. 2008;8:373–418.
51. Guttierrez J, Ramirez G, Rundek T, Sacco RL. Statin therapy in the prevention of recurrent cardiovascular events: a sex-based meta-analysis. Arch Intern Med. 2012;172:909–19.
52. Shepherd J, Blauw GJ, Murphy MB, Bollen EL, Buckley BM, Cobbe SM, et al. Pravastatin in elderly individuals at risk of vascular disease (PROSPER): a randomized controlled trial. Lancet. 2002;360:1623–30.
53. Weverling-Rijnsburger AW, Blauw GJ, Lagaay AM, Knook DL, Meinders AE, Westendorp RG. Total cholesterol and risk of mortality in the oldest old. Lancet. 1997;350:1119–23.
54. Ho JE, Paultre F, Mosca L. Is diabetes mellitus a cardiovascular disease risk equivalent for fatal stroke in women? Data from the Women's pooling project. Stroke. 2003;34:2812–6.
55. Sattar N, Preiss D, Murray HM, Welsh P, Buckley BM, de Craen AJ, et al. Statins and risk of incident diabetes: a collaborative meta-analysis of randomised statin trials. Lancet. 2010;375:735–42.
56. Golomb BA, Koperski S, White HL. Statins raise glucose preferentially among men who are older and at greater metabolic risk. Circulation. 2012;125:A055.
57. Davidson W, Molloy DW, Bédard M. Physician characteristics and prescribing for elderly people in New Brunswick: relation to patient outcomes. CMAJ. 1995;152:1227–34.
58. ALLHAT Officers and Coordinators for the ALLHAT Collaborative Research Group. Major outcomes in moderately hypercholseterolemic, hypertensive patients randomized to pravastatin vs usual care: the antihypertensive and lipid-lowering treatment to prevent heart attack trial (ALLHAT-LLT). JAMA. 2002;288:2998–3007.
59. Evans MA, Golomb BA. Statin-associated adverse cognitive effects: survey results from 171 patients. Pharmacotherapy. 2009;29:800–11.
60. Padala KP, Padala PR, McNeilly DP, Geske JA, Sullivan DH, Potter JF. The effect of HMG-CoAreductase inhibitors on cognition in patients with Alzheimer's dementia: a prospective withdrawal and rechallenge pilot study. Am J Geriatr Pharmacother. 2012;10:296–302.
61. Silver MA, Langsjoen PH, Szabo S, Patil H, Zelinger A. Effect of atorvastatin on left ventricular diastolic function and ability of coenzyme Q10 to reverse that dysfunction. Am J Cardiol. 2004;94:1306–10.
62. Amarenco P, Bogousslavsky J, Callahan A 3rd, Goldstein LB, Hennerici M, Rudolph AE, et al. High-dose atorvastatin after stroke or transient ischemic attack. N Engl J Med. 2006;355:549–59.
63. Kjekhus J, Apetrei E, Barrios V, Böhm M, Cleland JGF, Cornel JH, et al. Rosuvastatin in older patients with systolic heart failure. N Engl J Med. 2007;357:2248–61.

24

Receptor tyrosine kinase profiling of ischemic heart identifies ROR1 as a potential therapeutic target

Juho Heliste[1,2,3], Anne Jokilammi[1], Ilkka Paatero[1,4], Deepankar Chakroborty[1,2], Christoffer Stark[5], Timo Savunen[5], Maria Laaksonen[6] and Klaus Elenius[1,7,8*]

Abstract

Background: Receptor tyrosine kinases (RTK) are potential targets for the treatment of ischemic heart disease. The human RTK family consists of 55 members, most of which have not yet been characterized for expression or activity in the ischemic heart.

Methods: RTK gene expression was analyzed from human heart samples representing healthy tissue, acute myocardial infarction or ischemic cardiomyopathy. As an experimental model, pig heart with ischemia-reperfusion injury, caused by cardiopulmonary bypass, was used, from which phosphorylation status of RTKs was assessed with a phospho-RTK array. Expression and function of one RTK, ROR1, was further validated in pig tissue samples, and in HL-1 cardiomyocytes and H9c2 cardiomyoblasts, exposed to hypoxia and reoxygenation. ROR1 protein level was analyzed by Western blotting. Cell viability after ROR1 siRNA knockdown or activation with Wnt-5a ligand was assessed by MTT assays.

Results: In addition to previously characterized RTKs, a group of novel active and regulated RTKs was detected in the ischemic heart. ROR1 was the most significantly upregulated RTK in human ischemic cardiomyopathy. However, ROR1 phosphorylation was suppressed in the pig model of ischemia-reperfusion and ROR1 phosphorylation and expression were down-regulated in HL-1 cardiomyocytes subjected to short-term hypoxia in vitro. ROR1 expression in the pig heart was confirmed on protein and mRNA level. Functionally, ROR1 activity was associated with reduced viability of HL-1 cardiomyocytes in both normoxia and during hypoxia-reoxygenation.

Conclusions: Several novel RTKs were found to be regulated in expression or activity in ischemic heart. ROR1 was one of the most significantly regulated RTKs. The in vitro findings suggest a role for ROR1 as a potential target for the treatment of ischemic heart injury.

Keywords: Hypoxia, Ischemic cardiomyopathy, Myocardial ischemia, Myocardial infarction, Receptor tyrosine kinase

Background

Ischemic heart disease is the leading cause of death globally [1]. In the case of an acute myocardial infarction, myocardial damage caused by ischemia is exacerbated by oxygenized blood returning to the heart at reperfusion [2]. Approaches to treat infarction should both promote reperfusion and protect myocardium from the detrimental effects of ischemia and reperfusion.

Receptor tyrosine kinases (RTK) are cell surface receptors that mediate cellular survival, proliferation, and migration. A few RTKs have been shown to be necessary for development of the heart in gene-modified mouse models. Such examples include *Erbb2* [3, 4], *Erbb4* [5], *Ror1* [6], and *Ror2* [6, 7]. Understanding of the regulation of RTK activity and expression in ischemic heart is limited to few receptors. Expression of EGFR and ERBB2 have been demonstrated to be regulated in infarcted human heart [8, 9], and alterations in EGFR, ERBB2, ERBB4, VEGFR1, VEGFR2, IGF1R,

* Correspondence: klaele@utu.fi
[1]Institute of Biomedicine, University of Turku, Kiinamyllynkatu 10, FIN-20520 Turku, Finland
[7]Medicity Research Laboratories, University of Turku, Turku, Finland
Full list of author information is available at the end of the article

and INSR signaling have been observed in experimental ischemia-reperfusion models [8, 10–12].

Few RTKs have been investigated as targets for the treatment of experimental ischemia-reperfusion injury. Induction of constitutively active ERBB2 after infarction causes myocardial regeneration in mice [13]. Activating ERBB4 with its ligand neuregulin-1 reduces scar size in mouse [14] and rat [15] infarction models. Activation of INSR by insulin infusion during reperfusion has been shown to reduce infarction size in an ischemia-reperfusion rat heart model in Langendorff perfusion system [16]. Moreover, glucose-insulin-potassium infusion has been tested in clinical trials as a myocardial infarction treatment with mixed results [17].

Here, we used an in silico expression analysis and a phosphoarray analysis of an in vivo pig ischemia-reperfusion injury model to screen for changes in the expression and activity of RTKs in normal vs. ischemic heart. ROR1 was identified as a receptor demonstrating activity in both screens. We show that ROR1 was expressed in human heart, in pig myocardium and in cultured mouse cardiomyocytes and rat cardiomyoblasts. In cardiomyocytes in vitro, both ROR1 expression and phosphorylation were downregulated by hypoxia. We also demonstrate that ROR1 knockdown enhanced, and treatment with its ligand, Wnt-5a, reduced the viability of cardiomyocytes. These findings suggest that ROR1 signaling may suppress survival of cardiomyocytes and that ROR1 could be further tested as a potential treatment target for the myocardial ischemic injury.

Methods

In silico transcriptomics

Affymetrix gene expression data from IST Online database (ist.medisapiens.com; Medisapiens Ltd.) were analyzed to characterize RTK expression in samples representing healthy heart ($n = 62$), acute myocardial infarction ($n = 12$) or ischemic cardiomyopathy ($n = 63$). Out of the 55 RTKs listed by HUGO Gene Nomenclature Committee, data were available for 49 genes in acute myocardial infarction samples and for 52 genes in ischemic cardiomyopathy samples (Additional file 1). Data were normalized by array-generation-based gene centering method [18] and log2-transformed. Expression levels of RTKs demonstrating statistically significant differences in two-group comparisons were visualized as box plots and heatmaps using Pretty Heatmaps package (pheatmap) [19] in RStudio [20].

Pig model of heart ischemia-reperfusion injury

Animal experiments were approved by the Laboratory Animal Care and Use Committee of the State Provincial Office of Southern Finland (license number: ESAVI/1167/04.10.03/2011). The landrace pig myocardial samples ($n = 7$) were a kind gift from Drs. Christoffer Stark and Timo Savunen. Experimental procedure has been described in detail earlier [21]. Pigs weighed 29–43 kg. Myocardial ischemia-reperfusion injury was produced by exposing anesthetized pigs ($n = 4$) to cardiopulmonary bypass with aortic cross-clamping and cardioplegic arrest for 60 min, causing global myocardial ischemia. A pediatric membrane oxygenator (Dideco 905 Eos, Dideco) was used for the bypass. Procedures were performed in the laboratory of Research Center of Applied and Preventive Cardiovascular Medicine, University of Turku, Turku, Finland. For pre-anesthesia, an intramuscular injection of 100 mg xylazin (Rompun vet, Bayer Animal Health GmbH) and 25 mg midazolam (Midazolam Hameln, Hameln pharmaceuticals GmbH) was used. For anesthesia, 20 mg boluses of propofol (PropofolLipuro, B. Braun Melsungen AG) and 150 μg phentanyl (Fentanyl-Hameln, Hameln pharmaceuticals GmbH) were administered via a cannulated ear vein, and pigs were intubated and connected to a respirator (Dräger Oxylog 3000, Drägerwerk AG), the respiratory rate set to 18–22 times/min with a tidal volume of 8–10 ml/kg using 40% oxygen. Continuous infusion of propofol 15–30 mg/kg/h, phentanyl 1.5 μg/kg/h and midazolam 100 μg/kg/h was used to maintain anesthesia. A right sided thoracotomy was performed and the ascending aorta and right atrium cannulated for the bypass. 500 ml of cold (10 °C) Modified St Thomas Hospital No II cardioplegia was used to protect the hearts during the bypass, administered via a cannula to the aortic root at the time of cross-clamping and 30 min later. Antibiotic prophylaxis (Cefuroxime 750 mg, Orion Pharma) was given preoperatively and then every 8 h. 10,000 IU of heparin (Heparin, LEO Pharma) was administered as a bolus before cannulation of the heart and this was repeated every 30 min during extracorporeal circulation. 14,000 IU of protamine sulphate (Protamin, LEO Pharma) was used to neutralize the heparin. For thrombosis prophylaxis, 20 mg of enoxaparin (Klexane, Sanofi) was administered 1 and 12 h after the surgery. 100–150 mg of lidocaine (Lidocain, Orion Pharmaceuticals) and 150–225 mg of amiodarone (Cordarone, Sanofi) were used for rhythm disorders, and 5 mg boluses of ephedrine (Efedrin, Stragen Nordic) and noradrenaline infusion (80–160 μg/h) (Noradrenalin Hospira, Hospira) were used for post-operative hemodynamic support, when needed. For post-operative analgesia, 50 mg of bupivacaine (Bicain, Orion Pharmaceuticals) was infiltrated to the wound. For monitoring of adequate ventilation and perfusion, blood gases (i-STAT, Abbott Laboratories), invasive central venous pressure, ECG and oxygen saturation were followed throughout the procedure.

After the 60-min aortic cross-clamping, hearts were reperfused and the pigs were maintained anesthetized and mechanically ventilated for 29–31 h before sacrification with intravenous injection of potassium chloride.

Control samples ($n = 3$) were obtained from pigs used as blood donors for priming of the heart-lung machine. The control pigs underwent the same anesthetic protocol as the treatment group. Transmural left ventricle samples, collected after the sacrification, were snap-frozen and stored at – 80 °C. Troponin T levels were measured from plasma samples of ischemia-reperfusion-injured pigs, collected at the baseline and 6 and 24 h after reperfusion, by the laboratory of the Turku University Central Hospital using electrochemiluminescence immunoassay (Elecsys Troponin T high sensitive, Roche). Formalin-fixed, paraffin-embedded tissue samples were stained with hematoxylin and eosin and imaged with Zeiss AxioImager M1 microscope.

Phosphoarray analysis of RTK phosphorylation

Pig myocardial samples (280 to 460 mg) were homogenized and analyzed for phosphorylation status of 49 RTKs using the Proteome Profiler Human Phospho-RTK Array Kit (R&D Systems). Five hundred μg of protein was analyzed per sample. Receptors included in the analysis are listed in Additional file 2 B.

Array blot images were quantified by densitometry with NIH ImageJ v1.50i software. Intensity values were normalized by dividing each dot's intensity with the sum of intensities of the whole array, allowing comparison between different samples. Data were scaled to interval 0–1 by dividing all values with the highest value. Normalized values were visualized as a bargraph (mean (SD)) and as a heatmap with Pretty Heatmaps package [19]. Receptors with at least two quantifiable results in both sample groups were included. Receptors were clustered using maximum distance method.

Cell culture and Wnt-5a ligand treatment

HL-1 mouse atrial cardiomyocytes were a kind gift from Dr. Pasi Tavi (University of Eastern Finland). HL-1 cells were maintained in Claycomb medium (Sigma) supplemented with 10% FBS, 0.1 mM norepinephrine, 50 U/ml penicillin, 50 U/ml streptomycin, and 2 mM UltraGlutamine (Lonza). Culture plates were coated at 37 °C with a solution containing 0.02% gelatin and 10 μg/ml fibronectin. Seeding densities were 140,000 cells/6-well plate well, 100,000 cells/12-well plate well, and 5,000 cells/96-well plate well. H9c2 rat cardiomyoblasts were purchased from ATCC and maintained in DMEM with 1.5 g/l $NaHCO_3$, supplemented with 10% FBS, 50 U/ml penicillin, 50 U/ml streptomycin, and 2 mM UltraGlutamine. Seeding density was 100,000 cells/6-well plate well. Cells were routinely checked for mycoplasma infection using MycoAlert Mycoplasma Detection Kit (Lonza). For hypoxia-reoxygenation experiments, the cells were cultured in 1% O_2 in a hypoxic work station (InVivo$_2$, Ruskinn Technology Ltd.) for the indicated periods of time, and returned to normal cell incubator (21% O_2) for reoxygenation. In ROR1 ligand activation experiments, 200–400 ng/ml of recombinant human/mouse Wnt-5a (R&D Systems) was added to medium at the time of plating (for MTT assays) or 24 h after plating for 30–60 min (for Western analyses).

RNA interference

One day after plating, HL-1 cells were transfected with siRNAs (Qiagen) targeting *ROR1* (siRNA #1, SI01404655; siRNA #2, SI01404662), or *ROR2* (siRNA #1, SI01404683; siRNA #2, SI01404690) or with AllStars Negative Control siRNA at a concentration of 100 nM, using Lipofectamine 2000 (Invitrogen). Immediately prior to transfection, medium was changed to antibiotic- and norepinephrine-free Claycomb medium. Four to six hours after transfection, medium was replaced with antibiotic-free, norepinephrine-supplemented Claycomb medium.

RNA extraction and real-time RT-PCR

RNA was extracted from pig myocardium samples using TRIsure reagent (Bioline). Samples were treated with 10 units of DNAse I (Roche). cDNA was synthesized with SensiFAST cDNA Synthesis Kit (Bioline), using 1 μg of total RNA/sample. Real-time RT-PCR was carried out using QuantStudio 12 K Flex Real-Time PCR System thermal cycler (Thermo Fisher Scientific). For PCR reactions, 5 μl of TaqMan Universal Master Mix II (Thermo Fisher Scientific) and 10 ng of template cDNA were used in a reaction volume of 10 μl. Primer concentrations were 0.3 μM and probe concentration 0.1 μM. Primers were acquired from Eurofins Genomics and probes from Universal Probe Library (Roche). *GAPDH* was used as the reference gene [8]. *ROR1* was analyzed using the primers 5′-GCGGCTCGCAATATTCTC-3′ and 5′-GAAAGCCCAAGGTCTGAAATC-3′, and the probe #108. *GAPDH* was analyzed using the primers 5′-ACAGACAGCCGTGTGTTCC-3′ and 5′-ACCTTCACC ATCGTGTCTCA-3′, and the probe #28.

Western blotting and immunoprecipitation

Cells were lysed with lysis buffer [22] supplemented with Pierce Protease Inhibitor Mini Tablets (Thermo Fisher Scientific). Lysates were centrifuged for 15 min at 16,000 g and the supernatants were collected. Snap-frozen pig heart tissue samples were dissolved in ice-cold Lysis Buffer 17 supplied with the Proteome Profiler Human Phospho-RTK Array Kit. Samples were separated on 8–10% polyacrylamide gels. Protein amounts loaded on the gel were 20–35 μg for cell samples and 100 μg for pig tissue samples. Separated samples were transferred to nitrocellulose membrane which was blocked with 5% non-fat milk or bovine serum albumin in 10 mM Tris-HCl (pH 7.4), 150 mM NaCl and 0.05% Tween-20 (blocking solution) for 1 h at room temperature. Membranes were incubated with primary antibodies overnight at 4 °C in the blocking solution. The following primary antibodies and dilutions were used: anti-ROR1 (sc-83033 and sc-130386, Santa Cruz Biotechnology; 1:250 and 1:125, respectively), anti-actin (sc-1616, Santa Cruz Biotechnology; 1:1,000), anti-α-tubulin (sc-5546, Santa Cruz Biotechnology; 1:1,000), anti-phospho-Akt (#4060, Cell Signaling Technology; 1:1,000), anti-Akt (#9272, Cell Signaling Technology; 1:1,000), anti-phospho-p38 (#9211, Cell Signaling Technology; 1:500), anti-p38 (#9212, Cell Signaling Technology; 1:500), anti-phospho-tyrosine (4 g10, Upstate; 1:500), and anti-GAPDH (G8795, Sigma-Aldrich; 1:1,000). Incubation with secondary HRP-conjugated antibodies (Santa Cruz Biotechnology; 1:5,000) or IRDye secondary antibodies (LI-COR, 1:10,000) was carried out for 1 h at room temperature in the blocking solution. The immunosignals were visualized with WesternBright ECL HRP substrate reagent (Advansta) and imaged with ImageQuant LAS 4000 (GE Healthcare Life Sciences) or with Odyssey imaging system (LI-COR). Densitometric analysis of the Western signals was carried out with ImageJ.

For immunoprecipitation analyses, approximately 2 mg of total protein from HL-1 cell lysates was incubated overnight at 4 °C with 4 μg of mouse monoclonal anti-ROR1 antibody (sc-130386, Santa Cruz Biotechnology). Immunoprecipitated lysates were incubated with Protein G PLUS-Agarose beads (sc-2002, Santa Cruz Biotechnology) for one hour at 4 °C. After washing the beads three times with lysis buffer without protease inhibitors, samples from the supernatants were loaded onto 10% polyacrylamide gels for subsequent Western analysis.

MTT cell viability assay

CellTiter 96 Non-Radioactive Cell Proliferation Assay (MTT) (Promega) was used to measure viability of HL-1 cells. The assay was performed on 96-well plates with plating density of 5,000 cells/well. Before addition of the MTT dye solution, the culture medium was replaced by norepinephrine-free Claycomb medium (100 μl/well). Wells only containing the medium were used for background subtraction. Absorbances at 570 nm were detected with EnSight Multimode Plate Reader (PerkinElmer) and results were normalized to untreated control sample level.

Protein sequence alignment

Human and pig RTK protein sequences from UniProt database were aligned using EMBOSS Needle tool for global alignments and EMBOSS Water tool for local alignments by the European Bioinformatics Institute (http://www.ebi.ac.uk/Tools/psa/) [23]. The longest pig sequences available were used.

Statistical analyses

For in silico transcriptomics analyses, Student's t-test was used to assess the significance of differences between the expression levels of an RTK between sample groups. Correction for multiple testing was performed using false discovery rate (FDR) method [24]. Genes with significant differences in expression were selected for visualizations. Two-tailed Student's t-test was used for testing the significance of differences in phosphorylation array data (for RTKs with at least three quantifiable results in both treatments) and in expression levels in Western analyses. For in vitro experiments, data are represented as box plots depicting median (black horizontal line), first and third quartile (box) and the range of the data (whiskers). Multiple group comparisons were performed with Kruskal-Wallis test with Dunn's post-hoc test using FDR method for *P*-value adjustments. *P*-values < 0.05 were considered significant. Analyses were performed with RStudio.

Results

Regulation of RTK expression in ischemic human heart

Expression of human RTKs in healthy heart, heart with ischemic cardiomyopathy and heart with acute myocardial infarction was analyzed in silico using the IST Online database. Comparison of healthy samples to ischemic cardiopathy samples revealed a set of 14 receptors that were significantly differently expressed at the mRNA level (Fig. 1a). The most significantly up- and downregulated RTKs were *ROR1* and *EPHA2*, respectively, when ischemic cardiomyopathy was compared to normal heart (Fig. 1b). Interestingly, another ROR family member, *ROR2*, was downregulated in the ischemic cardiomyopathy samples (Fig. 1a). When comparing healthy hearts with hearts representing acute myocardial infarction, significant downregulation of *EGFR, ERBB2, ERBB3*, as well as *EPHA2*, was discovered in the infarcted heart, *ERBB2* demonstrating the greatest difference in expression (Fig. 1c and d). Statistical test values and differences in expression are shown in Additional file 1 and heatmaps generated from the data in Additional file 3.

RTK phosphorylation in experimental pig ischemia-reperfusion model

To experimentally address RTK activation in the ischemic heart, an ischemia-reperfusion model in pig, a relevant model animal close to human as a large mammal, was used. Pigs were subjected to ischemia-reperfusion injury by cardiopulmonary bypass and reperfusion, followed by phospho-RTK array analysis of myocardial samples. Increased amount of troponin T in the plasma (Additional file 4 A) and thinned cardiomyocytes with condensed nuclei as demonstrated by histological analysis (Additional file 4 B) indicated ischemic injury. The phosphoarray analysis was carried out after approximately 30 h of reperfusion. While

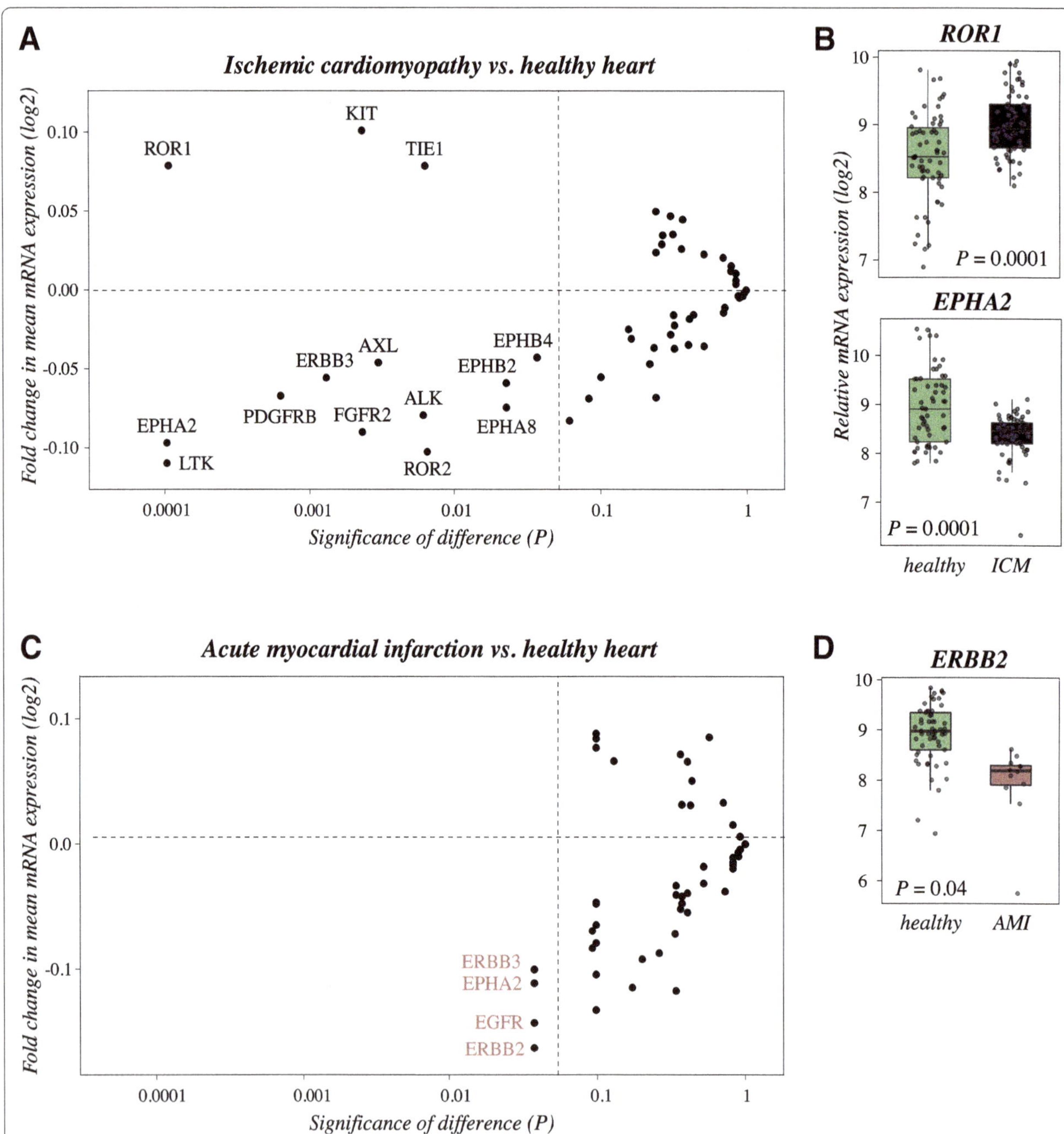

Fig. 1 Regulation of RTK expression in acute myocardial infarction and ischemic cardiomyopathy. Messenger RNA expression of 52 RTKs in human tissue samples representing healthy heart ($n = 62$), ischemic cardiomyopathy ($n = 63$), or acute myocardial infarction ($n = 12$) was analyzed in silico using IST Online database. **a** A dotplot presentation of FDR-corrected P values vs. the fold changes of RTK expression levels between samples representing ischemic cardiomyopathy or healthy heart. **b** A box plot presentation of expression levels of the most significantly up- or downregulated RTKs in ischemic cardiomyopathy vs. healthy heart. **c** A dotplot presentation of FDR-corrected P values vs. the fold changes of RTK expression levels between samples representing acute myocardial infarction or healthy heart. **d** A box plot presentation of expression level of the most significantly downregulated RTK in acute myocardial infarction vs. healthy heart. In A and C, the fold changes of means were calculated from log2-transformed Affymetrix expression values (arbitrary units). Vertical grey lines depict the threshold $P = 0.05$. RTKs not demonstrating significant ($P < 0.05$) changes in expression are only depicted by dots without labels

the observed phosphorylation-specific signal was relatively weak (possibly due to loss of phosphosignal during sample preparation and/or low cross-reactivity of the array antibodies between human and pig epitopes) (Additional file 2 A), the data indicated the presence of 23 activated RTKs in the heart. As expected, based on publications

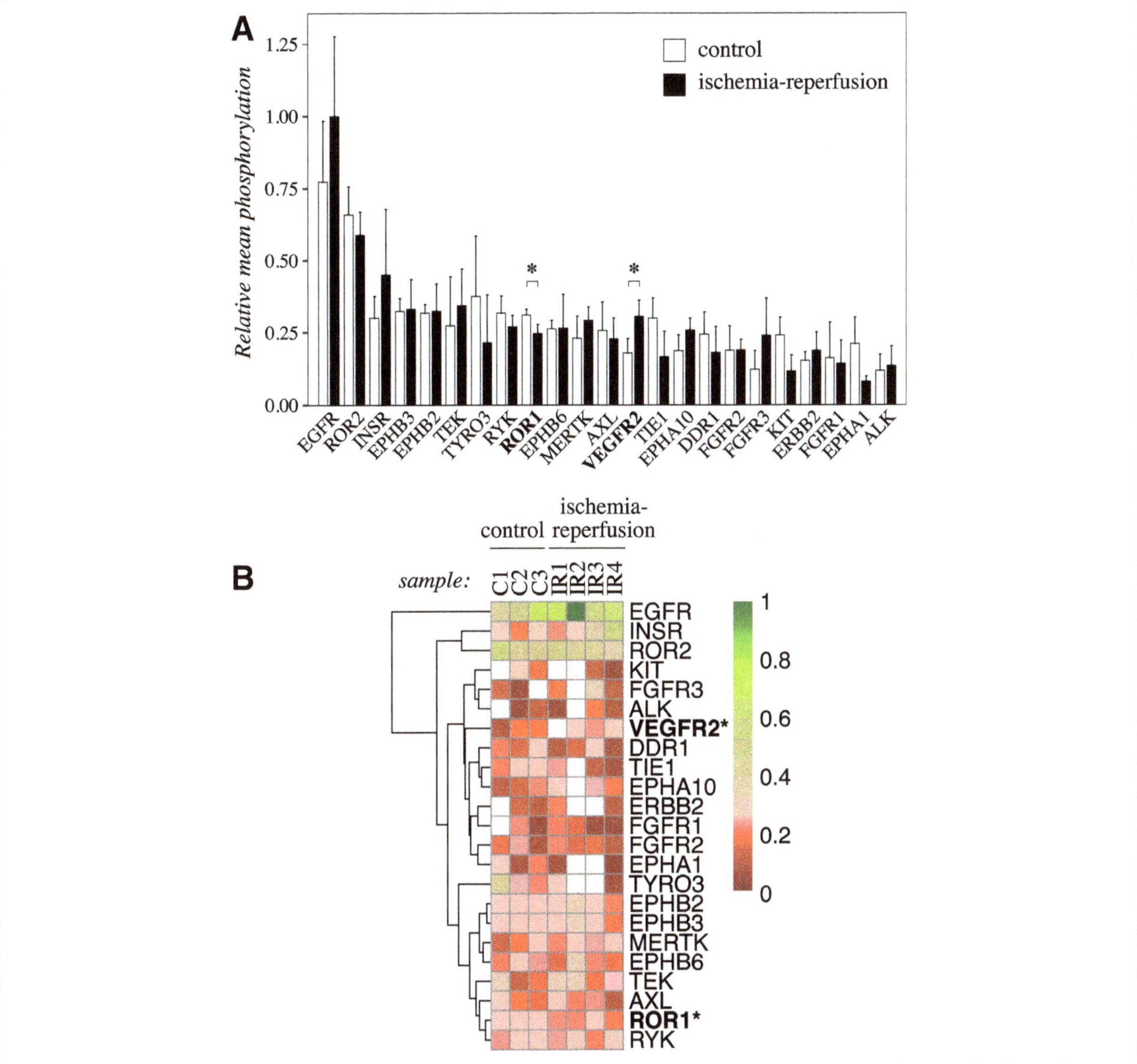

Fig. 2 RTK phosphorylation in a pig model of ischemia-reperfusion injury. A phospho-RTK array analysis addressing the phosphorylation of 49 RTKs was carried out for heart samples from a pig model of ischemia-reperfusion injury. Control pigs underwent the same anesthetic protocol as the ischema-reperfusion-injured pigs. **a** The intensity of the dots in the phospho-array were quantified by densitometry and normalized to each array's sum of intensities. The resulting values were scaled according to the highest value set to one. Normalized phosphorylation values of each receptor with at least two non-zero results per each treatment are shown (mean + SD). **b** The same set of normalized phospho-RTK dot intensities were visualized as a heatmap. Receptors with at least two samples with non-zero results per each treatment were included, and were clustered using the maximum distance method. White tiles depict missing data for few samples. Asterisk indicates significant difference in phosphorylation ($P < 0.05$) for comparison of control samples to ischemia-reperfusion samples

about RTK activity in the heart [8–12], the array identified phosphorylated EGFR, INSR, VEGFR2, and ERBB2 in both ischemic ($n = 4$) and control samples ($n = 3$) (Fig. 2a). Phosphorylation of a group of receptors, that to our knowledge have not previously been shown to be active or regulated in ischemic heart, was also detected. This group included both ROR receptors ROR1 and ROR2; the EPH receptors EPHB2, EPHB3, EPHB6, and EPHA10; TYRO3; RYK; FGFR3 and ALK (Fig. 2a).

Densitometric quantitation of the data indicated highest activity for EGFR, ROR2, INSR, EPHB3, EPHB2, TEK, TYRO3, RYK, ROR1 and EPHB6 (phosphosignal exceeding the 75th percentile of mean phosphorylation levels of all RTKs in all samples). Phosphorylation of ROR1 was significantly downregulated ($P = 0.022$), and phosphorylation of VEGFR2 significantly upregulated ($P = 0.043$), in ischemia-reperfusion-injured hearts. Unsupervised clustering of the RTKs on a heatmap grouped highly active EGFR, INSR and ROR2 together. ROR1 and RYK, demonstrating downregulation of phosphorylation by ischemia-reperfusion, were grouped together in the other end of the heatmap (Fig. 2b).

ROR1 is expressed in healthy and ischemic pig heart

As ROR1 was one of the most significantly regulated RTKs in the human heart expression analysis (Fig. 1b), and significantly downregulated in the ischemic pig heart (Fig. 2), it was selected for further validation. To confirm the presence of ROR1 in the heart in vivo, lysates from pig myocardium were analyzed by Western blotting with a polyclonal anti-ROR1 antibody. A band of the predicted size for full-length ROR1 protein (130 kDa) was detected in both control and ischemia-reperfusion-injured samples (Fig. 3a and b). The expression of *ROR1* mRNA was confirmed by RT-PCR (Fig. 3c). In both analyses, ROR1 expression did not demonstrate statistically significant difference between control and ischemia-reperfusion samples.

ROR1 expression and phosphorylation are downregulated by hypoxia-reoxygenation in cardiomyocytes in vitro

Analyses of the samples available from the IST Online database (Fig. 1) and the pig in vivo model (Figs. 2 and 3) indicated the presence of ROR1 in the heart tissue after ischemia and reperfusion, but did not allow for temporal analyses of ROR1 expression or activity at different time points after hypoxia and reoxygenation. To address the ROR1 regulation in vitro in cardiomyocytes under conditions simulating ischemia-reperfusion, HL-1 mouse atrial cardiomyocytes and H9c2 rat cardiomyoblasts were exposed to hypoxia (1% O_2) in a hypoxic workstation for 1, 3 or 24 h. Cells were subsequently either returned to normoxia for 3 or 24 h (hypoxia-reoxygenation), or directly lysed for expression analysis (hypoxia alone). ROR1 protein expression was analyzed by Western blotting.

In HL-1 cells, the total ROR1 protein level was significantly reduced by 1 h treatment in hypoxia ($P = 0.014$), remained low 3 h after reoxygenation, and was recovered with a high variation in expression after 24 h of reoxygenation (Fig. 4a and b). Treatment for 3 h in hypoxia also initially slightly reduced ROR1 protein expression, but the expression recovered already 3 h after reoxygenation (Fig. 4a and b). The longest time point of hypoxia analyzed, 24 h, did not result in changes in ROR1 protein levels (Fig. 4a and b). In H9c2 cells, downregulation of ROR1 was similarly observed in response to treatment for 1 h in hypoxia ($P = 0.002$), followed by a trend of expression returning back to the level of control samples after reoxygenation (Fig. 4c and d). In contrast to ROR1, ROR2 expression was not significantly regulated by hypoxia-reoxygenation (Additional file 5 A and B).

To address whether ROR1 phosphorylation was regulated in response to hypoxia, ROR1 was immunoprecipitated from HL-1 cell lysates followed by anti-phosphotyrosine Western

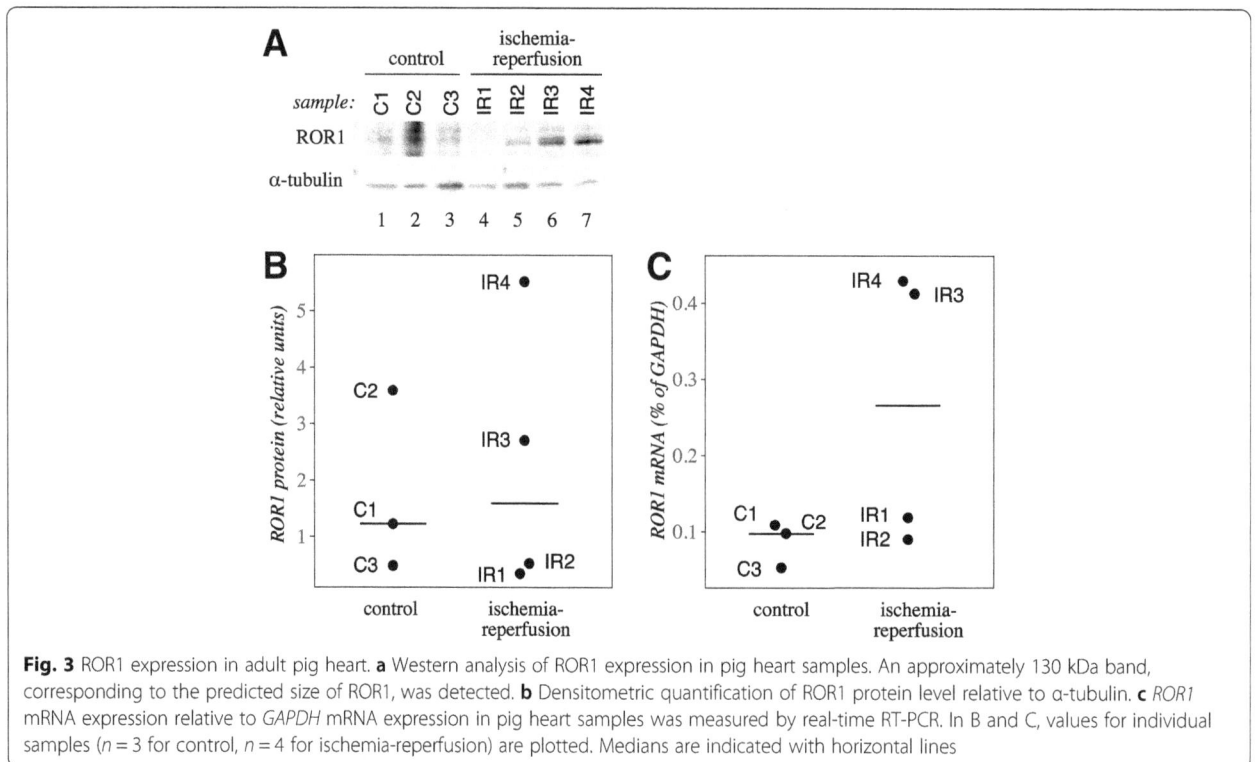

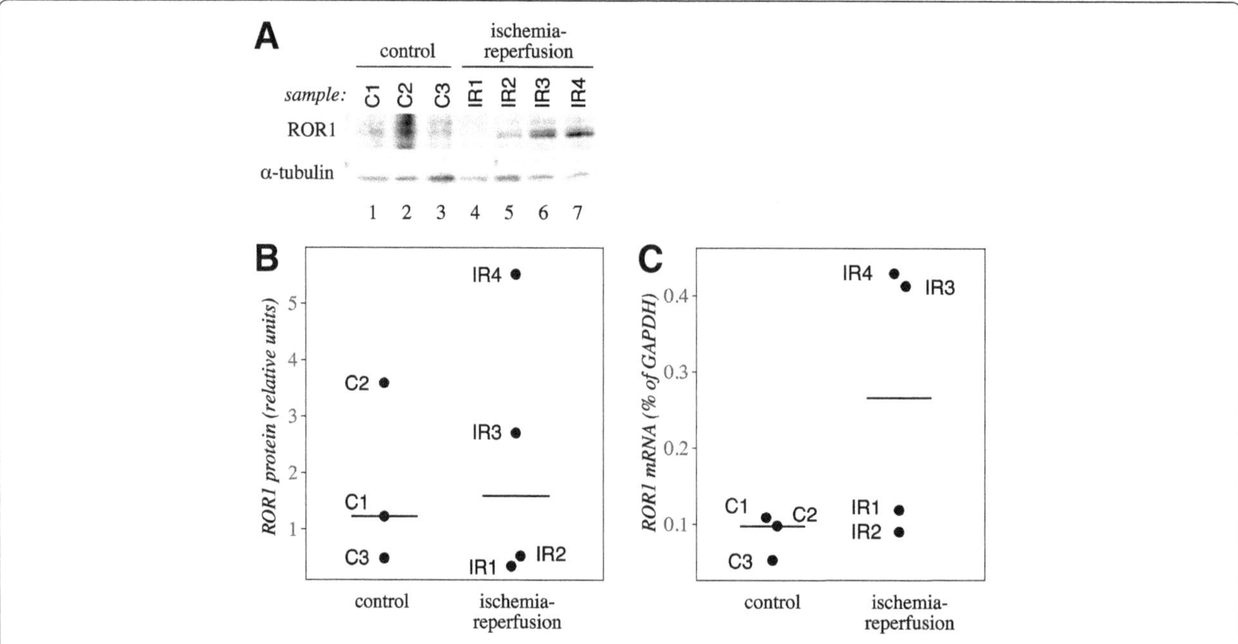

Fig. 3 ROR1 expression in adult pig heart. **a** Western analysis of ROR1 expression in pig heart samples. An approximately 130 kDa band, corresponding to the predicted size of ROR1, was detected. **b** Densitometric quantification of ROR1 protein level relative to α-tubulin. **c** *ROR1* mRNA expression relative to *GAPDH* mRNA expression in pig heart samples was measured by real-time RT-PCR. In B and C, values for individual samples ($n = 3$ for control, $n = 4$ for ischemia-reperfusion) are plotted. Medians are indicated with horizontal lines

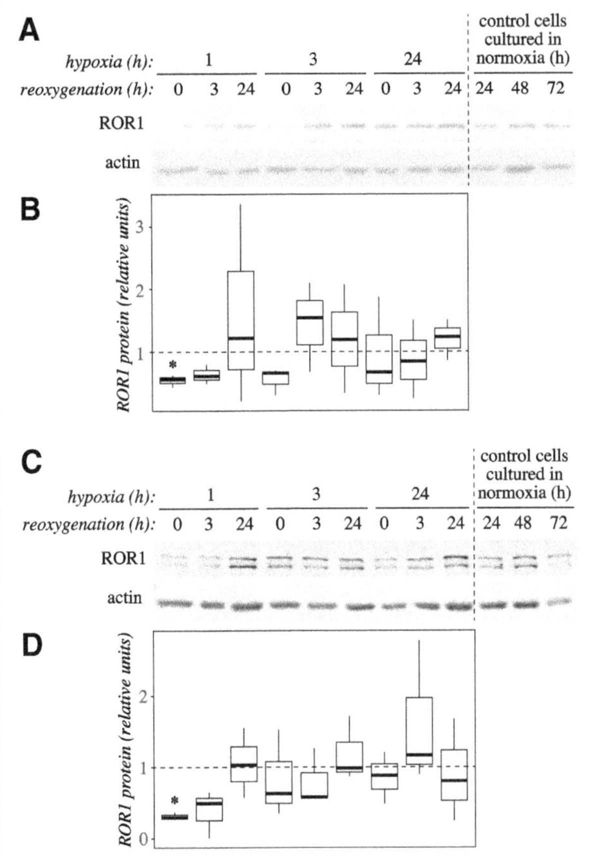

Fig. 4 ROR1 protein level is regulated in cardiomyocytes in response to hypoxia and reoxygenation. **a** A representative Western analysis of ROR1 protein level in HL-1 cardiomyocytes after treatment with hypoxia and reoxygenation. Cells were allowed to adhere for 24 h after plating in normoxia. This was followed by culturing the cells in a hypoxic work station at 1% O_2 (hypoxia) and subsequently again in the regular cell incubator in normoxia (reoxygenation) for the indicated periods of time. As time points were distributed over three days after plating, control samples cultured in normoxia for 24, 48 or 72 h were also analyzed. Time points (hypoxia+reoxygenation) 1 + 0, 1 + 3, 3 + 0 and 3 + 3 are comparable to the 24 h control (lane 10), time points 1 + 24, 3 + 24, 24 + 0 and 24 + 3 to the 48 h control (lane 11), and time points 24 + 24 to the 72 h control (lane 12). **b** A box plot presentation of quantitation of ROR1 bands from three Western blots similar to the one shown in panel A. ROR1 band intensities were normalized to each sample's actin level, and subsequently divided by the control sample value of the respective timepoint. **c** A representative Western analysis of ROR1 protein levels in H9c2 cardiomyoblasts after treatment with hypoxia and reoxygenation. Experiment was carried out as shown for HL-1 cells in panel A. The antibody recognized two bands between 130 and 180 kDa, that both were down-regulated by ROR1 siRNA knockdown (data not shown). **d** A box plot presentation of quantitation of ROR1 bands from three Western blots similar to the one shown in panel C. Data were normalized as for panel B. Asterisk indicates significant difference in expression
($P < 0.05$) as compared to control samples

analysis. The samples were collected at two time points: after one hour of hypoxia, a time point that demonstrated significant downregulation of total ROR1 protein level in both HL-1 and H9c2 cells (Fig. 4), and after one hour of hypoxia followed by 24 h of reoxygenation, a schedule chosen to reflect the ischemia-reperfusion treatment used for the in vivo analysis (Fig. 2). ROR1 phosphorylation was downregulated in response to both treatments (Additional file 6), suggesting that hypoxia alone is sufficient for the observed effect.

ROR1 knockdown increases the viability of cardiomyocytes in vitro

The regulation of ROR1 expression in both ischemia-reperfusion and hypoxia-reoxygenation models indicated functional relevance for ROR1 activity in the hypoxic heart. To address the contribution of ROR1 for the cardiomyocyte viability, expression of the receptor was knocked down in HL-1 cells by RNA interference, and the relative amount of viable cells was measured by MTT assay. Two *ROR1*-targeting siRNAs significantly enhanced the cellular viability both in normoxia ($P = 0.004$ and $P < 0.001$ for siRNAs #1 and #2, respectively; $n = 18$) and after 24 h of hypoxia followed by 24 h of reoxygenation ($P = 0.003$ and $P = 0.001$ for siRNAs #1 and #2, respectively; n = 18), when compared to negative control siRNAs (Fig. 5a and Additional file 5 E). Consistent with the expression data, knockdown of ROR2 expression did not significantly affect HL-1 cell viability (Additional file 5 C-E), suggesting that the effect was specific for ROR1 within the ROR subfamily of RTKs.

ROR1 promotes phosphorylation of Akt and p38

To study the downstream signaling effects of ROR1 knockdown, phosphorylation status of Akt and p38 was studied by Western blotting, as these pathways have been shown to be involved in ROR1 signaling [25, 26]. Phosphorylation of both Akt and p38 was decreased in HL-1 cells 24 h after siRNA transfection (Fig. 5b).

Wnt-5a is an activating ligand of ROR1 [27, 28] in addition to other receptor such as ROR2 [27–29], RYK [30] and Frizzled receptors [31]. Stimulation of HL-1 cells for 96 h with 200 or 400 ng/ml Wnt-5a significantly reduced the viability of the cells in both normoxia ($P = 0.012$ and $P = 0.015$, for 200 and 400 ng/ml, respectively; $n = 9$) and after 48-h hypoxia followed by 24 h of reoxygenation ($P = 0.006$ and $P < 0.001$, for 200 and 400 ng/ml, respectively; n = 9), as compared to non-treated controls (Fig. 5c). In accordance with the decrease in the level of phosphorylated Akt and p38 by ROR1-targeted RNA interference, phosphorylation of both Akt and p38 was enhanced in response to treatment with 400 ng/ml of Wnt-5a for 30 min (Fig. 5d).

Taken together, these results indicate that ROR1 expression and activity suppress cardiomyocyte viability in vitro, and that the pathways involved include Akt and p38.

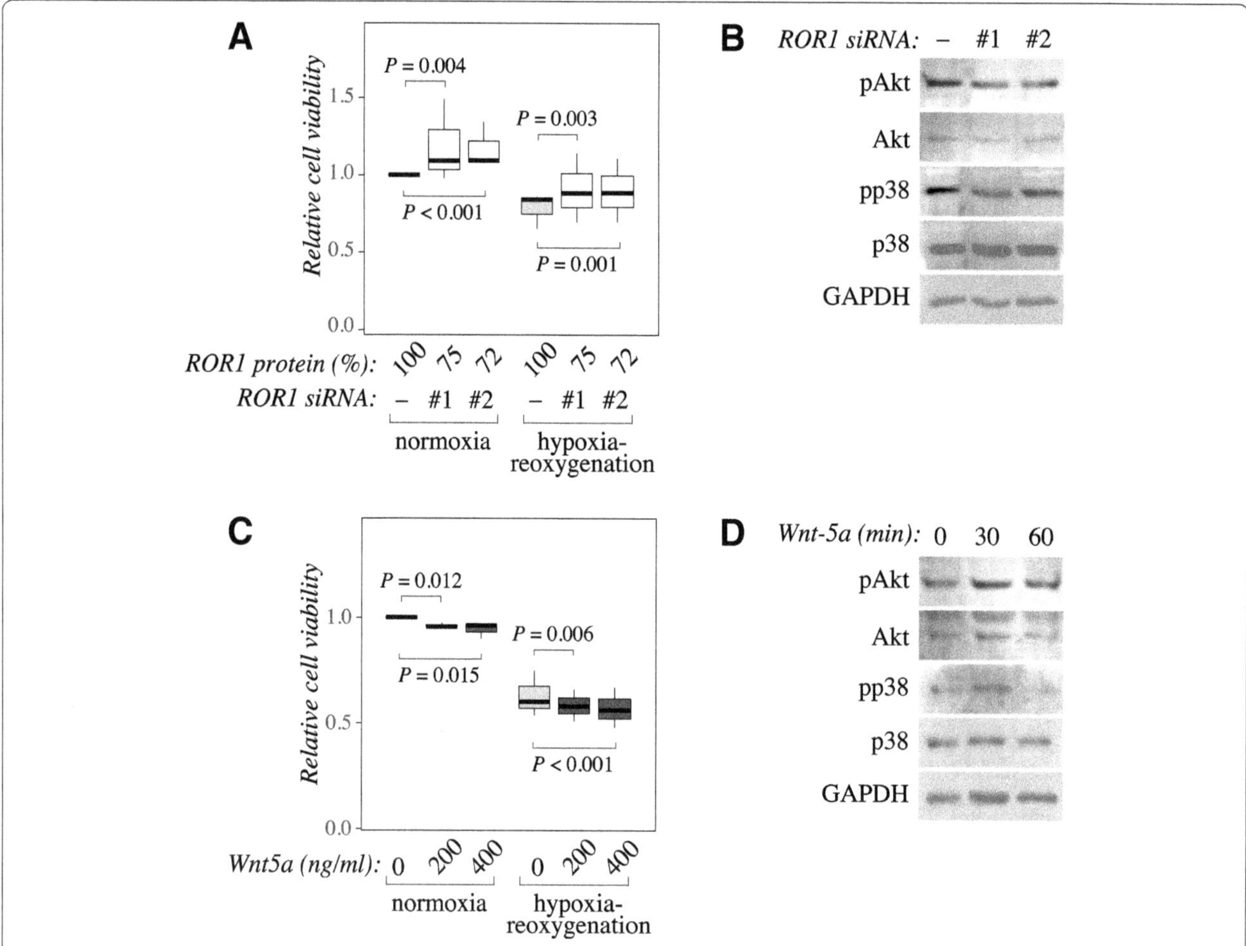

Fig. 5 ROR1 knockdown reduces but Wnt-5a ligand treatment increases cardiomyocyte viability under normoxia and hypoxia-reoxygenation. **a** HL-1 cells were transfected with two different siRNAs targeting ROR1 (*ROR1* siRNA #1 and #2) or negative control siRNA. Twenty-four hours after transfection, cells were either transferred into a hypoxic work station (1% O_2) or were maintained in normoxia as controls. After another 24 h, all cells were returned to normoxia for 24 h to allow for reoxygenation. Cell viability was analyzed using the MTT assay. A box plot presentation is shown indicating cell viability as normalized to negative control siRNA-treated cells cultured in normoxia. The efficacy of the *ROR1* siRNAs in down-regulating ROR1 expression is indicated (ROR1 protein %). Three independent experiments each including six replicates were carried out. **b** Western analysis of total and phosphorylated Akt and p38 in HL-1 cells lysed 48 h after siRNA transfection. **c** HL-1 cells were treated with the indicated concentrations of Wnt-5a since plating. Twenty-four hours after plating, cells were either transferred into a hypoxic work station (1% O_2) or were maintained in normoxia as controls. After another 48 h, all cells were returned to normoxia for 24 h to allow for reoxygenation. Cell viability was analyzed using the MTT assay. A box plot presentation is shown indicating cell viability as normalized to cells cultured in the absence of the ligand in normoxia. Three independent experiments each including three replicates were carried out. **d** Western analysis of total and phosphorylated Akt and p38 in HL-1 cells treated or not with 400 ng/ml of Wnt-5a for 30 or 60 min. Negative control cells were lysed at the same time as the 30-min sample

Discussion

To address the potential of RTKs as therapeutic targets in myocardial ischemia, expression and phosphorylation of RTKs was systematically analyzed in human and porcine ischemic heart samples. A subgroup of RTKs, both present in phosphorylated form in the ischemic myocardium, and differentially regulated at the expression level between the ischemic and normoxic samples, was identified. This subgroup included ALK, AXL, EGFR, EPHB2, ERBB2, FGFR2, KIT, ROR1, ROR2 and TIE1. As the role of ROR1 in ischemic heart has not previously been addressed, it was selected for further analyses. ROR1 expression and phosphorylation were found to be down-regulated in cardiomyocytes in response to hypoxia. Moreover, functional in vitro experiments with RNA interference and Wnt-5a stimulation indicated that targeting of ROR1 enhances cardiomyocyte viability.

Analysis of RTK expression in the acute myocardial infarction samples revealed 4 RTKs with significantly reduced expression (*EGFR*, *ERBB2*, *ERBB3* and *EPHA2*) when compared to healthy heart. Of these, *ERBB2* has also previously been shown to be downregulated in hypoxic human heart [8]. While the other two ERBB family members, *EGFR* and *ERBB3*, were down-regulated in our analyses, the previous report by Munk et al. [8] indicates upregulation of *EGFR* and no change for *ERBB3* expression in hypoxia. Interestingly, EPHA2 has been shown to have cardioprotective potential in mouse models of myocardial ischemia and ischemic cardiomyopathy [32, 33].

Analysis of RTK expression in the ischemic cardiomyopathy samples revealed 3 RTKs with significantly enhanced expression (*ROR1, KIT* and *TIE1*) and 11 with significantly reduced expression (*EPHA2, LTK, PDGFRB, ERBB3, FGFR2, AXL, ALK, ROR2, EPHA8, EPHB2* and *EPHB4*) when compared to healthy heart. *ROR1* expression was most significantly upregulated. However, the roles for most RTKs identified in our analyses in ischemic cardiomyopathy remain to be elucidated in future studies.

The phosphoarray analysis of porcine myocardial samples indicated the highest phosphorylation level for EGFR, ROR2, INSR, EPHB3, EPHB2, TEK, RYK, ROR1 and EPHB6. For ROR1 and VEGFR2, difference in phosphorylation between control and ischemia-reperfusion samples was statistically significant. While details about the antibodies included in the phospho-RTK array are not publicly available, the kit has been designed to detect human receptors. A conservation analysis between the human and porcine RTK protein sequences indicated high conservation for most receptors (median global similarity = 93.1%) and global similarity of 92.4% for ROR1 (Additional file 7). However, the specificity of the antibodies in the array could not be directly controlled and, especially, the phosphorylation status of ROR1 in ischemic heart remains to be studied in future analyses. Nevertheless, a reproducible set of active RTKs in the ischemic heart was detected, including both novel receptors (e.g. ROR1, ROR2) and ones formerly known to be active in the heart (EGFR, ERBB2, INSR, VEGFR2).

Both ROR1 expression and phosphorylation were found to be down-regulated in cardiomyocytes in vitro. Although ROR1 phosphorylation was downregulated also in the pig model of acute ischemia-reperfusion injury in vivo, *ROR1* expression in the pig model demonstrated a nonsignificant trend for increase. Moreover, *ROR1* mRNA expression was upregulated in the ischemic cardiomyopathy samples. These findings could reflect the intrinsic differences in measuring protein phosphorylation vs. expression, and the associated feed-back regulation, but also the duration of hypoxia in the different models. For example, ischemic cardiomyopathy is a chronic ischemic disease involving heart failure, while the ischemia-reperfusion-model in the pig and the in vitro analyses are models for more acute hypoxic conditions.

ROR1 signaling was demonstrated to inhibit cardiomyocyte survival, as its knockdown increased, while its ligand activation decreased, cellular viability. ROR1 and ROR2 comprise the Receptor tyrosine kinase-like Orphan Receptor (ROR) family. While ROR signaling in the ischemic heart has not previously been addressed, both receptors are known to regulate heart development during mouse embryogenesis [6, 7, 34]. Interestingly, in our in vitro analyses, hypoxia affected expression of ROR1, but not of ROR2, and knockdown of *ROR1*, but not of *ROR2*, enhanced cardiomyocyte viability, implying that the two receptors have overlapping but not fully redundant biological functions in these cells. The pathways regulating ROR1 functions in cardiomyocytes may involve p38, as our phospho-Western analyses indicated p38 regulation both in response to *ROR1* knockdown as well as to Wnt-5a ligand stimulation. Indeed, inhibition of p38 signaling has been shown to enable adult cardiomyocyte proliferation [35] and promote cardiac regeneration [36]. Interestingly, a ROR1-targeting monoclonal antibody, cirmtuzumab, has been developed for the treatment of chronic lymphatic leukemia [37] allowing future analysis of its effect on normal and ischemic heart.

Conclusions

In conclusion, we describe an RTK-proteome level approach to characterize RTK expression and activity in the ischemic heart. ROR1 was identified as one of the RTKs that was both present in the ischemic heart in an active form and regulated in expression in a manner that associated with clinical and experimental ischemia. Manipulation of ROR1 expression and activity in vitro indicated a functional role for ROR1 in suppressing cardiomyocyte viability. These findings warrant further studies addressing the targeting of ROR1 as an approach to treat ischemic heart disease.

Additional files

Additional file 1: RTKs included in in silico analysis of expression from IST Online data. Statistical analyses of differences in RTK mRNA expression between samples representing healthy human heart and ischemic cardiomyopathy or acute myocardial infarction. (XLSX 15 kb)

Additional file 2: Phospho-RTK array of ischemia-reperfusion-injured pig hearts. A) Representative phospho-RTK array blots from control and ischemia-reperfusion-injured pig heart samples. B) Array overlay and a corresponding coordinate table indicating the location of RTKs in the array. Each of the 49 RTKs included in the array are represented by two adjacent dots. (PDF 229 kb)

Additional file 3: Heatmaps of RTKs demonstrating significant changes in mRNA expression in either ischemic cardiomyopathy or acute myocardial infarction when compared to healthy heart. RTKs with significant expression level differences (FDR-corrected P values < 0.05) between pairwise group comparisons were selected for visualization. A) Ischemic cardiomyopathy vs. healthy heart. B) Acute myocardial infarction vs. healthy heart. The data represent normalized log2-transformed Affymetrix gene expression values from the IST Online database. (PDF 321 kb)

Additional file 4: Myocardial damage in ischemia-reperfusion-injured pig hearts. A) Plasma troponin T levels from four ischemia-reperfusion-injured pigs were collected at baseline, and 6 and 24 h after reperfusion. Medians are indicated with horizontal lines. B) Representative HE-stained images from a healthy and ischemia-reperfusion-injured pig heart (sample collected 31 h after reperfusion). (PDF 44885 kb)

Additional file 5: ROR2 in cardiomyocytes. A) A representative Western analysis of ROR2 protein level in HL-1 cardiomyocytes after treatment with hypoxia and reoxygenation. All cells were first allowed to adhere for 24 h after plating in normoxic conditions. This was followed by culturing the cells in a hypoxic work station at 1% O_2 (hypoxia) and subsequently again in the regular cell incubator in normoxia (reoxygenation) for the indicated periods of time. As different time points were distributed over three days after plating, control samples cultured in normoxia for 24, 48 or 72 h were also analyzed. Time points (hypoxia+reoxygenation) 1 + 0, 1 + 3, 3 + 0 and 3 + 3 are comparable to the 24 h control (lane 10), time points 1 + 24, 3 + 24, 24 + 0 and 24 + 3 to the 48 h control (lane 11), and time points 24 + 24 to the 72 h control (lane 12). B) A box plot presentation of densitometric quantitation of ROR1 bands from three replicate Western blots similar to the one shown in panel A. ROR1 band intensities were first normalized to each sample's actin level, and subsequently divided by the control sample value of the respective time point. C) Effect of ROR2 knockdown on cellular viability. HL-1 cells were transfected with two different siRNAs targeting ROR2 (ROR2 siRNA #1 and #2) or negative control siRNA. Twenty-four hours after transfection, cells were either transferred into a hypoxic work station (1% O_2) or were maintained in normoxia as controls. After another 24 h, all cells were returned to normoxia for 24 h to allow for reoxygenation. Cell viability was analyzed using the MTT assay. A box plot presentation is shown indicating cell viability as normalized to negative control siRNA-treated cells cultured in normoxia. Three independent experiments each including six replicates were carried out. D) Western analysis of ROR2 protein expression after ROR2 siRNA treatments. E) Western analyses of ROR1 and ROR2 protein expression after ROR1 siRNA treatment. (PDF 3815 kb)

Additional file 6: Analysis of ROR1 phosphorylation in HL-1 cardiomyocytes after hypoxia and reoxygenation. A) Western analysis of tyrosine phosphorylation after ROR1 immunoprecipitation. Cells were first allowed to adhere for 24 h after plating in normoxic conditions. This was followed by culturing the cells in a hypoxic work station at 1% O_2 (hypoxia) and subsequently again in the regular cell incubator in normoxia (reoxygenation) for the indicated periods of time. As different time points were distributed over two days after plating, control samples cultured in normoxia for 24 or 48 h were also analyzed. Time point of one hour of hypoxia (lane 1) is comparable to the 24 h control (lane 2) and time point of one hour of hypoxia and 24 h of reoxygenation (lane 3) is comparable to the 48 h control (lane 4). B) Quantitation of ROR1 phosphorylation relative to total protein. (PDF 179 kb)

Additional file 7: RTK similarity and identity between pig and human. (XLSX 12 kb)

Abbreviations

FDR: False discovery rate; ROR: Receptor tyrosine kinase-like Orphan Receptor; RTK: Receptor tyrosine kinase

Acknowledgements

We thank Maria Tuominen and Minna Santanen for excellent technical assistance, and Petra Miikkulainen and Heidi Högel for the maintenance of hypoxic workstation. The data were partially represented as a poster at AHA Scientific Sessions 2017.

Funding

This research was supported by grants from Academy of Finland [274728], Cancer Foundation of Finland, Sigrid Jusélius Foundation, Turku University Central Hospital and salary from Turku Doctoral Programme of Molecular Medicine.

Authors' contributions

JH, AJ, IP and KE designed and JH and AJ and performed the in vitro experiments. JH, DC and KE analyzed the data. CS and TS performed and provided the material of in vivo animal experiments. ML provided the in silico data and contributed to the data analyses. JH, IP and KE mainly wrote the manuscript. Every author read, revised and approved the manuscript.

Competing interests

JH is employed by and has ownership interest in Abomics Ltd. ML is employed by Medisapiens Ltd. KE has ownership interest in and is a board member of Abomics Ltd., and has ownership interest in Orion and Roche. IP, AJ, CS and TS have no competing interests.

Author details

[1]Institute of Biomedicine, University of Turku, Kiinamyllynkatu 10, FIN-20520 Turku, Finland. [2]Turku Doctoral Programme of Molecular Medicine, University of Turku, Turku, Finland. [3]Institute for Molecular Medicine Finland, University of Helsinki, Helsinki, Finland. [4]Turku Centre for Biotechnology, University of Turku and Åbo Akademi University, Turku, Finland. [5]Research Center of Applied and Preventive Cardiovascular Medicine, University of Turku, Turku, Finland. [6]Medisapiens Ltd., Helsinki, Finland. [7]Medicity Research Laboratories, University of Turku, Turku, Finland. [8]Department of Oncology, Turku University Hospital, Turku, Finland.

References

1. Global Health Estimates 2015. Deaths by Cause, Age, Sex, by Country and by Region, 2000-2015. Geneva: World Health Organization; 2016.
2. Hausenloy DJ, Yellon DM. Myocardial ischemia-reperfusion injury: a neglected therapeutic target. J Clin Invest. 2013;123(1):92–100.
3. Lee KF, Simon H, Chen H, Bates B, Hung MC, Hauser C. Requirement for neuregulin receptor erbB2 in neural and cardiac development. Nature. 1995; 378(6555):394–8.
4. Chan R, Hardy WR, Laing MA, Hardy SE, Muller WJ. The catalytic activity of the ErbB-2 receptor tyrosine kinase is essential for embryonic development. Mol Cell Biol. 2002;22(4):1073–8.
5. Gassmann M, Casagranda F, Orioli D, Simon H, Lai C, Klein R, et al. Aberrant neural and cardiac development in mice lacking the ErbB4 neuregulin receptor. Nature. 1995;378(6555):390–4.
6. Nomi M, Oishi I, Kani S, Suzuki H, Matsuda T, Yoda A, et al. Loss of mRor1 enhances the heart and skeletal abnormalities in mRor2-deficient mice: redundant and pleiotropic functions of mRor1 and mRor2 receptor tyrosine kinases. Mol Cell Biol. 2001;21(24):8329–35.
7. Takeuchi S, Takeda K, Oishi I, Nomi M, Ikeya M, Itoh K, et al. Mouse Ror2 receptor tyrosine kinase is required for the heart development and limb formation. Genes Cells. 2000;5:71–8.
8. Munk M, Memon AA, Goetze JP, Nielsen LB, Nexo E, Sorensen BS. Hypoxia Changes the Expression of the Epidermal Growth Factor (EGF) System in Human Hearts and Cultured Cardiomyocytes. Mohanraj R, editor. PLoS One. 2012;7(7):e40243.
9. Gordon LI, Burke MA, Singh ATK, Prachand S, Lieberman ED, Sun L, et al. Blockade of the erbB2 receptor induces cardiomyocyte death through mitochondrial and reactive oxygen species-dependent pathways. J Biol Chem. 2009;284(4):2080–7.
10. Infanger M, Faramarzi S, Grosse J, Kurth E, Ulbrich C, Bauer J, et al. Expression of vascular endothelial growth factor and receptor tyrosine

kinases in cardiac ischemia/reperfusion injury. Cardiovasc Pathol. 2007; 16(5):291–9.
11. Viswanath K, Bodiga S, Balogun V, Zhang A, Bodiga VL. Cardioprotective effect of zinc requires ErbB2 and Akt during hypoxia/reoxygenation. Biometals. 2011;24(1):171–80.
12. Beauloye C, Bertrand L, Krause U, Marsin AS, Dresselaers T, Vanstapel F, et al. No-flow ischemia inhibits insulin signaling in heart by decreasing intracellular pH. Circ Res. 2001;88(5):513–9.
13. D'Uva G, Aharonov A, Lauriola M, Kain D, Yahalom-Ronen Y, Carvalho S, et al. ERBB2 triggers mammalian heart regeneration by promoting cardiomyocyte dedifferentiation and proliferation. Nat Cell Biol. 2015;17(5): 627–38.
14. Bersell K, Arab S, Haring B, Kühn B. Neuregulin1/ErbB4 signaling induces cardiomyocyte proliferation and repair of heart injury. Cell. 2009;138(2): 257–70.
15. Liu X, Gu X, Li Z, Li X, Li H, Chang J, et al. Neuregulin-1/erbB-activation improves cardiac function and survival in models of ischemic, dilated, and viral cardiomyopathy. J Am Coll Cardiol. 2006;48(7):1438–47.
16. Jonassen AK, Sack MN, Mjøs OD, Yellon DM. Myocardial protection by insulin at reperfusion requires early administration and is mediated via Akt and p70s6 kinase cell-survival signaling. Circ Res. 2001;89(12):1191–8.
17. Grossman AN, Opie LH, Beshansky JR, Ingwall JS, Rackley CE, Selker HP. Glucose-insulin-potassium revived: current status in acute coronary syndromes and the energy-depleted heart. Circulation. 2013;127(9):1040–8.
18. Kilpinen S, Autio R, Ojala K, Iljin K, Bucher E, Sara H, et al. Systematic bioinformatic analysis of expression levels of 17,330 human genes across 9,783 samples from 175 types of healthy and pathological tissues. Genome Biol. 2008;9(9):R139.
19. Raivo Kolde (2015). pheatmap: Pretty Heatmaps. R package version 1.0.8. https://CRAN.R-project.org/package=pheatmap.
20. RStudio Team. RStudio: integrated development for R. Boston, MA: RStudio, Inc.; 2016. http://www.rstudio.com/
21. Stark CKJ, Tarkia M, Kentala R, Malmberg M, Vähäsilta T, Savo M, et al. Systemic dosing of thymosin beta 4 before and after ischemia does not attenuate global myocardial ischemia-reperfusion injury in pigs. Front Pharmacol. 2016;7(115).
22. Kainulainen V, Sundvall M, Ma JA, Santiestevan E, Klagsbrun M, Elenius K, et al. A natural ErbB4 isoform that does not activate phosphoinositide 3-kinase mediates proliferation but not survival or chemotaxis. J Biol Chem. 2000; 275(12):8641–9.
23. Rice P, Longden I, Bleasby A. EMBOSS: the European molecular biology open software suite. Trends Genet. 2000;16(6):276–7.
24. Benjamini Y, Hochberg Y. Controlling the false discovery rate: a practical and powerful approach to multiple testing. J R Stat Soc. 1995;57(1):289–300.
25. Fernández NB, Lorenzo D, Picco ME, Barbero G, Dergan-Dylon LS, Marks MP, et al. ROR1 contributes to melanoma cell growth and migration by regulating N-cadherin expression via the PI3K/Akt pathway. Mol Carcinog. 2016;55(11):1772–85.
26. Yamaguchi T, Yanagisawa K, Sugiyama R, Hosono Y, Shimada Y, Arima C, et al. NKX2–1/TITF1/TTF-1-Induced ROR1 Is Required to Sustain EGFR Survival Signaling in Lung Adenocarcinoma. Cancer Cell. 2012;21(3):348–61.
27. Fukuda T, Chen L, Endo T, Tang L, Lu D, Castro JE, et al. Antisera induced by infusions of autologous Ad-CD154-leukemia B cells identify ROR1 as an oncofetal antigen and receptor for Wnt5a. Proc Natl Acad Sci. 2008;105(8): 3047–52.
28. Yu J, Chen L, Cui B, li GFW, Shen Z, Wu R, et al. Wnt5a induces ROR1 / ROR2 heterooligomerization to enhance leukemia chemotaxis and proliferation. J Clin Invest. 2016;126(2):585–98.
29. Oishi I, Suzuki H, Onishi N, Takada R, Kani S, Shibuya H, et al. The receptor tyrosine kinase Ror2 is involved in non-canonical Wnt5a / JNK signalling pathway. Genes Cells. 2003;8(7):645–54.
30. Yoshikawa S, McKinnon RD, Kokel M, Thomas JB. Wnt-mediated axon guidance via the Drosophila derailed receptor. Nature. 2003;422(6932):583–8.
31. Park HW, Kim YC, Yu B, Moroishi T, Mo JS, Plouffe SW, et al. Alternative Wnt signaling activates YAP/TAZ. Cell. 2015;162(4):780–94.
32. O'Neal WT, Griffin WF, Kent SD, Faiz F, Hodges J, Vuncannon J, et al. Deletion of the EphA2 receptor exacerbates myocardial injury and the progression of ischemic cardiomyopathy. Front Physiol. 2014;24(5):132.
33. Dries JL, Kent SD, Virag JAI. Intramyocardial administration of chimeric ephrinA1-Fc promotes tissue salvage following myocardial infarction in mice. J Physiol. 2011;589(Pt 7):1725–40.
34. Matsuda T, Nomi M, Ikeya M, Kani S, Oishi I, Terashima T, et al. Expression of the receptor tyrosine kinase genes, Ror1 and Ror2, during mouse development. Mech Dev. 2001;105(1-2):153–6.
35. Engel FB, Schebesta M, Duong MT, Lu G, Ren S, Madwed JB, et al. p38 MAP kinase inhibition enables proliferation of adult mammalian cardiomyocytes. Genes Dev. 2005;19(10):1175–87.
36. Engel FB, Hsieh PCH, Lee RT, Keating MT. FGF1/p38 MAP kinase inhibitor therapy induces cardiomyocyte mitosis, reduces scarring, and rescues function after myocardial infarction. Proc Natl Acad Sci. 2006;103(42):15546–51.
37. Choi MY, li GFW, Wu CCN, Cui B, Lao F, Sadarangani A, et al. Pre-clinical specificity and safety of UC-961, a first-in-class monoclonal antibody targeting ROR1. Clin Lymphoma Myeloma Leuk. 2015;15(S1):S167–9.

Importance of iron deficiency in patients with chronic heart failure as a predictor of mortality and hospitalizations: insights from an observational cohort study

José González-Costello[1*], Josep Comín-Colet[1], Josep Lupón[3], Cristina Enjuanes[2], Marta de Antonio[3], Lara Fuentes[1], Pedro Moliner-Borja[2], Nuria Farré[2], Elisabet Zamora[3], Nicolás Manito[1], Ramón Pujol[4] and Antoni Bayés-Genis[3]

Abstract

Background: Iron deficiency (ID) in patients with chronic heart failure (CHF) is considered an adverse prognostic factor. We aimed to evaluate if ID in patients with CHF is associated with increased mortality and hospitalizations.

Methods: We evaluated ID in patients with CHF at 3 university hospitals. ID was defined as absolute (ferritin < 100 μg/L) or functional (transferrin Saturation index < 20% and ferritin between 100 and 299 μg/L). We excluded patients who received treatment with intravenous Iron or Erythropoietin during follow-up. We evaluated if ID was a predictor of death or hospitalization due to heart failure or any cause using univariate and multivariate cox regression analysis.

Results: We included 1684 patients, 65% males, 38% diabetics, median age of 72 years, 37% in functional class III-IV and 30% of patients with a left ventricular ejection fraction > 45%. Patients were well treated, with 87% and 88% of patients receiving renin-angiotensin inhibitors and beta-blockers, respectively. Median transferrin saturation index was 20%, median ferritin 155 ng/mL and median haemoglobin 13 g/dL. ID was present in 53% of patients; in 35% it was absolute and in 18% functional. Median follow-up was 20 months. ID was a predictor of death, hospitalization due to heart failure or to any cause in univariate analysis but not after multivariate analysis. No differences were found between absolute or functional ID regarding prognosis.

Conclusion: In a real life population of patients with CHF and a high prevalence of heart failure with preserved ejection fraction, ID did not predict mortality or hospitalizations after adjustment for comorbidities, functional class and neurohormonal treatment.

Keywords: Chronic heart failure, Iron deficiency, Mortality, Hospitalization

Background

Iron deficiency (ID) affects up to 50% of patients with chronic heart failure (HF) and has been identified as an adverse prognostic factor independently of the presence of anaemia and chronic kidney disease (CKD) [1, 2]. However, in another study of community-dwelling adults with self-reported heart failure there was no association between ID and all cause or cardiovascular mortality, but haemoglobin and C-reactive protein did predict worse survival [3]. ID frequently overlaps with anaemia and/or CKD in chronic HF and the presence of ID amplifies mortality risk, either alone or in combination with anaemia, CKD, or both [2].

Although the pathophysiology behind ID in patients with chronic HF is not fully understood and is considered multifactorial [4–6], treatment of ID in these patients has become a therapeutic goal. Oral iron is not associated with an increase in exercise capacity in patients with HF and systolic dysfunction [7]. Recent randomized trials have

* Correspondence: jgcostello@hotmail.com
[1]Area de Enfermedades del Corazón, Hospital Universitari de Bellvitge, IDIBELL, Universitat de Barcelona, L'Hospitalet de Llobregat, Feixa Llarga SN, 08907 Barcelona, Spain
Full list of author information is available at the end of the article

demonstrated how intravenous iron can improve exercise capacity, cardiac function, symptom severity and quality of life in patients with chronic HF and left ventricular systolic dysfunction [8–11]. In the most recent study, the CONFIRM-HF, the risk of hospitalization due to worsening heart failure was reduced in the ferric carboxymaltose arm vs. the placebo-treated arm. However, no study has evaluated the incidence of hospitalizations due to heart failure or to any cause in patients with chronic HF and ID.

Given the importance of reducing mortality and hospitalizations in patients with chronic HF and that treatment with intravenous iron may reduce hospitalizations, we aimed to evaluate the prognostic importance of ID in a large multicenter cohort of ambulatory patients with chronic HF, focusing on mortality and hospitalizations due to worsening heart failure or to any cause.

Methods

Study design

This is a retrospective observational cohort study of patients with heart failure in whom we evaluated the presence of ID and whether ID was associated with re-hospitalizations or mortality during follow-up.

Component population

The study population consisted of 2495 consecutive patients with stable chronic HF prospectively enrolled at 3 multidisciplinary heart failure (HF) units from 3 tertiary hospitals in Spain from 2005 to 2012. Patients had to be diagnosed of HF according to the European Society of Cardiology diagnostic criteria [12]. We defined HF with preserved LVEF (HFPEF) as the presence of symptoms of HF with a left ventricular ejection fraction ≥50% and an objective evidence of cardiac dysfunction (enlarged left atrium, diastolic dysfunction or elevated natriuretic peptides). We excluded patients without iron status assessed at entry and those with significant primary valvular or pericardial disease. Of the remaining 2172 patients, we excluded those who received treatment with intravenous iron or subcutaneous erythropoetin at any time point during follow-up, after review of the pharmacy records, as this treatment could influence outcomes. This left 1684 patients for analysis. Patients were treated according to the European Society of Cardiology guidelines [12].

Written informed consent was obtained from each patient. The investigation conforms with the principles outlined in the Declaration of Helsinki. The local ethic committees approved the study protocol.

Pooled methodology

The pooled data for the present study were assessed at a patient level and collected prospectively. The end points for the present study were all cause mortality, first hospitalization due to HF and first hospitalization due to any cause after inclusion in the HF unit. Vital status and hospitalizations were assessed by review of the clinical databases, hospital records or direct contact with patients or relatives. Follow-up duration was until death or up to the last visit in the out patient clinic before October 2015. For patients lost to follow-up, we contacted the patient or the family by telephone and determined vital status and hospitalizations. For patients that could not be contacted by telephone we accessed the electronic clinical history of the hospital and of the primary care health system and determined vital status and hospitalizations. If despite all these efforts, no information regarding hospitalizations and death could be obtained, end of follow-up was determined to be the last time the patient had been to the out patient clinic. Five patients received a heart transplant during follow-up and this was recorded as death and end of follow-up. No patient received a ventricular assist device.

Iron status and other laboratory measurements

The following blood biomarkers reflecting iron status were measured at study entry: Serum iron (ug/dL) was measured using spectrophotometry, serum ferritin (ng/mL) and transferrin (mg/dL) were measured using immunoturbidimetry. Transferrin saturation index (TSAT) was estimated using the formula: TSAT = serum iron (ug/dL)/[serum transferrin (mg/dL) × 1.25] [13]. ID was defined as absolute when ferritin < 100 ng/ml and functional when TSAT < 20% with ferritin 100–299 ng/ml [8].

Haemoglobin was measured using impedance laser colorimetry and anaemia was defined as Haemoglobin < 12 g/dL in women and Haemoglobin < 13 g/dL in men. Concentrations of N-terminal pro-brain-type natriuretic peptide (NT-proBNP) were measured using an immunoassay based on electrochemiluminescence on the Elecsys

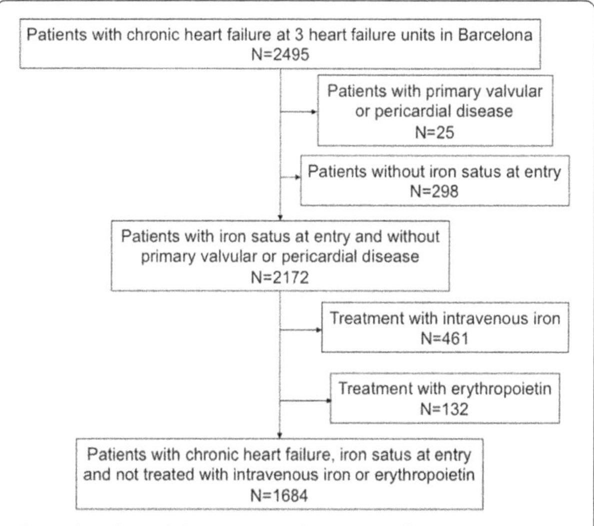

Fig. 1 Flowchart of the study population. 105 of patients treated with erythropoietin were also treated with intravenous iron

System (Roche Diagnostics, Basel, Switzerland). Renal function was assessed with the estimated glomerular filtration rate using the abbreviated Modification of Diet in Renal Disease equation.

Statistical analysis

Continuous variables were explored for normal distribution according to histograms and the Shapiro-Wilk test. The comparison of quantitative variables between the 2 groups was done using the Student-t test for normally distributed variables and the Mann-Whitney U test for non-normally distributed variables. The chi-square test was used for categorical variables and Fisher's exact test when cells had an expected count of less than 5.

The continuous variables that had a very skewed distribution, such as the TSAT, Ferritin and NT-proBNP underwent logarithmic transformation. The resulting variables are referred to as: logTSAT, logFerritin and logNT-proBNP. In order to assess if variables introduced in the multivariate regression analysis were highly correlated we evaluated collinearity using the variance inflation factor. The maximal variance inflation factor found

Table 1 Baseline variables according to iron deficiency

Variables	Overall *N* = 1684	No ID *N* = 786	ID *N* = 898	*P* value
Age (years)	72 (61–79)	70 (58–78)	73 (63–79)	< 0.0001
Female gender	588 (35)	207 (26)	381 (42)	< 0.0001
BMI (kg/m²)	27 (24–30)	30 (27–34)	31 (27–36)	0.011
Systolic BP (mm Hg)	120 (108–139)	118 (105–133)	125 (110–140)	< 0.0001
Heart rate (bpm)	70 (62–80)	70 (60–80)	70 (62–80)	0.398
NYHA Class III-IV	592 (35)	218 (28)	374 (42)	< 0.0001
LVEF (%)	35 (27–50)	35 (27–48)	36 (28–53)	0.032
HFPEF	428 (25)	182 (23)	246 (27)	0.046
Ischaemic aetiology	738 (44)	331 (42)	407 (45)	0.185
Hypertension	1136 (68)	492 (63)	644 (72)	< 0.0001
Diabetes Mellitus	639 (38)	262 (33)	377 (42)	< 0.0001
COPD	318 (19)	158 (20)	160 (18)	0.232
Treatment				
ACE-I or ARB	1457 (87)	695 (89)	762 (85)	0.019
Beta blockers	1474 (88)	690 (88)	784 (87)	0.766
MRAs	716 (43)	357 (45)	359 (40)	0.024
Digoxin	395 (23)	184 (23)	211 (24)	0.966
Oral anticoagulation	755 (45)	356 (45)	399 (44)	0.723
Antiplatelet	879 (52)	412 (52)	467 (52)	0.884
Diuretics	1458 (87)	661 (84)	797 (89)	0.001
ICD	136 (8)	64 (8)	72 (8)	0.933
Resynchronization	77 (5)	35 (5)	42 (5)	0.826
Laboratory values				
Haemoglobin (g/dL)	13.0 (11.7–14.3)	13.4 (12.0–14.7)	12.7 (11.5–13.9)	< 0.0001
eGFR (ml/min/1.73 m²)	53 (37–71)	56 (38–75)	52 (36–68)	0.032
Ferritin (ng/mL)	155 (72–276)	276 (172–435)	76 (43–141)	< 0.0001
Transferrin (mg/dL)	261 (224–313)	245 (213–288)	276 (239–330)	< 0.0001
Serum iron (ug/dL)	73 (51–99)	90 (71–116)	59 (44–79)	< 0.0001
TSAT (%)	20 (15–28)	26 (22–34)	16 (12–19)	< 0.0001
NTproBNP (ng/L)	1355 (536–3171)	1111 (488–2747)	1584 (609–3597)	< 0.0001
Sodium (mmol/L)	140 (138–142)	140 (138–142)	140 (138–142)	0.011

Continuous variables are expressed as median and interquartile range (IQR). Categorical variables are expressed as number and percentage
ID Iron deficiency, *BMI* Body mass index, *NYHA* New York Heart Association, *LVEF* Left ventricular ejection fraction, *HFPEF* Heart failure with preserved ejection fraction, *COPD* Chronic obstructive pulmonary disease, *ACE-I* Angiotensin converting enzyme inhibitor, *ARB* Angiotensin II receptor blocker, *MRA* Mineralocorticoid receptor antagonist, *ICD* Implantable cardioverter defibrillator, *eGFR* estimated glomerular filtration rate, *TSAT* Transferrin saturation, *NTproBNP* N-terminal pro-brain natriuretic peptide

among baseline variables was 1.5, indicating a low degree of collinearity.

To evaluate predictors of ID we used multivariate logistic regression analysis. All baseline variables with a significant univariate association ($p < 0.10$) or deemed to be clinically relevant were entered in a step-wise backward multivariable model with an exclusion criteria of $p > 0.10$. Additional bootstrap analysis (1000 cycles) of the multivariate model was performed to measure accuracy of the estimated model. The R2 value for the multivariate model was also calculated.

Incidence ratio of death and hospitalizations due to HF or any cause were determined dividing the incidence rate of events in patients with ID vs. without ID. Significance was assessed using the Mantel-Haenszel Chi square test.

Survival and time to first hospitalization due to heart failure or any cause were evaluated using Kaplan Meier survival curves. We evaluated if ID was a predictor of survival or hospitalization using univariate Cox proportional hazard regression analysis. With the variables that were significant in the univariate analysis ($p < 0.10$) and those that were deemed to be clinically relevant, we then performed backward step multivariate Cox proportional hazard analysis with an exclusion criteria of $p > 0.10$. ID is forced in to the final multivariate model given that it is the purpose of our study. The proportionality assumption for the Cox regression analysis was evaluated using residual analysis. Significance was set at $p < 0.05$ (2 tailed) and SPSS version 18 and Stata 14 were used to perform all statistical evaluations.

Results

We included 1684 patients in the analysis (see flowchart in Fig. 1), whose baseline characteristics are shown in Table 1. ID was present at inclusion in 898 (53%) patients. In 35% it was absolute ID and in 18% functional ID. There were 953 (57%) patients who were not

Table 2 Predictors of iron deficiency using logistic regression analysis

Variables	Univariate OR	*P* value	Multivariate OR	*P* value
Age (per 5 years)	1.09 (1.05–1.13)	< 0.001		
Female sex	2.05 (1.67–2.53)	0.396	1.62 (1.29–2.03)	< 0.001
Hypertension	1.50 (1.23–1.85)	< 0.001		
Diabetes Mellitus	1.44 (1.18–1.76)	< 0.001		
COPD	0.86 (0.67–1.10)	0.223		
HFPEF	1.25 (1.00–1.56)	0.047		
Ischaemic aetiology	1.15 (0.94–1.39)	0.175		
NYHA class III-IV	1.84 (1.50–2.26)	< 0.001	1.50 (1.20–1.88)	< 0.001
Systolic BP (per 10 mmHg)	1.11 (1.06–1.16)	< 0.001	1.09 (1.04–1.14)	< 0.001
Heart rate (per 10 bpm)	1.03 (0.97–1.10)	0.379		
BMI (1 kg/m^2)	1.03 (1.01–1.04)	0.008	1.03 (1.00–1.05)	0.018
ACE-I or ARB	0.71 (0.53–0.95)	0.021		
Beta blockers	0.96 (0.72–1.28)	0.781		
Diuretics	1.50 (1.13–1.98)	0.005		
MRAs	0.81 (0.66–0.98)	0.028		
Digoxin	1.00 (0.80–1.26)	0.988		
Oral anticoagulants	0.96 (0.79–1.17)	0.690		
Antiplatelet	0.99 (0.82–1.20)	0.921		
ICD	1.02 (0.71–1.44)	0.94		
Haemoglobin (per 1 g/dL)	0.82 (0.78–0.87)	< 0.001	0.87 (0.82–0.92)	< 0.001
Log NT-proBNP (per 1 SD)	1.20 (1.09–1.33)	< 0.001	1.12 (0.99–1.25)	0.051
Sodium (per 5 mmol/L)	1.17 (1.02–1.34)	0.030		
eGFR (per 5 ml/min/1.73m^2)	0.98 (0.96–0.99)	0.016		

OR Odds Ratio, *COPD* Chronic Obstructive Pulmonary Disease, *HFPEF* Heart failure with preserved ejection fraction, *NYHA* New York Heart Association, *BP* Blood pressure, *BMI* Body mass index, *ACE-I* Angiotensin converting enzyme inhibitor, *ARB* Angiotensin II receptor blocker, *MRAs* Mineralocorticoid receptor antagonists, *ICD* Implantable cardioverter defibrillator, *Log* Logarithmic transformation, *NTproBNP* N-terminal pro-brain natriuretic peptide, *SD* Standard deviation, *eGFR* Estimated glomerular filtration rate

Variables introduced in the multivariate model were: Age, gender, hypertension, diabetes mellitus, COPD, HFPEF, NYHA functional class III-IV, systolic BP, heart rate, BMI, haemoglobin, logNT-proBNP, eGFR, sodium, treatment with beta blockers, ACE-i/ARBs, diuretics and MRAs

anaemic and ID was present in 460 (48%) of these. Of the 731 patients with anaemia, ID was present in 438 (60%).

Predictors of ID after multivariate analysis are shown in Table 2. The R2 for the multivariate model was 0.05 (5%). Median follow-up was 20 (interquartile range: 12–47) months.

Iron deficiency and mortality

Patients with ID had 307 (34%) deaths with an incidence rate of 0.134 per year compared with those without ID, who had 212 (27%) deaths, with an Incidence Rate of 0.101 per year. The incidence ratio was 1.32 (95% confidence interval: 1.11–1.57; $p = 0.0017$). Both absolute and functional ID had similar mortality rates of 0.145 and 0.128 per year, respectively, $p = 0.29$. When we analysed both components of the definition of ID, lower logTSAT predicted mortality but not logFerritin. ID was not a predictor of mortality in multivariate analysis. Table 3 shows the hazard ratios for mortality in our cohort of patients using univariate and multivariate cox regression analysis. When we introduced logTSAT in the multivariate model, instead of the usual definition of ID, it also was not a significant predictor of mortality. Figure 2 shows no differences in the survival curves stratified for ID after adjustment for the covariates that were significant in the multivariate model.

Iron deficiency and hospitalizations due to heart failure

Patients with ID had 246 (27%) hospitalizations due to HF with an incidence rate of 0.121 per year compared with those without ID, who had 182 (23%) hospitalizations due HF, with an incidence rate of 0.097 per year. The incidence ratio was 1.24 (95% confidence interval: 1.03–1.51; $p = 0.025$). There was no significant difference in the incidence rate of hospitalizations due to heart failure between patients with functional or absolute ID: 0.110 and 0.125 per year respectively, $p = 0.37$. ID was not a predictor of hospitalization due to heart failure after multivariate analysis. Table 4 shows predictors of hospitalization due to HF after univariate and multivariate adjustment. Figure 3 shows the survival curves for

Table 3 Predictors of mortality using cox regression analysis

Variables	Univariate HR	*P* value	Multivariate HR	*P* value
Age (per 5 years)	1.36 (1.30–1.42)	< 0.001	1.21 (1.16–1.27)	< 0.001
Female sex	1.08 (0.90–1.30)	0.39	0.65 (0.54–0.79)	< 0.001
Hypertension	1.35 (1.12–1.63)	0.002		
Diabetes Mellitus	1.51 (1.27–1.80)	< 0.001	1.30 (1.08–1.55)	0.005
COPD	1.63 (1.33–1.99)	< 0.001		
HFPEF	1.11 (0.90–1.36)	0.34		
Ischaemic aetiology	1.09 (0.92–1.30)	0.33		
NYHA class III-IV	3.14 (2.63–3.74)	< 0.001	1.85 (1.53–2.24)	< 0.001
Systolic BP (per 10 mmHg)	0.97 (0.93–1.01)	0.112		
Heart rate (per 10 bpm)	1.09 (1.03–1.16)	0.004		
BMI (1 kg/m^2)	0.96 (0.95–0.98)	< 0.001		
ACE-I or ARB	0.37 (0.29–0.46)	< 0.001	0.70 (0.55–0.89)	0.004
Beta blockers	0.41 (0.33–0.51)	< 0.001	0.59 (0.47–0.74)	< 0.001
Diuretics	2.46 (1.77–3.42)	< 0.001	1.66 (1.19–2.31)	0.005
MRAs	0.97 (0.82–1.16)	0.77		
Digoxin	1.26 (1.05–1.52)	0.015		
ICD	0.72 (0.52–0.98)	0.039		
Iron deficiency	1.32 (1.11–1.57)	0.002	1.09 (0.91–1.31)	0.337
Haemoglobin (per 1 g/dL)	0.78 (0.75–0.82)	< 0.001	0.90 (0.85–0.95)	< 0.001
Log NT-proBNP (per 1 SD)	1.93 (1.76–2.11)	< 0.001	1.49 (1.34–1.66)	< 0.001
Sodium (per 5 mmol/L)	0.78 (0.69–0.88)	< 0.001	0.96 (0.94–0.99)	0.003
eGFR (per 5 ml/min/1.73m^2)	0.89 (0.87–0.91)	< 0.001		

HR Hazard Ratio, *COPD* Chronic Obstructive Pulmonary Disease, *HFPEF* Heart failure with preserved ejection fraction, *NYHA* New York Heart Association, *BP* Blood pressure, *BMI* Body mass index, *ACE-I* Angiotensin converting enzyme inhibitor, *ARB* Angiotensin II receptor blocker, *MRAs* Mineralocorticoid receptor antagonists, *ICD* Implantable cardioverter defibrillator, *Log* Logarithmic transformation, *NTproBNP* N-terminal pro-brain natriuretic peptide, *SD* Standard deviation, *eGFR* Estimated glomerular filtration rate

Variables introduced in the multivariate model were: Age, gender, ischaemic aetiology, systolic BP, HFPEF, diabetes mellitus, hypertension, COPD, BMI, NYHA functional class III-IV, haemoglobin, logNT-proBNP, eGFR, sodium, heart rate, treatment with beta blockers, ACE-i/ARBs, diuretics, digoxin and an ICD

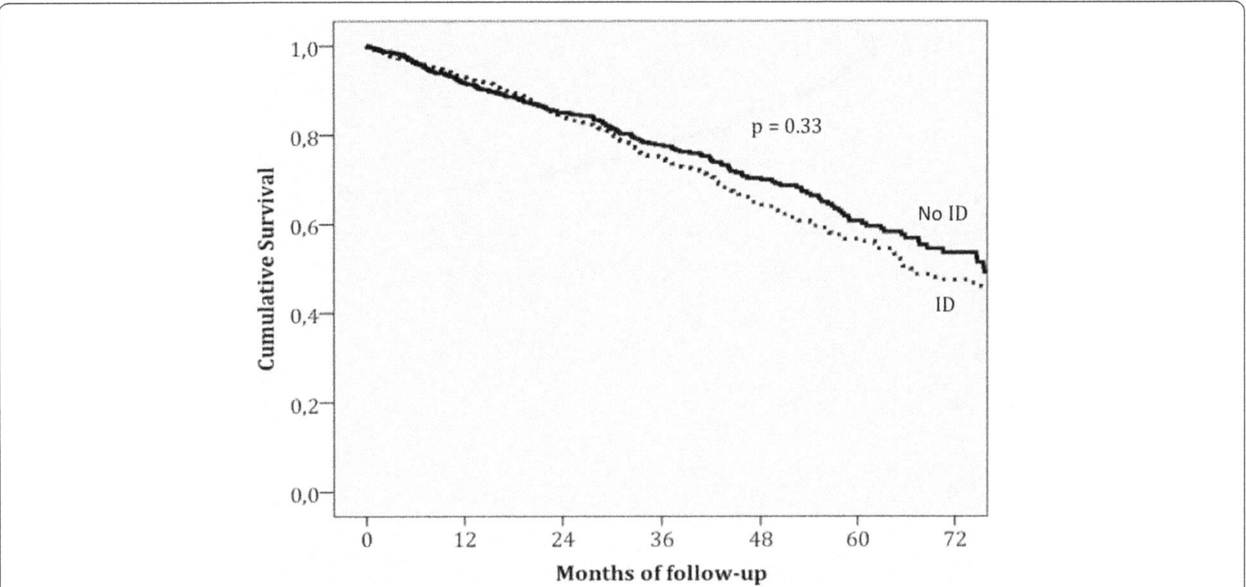

Fig. 2 Survival curves stratified for ID after adjustment for the covariates that are significant in the multivariate model: Age, sex, diabetes mellitus, New York Heart Association class III-IV, haemoglobin, logarithmic transformation of N-terminal pro-brain natriuretic peptide, serum sodium, and treatment with an angiotensin converting enzyme inhibitor or angiotensin II receptor blocker, beta blockers and diuretics

Table 4 Predictors of heart failure hospitalization using Cox regression analysis

Variables	Univariate HR	*P* value	Multivariate HR	*P* value
Age (per 5 years)	1.23 (1.18–1.29)	< 0.001	1.11 (1.05–1.17)	< 0.001
Female sex	1.50 (1.25–1.83)	< 0.001		
Hypertension	1.47 (1.19–1.81)	< 0.001		
Diabetes Mellitus	1.46 (1.20–1.77)	< 0.001	1.26 (1.03–1.54)	0.026
COPD	1.76 (1.41–2.19)	< 0.001	1.63 (1.28–2.07)	< 0.001
HFPEF	1.60 (1.30–1.97)	< 0.001	1.67 (1.31–2.18)	< 0.001
Ischaemic aetiology	1.14 (0.95–1.38)	0.166	1.40 (1.12–1.73)	0.003
NYHA class III-IV	2.55 (2.10–3.09)	< 0.001	1.64 (1.33–2.03)	< 0.001
Systolic BP (per 10 mmHg)	0.97 (0.93–1.01)	0.123		
Heart rate (per 10 bpm)	1.09 (1.03–1.16)	0.005		
BMI (per 1 kg/m^2)	0.99 (0.97–1.01)	0.21		
ACE-I or ARB	0.47 (0.37–0.61)	< 0.001		
Beta blockers	0.46 (0.36–0.58)	< 0.001	0.71 (0.54–0.93)	0.013
Diuretics	3.47 (2.28–5.28)	< 0.001	2.53 (1.64–3.91)	< 0.001
MRAs	1.10 (0.91–1.33)	0.327		
Digoxin	1.13 (0.91–1.40)	0.263		
ICD	0.91 (0.66–1.27)	0.581		
Iron deficiency	1.21 (1.00–1.47)	0.047	0.96 (0.78–1.17)	0.677
Haemoglobin (per 1 g/dL)	0.84 (0.80–0.89)	< 0.001		
Log NT-proBNP (per 1 SD)	2.00 (1.87–2.15)	< 0.001	1.49 (1.32–1.68)	< 0.001
Sodium (per 5 mmol/L)	0.93 (0.81–1.07)	0.328		
eGFR (per 5 ml/min/1.73m^2)	0.95 (0.93–0.97)	< 0.001		

HR Hazard Ratio, *COPD* Chronic Obstructive Pulmonary Disease, *HFPEF* Heart failure with preserved ejection fraction, *NYHA* New York Heart Association, *BP* Blood pressure, *BMI* Body mass index, *ACE-I* Angiotensin converting enzyme inhibitor, *ARB* Angiotensin II receptor blocker, *MRAs* Mineralocorticoid receptor antagonists, *ICD* Implantable cardioverter defibrillator, *Log* Logarithmic transformation, *NTproBNP* N-terminal pro-brain natriuretic peptide, *SD* Standard deviation, *eGFR* Estimated glomerular filtration rate

Variables introduced in the multivariate model were gender, age, diabetes mellitus, hypertension, BMI, ischaemic aeetiology, systolic blood pressure, COPD, HFPEF, heart rate, NYHA functional class III-IV, haemoglobin, logNT-proBNP, eGFR and treatment with ACE-i/ARBs, beta blockers, diuretics and MRAs

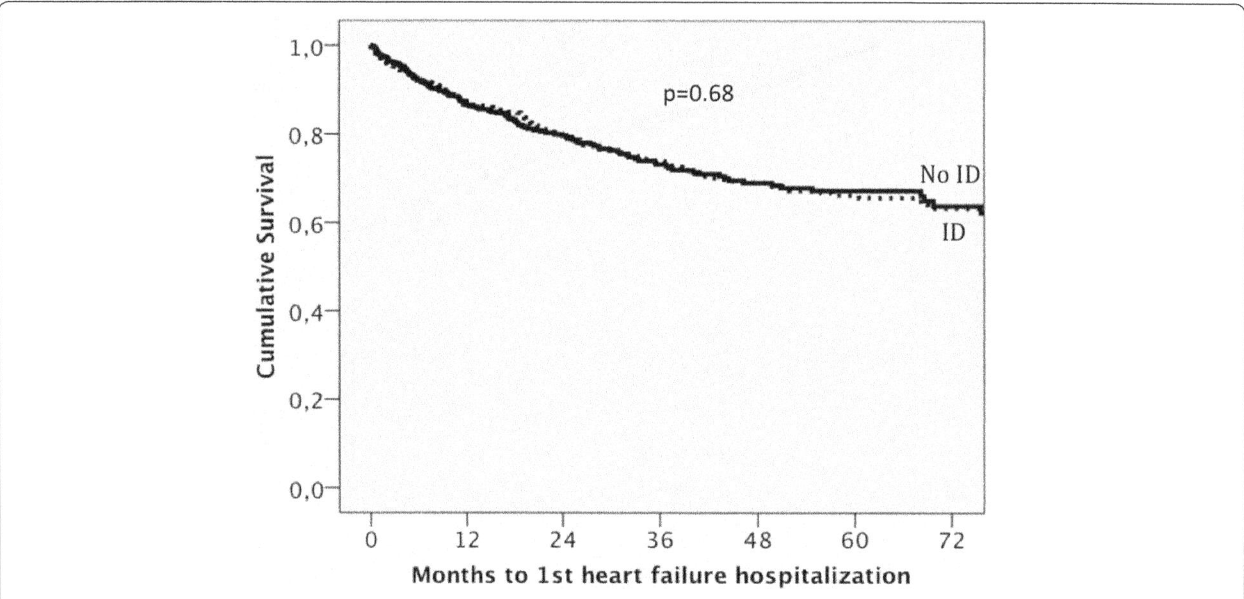

Fig. 3 Survival curves for hospitalization due to HF stratified for ID after adjustment for the covariates that are significant in the multivariate model: Age, diabetes mellitus, chronic pulmonary obstructive disease, heart failure with preserved ejection fraction, ischaemic aetiology, New York Heart Association class III-IV, logarithmic transformation of N-terminal pro-brain natriuretic peptide, and treatment with an angiotensin converting enzyme inhibitor or angiotensin II receptor blocker, beta blockers and diuretics

hospitalization due to HF stratified for ID and adjusted for the covariates that were significant in the multivariate model.

Iron deficiency and hospitalizations due to any cause

Patients with ID had 465 (52%) hospitalizations due to any cause with an Incidence Rate of 0.284 per year compared with those without ID, who had 363 (46%) hospitalizations due to any cause, with an incidence rate of 0.226 per year. The incidence ratio was 1.26 (95% confidence interval: 1.09–1.44; $p = 0.001$).

Patients with functional ID had a rate of hospitalizations due to any cause of 0.266 per year compared with 0.290 per year in those with absolute ID, $p = 0.36$. ID was not a predictor of hospitalization due to any cause after multivariate analysis. Table 5 shows the predictors of hospitalization due to any cause after univariate and multivariate adjustment. Figure 4 shows the survival curves for hospitalization due to any cause stratified for ID and adjusted for the covariates that were significant in the multivariate model.

Discussion

The main findings of our study are:

1. ID was present in more than half of a large cohort of ambulatory patients with chronic HF.
2. ID did not predict mortality after multivariate adjustment.
3. ID did not predict increased hospitalizations due to heart failure or due to any cause after multivariate adjustment.

ID was very prevalent in our cohort of patients with chronic HF and most of it was due to absolute ID. Predictors of ID after multivariate analysis were female gender, a higher body mass index, more advanced functional class, increased systolic blood pressure and lower haemoglobin values. These findings are comparable to previous findings from other groups [1–3, 14].

Iron deficiency and mortality

ID has been shown to be a marker of increased mortality independently of anaemia and CKD [1, 2, 14], but in our study we were not able to demonstrate it after multivariate analysis. However haemoglobin remained a significant predictor of mortality, as in the study by Parikh et al. [3]. We can only hypothesize why this is, but one major difference is that in our study the number of patients with HFPEF was significant compared with none in the study by Jankowska et al. [1] and 13% in the study by Klip et al. [14]. In the study by Parikh et al. [3] this data is unknown but given the relatively high mean systolic blood pressure, large proportion of women and age of the population it is likely that many of the participants had HFPEF. When we analyzed if ID was a predictor of mortality only in patients with systolic dysfunction, in our cohort it was not significant in

Table 5 Predictors of hospitalization due to any cause using Cox regression analysis

Variables	Univariate HR	*P* value	Multivariate HR	*P* value
Age (per 5 years)	1.17 (1.13–1.20)	< 0.001	1.06 (1.02–1.09)	0.001
Female sex	1.29 (1.12–1.45)	< 0.001		
Hypertension	1.42 (1.22–1.65)	< 0.001		
Diabetes Mellitus	1.46 (1.27–1.68)	< 0.001	1.23 (1.06–1.42)	0.006
COPD	1.56 (1.32–1.84)	< 0.001	1.44 (1.21–1.71)	< 0.001
HFPEF	1.40 (1.20–1.63)	< 0.001	1.44 (1.21–1.73)	< 0.001
Ischaemic aetiology	1.16 (1.01–1.33)	0.032	1.32 (1.14–1.54)	< 0.001
NYHA class III-IV	2.03 (1.77–2.34)	< 0.001	1.40 (1.20–1.64)	< 0.001
Systolic BP (per 10 mmHg)	1.01 (0.98–1.04)	0.522		
Heart rate (per 10 bpm)	1.13 (1.08–1.19)	< 0.001	1.07 (1.02–1.12)	0.006
BMI (per 1 kg/m^2)	0.99 (0.97–0.99)	0.033		
ACE-I or ARB	0.50 (0.41–0.61)	< 0.001	0.80 (0.65–0.98)	0.030
Beta blockers	0.51 (0.43–0.62)	< 0.001	0.69 (0.57–0.86)	0.001
Diuretics	1.70 (1.36–2.12)	< 0.001	1.31 (1.04–1.65)	0.022
MRAs	0.95 (0.83–1.09)	0.488		
Digoxin	1.01 (0.86–1.18)	0.940		
ICD	0.88 (0.69–1.12)	0.284		
Iron deficiency	1.21 (1.05–1.39)	0.007	0.99 (0.86–1.14)	0.857
Haemoglobin (per 1 g/dL)	0.85 (0.81–0.88)	< 0.001	0.94 (0.90–0.98)	0.002
LogNT-proBNP (per 1 SD)	1.53 (1.42–1.64)	< 0.001	1.31 (1.20–1.42)	< 0.001
Sodium (per 5 mmol/L)	0.89 (0.80–0.98)	0.023		
eGFR (per 5 ml/min/1.73m^2)	0.95 (0.94–0.96)	< 0.001		

HR Hazard Ratio, *COPD* Chronic Obstructive Pulmonary Disease, *HFPEF* Heart failure with preserved ejection fraction, *NYHA* New York Heart Association, *BP* Blood pressure, *bpm* beats per minute, *BMI* Body mass index, *ACE-I* Angiotensin converting enzyme inhibitor, *ARB* Angiotensin II receptor blocker, *MRAs* Mineralocorticoid receptor antagonists, *ICD* Implantable cardioverter defibrillator, *Log* Logarithmic transformation, *NTproBNP* N-terminal pro-brain natriuretic peptide, *SD* Standard deviation, *eGFR* Estimated glomerular filtration rate

We included the following variables in the multivariate analysis: Haemoglobin, sex, age, HFPEF, BMI, Diabetes Mellitus, Hypertension, COPD, ischaemic aetiology, logNTproBNP, eGFR, serum sodium, systolic BP, heart rate, NYHA functional class III-IV and treatment with ACE-I/ARB, Beta-blockers and diuretics

multivariate analysis. Our patients were more likely to be older and had more CKD and anaemia compared to those studied in the 3 previously mentioned cohorts and this may imply that other factors besides ID may be more important in predicting mortality in our patients. The variables that predicted mortality in our patients are otherwise not different from those previously described in the literature [9, 15].

We used the definition of ID according to the FAIR-HF trial [8]. However, diagnosis based on TSAT and ferritin may be inadequate in advanced disease or acute HF, where ferritin becomes an unreliable marker [16]. In our cohort of ambulatory patients with chronic HF, ferritin did not predict mortality in univariate analysis and the driver of adverse prognosis was the TSAT.

Iron deficiency and hospitalizations

Hospitalizations due to HF are frequent in patients with chronic HF and linked with increased mortality [17], impairment of patient's quality of life and an economic burden for the health system [18]. Although ID has been shown to be a key determinant of health-related quality of life in patients with chronic HF [19], we are not aware that the association between ID and increased risk of hospitalizations due to HF or due to any cause has been studied in patients with chronic HF. Our study is the first to do so, and we have shown that ID was associated with hospitalizations due to HF in univariate analysis but not after multivariate analysis. When we looked at predictors of hospitalization due to HF we found that they were very similar to those that predicted mortality. The only difference being that lower serum sodium and lower haemoglobin predicted mortality but not hospitalizations due to HF. On the other hand, chronic obstructive pulmonary disease, HFPEF and ischaemic etiology were associated with increased risk of hospitalization due to HF but not with mortality. Patients with chronic HF such as those seen in our study and in recent registries have many comorbidities [20], and hospitalizations may be related to these comorbidities. Therefore, we thought it would be interesting to look at hospitalizations due to any cause. ID was a predictor of hospitalizations due to any cause in

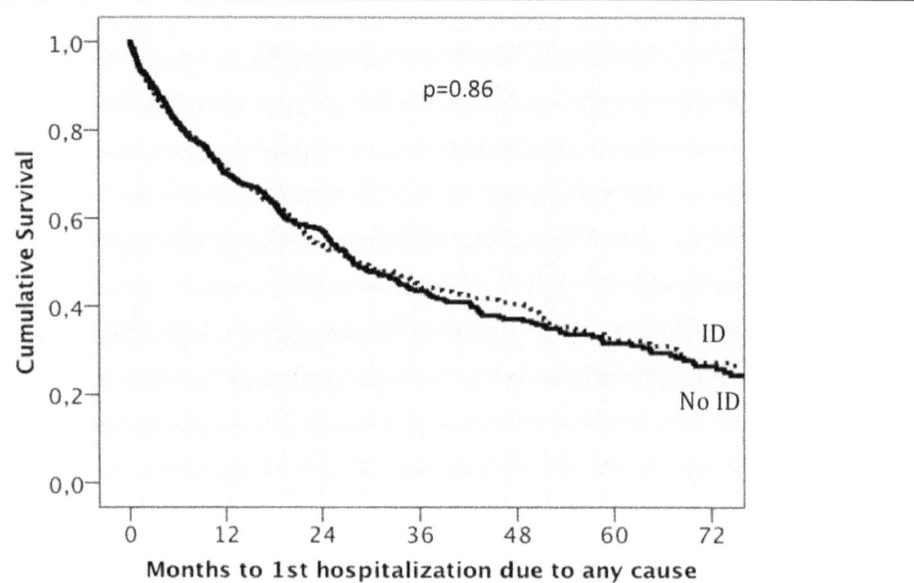

Fig. 4 Survival curves for hospitalization due to any cause stratified for ID after adjustment for the covariates that are significant in the multivariate model: Age, diabetes mellitus, chronic pulmonary obstructive disease, heart failure with preserved ejection fraction, New York Heart Association class III-IV, heart rate, haemoglobin, logarithmic transformation of N-terminal pro-brain natriuretic peptide, and treatment with an angiotensin converting enzyme inhibitor or angiotensin II receptor blocker, beta blockers and diuretics

univariate analysis, but again not after multivariate analysis. Predictors of hospitalization due to any cause were multiple and included all that predicted mortality and all that predicted hospitalizations due to HF, except for female sex and serum sodium, but with the addition of heart rate. What stands out from our analysis is that HFPEF was associated with a higher risk of hospitalizations due to heart failure or to any cause, and this may be related not so much to heart failure itself but to the increased cardiovascular and non-cardiovascular comorbidities of patients with HFPEF [21]. One comorbidity that is particularly prevalent in HFPEF is chronic pulmonary obstructive disease [22], and it is notable that in our cohort it was strongly associated with increased hospitalizations due to HF and to any cause but not with mortality, as has been shown in previous studies of patients with HF [23, 24].

It is plausible that in our cohort, other factors might diminish the importance of ID as a predictor of hospitalizations. However, our patient population clearly resembles the usual patients seen in clinical practice [18] and our results issue a word of caution in extrapolating that ID is linked with increased hospitalizations either due to HF or to any cause. Therefore, further studies are needed to evaluate this association, and in this direction, a report linking ID with 30 days readmission in patients with acute heart failure was recently published [25].

Iron deficiency in non-anaemic patients

In the FAIR-HF trial, treatment of ID with ferric carboximaltose in patients with chronic HF was equally efficacious in anaemic and in non-anaemic patients [26]. Given the fact that in our study, anaemia but not ID predicted mortality, we explored the association of ID with prognosis in non-anaemic patients. Although ID predicted increased mortality and hospitalizations in univariate analysis, this association did not hold up in multivariate analysis.

Limitations

We did not measure other markers of ID, such as the soluble transferrin receptor, hepcidin or the ferritin index that may better evaluate iron metabolism in patients with chronic heart failure [5, 27, 28]. We also did not assess C-reactive protein, high-sensitivity cardiac troponin T, and high-sensitivity soluble ST2, which have been associated with increased mortality in patients with chronic HF [3, 15]. We had no information regarding other non-cardiovascular comorbidities such as cancer or liver disease that could be potential confounders of outcomes in such an elderly population.

We excluded from the analysis patients that received treatment with intravenous iron or erythropoietin, creating a possible bias. However, this treatment was not approved by the guidelines at the time the study was performed and given that both these treatments could influence ID, we preferred to exclude these patients.

When assessing hospitalizations we did not look at recurrent number of hospitalizations, and this is also an important outcome that influences quality of life in patients with HF.

Conclusions

In a contemporary cohort of patients with chronic HF, ID was present in more than half of the patients. However, its presence was not a predictor of mortality or hospitalizations due to HF or to any cause after multivariate adjustment. Further studies are needed to assess the prognostic significance of ID in real life patients with chronic HF and where HFPEF is increasingly prevalent.

Abbreviations

CKD: Chronic kidney disease; HF: Heart failure; HFPEF: Heart failure with preserved ejection fraction; ID: Iron deficiency; NT-proBNP: N-terminal pro-brain-type natriuretic peptide; TSAT: Transferrin saturation index

Acknowledgments

We would like to thank Dr. Julián Rodríguez Larrea for support in performing the statistical analysis and the CERCA Programme/Generalitat de Catalunya for institutional support.

Funding

The design and collection of the data by the investigators from Hospital Germans Trias i Pujol was supported by Red de Investigación Cardiovascular – RIC (RD12/0042/0047) and Fondo de Investigación Sanitaria, Instituto de Salud Carlos III (FIS PI14/01682) projects as part of the Plan Nacional de I + D + I and cofounded by ISCIII-Subdirección General de Evaluación y el Fondo Europeo de Desarrollo Regional (FEDER).

Authors' contributions

JGC, JCC, JL and ABG devised the study and developed it. JGC, CE, MDA, LF, PMB, NF and EZ collected data, JGC analyzed the data and wrote the manuscript. JCC, JL, NM, RP and ABG contributed to the manuscript review process, including analysis and interpretation of the data and provided significant ideas for the execution of the study. All authors critically reviewed the manuscript for important intellectual content, approved the final manuscript and agree to be accountable for all aspects of the work.

Competing interests

JCC has received speaking fees from Vifor Pharma and was a member of the steering committee of the FAIR-HF and CONFIRM-HF studies. None of the other authors have any conflicts of interest.

Author details

[1]Area de Enfermedades del Corazón, Hospital Universitari de Bellvitge, IDIBELL, Universitat de Barcelona, L'Hospitalet de Llobregat, Feixa Llarga SN, 08907 Barcelona, Spain. [2]Servicio de Cardiología, Hospital del Mar, IMIM, Universitat Autònoma de Barcelona, Barcelona, Spain. [3]Unidad de Insuficiencia Cardíaca, Hospital Universitari Germans Trias i Pujol, Universitat Autònoma de Barcelona, Badalona, Barcelona, Spain. [4]Servicio de Medicina Interna, Hospital Universitari de Bellvitge, IDIBELL, University of Barcelona, L'Hospitalet de Llobregat, Barcelona, Spain.

References

1. Jankowska EA, Rozentryt P, Witkowska A, Nowak J, Hartman O, Ponikowska B, et al. Iron deficiency: an ominous sign in patients with systolic chronic heart failure. Eur Heart J. 2010;31:1872–80.
2. Klip IT, Jankowska EA, Enjuanes C, Voors AA, Banasiak W, Bruguera J, et al. The additive burden of iron deficiency in the cardiorenal-anaemia axis: scope of a problem and its consequences. Eur J Heart Fail. 2014;16:655–62.
3. Parikh A, Natarajan S, Lipsitz SR, Katz SD. Iron deficiency in community-dwelling US adults with self-reported heart failure in the National Health and nutrition examination survey III. Prevalence and association with anaemia and inflammation. Circ Heart Fail. 2011;4:599–606.
4. González-Costello J, Comin-Colet J. Iron deficiency and anaemia in heart failure: understanding the FAIR-HF trial. Eur J Heart Fail. 2010;12:1159–62.
5. Jankowska EA, Malyszko J, Ardehali H, Koc-Zorawska E, Banasiak W, von Haehling S, et al. Iron status in patients with chronic heart failure. Eur Heart J. 2013;34:827–34.
6. Haddad S, Wang Y, Galy B, Korf-Klingebiel M, Hirsch V, Baru AM, et al. Iron-regulatory proteins secure iron availability in cardiomyocytes to prevent heart failure. Eur Heart J. 2017;38:362–72.
7. Lewis GD, Malhotra R, Hernandez AF, McNulty SE, Smith A, Felker M, et al. Effect of oral iron repletion on exercise capacity in patients with heart failure with reduced ejection fraction and iron deficiency. The IRONOUT HF randomized clinical trial. JAMA. 2017;317:1958–66.
8. Anker SD, Colet JC, Filippatos G, Willenheimer R, Dickstein K, Drexler H, et al. Ferric carboxymaltose in patients with heart failure and iron deficiency. N Engl J Med. 2009;361:2436–48.
9. Ponikowski P, van Veldhuisen DJ, Comin-Colet J, Ertl G, Komajda M, Mareev V, et al. Beneficial effects of long-term intravenous iron therapy with ferric carboxymaltose in patients with symptomatic heart failure and iron deficiency. Eur Heart J. 2014;36:657–68.
10. Jankowska EA, Tkaczyszyn M, Suchocki T, Drozd M, von Haeling S, Doehner W, et al. Effects of intravenous iron therapy in iron-deficient patients with systolic heart failure: a meta-analysis of randomized controlled trials. Eur J Heart Fail. 2016;18:786–95.
11. Van Veldhuisen DJ, Ponikowski P, van der Meer P, Metra M, Bohm M, Doletsky A, et al. Effect of ferric carboxymaltose on exercise capacity in patients with chronic heart failure and iron deficiency. Circulation. 2017;136: 1374–83.
12. Ponikowski P, Voors AA, Anker SD, Bueno H, Cleland JGF, Coats AJS, et al. Guidelines for the diagnosis and treatment of acute and chronic heart failure. The task force for the diagnosis and treatment of acute and chronic heart failure of the European Society of Cardiology. Developed with the special contribution of the heart failure association (HFA) of the ESC. Eur Heart J. 2016;37:2129–200.
13. Wu A. Tietz Clinical Guide to Laboratory Tests. 4th ed. St Louis, MO: Saunders Elsevier; 2006. p. 56–61.
14. Klip IT, Comin-Colet J, Voors AA, Ponikowski P, Enjuanes C, Banasiak W, et al. Iron deficiency in chronic heart failure: an international pooled analysis. Am Heart J. 2013;165:575–82.
15. Lupón J, de Antonio M, Vila J, Peñafiel J, Galán A, Zamora E, et al. Development of a novel heart failure risk tool: the Barcelona bio-heart failure risk calculator (BCN bio-HF calculator). PLoS One. 2014;9:e85466.
16. Jankowska EA, Kasztura M, Sokolski M, Bronisz M, Nawrocka S, Oleskowska-Florek W, et al. Iron deficiency defined as depleted iron stores accompanied by unmet cellular iron requirements identifies patients at the highest risk of death after an episode of acute heart failure. Eur Heart J. 2014;35:2468–76.
17. Fang J, Mensah GA, Croft JB, Keenan NL. Heart failure-related hospitalization in the U.S., 1979 to 2004. J Am Coll Cardiol. 2008;52:428–34.
18. Berry C, Murdoch DR, McMurray JJ. Economics of chronic heart failure. Eur J Heart Fail. 2001;3:283–91.
19. Comin-Colet J, Enjuanes C, Gonzalez G, Torrens A, Cladellas M, Meroño O, et al. Iron deficiency is a key determinant of health-related quality of life in patients with chronic heart failure regardless of anaemia status. Eur J Heart Fail. 2013;15:1164–72.
20. Crespo-Leiro MG, Segovia-Cubero J, González-Costello J, Bayes-Genis A, López-Fernández S, Roig E, et al. Adherence to the ESC Heart Failure Treatment Guidelines in Spain: ESC Heart Failure Long-term Registry. Rev Esp Cardiol. 2015;68:785–93.
21. Lund LH, Donal E, Oger E, Hage C, Persson H, Haugen-Löfman I, et al. Association between cardiovascular vs. non-cardiovascular co-morbidities and outcomes in heart failure with preserved ejection fraction. Eur J Heart Fail. 2014;16:992–1001.
22. Iversen KK, Kjaergaard J, Akkan D, Kober L, Torp-Pedersen C, Hassager C, et al. Chronic obstructive pulmonary disease in patients admitted with heart failure. J Intern Med. 2008;264:361–9.
23. Rusinaru D, Saaidi I, Godard S, Mahjoub H, Battle C, Tribouilloy C. Impact of chronic obstructive pulmonary disease on long-term outcome of patients hospitalized for heart failure. Am J Cardiol. 2008;101:353–8.

26

Using an introduced index to assess the association between food diversity and metabolic syndrome and its components in Chinese adults

Wenzhi Zhao, Jian Zhang, Ai Zhao, Meichen Wang, Wei Wu, Shengjie Tan, Mofan Guo and Yumei Zhang*

Abstract

Background: It is reported that an increase in food diversity would lower the risk of cardiac–cerebral vascular diseases.

Methods: A new index was introduced to develop a Chinese healthy food diversity (HFD) index, exploring the association with metabolic syndrome (MetS) and its components among Chinese adults. Two sets of data were used. The primary data were from a cross-sectional survey conducted in 2016 called the Chinese Urban Adults Diet and Health Study (CUADHS); the verification data were from the China Health and Nutrition Survey (CHNS) of 2009. The Chinese HFD index was developed according to the Chinese Dietary Guideline, with food consumption information from 24-h dietary recalls. The association between the index and MetS and its components was explored in logistic regression models.

Results: Among 1520 participants in the CUADHS, the crude prevalence of MetS was 36.4%, which was 29.0% after the standardisation of age and gender by the 2010 Chinese national census. In the CUADHS, the HFD index ranged from 0.04 to 0.63. The value of the index among participants who are male, young, poorly educated, drinking or smoking, and with high energy intakes was significantly lower than that of their counterparts. In the verification dataset of the CHNS, there were 2398 participants, and the distribution of different genders and age groups was more balanced. The crude prevalence of MetS in the CHNS was 27.3% and the standardised prevalence was 19.5%. The Chinese HFD index ranged from 0.02 to 0.62. In the CUADHS, the Chinese HFD index was not significantly associated with MetS in covariate-adjusted models or with its components. In the CHNS, the Chinese HFD index had a significantly negative correlation with MetS and its components (i.e., elevated fasting glucose and elevated waist circumference) in covariate-adjusted models.

Conclusions: Increased food diversity may decrease the risk of MetS, which is important in dietary interventions of cardiac–cerebral vascular disease. This underscores the necessity of continued investigation into the role of HFD in the prevention of MetS and provides an integral framework for ongoing research.

Keywords: Metabolic syndrome, Diet, Healthy food diversity, Adult

* Correspondence: zhangyumei@bjmu.edu.cn
Department of Nutrition and Food Hygiene, School of Public Health, Peking University Health Science Center, Xueyuan Road 38, Haidian District, 100191 Beijing, China

Background

Metabolic syndrome (MetS) is a clustering of risk factors for cardiovascular disease (CVD) and type 2 diabetes and has been a public health challenge globally [1–3]. People diagnosed with MetS have a five-time higher risk of developing type 2 diabetes and are twice as likely to develop CVD within the next 5–10 years [4, 5]. It has been reported that the occurrence of MetS increases total mortality by 1.5 times and cardiovascular death by 2.5 times [5, 6]. The prevalence of MetS is striking in both developed and developing countries. The National Health and Nutrition Examination Survey (NHANES) of the United States showed that the prevalence of MetS among adults increased from 25.3% in 1988–1994 to 34.2% in 2007–2012. The Korean National Health and Nutrition Examination Survey (KNHANES) from 2008 to 2013 found a stable prevalence of 28.9%. In China's most recent national survey in 2009, a prevalence of 21.3% was reported [6–8]. It should be noticed that the prevalence of MetS in different areas of China was largely altered, ranging from 20 to 45% [9–11].

Environmental factors, including diet, exercise, stress, and certain addictions (tobacco or alcohol), as well as genetic factors are crucial in the development of MetS [12–14]. Lifestyle modification, such as dietary intervention, is recommended to manage MetS. Studies have reported that some dietary components influence MetS directly, as either protective factors or risk factors [15–19]. There are many researches focusing on the association between dietary pattern or kinds of indices evaluating dietary quality and MetS. However, it is difficult for most people to develop and sustain healthful dietary patterns with individual knowledge and self-control, particularly given that transformations in diet environments have expanded access to all kinds of food [12, 20–22]. The increasing dietary variety comes with benefits and challenges. On the one hand, it avoids malnutrition; on the other hand, it may result in overweight and obesity [23–25].

Dietary guidelines recommended by government institutions or national nutrition associations provide guidance to the public and serve as referential files when designing dietary and nutritional interventions. Researchers in Germany and the US developed and validated a healthy food diversity (HFD) index based on actual food guidelines and explored the correlation between HFD and body adiposity and MetS [26–28]. The US researchers found that the HFD index values were inversely associated with indicators of body adiposity; the odds of obesity and android-to-gynoid ratio > 1 are lower among those with a higher US HFD index [26]. In a randomised-controlled clinical weight-loss trial, participants with a higher US HFD index had greater weight loss and waist circumference (WC) reduction [29]. Besides, the US HFD index was inversely associated with components of MetS, including elevated WC and low HDL cholesterol [27].

The latest version of the dietary guidelines in China was released in 2016, and up to now there is no study introducing the Chinese HFD index. It is necessary and meaningful to develop and evaluate an index considering food type, quality, and consumption amounts simultaneously, and to explore its association with health conditions in Chinese adults in order to guide dietary interventions.

In this study, we developed the Chinese HFD index based on the Dietary Guidelines for Chinese Residents and then examined its associations with MetS and its components in urban adults.

Methods

Study design and participants

There were two sets of data in the analysis. The primary data were from a cross-sectional survey designed and conducted by our team, the Chinese Urban Adults Diet and Health Study (CUADHS), conducted from March to July 2016, in which a multi-stage sampling method was utilised to recruit adult subjects. Firstly, eight cities were selected based on geographical location and economic status, including two first-tier cities with higher economic performance. Secondly, two communities from each first-tier city and one community from each non-first-tier city were chosen by convenience sampling. In the last step, subjects were recruited by age groups, with at least 60 people from the age group of 18–44 years, 60 from 45 to 64 years, and 50 from over 65 years in each community. The study recruited 1806 subjects, and those with a physical disability, mental illness, or memory problems and women who were pregnant were excluded from analysis. In the end, a total of 1520 subjects were considered eligible for this study. We obtained a formal written agreement from each participant.

The verification data were from the China Health and Nutrition Survey (CHNS) of 2009. The CHNS is an international collaborative project between the National Institute for Nutrition and Food Safety of the Chinese Centre for Disease Control and Prevention, and the University of North Carolina at Chapel Hill. As a longitudinal, household-based survey, it was conducted in 1989, 1991, 1993, 1997, 2000, 2004, 2006, 2009, and 2011 in sequence. Only the survey conducted in 2009 contained information about blood biochemical examination. Details are provided elsewhere [30]. Questionnaires and blood biochemical tests were used to collect information of adults (except pregnant women) living in urban areas (i.e., residence in city and town or county capital city). In this study, we analysed 2398 individuals from the CHNS who met our inclusion criteria described in the data collection section.

Data collection

In the CUADHS, the interviewer-administered questionnaires contained questions about socio-demographic characteristics, lifestyles, disease history, health literacy, dietary intakes, and physical examination. Anthropometry measurement and blood tests were also conducted. The food frequency questionnaire (FFQ) and 24-h dietary recall for 1 day were used in this study to collect dietary intake information. The FFQ was a semi-quantitative questionnaire, in which 41 groups of food were asked about regarding the frequency and amount of consumption within the past month. Intakes of different kinds of alcohol and beverages were included. One-time 24-h dietary recall was used to obtain the data on food intakes, and then nutrient intakes were calculated based on it. About 1/8 (205 adults) of the subjects were invited to complete the 24-h dietary recall for 3 days to evaluate the representativeness of one-time 24-h dietary recall. Energy and nutrient intakes were calculated and analysed based on the Chinese Food Composition Tables (CFCT) of 2004 and 2009 (CFCT, National Institute of Nutrition and Food Safety, China CDC), the Standard Tables of Food Composition in Japan (2010), and the nutrient composition table on the food packaging. Training of the interviewers and a pilot investigation were completed prior to data collection.

Questionnaire information and blood biochemical indices of the CHNS 2009 were downloaded from the official website of the CHNS, and information was gathered about socio-demographic characteristics, lifestyles, disease history, 24-h dietary recalls for 3 days, consumption of household food inventory, energy and macronutrient intakes, anthropometry information, and blood biochemical indices labelled by specimen collection and processing by the China–Japan Friendship Hospital (CJFH).

Assessment of diet factors and development of the Chinese HFD index

For the CUADHS, we calculated energy and nutrient intakes based on CFCT, Standard Tables of Food Composition in Japan [31], and ingredient lists of common supplements. Then we computed the absorbed amount of special micronutrients by bioavailability adjustment, the detailed processing procedure of which is described elsewhere [32]. We referred to the FAO protocol [33] to calculate the probabilities of nutrient adequacy (PA) of some nutrients based on Chinese Dietary Reference Intakes (DRIs) 2013 edition, which included definitions and specified values for estimated average requirements (EAR) and recommended nutrient intakes (RNI). The equation was PA = Probnorm [(estimated intakes-EAR)/CV] for most nutrients except iron; the CV was set to 10% of EAR for all nutrients except vitamin A (20%), niacin (15%), and zinc (25%).

For iron, since its distribution was not normal, we used the eq. PA = estimated participant's intake/RNI. PA was defined as the ratio of a certain nutrient intake to its recommended allowance, and when intakes of a certain nutrient exceeded requirement, the value should be capped at 1, indicating 100% adequacy. We calculated the PA of protein, carbohydrates, vitamin A, niacin, vitamin B6, vitamin B1, vitamin B2, vitamin B12, vitamin C, folate, calcium, iron, and zinc. We then calculated the mean probability of adequacy (MPA) of micronutrients by applying equal weight to every individual micronutrient.

We evaluated the representativeness of one-time 24-h dietary recall in the CUADHS, and the results are showed in Additional file 1: Table S1. There were no significant differences in energy and macronutrient intakes between one-time 24-h dietary recall and three-day 24-h dietary recall. We decided that one-time 24-h dietary recall was able to represent the results of 24-h dietary recall for 3 days, which was similar to other studies [34–36].

In the CHNS the food intakes of every participant were the summation of two parts. Firstly, daily average food intake was calculated from three-day 24-h dietary recalls. Secondly, for food consumed at home, the daily amount of each ingredient from the household food inventory consumed by each individual was estimated based on his/her respective proportion of energy intake in the whole family.

For the two studies, all of the food items were divided into 15 groups according to the Dietary Guideline and Balance Diet Pagoda for Chinese Residents (as showed in Table 1), and, subsequently, the consumption of each food group was calculated, respectively. Though there were only 12 food groups in the Balance Diet Pagoda, in the detailed Dietary Guidelines there were precise recommended daily/weekly intakes of 15 food groups, in which cereals, tubers, and beans were divided into three groups: whole grains and legumes, tubers, and refined grains. Soya and nuts were divided into two groups: soya products and nuts and seeds [37]. According to similar research [28, 38], weight based on the recommended proportions of each food group at the 2000-kcal level in the Dietary Guideline and Balance Diet Pagoda for Chinese Residents was selected to build the Chinese HFD index (Table 1). There was no precise definition for dark green and yellow or orange vegetables in the recommendation, so we redefined them as vegetables rich in vitamin A (content of vitamin A ≥ 150 RAE/100 g; RAE = retinol equivalent) or vitamin C (content of vitamin C ≥ 50 mg/100 g). The Chinese HFD index values were calculated using the following algorithm:

Table 1 Development of health factors (hf) for each food group according to recommendations based on the energy intake of 2000 kcal

Food groups	Recommended amount (g)	Share of food group (broad or single)	hf
Emphases	1300	0.81	
Whole grains and legumes	100	0.08	0.06
Tubers	75	0.06	0.05
Other vegetables	225	0.17	0.14
Vitamin A- or vitamin C-rich vegetables[a]	225	0.17	0.14
Fruits	300	0.23	0.19
Dairy[b]	300	0.23	0.19
Soya products[c]	15	0.01	0.01
Nuts and seeds	10	0.01	0.01
Aquatic products	50	0.04	0.03
Includes	275	0.17	
Refined grains	150	0.55	0.09
Meat and poultry	50	0.18	0.03
Eggs	50	0.18	0.03
Oil	25	0.09	0.02
Limits	31	0.02	
Salt	6	0.19	0.00
Added sugar	25	0.81	0.02

Note: [a] = dark green and yellow or orange vegetables in the Dietary Guideline and Balance Diet Pagoda for Chinese Residents;
[b]= liquid milk based on food exchanging of all kinds of dairy
[c]= soybean based on food exchanging of all kinds of soy foods

Chinese HFD index=$(1-\sum S_i^2) \times$ hv,
in which $S_i = \frac{\textit{Amount of recommended food group i by weight}}{\textit{Amount of 15 food groups by weight}}$,
hv = $\sum hf_i \times S_i$, hf_i = *Broad food share* × *share of food group*,
where S_i is the quantitative share of a single food group; hv is the health value; and hf_i is health factors.

Theoretically, the range of the Chinese HFD index is between 0 (i.e., a diet with a single food group) and nearly 1 (i.e., a more balanced diet). In fact, the maximum hv that can be achieved according to the recommendation at the 2000-kcal level is 0.187, and the Chinese HFD index was calibrated by dividing hv by its maximum. Then, the Chinese HFD index values and energy intakes were equally divided into four groups (Q1, Q2, Q3, and Q4).

Assessment of non-dietary factors

We categorised age groups as 18~ 44.9 years old, 45~ 54.9 years old, 55~ 64.9 years old, and ≥ 65 years old. Smoking status was classified as never smoked, former smoker, and current smoker. Drinking behaviours were defined as not drinking and drinking now. Physical activity (PA) levels calculated from a PA questionnaire were trisected from the smallest to the highest and marked as T1, T2, and T3, which were expressed as metabolic equivalents (MET)/d; subjects who only reported sedentary behaviours were classified as a separate group. Educational background was classified as illiterate, middle school or lower, high school or professional training, undergraduate, and postgraduate student or higher. Body mass index (BMI) was defined as weight (in kilograms) divided by the squared height (in metres). Consistent with the WHO criteria, obesity, overweight, normal, and underweight were defined as BMI ≥28 kg/m^2, BMI ≥24 kg/m^2 and < 28 kg/m^2, BMI ≥18.5 kg/m^2 and < 24 kg/m2, and BMI<18.5 kg/m^2, respectively [39].

Diagnostic criteria of MetS

The definition of MetS was consistent with the most recent Joint Interim Statement (JIS) by adopting the Asian criteria for WC recommended by the International Diabetes Federation. Indicators of MetS are shown in Table 2, and subjects were diagnosed as patients if they had at least three of the indicators [5]. The methods of measuring anthropometry indicators and blood biochemical indices are presented in Additional file 2: Table S2.

Statistical analysis

Normality was examined before the related analysis. Values were presented as mean ± standard deviation ($\overline{x} \pm SD$) for continuous variables or as number (percentage) for

Table 2 Criteria for clinical diagnosis of metabolic syndrome

No.	Measure	Categorical Cut Points
1	Elevated waist circumference (WC)	≥90 cm in males; ≥85 cm in females
2	Elevated triglycerides (TC) (drug treatment for elevated triglycerides is an alternate indicator)	≥150 mg/dL (1.7 mmol/L)
3	Reduced high-density lipoprotein cholesterol (HDL-C) (drug treatment for reduced HDL-C is an alternate indicator)	<40 mg/dL (1.0 mmol/L) in males;<50 mg/dL (1.3 mmol/L) in females
4	Elevated blood pressure (antihypertensive drug treatment in a patient with a history of hypertension is an alternate indicator)	Systolic ≥130 and/or diastolic ≥85 mmHg
5	Elevated fasting glucose (drug treatment of elevated glucose is an alternate indicator)	≥100 mg/dL

categorical variables. Student t tests or one-way ANOVA were performed to compare means between different groups. Chi-square tests or trend Chi-square tests were performed to compare the distribution of categorical variables. Kendall's tau-b correlation was tested between PA/MPA and the Chinese HFD index, with energy intake as a covariate. Binominal unconditional logistic regression models were used to estimate the effects of factors on MetS and the regression coefficients (ORs), and their 95% confidence interval (CI) was obtained. All statistical analyses were performed using the Statistic Package for Social Science (SPSS) version 20.0 (SPSS Inc., Chicago, IL, USA). *P* values lower than 0.05 were considered statistically significant.

Results

Demographic characteristics and the prevalence of MetS and its components

There were 1520 adults analysed in the CUADHS, of which 527 were male. Those who were 18~ 44.9 years old and older than 65 years accounted for about 1/3 of the total, respectively. The educational attainment of about 70% participants was high school or lower. About half of the participants never smoked and were non-drinking now. The prevalence of overweight and obesity was 35.4% and 11.0%, respectively. The detailed distribution of demographic characteristics is showed in Table 3.

Table 3 also shows that in the CUADHS the prevalence of MetS was 36.4%, which was 29.0% after standardisation of age and gender by the 2010 Chinese national census. Significant differences in the prevalence of MetS were found between different groups of gender, age, education, smoking behaviour, BMI, and HFD index. The prevalence of MetS and its five components was significantly higher in participants who are male, older, poorly educated, a former or current smoker, and overweight or obese.

In the verification data of the CHNS, 2398 participants were analysed, and the distribution of gender (47.9% male) and age groups (30.9%, 25.4%, 20.7%, and 23.0%, respectively) was more balanced than that of the CUADHS. For the educational attainment, more than 85% of the participants were high school or lower. About 70% of the participants never smoked and were non-drinking now. The prevalence of overweight and obesity was 32.7% and 11.1%, respectively. Detailed information is shown in Table 4.

The crude prevalence of MetS in the CHNS was 27.3%, and the standardised prevalence was 19.5%. The prevalence of MetS was significantly higher in participants who are older, poorly educated, overweight or obese, and lack PA, while no similar trend was found in the five components of MetS.

Distribution of the Chinese HFD index and its correlations with nutrients

In the CUADHS, the Chinese HFD index ranged from 0.04 to 0.63. The values of the index were significantly lower in participants who are male, young, poorly educated, drinking or smoking now, and with high energy intakes (Table 5).

To validate the Chinese HFD index, correlations between the Chinese HFD index and PA of nutrients were analysed, and the results are showed in Table 6. The Chinese HFD index was positively correlated with PA of carbohydrates, vitamin B2, niacin, vitamin B6, folate, vitamin A, vitamin C, and MPA of micronutrients after adjusting for energy.

In the verification study, the Chinese HFD index ranged from 0.02 to 0.62, as showed in Table 5. Participants who were male, young, poorly educated, drinking or smoking now, obese, and with the highest energy intakes had a significantly lower Chinese HFD index.

Regression analysis of the Chinese HFD index and MetS and its components

As shown in Table 7, in the CUADHS the Chinese HFD index was not significantly associated with MetS in covariate-adjusted models or its components. Only in an unadjusted model was the Chinese HFD index positively correlated with elevated fasting glucose and reduced HDL.

In the verification data of the CHNS, the results were different, as shown in Table 8. The Chinese HFD index was significantly negatively correlated with MetS and its components of elevated fasting glucose and elevated WC in covariate-adjusted models. It indicated that a higher Chinese HFD index decreased the risk of MetS.

Discussion

This study was conducted to analyse the associations between MetS and food diversity in Chinese urban adults, and the analysis was repeated in a representative sample for validation. In the two studies, the prevalence of MetS was within the range of contemporaneous researches. In this study, a multi-dimensional food diversity index in consideration of dietary quality and proportionality was applied to evaluate the associations between food diversity and MetS and its components in Chinese adults. The Chinese HFD index was positively correlated with carbohydrates and micronutrients, meaning that if one had a higher HFD index, he/she was more likely to have adequate nutrient intakes. In comparison, the correlations between the Chinese HFD index and PA of most nutrients were weaker than those of the German population (except vitamin A) and US

Table 3 General characteristics of participants and the distribution of MetS and its components of CUADHS

Factor	Group	N	Elevated WC		Elevated fasting glucose		Elevated blood pressure		Elevated TC	Reduced HDL			MetS	
			%	P	%	P	%	P	%	P	%	P	%	P
Total		1520,100	35.3		32.9		37		40.9		43.6		36.4	
Gender	Male	527,34.7	41.2	<0.001	41.7	<0.001	46.1	<0.001	47.2	<0.001	42.5	0.548	43.5	<0.001
	Female	993,65.3	32.1		28.2		32.2		37.5		44.1		32.7	
Age	18~ 44.9 years	547,36	17.6	<0.001	13.7	<0.001	9.7	<0.001	20.8	<0.001	30.2	<0.001	14.6	<0.001
	45~ 54.9 years	260,17.1	36.2		24.6		26.9		40		43.5		29.2	
	55~ 64.9 years	272,17.9	48.2		46		55.5		56.6		56.3		52.6	
	≥65 years	441,29.0	48.8		53.5		65.5		56.5		52.4		57.8	
Educational attainment	Illiterate	66,4.3	63.6	<0.001	47	<0.001	69.7	<0.001	62.1	<0.001	60.6	<0.001	69.7	<0.001
	Middle school or lower	445,29.3	46.5		45.4		51.9		49.4		47.4		46.3	
	High school or professional training education	627,41.3	32.7		28.4		32.4		40.4		46.1		34	
	Undergraduate education or higher	378,24.9	21.2		23		21.2		28.3		32.3		23	
Drinking behavior	No	942,68.5	36.3	0.427	34.9	0.594	41.3	0.027	44.8	0.188	45.8	0.315	39.7	0.212
	Yes	434,31.5	34.1		36.4		35		41		42.9		36.2	
Smoking behavior	Never smoked	1145,75.3	32.3	<0.001	30.2	<0.001	34.4	<0.001	38.4	0.002	42.4	0.066	33.1	<0.001
	Former smoker	165,10.9	46.1		46.7		53.3		44.8		42.4		46.1	
	Current smoker	210,13.8	42.9		36.7		38.6		51		51		47.1	
BMI	<18.5 kg/m2	74,4.9	0	<0.001	9.5	<0.001	5.4	<0.001	4.1	<ss0.001	12.2	<0.001	4.1	<0.001
	18.5~ 24.0 kg/m2	739,48.6	7		26		26.9		29.8		33		18.3	
	24.0~ 28.0 kg/m2	538,35.4	60.8		41.4		48.1		53.9		56.1		53.9	
	≥28.0 kg/m2	168,11.1	92.9		46.4		60.1		64.3		63.7		75	
Physical activity	Sedentary group	119,7.8	38.7	0.095	33.6	0.008	32.8	0.001	45.4	0.132	50.4	0.169	40.3	0.092
	T1	468,30.8	30.8		28.6		31		36.5		41		31.8	
	T2	466,30.7	36.3		31.1		38		42.7		45.9		38.6	
	T3	467,30.7	37.9		38.8		43.3		42.2		42		37.9	
Energy intake	Q1	380,25.0	35.8	0.964	30.3	0.121	35.3	0.647	37.6	0.485	41.3	0.71	33.7	0.639
	Q2	380,25.0	35.8		35.5		35.8		41.8		44.5		37.1	
	Q3	380,25.0	34.2		29.7		37.9		42.9		45.3		37.4	
	Q4	380,25.0	35.3		36.1		39.2		41.1		43.2		37.6	
HFD-index	Q1	368,24.2	33.2	0.764	29.9	0.166	36.1	0.295	38.6	0.196	37.5	0.014	35.3	0.035
	Q2	410,27.0	36.6		36.8		39		41.2		46.1		37.1	
	Q3	368,24.2	35.1		27.4		33.4		38.3		41.8		31.5	
	Q4	374,24.6	36.1		36.9		39.3		45.2		48.4		41.7	

Note: [a]Subjects who only reported sedentary behaviors were classified as Sedentary group, the others were trisected into three groups (T1, T2 and T3) according to the calculated metabolic equivalents (MET)/d from the smallest to the highest;
[b]Energy intakes were quadrisected into four groups (Q1, Q2, Q3 and Q4) from the smallest to the highest;
[c]Chinese HFD-Index values were quadrisected into four groups (Q1, Q2, Q3 and Q4) from the smallest to the highest

population (except vitamin C), despite the fact that the two foreign studies neglected bioavailability adjustment of minerals [28, 38]. The Chinese HFD index could reflect dietary quality to some extent.

The mean and range of the Chinese HFD index of participants in the two studies were similar, and the trend by grouping factors was also similar. The Chinese HFD index values in the two studies were comparable with

Table 4 General characteristics of participants and the distribution of MetS and its components of CHNS

Factor	Group	N	Elevated WC		Elevated fasting glucose		Elevated blood pressure		Elevated TC		Reduced HDL		MetS	
			%	P	%	P	%	P	%	P	%	P	%	P
Total		2398	36.2		33.1		33.3		36.2		28.1		27.3	
Gender	Male	1106	37	0.485	35.5	0.018	36.7	<0.001	42	<0.001	21.3	<0.001	28.7	0.171
	Female	1292	35.6		31		30.3		31.2		33.9		26.2	
Age	18~ 44.9 years	742	22.8	<0.001	20.1	<0.001	10	<0.001	32.1	0.014	28	0.935	14.3	<0.001
	45~ 54.9 years	608	33.7		31.7		27.1		36.3		27.6		23.8	
	55~ 64.9 years	496	45.4		40.7		42.5		40.9		29.2		35.9	
	≥65 years	552	48.9		45.1		63		37.3		27.7		40.9	
Educational attainment	Illiterate	192	52.1	<0.001	42.7	<0.001	61.5	<0.001	32.8	0.311	29.2	0.929	40.6	<0.001
	Middle school or lower	1145	40.1		37.7		36		37.8		28.6		30.9	
	High school or professional training education	755	28.1		26		27.3		34.3		27.7		20.4	
	Undergraduate education or higher	303	32.3		27.1		20.1		37.3		27.1		22.8	
Drinking behavior	No	1646	36.6	0.614	33.4	0.661	33.8	0.441	34	<0.001	30.9	<0.001	27.7	0.527
	Yes	752	35.5		32.4		32.2		41		21.9		26.5	
Smoking behavior	Never smoked	1735	36.7	0.788	32	0.226	31.9	<0.001	33.8	<0.001	30.5	<0.001	26.5	0.332
	Former smoker	83	34.9		36.1		55.4		38.6		19.3		31.3	
	Current smoker	580	35.2		35.7		34.1		42.9		22.1		29.1	
BMI	<18.5 kg/m2	116	2.6	<0.001	17.2	<0.001	15.5	<0.001	9.5	<0.001	17.2	<0.001	2.6	<0.001
	18.5~ 24.0 kg/m2	1221	14.2		26.9		25.6		28.3		23.8		14.9	
	24.0~ 28.0 kg/m2	779	56.6		38.5		41.1		45.7		30.8		37.7	
	≥28.0 kg/m2	264	92.8		53		52.7		55.7		44.7		64.8	
Physical activity[a]	Sedentary group	1132	43.3	<0.001	38.3	<0.001	42.8	<0.001	38.1	0.356	29.2	0.225	33.9	<0.001
	T1	463	31.3		29.8		30.9		34.8		27.6		24.4	
	T2	544	28.5		27.6		20.6		34.4		28.7		20.4	
	T3	258	30.6		27.9		22.9		34.5		22.9		18.2	
Energy intake[b]	Q1	691	35.6	0.442	34.6	0.622	37.5	0.023	34.7	0.152	30	0.093	28.7	0.752
	Q2	678	37.5		32		33.3		35.3		28.6		26.5	
	Q3	580	34		33.8		29.8		40.2		29		27.6	
	Q4	449	38.3		31.4		31.2		34.7		23.4		26.1	
HFD-index[c]	Q1	479	40.3	0.013	36.1	0.141	31.9	0.668	39.2	0.265	25.9	0.275	28.8	0.046
	Q2	519	39.5		35.3		35.1		37.6		27.6		30.3	
	Q3	579	35.1		31.8		34		35.2		31.1		28.3	
	Q4	821	32.6		30.8		32.4		34.2		27.6		23.9	

Note:[a]Subjects who only reported sedentary behaviors were classified as Sedentary group, the others were trisected into three groups (T1, T2 and T3) according to the calculated metabolic equivalents (MET)/d from the smallest to the highest;

[b]Energy intakes were quadrisected into four groups (Q1, Q2, Q3 and Q4) from the smallest to the highest;

[c]Chinese HFD-Index values were quadrisected into four groups (Q1, Q2, Q3 and Q4) from the smallest to the highest

the studies conducted in the US and Germany [27–29, 38]. They were also the same as former studies in which the participants who are old, female, and with higher educational attainment were more likely to have a higher HFD index value [26, 27]. Considering that the CUADHS and the CHNS were two independent surveys, the comparable results indicated the feasibility and applicability of the methods in the Chinese population.

Currently, economic growth and globalisation have increased access to seasonal, animal-source, and processed foods, which may result in the intake of both high- and low-quality foods. Health effects of food variety or diversity are controversial; for example, some researches have

Table 5 Distribution of Chinese HFD-index in participants of two studies

Factor	Group	CUADHS		CHNS	
		$\bar{x} \pm s$	P	$\bar{x} \pm s$	P
Total		0.41 ± 0.10		0.38 ± 0.06	
Gender	Male	0.38 ± 0.10	<0.001	0.37 ± 0.06	<0.001
	Female	0.42 ± 0.10		0.38 ± 0.06	
Age	18~ 44.9 years	0.39 ± 0.10	<0.001	0.37 ± 0.06	0.001
	45~ 54.9 years	0.41 ± 0.10		0.38 ± 0.06	
	55~ 64.9 years	0.40 ± 0.10		0.38 ± 0.06	
	≥65 years	0.42 ± 0.10		0.38 ± 0.07	
Educational attainment	Illiterate	0.39 ± 0.09	0.018	0.36 ± 0.06	<0.001
	Middle school or lower	0.40 ± 0.10		0.37 ± 0.06	
	High school or professional training education	0.42 ± 0.10		0.39 ± 0.07	
	Undergraduate education or higher	0.41 ± 0.10		0.41 ± 0.07	
Drinking behavior	Yes	0.40 ± 0.10	0.001	0.37 ± 0.06	<0.001
	No	0.42 ± 0.10		0.38 ± 0.06	
Smoking behavior	Never smoked	0.42 ± 0.10	<0.001	0.38 ± 0.06	<0.001
	Former smoker	0.39 ± 0.11		0.38 ± 0.07	
	Current smoker	0.37 ± 0.09		0.37 ± 0.06	
BMI	<18.5 kg/m2	0.40 ± 0.09	0.367	0.38 ± 0.06	0.875
	18.5~ 24.0 kg/m2	0.41 ± 0.10		0.38 ± 0.06	
	24.0~ 28.0 kg/m2	0.41 ± 0.10		0.38 ± 0.06	
	≥28.0 kg/m2	0.40 ± 0.10		0.37 ± 0.07	
Physical activity[a]	Sedentary group	0.40 ± 0.09	0.443	0.38 ± 0.06	<0.001
	T1	0.41 ± 0.10		0.38 ± 0.06	
	T2	0.41 ± 0.10		0.38 ± 0.06	
	T3	0.41 ± 0.10		0.37 ± 0.06	
Energy intake[b]	Q1	0.41 ± 0.10	<0.001	0.38 ± 0.07	<0.001
	Q2	0.42 ± 0.10		0.38 ± 0.06	
	Q3	0.41 ± 0.09		0.38 ± 0.06	
	Q4	0.39 ± 0.10		0.36 ± 0.06	

Note:[a]Subjects who only reported sedentary behaviors were classified as Sedentary group, the others were trisected into three groups (T1, T2 and T3) according to the calculated metabolic equivalents (MET)/d from the smallest to the highest;
[b]Energy intakes were quadrisected into four groups (Q1, Q2, Q3 and Q4) from the smallest to the highest

showed that greater food variety resulted in increased food consumption and obesity [23, 40, 41], while others have indicated beneficial effects of food variety on weight control [42, 43]. However, the difference in definition of food variety between studies should be noticed. The Chinese HFD index was based on recommended food groups for adults to keep healthy, and it considered three aspects comprehensively: type, amount, and health value of consumed food. Participants with higher Chinese HFD index values showed better adherence to the Dietary Guideline and Balance Diet Pagoda for Chinese Residents, and our assumption was that the higher Chinese HFD index values would favourably influence MetS and its components.

In CUADHS data, we did not find that a higher Chinese HFD index influenced the risk of MetS and its components. In CHNS data, it is significant that the Chinese HFD index was negatively correlated with MetS and its components of elevated fasting glucose and elevated WC, suggesting favourable effects of food diversity on MetS and its components. The Chinese HFD index was negatively correlated with elevated WC, and it was similar with the results of articles exploring the influence of HFD on MetS or obesity [26, 27]. The protective effect of food diversity on weight control was proved in some studies [44–46], and it was supposed that diversified diets would provide adequate vitamins, minerals, and bioactive substances but moderate or restricted energy, leading to more balanced and healthier diets. In our research, we verified that those people with the lowest Chinese HFD index had the highest energy intakes.

Table 6 Correlations between Chinese HFD-index and nutrients

Nutrients		Correlation coefficient	
		Crude	Energy adjusted
Macronutrient	PA(Protein)	−0.027	0.047
	PA(Carbohydrates)	−0.03	0.078**
Micronutrient	PA(VitaminB1)	0.016	0.044
	PA(VitaminB2)	0.288**	0.280**
	PA(Niacin)	−0.032	0.054*
	PA(VitaminB6)	0.172**	0.072**
	PA(VitaminB12)	0.034	0.037
	PA(Folate)	0.179**	0.206**
	PA(VitaminA)	0.293**	0.249**
	PA(VitaminC)	0.381**	0.296**
	PA(Zn)	0.075**	0.015
	PA(Ca)	0.378**	0.018
	PA(Fe)	−0.043	−0.009
	MPA	0.141**	0.271**

Note: *,$P<0.05$;**,$P<0.01$

There are researches exploring the correlations between food diversity and glucose homeostasis, suggesting that higher food diversity decreased the risk of diabetes or impaired glucose homeostasis [44, 47, 48]. The protection mechanism was partly attributed to its favourable effects on weight control, and further research was needed to explore the mechanism accurately.

Our research showed that the Chinese HFD index was negatively correlated with MetS and some of its components, indicating that the increase in food diversity would decrease the risk of MetS. Although we failed to find correlations between the Chinese HFD index and hypertension or dyslipidemia, results of other researches support the premises that higher food diversity lowers cardiovascular risk and an increase in food diversity is important in dietary interventions against chronic non-communicable diseases [47].

There were some limitations of our analysis that cannot be ignored. Firstly, we failed to incorporate family medical history or genetic factors into the analysis. Secondly, we applied one-day or three-day 24-h dietary

Table 7 Odds of MetS and its components across quartiles of the Chinese HFD-index among participants of CUADHS, OR(95%CI)

Item	Q1[3]	Q2[3]	Q3[3]	Q4[3]	P-trend
Elevated WC					
Crude	1	1.163 (0.865,1.564)	1.088 (0.802,1.476)	1.139 (0.841,1.542)	0.486
Model 1[a]	1	1.047 (0.766,1.431)	1.069 (0.773,1.477)	1.002 (0.723,1.387)	0.951
Model 2[b]	1	1.107 (0.796,1.539)	0.996 (0.705,1.405)	0.967 (0.684,1.367)	0.726
Elevated fasting glucose					
Crude	1	1.367 (1.013,1.846)	0.887 (0.644,1.222)	1.371 (1.009,1.863)	0.272
Model 1[a]	1	1.244 (0.898,1.724)	0.878 (0.621,1.243)	1.221 (0.869,1.715)	0.628
Model 2[b]	1	1.270 (0.906,1.780)	0.844 (0.589,1.210)	1.216 (0.855,1.730)	0.726
Elevated blood pressure					
Crude	1	1.131 (0.845,1.513)	0.887 (0.655,1.202)	1.144 (0.85,1.540)	0.728
Model 1[a]	1	0.901 (0.640,1.268)	0.799 (0.559,1.142)	0.84 (0.589,1.198)	0.258
Model 2[b]	1	0.908 (0.636,1.297)	0.764 (0.526,1.110)	0.812 (0.56,1.177)	0.183
Elevated blood pressure					
Crude	1	1.116 (0.837,1.488)	0.989 (0.735,1.330)	1.312 (0.979,1.758)	0.144
Model 1[a]	1	0.992 (0.730,1.349)	0.963 (0.701,1.325)	1.162 (0.845,1.598)	0.427
Model 2[b]	1	0.931 (0.675,1.283)	0.932 (0.669,1.299)	1.127 (0.808,1.573)	0.52
Reduced HDL					
Crude	1	1.425 (1.070,1.899)	1.199 (0.892,1.612)	1.563 (1.166,2.095)	0.012
Model 1[a]	1	1.302 (0.969,1.749)	1.13 (0.832,1.534)	1.356 (0.998,1.843)	0.112
Model 2[b]	1	1.251 (0.914,1.713)	1.096 (0.792,1.517)	1.355 (0.978,1.878)	0.134
MetS					
Crude	1	1.079 (0.805,1.446)	0.843 (0.620,1.145)	1.31 (0.974,1.762)	0.244
Model 1[a]	1	0.913 (0.661,1.259)	0.788 (0.562,1.104)	1.091 (0.783,1.522)	0.848
Model 2[b]	1	0.884 (0.631,1.239)	0.754 (0.529,1.073)	1.074 (0.757,1.523)	0.936

Note: [a]regression model adjusted age and gender;
[b]regression model adjusted age, gender, drinking behavior, smoking behavior, BMI, physical activity and energy intakes;
[c]Chinese HFD-Index values were quadrisected into four groups (Q1, Q2, Q3 and Q4) from the smallest to the highest

Table 8 Odds of MetS and its components across quartiles of the Chinese HFD-index among participants of CHNS, OR(95%CI)

Item	Q1[3]	Q2[3]	Q3[3]	Q4[3]	P-trend
Elevated WC					
Crude	1	0.846 (0.672,1.067)	0.710 (0.562,0.899)	0.664 (0.524,0.841)	<0.001
Model 1[a]	1	0.801 (0.631,1.017)	0.650 (0.510,0.829)	0.579 (0.453,0.740)	<0.001
Model 2[b]	1	0.811 (0.638,1.031)	0.671 (0.525,0.858)	0.603 (0.470,0.773)	<0.001
Elevated fasting glucose					
Crude	1	0.893 (0.704,1.132)	0.752 (0.591,0.958)	0.820 (0.645,1.041)	0.077
Model 1[a]	1	0.859 (0.673,1.096)	0.704 (0.549,0.903)	0.744 (0.581,0.954)	0.013
Model 2[b]	1	0.856 (0.671,1.094)	0.701 (0.545,0.901)	0.747 (0.582,0.960)	0.016
Elevated blood pressure					
Crude	1	1.244 (0.98,1.579)	0.965 (0.756,1.232)	1.066 (0.837,1.358)	0.909
Model 1[a]	1	1.214 (0.931,1.584)	0.839 (0.639,1.101)	0.883 (0.674,1.157)	0.101
Model 2[b]	1	1.230 (0.942,1.606)	0.870 (0.661,1.146)	0.908 (0.691,1.194)	0.165
Elevated blood pressure					
Crude	1	0.973 (0.772,1.227)	0.720 (0.568,0.914)	0.837 (0.662,1.059)	0.056
Model 1[a]	1	0.985 (0.779,1.245)	0.733 (0.576,0.933)	0.869 (0.684,1.104)	0.117
Model 2[b]	1	0.977 (0.772,1.236)	0.717 (0.563,0.915)	0.856 (0.672,1.091)	0.096
Reduced HDL					
Crude	1	1.197 (0.927,1.544)	1.190 (0.921,1.537)	1.229 (0.952,1.586)	0.161
Model 1[a]	1	1.157 (0.894,1.497)	1.125 (0.868,1.457)	1.117 (0.862,1.448)	0.53
Model 2[2]	1	1.161 (0.896,1.503)	1.095 (0.844,1.422)	1.094 (0.842,1.422)	0.677
MetS					
Crude	1	1.008 (0.787,1.292)	0.827 (0.641,1.067)	0.791 (0.612,1.022)	0.033
Model 1[a]	1	0.962 (0.744,1.244)	0.758 (0.582,0.987)	0.692 (0.530,0.904)	0.002
Model 2[b]	1	0.964 (0.745,1.247)	0.757 (0.580,0.987)	0.698 (0.533,0.914)	0.003

Note:[a] regression model adjusted age and gender;
[b]regression model adjusted age, gender, drinking behavior, smoking behavior, BMI, physical activity and energy intakes;
[c]Chinese HFD-Index values were quadrisected into four groups (Q1, Q2, Q3 and Q4) from the smallest to the highest

recall to represent the general condition of food intakes, and the representativeness was limited and recall bias was unavoidable. Thirdly, in a cross-sectional study we can only prove association rather than causal relationship between the Chinese HFD index and MetS and its components. However, this was the first analysis based on the Dietary Guideline and Balance Diet Pagoda for Chinese Residents regarding HFD and MetS in Chinese urban adults. The Chinese HFD index developed by this study was comparable to that of other countries and made it possible to measure compliance with dietary guidelines quantitatively.

Conclusions

This study quantitatively described the status of MetS and the Chinese HFD index, and found that the Chinese HFD index was negatively associated with MetS and some of its components, such as elevated WC and elevated fasting glucose. Increased food diversity may lower the risk of MetS, which is important in designing dietary interventions for cardiac–cerebral vascular diseases. The study underscores the necessity of continued investigation into the role of healthful food diversity in the prevention of MetS and provides an integral framework for ongoing research.

Abbreviations

ANOVA: analysis of variance; BMI: body mass index; CFCT: Chinese Food Composition Tables; CHNS: China Health and Nutrition Survey; CI: confidence interval; CJFH: specimen collection and processing by the China–Japan Friendship Hospital; CUADHS: Chinese Urban Adults Diet and Health Study; CV: coefficient of variation; CVD: cardiovascular disease; DBP: diastolic blood pressure; DRIs: Dietary Reference Intakes; EAR: estimated average requirements; FAO: Food and Agriculture Organisation of the United Nations; FFQ: food frequency questionnaire; FSG: fasting serum glucose; HDL: high-density lipoprotein; HFD: healthful food diversity; KNHANES: Korean National Health and Nutrition Examination Survey; MET: metabolic equivalents; MetS: metabolic syndrome; MPA: mean probability of adequacy; NHANES: National Health and Nutrition Examination Survey; PA: probabilities of nutrient adequacy; RNI: recommended nutrient intakes; SBP: systolic blood pressure; TC: total cholesterol; TG: triglyceride; WC: waist circumference

Acknowledgements
The authors thank the data share of the CHNS work team.

Funding
This research received no specific grant from any funding agency in the public, commercial, or not-for-profit sectors.

Authors' contributions
The research question and study design were formulated by WZ and JZ. The study was carried out by WZ, JZ, AZ, MW, WW, ST, MG, and YZ. Data analysis was carried out by WZ and JZ. The article was written by all authors, with editing by WZ, AZ, and YZ.

Competing interests
None.

References
1. de Carvalho VF, Bressan J, Babio N, Salas-Salvado J. Prevalence of metabolic syndrome in Brazilian adults: a systematic review. BMC Public Health. 2013; 13:1198.
2. Beltran-Sanchez H, Harhay MO, Harhay MM, McElligott S. Prevalence and trends of metabolic syndrome in the adult U.S. population, 1999-2010. J Am Coll Cardiol. 2013;62(8):697–703.
3. Yeh CJ, Chang HY, Pan WH. Time trend of obesity, the metabolic syndrome and related dietary pattern in Taiwan: from NAHSIT 1993-1996 to NAHSIT 2005-2008. Asia Pac J Clin Nutr. 2011;20(2):292–300.
4. Eckel RH, Alberti KG, Grundy SM, Zimmet PZ. The metabolic syndrome. Lancet. 2010;375(9710):181–3.
5. Alberti KG, Eckel RH, Grundy SM, Zimmet PZ, Cleeman JI, Donato KA, Fruchart JC, James WP, Loria CM, Smith SJ. Harmonizing the metabolic syndrome: a joint interim statement of the international diabetes federation task force on epidemiology and prevention; National Heart, Lung, and Blood Institute; American Heart Association; world heart federation; international atherosclerosis society; and International Association for the Study of obesity. Circulation. 2009;120(16):1640–5.
6. Moore JX, Chaudhary N, Akinyemiju T. Metabolic syndrome prevalence by race/ethnicity and sex in the United States, National Health and nutrition examination survey, 1988-2012. Prev Chronic Dis. 2017;14:E24.
7. Tran BT, Jeong BY, Oh JK. The prevalence trend of metabolic syndrome and its components and risk factors in Korean adults: results from the Korean National Health and nutrition examination survey 2008-2013. BMC Public Health. 2017;17(1):71.
8. Xi B, He D, Hu Y, Zhou D. Prevalence of metabolic syndrome and its influencing factors among the Chinese adults: the China health and nutrition survey in 2009. Prev Med. 2013;57(6):867–71.
9. Xiao J, Wu CL, Gao YX, Wang SL, Wang L, Lu QY, Wang XJ, Hua TQ, Shen H, Cai H. Prevalence of metabolic syndrome and its risk factors among rural adults in Nantong, China. Sci Rep. 2016;6:380–9.
10. Xiao J, Wu C, Xu G, Huang J, Gao Y, Lu Q, Hua T, Cai H. Association of physical activity with risk of metabolic syndrome: findings from a cross-sectional study conducted in rural area, Nantong, China. J Sports Sci. 2016;34(19):1839–48.
11. Song QB, Zhao Y, Liu YQ, Zhang J, Xin SJ, Dong GH. Sex difference in the prevalence of metabolic syndrome and cardiovascular-related risk factors in urban adults from 33 communities of China: the CHPSNE study. Diab Vasc Dis Res. 2015;12(3):189–98.
12. Park JH, Kim SH, Lee MS, Kim MS. Epigenetic modification by dietary factors: implications in metabolic syndrome. Mol Asp Med. 2017;54: 58–70.
13. de la Iglesia R, Loria-Kohen V, Zulet MA, Martinez JA, Reglero G, Ramirez DMA. Dietary strategies implicated in the prevention and treatment of metabolic syndrome. Int J Mol Sci. 2016;17(11):1877.
14. Lucke-Wold B, Shawley S, Ingels JS, Stewart J, Misra R. A critical examination of the use of trained health coaches to decrease the metabolic syndrome for participants of a community-based diabetes prevention and management program. J Health Commun. 2016;1(4):38.
15. Baik I, Lee M, Jun NR, Lee JY, Shin C. A healthy dietary pattern consisting of a variety of food choices is inversely associated with the development of metabolic syndrome. Nutr Res Pract. 2013;7(3):233–41.
16. de Oliveira EP, McLellan KC, Vaz DASL, Burini RC. Dietary factors associated with metabolic syndrome in Brazilian adults. Nutr J. 2012;11:13.
17. Kastorini CM, Milionis HJ, Esposito K, Giugliano D, Goudevenos JA, Panagiotakos DB. The effect of Mediterranean diet on metabolic syndrome and its components: a meta-analysis of 50 studies and 534,906 individuals. J Am Coll Cardiol. 2011;57(11):1299–313.
18. Azadbakht L, Esmaillzadeh A. Red meat intake is associated with metabolic syndrome and the plasma C-reactive protein concentration in women. J Nutr. 2009;139(2):335–9.
19. Aleixandre A, Miguel M. Dietary fiber in the prevention and treatment of metabolic syndrome: a review. Crit Rev Food Sci Nutr. 2008;48(10):905–12.
20. Chung SJ, Lee Y, Lee S, Choi K. Breakfast skipping and breakfast type are associated with daily nutrient intakes and metabolic syndrome in Korean adults. Nutr Res Pract. 2015;9(3):288–95.
21. Nazare JA, Smith J, Borel AL, Almeras N, Tremblay A, Bergeron J, Poirier P, Despres JP. Changes in both global diet quality and physical activity level synergistically reduce visceral adiposity in men with features of metabolic syndrome. J Nutr. 2013;143(7):1074–83.
22. McCrory MA, Burke A, Roberts SB. Dietary (sensory) variety and energy balance. Physiol Behav. 2012;107(4):576–83.
23. Raynor HA. Can limiting dietary variety assist with reducing energy intake and weight loss? Physiol Behav. 2012;106(3):356–61.
24. Ruel MT. Operationalizing dietary diversity: a review of measurement issues and research priorities. J Nutr. 2003;133(11 Suppl 2):3911S–26S.
25. Tiew KF, Chan YM, Lye MS, Loke SC. Factors associated with dietary diversity score among individuals with type 2 diabetes mellitus. J Health Popul Nutr. 2014;32(4):665–76.
26. Vadiveloo M, Parekh N, Mattei J. Greater healthful food variety as measured by the US healthy food diversity index is associated with lower odds of metabolic syndrome and its components in US adults. J Nutr. 2015;145(3): 564–71.
27. Vadiveloo M, Dixon LB, Mijanovich T, Elbel B, Parekh N. Dietary variety is inversely associated with body adiposity among US adults using a novel food diversity index. J Nutr. 2015;145(3):555–63.
28. Drescher LS, Thiele S, Mensink GB. A new index to measure healthy food diversity better reflects a healthy diet than traditional measures. J Nutr. 2007;137(3):647–51.
29. Vadiveloo M, Sacks FM, Champagne CM, Bray GA, Mattei J. Greater healthful dietary variety is associated with greater 2-year changes in weight and adiposity in the preventing overweight using novel dietary strategies (POUNDS lost) trial. J Nutr. 2016;146(8):1552–9.
30. Popkin BM, Du S, Zhai F, Zhang B. Cohort profile: the China health and nutrition survey: monitoring and understanding socio-economic and health change in China, 1989-2011. Int J Epidemiol. 2010;39(6):1435–40.
31. Standard Tables of Food Composition in Japan. Tokyo: Ishiyaku Publishers, Inc; 2010.
32. Zhao W, Yu K, Tan S, Zheng Y, Zhao A, Wang P, Zhang Y. Dietary diversity scores: an indicator of micronutrient inadequacy instead of obesity for Chinese children. BMC Public Health. 2017;17(1):440.
33. Kennedy G, Nantel G. Basic guidelines for validation of a simple dietary score as an indicator of dietary nutrient adequacy for non-breastfeeding children 2–6 years. ftp://ftp.fao.org/ag/agn/nutrition/dds_validation.pdf. Accessed 15 Apr 2006.
34. Frankenfeld CL, Poudrier JK, Waters NM, Gillevet PM, Xu Y. Dietary intake measured from a self-administered, online 24-hour recall system compared with 4-day diet records in an adult US population. Jacad Nutr Diet. 2012; 112(10):1642–7.
35. Xue H, Yang M, Liu Y, Duan R, Cheng G, Zhang X. Relative validity of a 2-day 24-hour dietary recall compared with a 2-day weighed dietary record among adults in South China. Nutr Diet. 2017;74(3):298–307.
36. Nightingale H, Walsh KJ, Olupot-Olupot P, Engoru C, Ssenyondo T, Nteziyaremye J, Amorut D, Nakuya M, Arimi M, Frost G, et al. Validation of triple pass 24-hour dietary recall in Ugandan children by simultaneous weighed food assessment. BMC Nutr. 2016;2:56.

37. Chinese Nutrition Society. Chinese dietary guidelines summary (2016). Beijing: People's Medical Publishing House; 2017.
38. Vadiveloo M, Dixon LB, Mijanovich T, Elbel B, Parekh N. Development and evaluation of the US healthy food diversity index. Br J Nutr. 2014;112(9): 1562–74.
39. World Health Organization. Regional Office for the Western Pacific. The Asia-Pacific perspective: redefining obesity and its treatment. Sydney: Health Communications Australia; 2000.
40. Remick AK, Polivy J, Pliner P. Internal and external moderators of the effect of variety on food intake. Psychol Bull. 2009;135(3):434–51.
41. Epstein LH, Robinson JL, Temple JL, Roemmich JN, Marusewski AL, Nadbrzuch RL. Variety influences habituation of motivated behavior for food and energy intake in children. Am J Clin Nutr. 2009;89(3):746–54.
42. Lassale C, Fezeu L, Andreeva VA, Hercberg S, Kengne AP, Czernichow S, Kesse-Guyot E. Association between dietary scores and 13-year weight change and obesity risk in a French prospective cohort. Int J Obes. 2012; 36(11):1455–62.
43. Gregory CO, McCullough ML, Ramirez-Zea M, Stein AD. Diet scores and cardio-metabolic risk factors among Guatemalan young adults. Br J Nutr. 2009;101(12):1805–11.
44. Azadbakht L, Mirmiran P, Azizi F. Dietary diversity score is favorably associated with the metabolic syndrome in Tehranian adults. Int J Obes. 2005;29(11):1361–7.
45. Vadiveloo MK, Parekh N. Dietary variety: an overlooked strategy for obesity and chronic disease control. Am J Prev Med. 2015;49(6):974–9.
46. Vadiveloo M, Dixon LB, Parekh N. Associations between dietary variety and measures of body adiposity: a systematic review of epidemiological studies. Br J Nutr. 2013;109(9):1557–72.
47. Azadbakht L, Mirmiran P, Esmaillzadeh A, Azizi F. Dietary diversity score and cardiovascular risk factors in Tehranian adults. Public Health Nutr. 2006;9(6): 728–36.
48. Danquah I, Galbete C, Meeks K, Nicolaou M, Klipstein-Grobusch K, Addo J, Aikins AD, Amoah SK, Agyei-Baffour P, Boateng D, et al. Food variety, dietary diversity, and type 2 diabetes in a multi-center cross-sectional study among Ghanaian migrants in Europe and their compatriots in Ghana: the RODAM study. Eur J Nutr. 2017; https://doi.org/10.1007/s00394-017-1538-4.

Risk factors for prehypertension and their interactive effect

Jian Song[1†], Xue Chen[1†], Yingying Zhao[2], Jing Mi[1], Xuesen Wu[1*] and Huaiquan Gao[1*]

Abstract

Background: Individuals with prehypertension are at higher risk of developing hypertension and cardiovascular diseases, while the interaction between factors may aggravate prehypertension risk. Therefore, this study aimed to evaluate the risk factors for prehypertension in Chinese middle-aged and elderly adults, and explore the potentially interactive effect of evaluated factors.

Methods: All the participants that came from a community based cross-sectional survey were investigated in Bengbu, China, by being interviewed with a questionnaire. Body mass index (BMI), Waist circumference (WC) and lipid accumulation product (LAP) that reflect participants' obesity were also calculated. In addition, logistic regression model was applied to explore the risk factors of prehypertension, followed by the assessment of the interactive effects between risk factors on prehypertension by the relative excess risk due to interaction (RERI), attributable proportion due to interaction (AP) and synergy index (SI).

Results: A total of 1777 participants were enrolled in this study, among which the prevalence of normtension, prehypertension and hypertension were 41.70%, 33.93% and 24.37% respectively. According to the multivariate logistic regression analysis, age (OR: 1.01, 95%CI: 1.00–1.02), smoking (OR: 1.67, 95%CI: 1.22–2.29), family history of cardiovascular diseases (OR: 1.52, 95%CI: 1.14–2.02), general obesity (OR: 1.51, 95%CI: 1.15–1.97) and LAP (OR: 2.58, 95%CI: 1.76–3.80) were all defined as the major factors that significantly related with the risk of prehypertension. When identifying prehypertension risk, the receiver-operating characteristics (ROC) curves (AUC) analysis indicated that LAP performed better than BMI in males ($Z = 2.05$, $P = 0.03$) and females ($Z = 2.12$, $P = 0.03$), but was superior to WC only in females ($Z = 2.43$, $P = 0.01$). What is more, there were significant interactive effects of LAP with family history of cardiovascular diseases (RERI: 1.88, 95%CI: 0.25–3.51; AP: 0.44, 95%CI: 0.20–0.69; SI: 2.37, 95%CI: 1.22–4.60) and smoking (RERI: 1.99, 95%CI: 0.04–3.93; AP: 0.42, 95%CI: 0.17–0.67; SI: 2.16, 95%CI: 1.68–4.00) on prehypertension risk. The value of AP (0.40, 95%CI: 0.03–0.77) also indicated a significant interaction between family history of cardiovascular diseases and smoking on prehypertension.

Conclusion: Prehypertension is currently prevalent in Chinese adults. This study indicated that age, family history of cardiovascular diseases, smoking, general obesity and LAP were significantly related with prehypertension risk. Furthermore, interactive effects on risk of prehypertension had been demonstrated in this study as well, which would help researchers to build strategy against prehypertension more comprehensively and scientifically.

Keywords: Prehypertension, Visceral obesity, LAP, Interaction

* Correspondence: xuesenwu@163.com; ghqbbmc@sina.com
†Jian Song and Xue Chen contributed equally to this work.
[1]School of public health, Bengbu medical college, 2600 Donghai Road, Bengbu 233000, Anhui Province, China
Full list of author information is available at the end of the article

Background

Elevated blood pressure is a common and serious public issue [1, 2], which was significantly related to incidence of gout [3], Parkinson's disease [4] and even prognosis in patients with systemic lupus erythematosus [5]. In 2003, the definition of prehypertension was first proposed in the Seventh Report of the Joint National Committee on Prevention, Detection, Evaluation, and Treatment of High Blood Pressure (JNC-7) [6]. According to JNC-7, prehypertension was more likely to develop hypertension than normotension [6]. Soon afterwards, relevant studies have demonstrated that the interventions against prehypertension may bring new breakthroughs in the prevention of hypertension [7, 8]. With the social development and acceleration of the population aging in China, the prevalence of prehypertension and hypertension has significantly increased. As indicated in a large-scale multi- ethnic population survey with 47,495 adult participants in China, the prevalence of prehypertension was up to 36.4% [9]. Moreover, a clustering of cardiovascular disease risk factors was also observed in the prehypertension population of Han and Mongolian adults [10]. A four-year follow-up study indicated that prehypertension significantly increased the occurrence of chronic kidney disease in Chinese adults [11]. Meta-analyses have demonstrated that prehypertension, as well as hypertension and diabetes, are significantly associated with the risk of cardiovascular events including coronary heart disease, stable angina and stroke. [12–14]. Most importantly, the earlier the effective interventions had been performed, the more significant the risk of cardiovascular disease and death would be reduced, with a reduction up to 15% [15].

Increased blood pressure is caused by a variety of factors, among which obesity is increasingly proved to be closely related to hypertension by accumulating evidence [16]. Previous studies mostly assessed obesity by using body mass index (BMI) and waist circumference (WC), however, obesity not only refers to excessive fat accumulation, but also implies the abnormal distribution of fat, and there are significant differences in morphology and function between subcutaneous adipose tissue (SAT) and visceral adipose tissue (VAT) [17]. Lipid accumulation product (LAP), as a combination of WC and triglycerides (TG), was proved to be an available indicator that reflects visceral obesity, and it was significant associated with total cholesterol, lipoproteins, and glucose [18, 19]. Higher LAP significantly increased the risk of hyperuricemia among Chinese rural population [20]. LAP was also proved to be significantly associated with insulin resistance, which involved in the development of a series of metabolic-related diseases [21]. Furthermore, LAP performed superior to BMI and WC as a predictor of metabolic syndrome [22]. However, to our best of knowledge, few articles applied LAP to assess obesity when analyzing the risk factors of prehypertension. Meanwhile, whether LAP performs better than other obesity indices for discriminating prehypertension has not been confirmed. Additionally, numerous studies have demonstrated that the interaction between environmental-genetic and environmental-environmental may be related to the occurrence of chronic diseases [23, 24]. For instance, the interaction between smoking and obesity has remarkable effects on type 2 diabetes risk in Chinese adults [23]. Therefore, the interaction between risk factors may aggravate the risk of prehypertension. However, most of previous studies only analyzed the risk factors for prehypertension, and rarely further explored their interactive effects.

This study, firstly, investigated the epidemiological characteristics of prehypertension and its associated factors. Secondly, the abilities of BMI, WC and LAP in predicting prehypertension risk were compared. Finally, we assessed the possibly interactive effects between various factors on prehypertension risk.

Methods

Study design

This community-based cross-sectional survey on the basis of the project called "creating a provincial demonstration area of chronic diseases management in community" was conducted in Longzihu, Bengbu, China. The project mainly aimed to investigate the epidemiological situation of main chronic diseases among residents living in Longzihu, Bengbu, China, and attempted to create a provincial demonstration community of chronic diseases management. Participants were selected through a multistage random sampling, which excluded individuals who had no abilities to communicate with investigators normally or finish the overall survey independently due to inconvenience or serious illness. After the screening, selected individuals were required to complete relevant survey and health checks in community clinics. All participants signed the informed consent. The Ethics Committee of Bengbu medical college approved this study.

Questionnaire survey

A self-designed questionnaire as shown in Additional file 1 was completed for each participant by qualified staffs through face-to-face interview. The relevant definitions or grouping methods of sociodemographic variables were as followings: (1) Educational level: classified as "elementary school or lower", "middle school graduate" and "high school graduate or higher"; (2) Monthly income: grouped as "0–2000", "2000-" and "4000-" (yuan); (3) Marital status: categorized as "currently married" and "currently not married" (including single or divorced); (4) Smoking: defined by the status of pre-smoking or current-smoking; (5) Positive family history of cardiovascular diseases: refers to the individuals who had at least one parent or sibling with cardiovascular diseases [9]. Once the questionnaire survey was completed, the information was entered into Epidata software by using double entry approach.

Blood pressure measurement

Before taking measuring blood pressure measurements, the participants were required to take a rest for 5 to 10 min. Afterwards, mercury sphygmomanometer was applied to measure blood pressure three times for each participant and the average one was calculated. Hypertension was defined as systolic blood pressure (SBP) ≥ 140 mmHg, or diastolic blood pressure (DBP) ≥ 90 mmHg, or the subject reported antihypertensive medication having been prescribed [25]. Individuals had SBP of 120–139 mmHg and/or DBP of 80–89 mmHg without antihypertensive medication were regarded as prehypertension [6], while those with SBP and DBP less than 120 mmHg and 80 mmHg respectively were defined as normotension [6].

Anthropometric tests and laboratory examinations

Height, weight and WC were examined by trained investigators using uniform instruments. When measuring height and weight, the participants were required to take off their shoes and wear light clothes for obtaining more accurate measurements. BMI was calculated as weight(kg)/height(m)^2. According to the recommendation given by the Working Group on Obesity in China, BMI ≥ 28 kg/m^2 was defined as general obesity [26], WC ≥ 90 cm for males and WC ≥ 85 cm for females were regarded as abdominal obesity, respectively [27]. Meanwhile, all participants had blood samples taken after fasting for more than 8 h overnight. LAP was calculated as [WC (cm)-65] × [TG(mmol/L)] for males, and [WC (cm)-58] × [TG(mmol/L)] for females [18].

Statistical methods

Firstly, the basic characteristics of enrolled participants were presented, and quantitative data and categorical variables were respectively described using mean ± SD (standard deviation) and percentages. Furthermore, the differences in categorical variables between normotension, prehypertension and hypertension individuals were compared by Chi-squared test or Kruskal-Wallis H test. LAP was divided into four groups (Q1, Q2, Q3, and Q4) in accordance with quartiles. Secondly, univariate and multivariate logistic regression model was applied to evaluate the risk factors for prehypertension, followed by the calculation of odds ratio (OR) with corresponding 95% confidence interval (95%CI). A stepwise backward selection procedure was used in multivariate analysis. Thirdly, the abilities of BMI, WC and LAP in predicting prehypertension risk were compared by the area under the receiver-operating characteristics (ROC) curves (AUC) analysis. Finally, the interaction between various factors on prehypertension was assessed by the following indicators: (1) the relative excess risk due to interaction (RERI = RR_{11}- RR_{10}-RR_{01} + 1); (2) the attributable proportion due to interaction (AP = RERI/RR_{11}); (3) the synergy index (SI = (RR_{11}−1)/ (RR_{01}−1) + (RR_{10}−1)) [28, 29]. All p values were two-sided, and $p < 0.05$ was considered statistically significant. R and Medcalc software were applied to complete all statistical calculations.

Results

Baseline characteristics

Totally, 1777 middle-aged and elderly participants with average age of 60.82 were enrolled in this study, including 748 males (42.09%) and 1029 females (57.91%). The total prevalence of normtension, prehypertension and hypertension was 41.70%, 33.93% and 24.37% respectively, while male had a higher prevalence of prehypertension (37.43%) than female (31.39%). The mean age for normtension, prehypertension and hypertension members were 59.67 ± 11.34, 61.15 ± 11.41 and 62.31 ± 10.64 years old separately, with $p < 0.01$. Significant differences were presented in educational level ($p = 0.03$), smoking ($p < 0.01$), family history of cardiovascular diseases ($p < 0.01$), general obesity ($p < 0.01$) and abdominal obesity ($p < 0.01$) between normtension, prehypertension and hypertension individuals, among which the prehypertension members had the highest smoking rate (34.66%), intermediate prevalence of general obesity and abdominal obesity. However, no significant differences in marital status ($p = 0.73$) and income ($p = 0.26$) between groups were observed. As for LAP, a significant difference was obtained in LAP quartiles between three groups ($p < 0.01$), and the prevalence of prehypertension gradually increased ($p < 0.01$, trend Chi-square test) across LAP quartiles, as demonstrated in Fig. 1. All of the detailed information was presented in Table 1.

Analyses of risk factors for prehypertension

The results of univariate and multivariate logistic regression analysis were introduced in Table 2. Male had a higher risk of prehypertension than female in univariate analysis (OR: 1.65, 95%CI: 1.32–2.06), but no association of importance was observed after controlling other factors (OR: 1.16, 95%CI: 0.85–1.58). Besides, both univariate and multivariate analysis indicated that individuals had a higher risk of being prehypertension with aging (OR: 1.01, 95%CI: 1.00–1.02). No statistically significant relationship between educational level, income and marital status with prehypertension risk were observed. Compared with non-smoker, smokers had 1.67 fold risks in getting prehypertension, testified by multivariate analysis (OR: 1.67, 95%CI: 1.22–2.29). Members with positive family history of cardiovascular diseases were similarly effected in prehypertension (OR: 1.52, 95%CI: 1.14–2.02). In terms of obesity indices, a

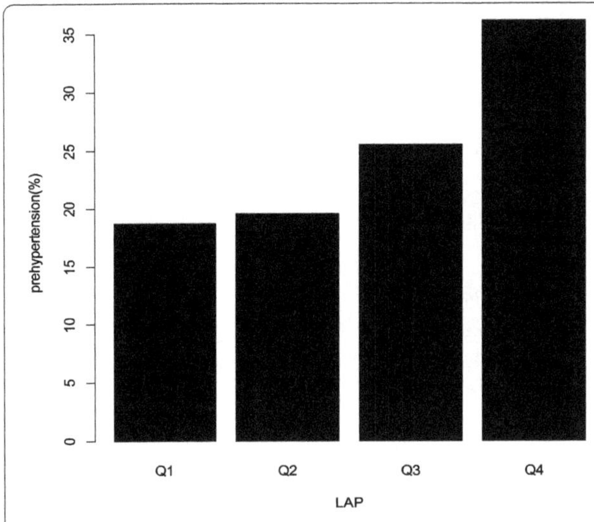

Fig. 1 The prevalence of prehypertension across LAP quartiles (*P* for trend< 0.001)

significant association between general obesity and increased risk of prehypertension were detected using both univariate (OR: 1.58, 95%CI: 1.15–2.17) and multivariate analysis (OR: 1.51, 95%CI: 1.15–1.97). However, in univariate analysis, abdominal obesity was significantly related to prehypertension (OR: 2.08, 95%CI: 1.67–2.60), while in multivariate analysis, there was no correlation worth of attention (OR: 1.94, 95%CI: 0.89–1.60).The risk of prehypertension significantly increased with LAP levels in the fourth quartile as compared with the bottom quartile (crude OR: 3.70, 95%CI: 2.69–5.08; adjusted OR: 2.58, 95% CI: 1.76–3.80).

Comparisons between LAP, BMI and WC

The ROC curves analyses were presented in Table 3 and Figs. 2 and 3. Overall, the AUC with corresponding 95%CI of BMI, WC and LAP were 0.60(0.57–0.63), 0.63(0.60–0.65) and 0.65 (0.62–0.68) respectively. LAP performed better than BMI ($Z = 3.52$, $P < 0.01$) and WC ($Z = 2.05$, $P = 0.04$) in discriminating prehypertension risk. Moreover, when grouped by gender, although LAP still performed better than BMI in male ($Z = 2.05$, $P = 0.03$) and female ($Z = 2.12$, $P = 0.03$), its AUC was significant higher than that of WC only in female ($Z = 2.43$, $P = 0.01$), but not in men ($Z = 1.77$, $P = 0.07$). The AUC with corresponding 95%CI of BMI, WC, LAP were 0.59(0.54–0.63), 0.60(0.55–0.64), 0.63(0.59–0.67) in males, and 0.61(0.58–0.65), 0.61(0.58–0.65), 0.65(0.62–0.68) in females respectively.

Interaction analysis

Finally, the interaction analyses were conducted by relevant indicators as shown in Table 4, and the interaction between LAP and family history of cardiovascular diseases on prehypertension risk was found to be significant (RERI: 1.88, 95%CI: 0.25–3.51; AP: 0.44, 95%CI: 0.20–0.69; SI: 2.37, 95%CI: 1.22–4.60). According to the results of RERI (1.99, 95%CI: 0.04–3.93), AP (0.42, 95%CI: 0.17–0.67) and SI (2.16, 95%CI: 1.68–4.00), LAP also considerably associated with smoking in prehypertension risk. The value of AP (0.40, 95%CI: 0.03–0.77) indicated a significant interaction of family history of cardiovascular diseases and smoking on prehypertension, while neither RERI (1.32, 95%CI:-0.60–3.23) nor SI did (2.37, 95% CI: 0.87–6.44).

Discussion

With the rapid economic and social development, the number of Chinese adults with prehypertension has become considerably massive [30–34]. The prevalence of prehypertension (33.93%) in this study was consistent with the survey conducted in Taiwanese adults (34.0%) [30], higher than that of adults living in Inner Mongolia (28.77%) [10], Jiangxi province (32.3%) [31] and Zhejiang province (32.1%) [32], but lower than the rate in Hubei Province (42.2%) [33] and Qinghai Province (41.3%) [34]. China is a vast multi-ethnic country, consequently, the specific life styles and distinct socioeconomic status may influence the epidemic of prehypertension. In other Asian countries, the National Adult Overweight Survey 2005 in Vietnam reported a prehypertension prevalence rate of 41.8% in 17,199 adults [35]. Moreover, Lifestyle Promotion Project (LPP) in Iranian population announced that the prevalence of prehypertension was as high as 47.3% [36], while Korean National Health and Nutrition Examination Survey (KNHANES) demonstrated a similar rate of prehypertension (33.3%) with our research [37]. In the United States, a cohort study named Reasons for Geographic and Racial Differences in Stroke (REGARDS) reported an amazing prevalence of prehypertension of 62.9% in black and 54.1% in white participants [38]. Numerous researches have demonstrated that prehypertension has serious effects on human health such as carotid atherosclerotic plaque [39], stroke [14] and even mortality [40]. Thus, prehypertension is a prevalent public health problem that worth attention worldwide. The present study also revealed that the prevalence of prehypertension significantly increased with aging, suggesting that the prevention of prehypertension should be carried out as early as possible. Similarly, Liu et al. [41] conducted a survey with 3891 Chinese adults, and the results also demonstrated that age was a significant risk factor of prehypertension in both genders. In contrast with the univariate analysis, the risk of prehypertension in male was not significantly higher than female, proposing that the influence of gender on prehypertension remains inconsistent, with several studies reporting a significant relationship [6, 38], while others did not [31]. This may be resulted by the differences in ethnic group and various adjusted variables in different studies.

The commonness of obesity in China has increased dramatically in recent years [42]. Extensive studies have proved

Table 1 Basic characteristic of participants in this study

Variables	Normotension ($N = 741$)	Prehypertension ($N = 603$)	Hypertension ($N = 433$)	P^a
Gender (%)				< 0.01[b]
Male	255(34.41)	280(46.43)	213(49.19)	
Female	486(65.59)	323(53.57)	220(50.81)	
Age (years)	59.67 ± 11.34	61.15 ± 11.41	62.31 ± 10.64	< 0.01[c]
Educational level (%)				0.03[c]
Elementary level or lower	233(31.44)	189(31.34)	168(38.80)	
Middle school graduate	276(37.25)	221(36.65)	146(33.72)	
High school graduate or higher	232(31.31)	193(32.01)	119(27.48)	
Marital status (%)				0.73[b]
Currently married	621(83.81)	506(83.91)	370(85.45)	
Currently not married	120(16.19)	97(16.09)	63(14.55)	
Income (yuan) (%)				0.26[c]
0–2000	419(56.55)	315(52.24)	230(53.12)	
2000–4000	288(38.87)	256(42.45)	185(42.73)	
> 4000	34(4.58)	32(5.31)	18(4.15)	
Smoking (%)				< 0.01[b]
No	573(77.33)	394(65.34)	284(65.59)	
Yes	168(22.67)	209(34.66)	149(34.41)	
Family history of cardiovascular diseases (%)				< 0.01[b]
No	608(82.1)	458(75.95)	322(74.36)	
Yes	133(17.9)	145(24.05)	111(25.64)	
General obesity (%)				< 0.01[b]
No	660(89.05)	505(83.75)	324(74.83)	
Yes	81(10.95)	98(16.25)	109(25.17)	
Abdominal obesity (%)				< 0.01[b]
No	502(67.75)	304(50.41)	151(34.87)	
Yes	238(32.25)	299(49.59)	282(65.13)	
LAP (%)				< 0.01[c]
Q1	226(30.50)	113(18.74)	42(9.70)	
Q2	215(29.01)	118(19.57)	92(21.25)	
Q3	182(24.56)	154(25.54)	119(27.48)	
Q4	118(15.93)	218(36.15)	180(41.57)	

a:Comparisons of variables between normotension, prehypertension and hypertension members
b:Chi-squared test
c: Kruskal-Wallis H test

that obesity, especially visceral obesity, plays an essential role in the increase of blood pressure [16]. Visceral fat can activate the renin-angiotensin-aldosterone system [43]. The aldosterone concentration is positively correlated with the amount of visceral adipose tissue as VAT can stimulate the release of aldosterone from adrenal cells [44]. Insulin metabolism may be affected by visceral fat through releasing free fatty acids. Meanwhile, visceral fat is capable to promote inflammations process through a source of adipokines, such as tumor necrosis factor-alpha (TNF-alpha), plasminogen activator inhibitor-1 and angiotensinogen and C-reactive protein [45].

Traditional obesity indices, including BMI and WC, have certain limitations. For instance, BMI is unable to distinguish between fat and muscle, and is not suitable to evaluate the people whose muscle accounts for a larger proportion of the body composition. Recently, "Obesity paradox" has attained notable attention. Heart failure, chronic kidney disease, or cancer patients with obesity defined by BMI have even a better prognosis than those with

Table 2 Logistic regression model for risk factors associated with prehypertension

Variables	Univariate analysis		Multivariate analysis	
	OR	95%CI	OR	95%CI
Gender				
Female	1.00(ref.)	–	1.00(ref.)	–
Male	1.65	1.32–2.06	1.16	0.85–1.58
Age (years)	1.01	1.00–1.02	1.01	1.00–1.02
Educational level				
Elementary level or lower	1.00(ref.)	–	1.00(ref.)	–
Middle school graduate	0.99	0.76–1.28	0.99	0.74–1.33
High school graduate or higher	1.03	0.78–1.34	1.24	0.90–1.69
Marital status				
Currently married	1.00(ref.)	–		
Currently not married	0.99	0.74–1.33	0.99	0.72–1.37
Income (yuan)				
0–2000	1.00(ref.)	–	1.00(ref.)	–
2000–4000	1.18	0.95–1.48	0.98	0.76–1.27
> 4000	1.25	0.76–2.07	0.87	0.49–1.53
Smoking	1.81	1.42–2.30	1.67	1.22–2.29
Family history of cardiovascular diseases	1.45	1.11–1.89	1.52	1.14–2.02
General obesity	1.58	1.15–2.17	1.51	1.15–1.97
Abdominal obesity	2.08	1.67–2.60	1.94	0.89–1.60
LAP				
Q1	1.00(ref.)	–	1.00(ref.)	–
Q2	1.10	0.88–1.51	0.96	0.68–1.34
Q3	1.69	1.24–2.31	1.32	0.93–1.87
Q4	3.70	2.69–5.08	2.58	1.76–3.80

normal weight [46–48]. WC can accurately reflect abdominal obesity, but is unable to distinguish between subcutaneous fat and visceral fat. Importantly, visceral and subcutaneous adipose depots play differential roles in human health [17, 49]. Substantial evidence have suggested that visceral obesity may be more closely related with adverse outcomes such as cardiovascular diseases and death, and higher VAT significantly reduced the probability of conversion of prehypertension transforming to normotension [49–52]. Compared with SAT, VAT adipocytes are more metabolically active and less sensitive to insulin than SAT, it also can generate more free fatty acids and has a

Table 3 the comparisons of obesity indices in predicting prehypertension risk

		Cut-off value	Sensitivity (%)	Specificity (%)	AUC(95%CI)	Z	P^a
All	BMI	23.99	61.03	57.09	0.60(0.57–0.63)	3.52	< 0.01
	WC	86.50	52.40	68.83	0.63(0.60–0.65)	2.05	0.04
	LAP	38.22	56.22	66.80	0.65(0.62–0.68)	–	–
Male	BMI	24.00	62.50	56.08	0.59(0.54–0.63)	2.05	0.03
	WC	88.00	53.21	65.10	0.60(0.55–0.64)	1.77	0.07
	LAP	48.18	49.29	76.47	0.63 (0.59–0.67)	–	–
Female	BMI	23.95	59.75	57.61	0.61(0.58–0.65)	2.12	0.03
	WC	86.50	44.58	76.95	0.61(0.58–0.65)	2.43	0.01
	LAP	26.40	74.30	50.21	0.65 (0.62–0.68)	–	–

[a]compared with AUC

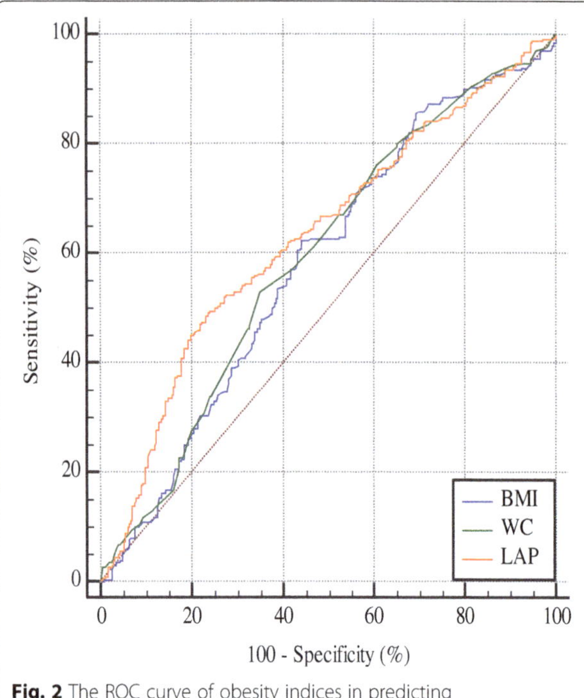

Fig. 2 The ROC curve of obesity indices in predicting prehypertension risk in males

greater ability to uptake glucose [53]. The Framingham Heart study with a follows up lasted for 6.2 years demonstrated that the effect of SAT on metabolic risk factors was less striking than that of VAT [50]. Tang et al. [51] measured VAT and SAT among 1449 Chinese adults by MRI, and the results also indicated that VAT was more strongly associated with cardiometabolic risk factors than SAT. High

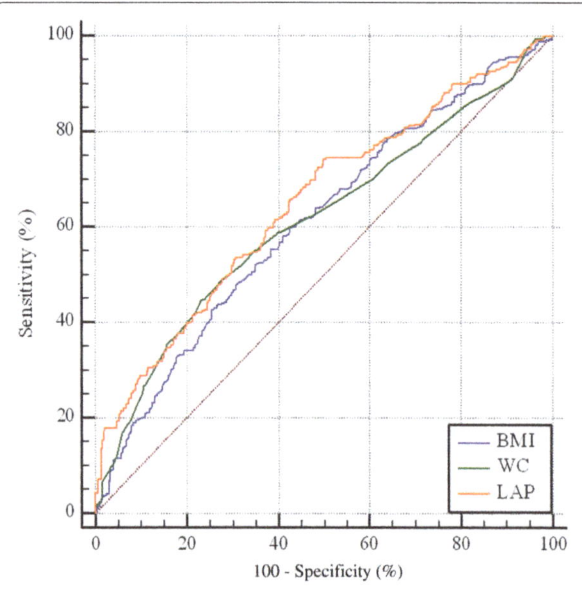

Fig. 3 The ROC curve of obesity indices in predicting prehypertension risk in females

visceral fat with low subcutaneous fat accumulation was significantly related with atherosclerosis in type 2 diabetes patients, suggesting that SAT may be a protective role against atherosclerosis [54]. Compared with epicardial fat volume and SAT, VAT had the strongest effect on cardiometabolic diseases [55]. Madero et al. [56] compared the value of different measures of body fat, including SAT, VAT, BMI and WC in predicting the incidence of chronic kidney diseases, and only VAT remained a decisive factor in multivariable analysis. Unfortunately, neither of BMI nor WC can distinguish between subcutaneous fat and visceral fat. Meanwhile, computed tomography (CT) and magnetic resonance imaging (MRI), as the gold standards to evaluate visceral fat, are not appropriate for widespread promotion and use in large-scale epidemiological survey because of their high costs and radiation exposure. Consequently, an inexpensive, efficient and available indicator that reflects visceral obesity is urgently needed.

LAP, as a combination of WC and TG, can reflect anatomic and physiologic changes and has theoretical basis to evaluate visceral obesity [18]. TG can reflect the degree of visceral fat accumulation caused by metabolic disorders, and significant relationships had been found between WC and insulin resistance, hypertension and metabolic syndrome [57–59]. Moreover, a cross-sectional study in China demonstrated that higher TG was the main risk factor of prehypertension [41]. Surprisingly, no significant relationship was found between WC and prehypertension risk in multivariable model, which was consistent with a published study [31]. This may be explained by the fact that most of individuals with abdominal obesity would progress to actual hypertension [31]. A strong correlation between LAP and area of visceral adipose tissue measured by CT were observed, suggesting that LAP was an effective marker discriminating visceral obesity [60]. "Hypertriglyceridemic waist (HTGW)", the combination of WC and TG, is a dichotomous indicator, while LAP is developed to express as a continuous indicator. A growing number of evidence has proved that LAP may be more reasonable and scientific than HTGW, as obesity itself is a continuous process [18]. As a result, LAP was applied as a visceral obesity indicator rather than HTGW in this study.

The results obtained in this study indicated that higher LAP significantly increased the risk of prehypertension, and it is superior to BMI and WC for discriminating prehypertension risk. However, when grouped by gender, LAP was only better than WC in female. With aging, the patterns of lipid over accumulation in men and women became more and more distinct, as LAP got higher or stayed the same level in women with aging, while it reduced gradually in men at older age [61]. At the same BMI level, female have more body fat than male [62]. In addition to the greater impact of Hyper-TG on cardiovascular diseases in female than male [63], VAT was reported to be more strongly associated

Table 4 the interaction analysis for prehypertension risk

Variable		Interaction analysis[b]		
		RERI	AP	SI
LAP[a]	Family history	1.88(0.25–3.51)[3]	0.44(0.20–0.69)[3]	2.37(1.22–4.60)[3]
LAP[a]	Smoking	1.99(0.04-3.93)[3]	0.42(0.17-0.67)[3]	2.16(1.68–4.00)[3]
Family history	Smoking	1.32(−0.60–3.23)[4]	0.40(0.03-0.77)[3]	2.37(0.87-6.44)[4]

[a]: grouped by cut-off values in Table 2
[b]: adjust for age, sex, educational level, marital status and monthly income
[3]: $P<0.05$
[4]: $P>0.05$

with cardiometabolic risk factors in obese female than male as well [64]. In men, SAT and VAT had similar effects on insulin resistance, while in female, only VAT was associated with insulin resistance [65]. Similar to our study, LAP seemed to increase diabetes risk stronger in female than male in Japanese [66]. What is more, a hospital-based cross-sectional survey in China indicated that LAP was significantly associated with intracranial atherosclerotic stenosis in middle-aged and elderly female, but not in male [67]. Compared with BMI, LAP performed better in identifying chronic kidney disease in female living in the rural of Northeast China, but less well in male [68]. Therefore, LAP may have a more excellent value in female and the gender-specific differences need to be further explored. Additionally, several studies have also demonstrated that the relationship between LAP and diseases risk may be influenced by age, which was then proved by the analysis of the relationship between LAP and risk of non-alcoholic fatty liver disease in Chinese adults, indicating that the diagnostic ability of LAP was higher in younger adults [69]. A cohort study with 6-years follow-up further explored that LAP was superior to BMI in predicting incident diabetes only in young men [70]. A given WC represented differential amount of visceral fat in older subjects and younger subjects [71]. However, in this study, the mean age of participants was 60.82, for that reason, the effect of LAP on prehypertension in younger groups should be further investigated.

Biological interaction refers to the mutual influence of two pathogenic factors on the pathogenesis of the diseases. We demonstrated significant interactions between LAP and family of cardiovascular diseases, LAP and smoking, family of cardiovascular diseases and smoking on prehypertension risk, separately. Family history of cardiovascular diseases is considered to be an indicative sign of genetic susceptibility. The present study, as well as other research [9], announced a significant relationship between family of cardiovascular diseases and prehypertension risk. Laboratory stressor tests showed that healthy subjects with family history of cardiovascular diseases had a more positive hemodynamic responsiveness to stressor tests [72]. Our results demonstrated that smokers had 1.67 fold risks in getting prehypertension, while other researchers failed to report a significant relationship [31, 34]. This may be due to the various standards of smoking. It was suggested by JNC-7 that lifestyle modifications, including quitting smoking, might be beneficial to the prevention of prehypertension. Furthermore, relevant research had indicated that obesity and smoking have several common mechanisms to increase blood pressure, such as inhibiting vascular reflex vasodilation and increasing oxidative stress [73]. Smoking was interacted with obesity on diabetes risk [23]. There was also a significant interaction of passive smoking with pregnancy obesity on risk of gestational diabetes mellitus in Chinese adults [74]. So far, there are few articles exploring the interaction of risk factors on prehypertension risk, and the interactive mechanisms between factors needs to be further studied in the future.

There are several limitations of this study in the following aspects. Firstly, as a cross-sectional survey, it failed to infer causality in its results. Secondly, there were ethnic and racial differences in body composition [75], therefore the relationship between LAP and prehypertension was not clear in other ethnic individuals. Thirdly, whether participated individuals had taken lipid lowering drugs was not investigated.

Conclusion

In conclusion, prehypertension is prevalent in Chinese adults. This study indicated that age, family history of cardiovascular diseases, smoking and LAP were significantly related to prehypertension risk. Furthermore, we demonstrated significant interactions between risk factors on prehypertension risk, which would help us to establish strategy against prehypertension more comprehensively and scientifically. Further studies should pay more attention to the gender-difference of LAP and the underlying mechanisms of interactive effect on prehypertension risk.

Abbreviations

BMI: Body mass index; CT: Computed tomography; LAP: Lipid accumulation product; MRI: Magnetic resonance imaging; SAT: Subcutaneous adipose tissue; VAT: Visceral adipose tissue; WC: Waist circumference

Acknowledgments

We are grateful to all professionals and participants of the study.

Funding

Our work was financed by the National Natural Science Foundation of China (number: 81373100) and Bengbu health board, China. The funders had no part in the study design, data collection, data analysis, interpretation of data or in writing the manuscript.

Authors' contributions

GHQ and WXS designed the conception of the study. SJ, ZYY, MJ, CX were responsible for the acquisition of data. WXS and SJ contributed to statistical analysis. SJ and CX contributed to the interpretation of data. SJ drafted the manuscript. All authors revised it critically and approved the final version.

Competing interests

The authors declare that they have no competing interests.

Author details

[1]School of public health, Bengbu medical college, 2600 Donghai Road, Bengbu 233000, Anhui Province, China. [2]Bengbu health board, 568 Nanhu Road, Bengbu 233000, Anhui Province, China.

References

1. Lackland DT, Beilin LJ, Campbell NRC, Jaffe MG, Orias M, Ram CV, et al. Global implications of blood pressure thresholds and targets: guideline conversations from the world hypertension league. Hypertension. 2018;71(6):985–7.
2. Vaduganathan M, Pareek M, Qamar A, Pandey A, Olsen MH, Bhatt DL. Baseline Blood Pressure, the 2017 ACC/AHA High Blood Pressure Guidelines, and Long- Term Cardiovascular Risk in SPRINT. Am J Med. 2018.
3. Evans PL, Prior JA, Belcher J, Mallen CD, Hay CA, Roddy E. Obesity, hypertension and diuretic use as risk factors for incident gout: a systematic review and meta-analysis of cohort studies. Arthritis Res Ther. 2018;20(1):136.
4. Hou L, Li Q, Jiang L, Qiu H, Geng C, Hong JS, et al. Hypertension and diagnosis of Parkinson's disease: a meta-analysis of cohort studies. Front Neurol. 2018;9:162.
5. Ballocca F, D'Ascenzo F, Moretti C, Omede P, Cerrato E, Barbero U, et al. Predictors of cardiovascular events in patients with systemic lupus erythematosus (SLE): a systematic review and meta-analysis. Eur J Prev Cardiol. 2015;22(11):1435–41.
6. Chobanian AV, Bakris GL, Black HR, Cushman WC, Green LA, et al. The seventh report of the joint National Committee on prevention, detection, evaluation, and treatment of high blood pressure: the JNC 7 report. JAMA. 2003;289(19):2560–72.
7. Fuchs FD, De Mello RB, Fuchs SC. Preventing the progression of prehypertension to hypertension: role of antihypertensives. Curr Hypertens Rep, 2015,17(1):505.
8. Tseng CD, Yen AM, Chiu SY, et al. A predictive model for risk of prehypertension and hypertension and expected benefit after population-based life-style modification (KCIS no. 24). Am J Hypertens. 2012;25(2):171–9.
9. Xu T, Liu J, Zhu G, Liu J, Han S. Prevalence of prehypertension and associated risk factors among Chinese adults from a large-scale multi-ethnic population survey. BMC Public Health. 2016;16(1):775.
10. Li G, Guo G, Wang W, Wang K, Wang H, Dong F, et al. Association of prehypertension and cardiovascular risk factor clustering in Inner Mongolia: a cross-sectional study. BMJ Open. 2017;7(6):e015340.
11. Xue H, Wang J, Hou J, Li J, Gao J, Chen S, et al. Prehypertension and chronic kidney disease in Chinese population: four-year follow-up study. PLoS One. 2015;10(12):e0144438.
12. Huang Y, Cai X, Liu C, Zhu D, Hua J, Hu Y, et al. Prehypertension and the risk of coronary heart disease in Asian and Western populations: a meta-analysis. J Am Heart Assoc. 2015;4:2.
13. Barbero U, D'Ascenzo F, Nijhoff F, Moretti C, Biondi-Zoccai G, Mennuni M, Capodanno D, et al. Assessing Risk in Patients with Stable Coronary Disease: When Should We Intensify Care and Follow-Up? Results from a Meta-Analysis of Observational Studies of the COURAGE and FAME Era. Scientifica (Cairo). 2016;2016:3769152.
14. Huang Y, Cai X, Li Y, Su L, Mai W, Wang S, et al. Prehypertension and the risk of stroke: a meta-analysis. Neurology. 2014;82(13):1153–61.
15. Egan BM, Stevens-Fabry S. Prehypertension–prevalence, health risks, and management strategies. Nat Rev Cardiol. 2015;12(5):289–300.
16. Stabouli S, Papakatsika S, Kotsis V. The role of obesity, salt and exercise on blood pressure in children and adolescents. Expert Rev Cardiovasc Ther. 2011;9(6):753–61.
17. Ibrahim MM. Subcutaneous and visceral adipose tissue: structural and functional differences. Obes Rev. 2010;11(1):11–8.
18. Kahn HS. The "lipid accumulation product" performs better than the body mass index for recognizing cardiovascular risk: a population-based comparison. BMC Cardiovasc Disord. 2005;5:26.
19. Cartolano FC, Pappiani C, Freitas MCP, Figueiredo Neto AM, Carioca AAF, Damasceno NRT. Is lipid accumulation product associated with an Atherogenic lipoprotein profile in Brazilian subjects? Arq Bras Cardiol. 2018;110(4):339–47.
20. Wang H, Sun Y, Wang S, Qian H, Jia P, Chen Y, et al. Body adiposity index, lipid accumulation product, and cardiometabolic index reveal the contribution of adiposity phenotypes in the risk of hyperuricemia among Chinese rural population. Clin Rheumatol. 2018. https://doi.org/10.1007/s10067-018-4143-x.
21. Mazidi M, Kengne AP, Katsiki N, Mikhailidis DP, Banach M. Lipid accumulation product and triglycerides/glucose index are useful predictors of insulin resistance. J Diabetes Complicat. 2018;32(3):266–70.
22. Ray L, Ravichandran K, Nanda SK. Comparison of lipid accumulation product index with body mass index and waist circumference as a predictor of metabolic syndrome in Indian population. Metab Syndr Relat Disord. 2018;16(5):240–5.
23. Luo W, Guo Z, Wu M, Hao C, Zhou Z, Yao X. Interaction of smoking and obesity on type 2 diabetes risk in a Chinese cohort. Physiol Behav. 2015;139:240–3.
24. Barbero U, Destefanis P. An Indian-look right into restrictive cardiomyopathies. Indian Heart J. 2015;67(6):512–3.
25. Writing Group of 2010 Chinese guidelines for the Management of Hypertension. 2010 Chinese guidelines for the management of hypertension. Chine J Cardiol. 2011;39:579–616 (In Chinese).
26. Chen C, Lu FC, Department of Disease Control Ministry of Health, PR China. The guidelines for prevention and control of overweight and obesity in Chinese adults. Biomed EnvironSci. 2004, 17 Suppl: 1–36.
27. Chu JR, Gao JL, Zhao SP, et al. Blood lipid abnormity prevention guidance in Chinese adult. Chin Circ J. 2016;31(10):937–53.
28. Andersson T, Alfredsson L, Kallberg H, et al. Calculating measures of biological interaction. Eur J Epidemiol. 2005;20:575–9.
29. Knol MJ, Vander Weele TJ, Groenwold RH, et al. Estimating measures of interaction on an additive scale for preventive exposures. Eur J Epidemiol. 2011;26(6):433–8.
30. Tsai PS, Ke TL, Huang CJ, Tsai JC, Chen PL, Wang SY, et al. Prevalence and determinants of prehypertension status in the Taiwanese general population. J Hypertens. 2005;23:1355–60.
31. Hu L, Huang X, You C, Li J, Hong K, Li P, et al. Prevalence and Risk Factors of Prehypertension and Hypertension in Southern China. PLoS One. 2017;12(1):e 0170238.
32. Yang L, Yan J, Tang X, Xu X, Yu W, Wu H. Prevalence, awareness, treatment, control and risk factors associated with hypertension among adults in southern China, 2013. PLoS One. 2016;11:e146181.
33. Ma M, Tan X, Zhu S. Prehypertension and its optimal indicator among adults in Hubei Province, Central China, 2013-2015. Clin Exp Hypertens. 2017;39(6):532–8.

34. Shen Y, Chang C, Zhang J, Jiang Y, Ni B, Wang Y. Prevalence and risk factors associated with hypertension and prehypertension in a working population at high altitude in China: a cross-sectional study. Environ Health Prev Med. 2017;22(1):19.
35. Do HT, Geleijnse JM, Le MB, Kok FJ, Feskens EJ. National prevalence and associated risk factors of hypertension and prehypertension among Vietnamese adults. Am J Hypertens. 2015;28(1):89–97.
36. Tabrizi JS, Sadeghi-Bazargani H, Farahbakhsh M, Nikniaz L, Nikniaz Z. Prevalence and Associated Factors of Prehypertension and Hypertension in Iranian Population: The Lifestyle Promotion Project (LPP). PLoS One. 2016;11(10):e01652 64.
37. Lee W, Yoon JH, Roh J, Lee S, Seok H, Lee JH, et al. The association between low blood lead levels and the prevalence of prehypertension among nonhypertensive adults in Korea. Am J Hum Biol. 2016;28(5):729–35.
38. Glasser SP, Judd S, Basile J, Lackland D, Halanych J, Cushman M, et al. Prehypertension, racial prevalence and its association with risk factors: analysis of the REasons for geographic and racial differences in stroke (REGARDS) study. Am J Hypertens. 2011;24(2):194–9.
39. Hong H, Wang H, Liao H. Prehypertension is associated with increased carotid atherosclerotic plaque in the community population of southern China. BMC Cardiovasc Disord. 2013;13:20.
40. Lorenzo C, Aung K, Stern MP, Haffner SM. Pulse pressure, prehypertension, and mortality: the San Antonio heart study. Am J Hypertens. 2009;22(11):1219–26.
41. Liu B, Dong X, Xiao Y, et al. Variability of metabolic risk factors associated with prehypertension in males and females: a cross-sectional study in China. Arch Med Sci. 2018;14(4):766–72.
42. Wu J, Xu H, He X, et al. Six-year changes in the prevalence of obesity and obesity-related diseases in northeastern China from 2007 to 2013. Sci Rep. 2017;7:41518.
43. Boscaro M, Giacchetti G, Ronconi V. Visceral adipose tissue: emerging role of gluco-and mineralocorticoid hormones in the setting of cardiometabolic alterations. Ann N Y Acad Sci. 2012;1264:87–102.
44. Kawarazaki W, Fujita T. The role of aldosterone in obesity-related hypertension. Am J Hypertens. 2016;29(4):415–23.
45. Lovren F, Teoh H, Verma S. Obesity and atherosclerosis:mechanistic insights. Can J Cardiol. 2015;31(2):177–83.
46. Horwich TB, Fonarow GC, Clark AL. Obesity and the Obesity Paradox in Heart Failure. Prog Cardiovasc Dis. 2018.
47. Cespedes Feliciano EM, Kroenke CH, Caan BJ. The obesity paradox in Cancer: how important is muscle? Annu rev Nutr. 2018;38:357–79.
48. Lin TY, Lim PS, Hung SC. Impact of misclassification of obesity by body mass index on mortality in patients with CKD. Kidney Int Rep. 2017;3(2):447–55.
49. Sam S. Differential effect of subcutaneous abdominal and visceral adipose tissue on cardiometabolic risk. Horm Mol Biol Clin Investig. 2018;33:1.
50. Abraham TM, Pedley A, Massaro JM, Hoffmann U, Fox CS. Association between visceral and subcutaneous adipose depots and incident cardiovascular disease risk factors. Circulation. 2015;132(17):1639–47.
51. Tang L, Zhang F, Tong N. The association of visceral adipose tissue and subcutaneous adipose tissue with metabolic risk factors in a large population of Chinese adults. Clin Endocrinol. 2016;85(1):46–53.
52. Hwang YC, Fujimoto WY, Kahn SE, Leonetti DL, Boyko EJ. Greater visceral abdominal fat is associated with a lower probability of conversion of prehypertension to normotension. J Hypertens. 2017;35(6):1213–8.
53. Viljanen AP, Lautamaki R, Jarvisalo M, et al. Effects of weight loss on visceral and abdominal subcutaneous adipose tissue blood flow and insulin-mediated glucose uptake in healthy obese subjects. Ann Med. 2009;41:152–60.
54. Bouchi R, Takeuchi T, Akihisa M, Ohara N, Nakano Y, Nishitani R, et al. High visceral fat with low subcutaneous fat accumulation as a determinant of atherosclerosis in patients with type 2 diabetes. Cardiovasc Diabetol. 2015;14:136.48.
55. Sato F, Maeda N, Yamada T, Namazui H, Fukuda S, Natsukawa T, et al. Association of Epicardial, visceral, and subcutaneous fat with Cardiometabolic diseases. Circ J. 2018;82(2):502–8.
56. Madero M, Katz R, Murphy R, Newman A, Patel K, Ix J, et al. Comparison between different measures of body fat with kidney function decline and incident CKD. Clin J Am Soc Nephrol. 2017;12(6):893–903.
57. Wolfgram PM, Connor EL, Rehm JL, et al. In nonobese girls, waist circumference as a predictor of insulin resistance is comparable to MRI fat measures and superior to BMI. Horm Res Paediatr. 2015;84(4):258–65.
58. Nurdiantami Y, Watanabe K, Tanaka E, et al. Association of general and central obesity with hypertension. Clin Nutr. 2017.
59. Owolabi EO, Ter Goon D, Adeniyi OV, Ajayi AI. Optimal waist circumference cut-off points for predicting metabolic syndrome among low-income black south African adults. BMC Res Notes 2018, 11(1):22.
60. Roriz AK, Passos LC, de Oliveira CC, Eickemberg M, Moreira Pde A, Sampaio LR. Evaluation of the accuracy of anthropometric clinical indicators of visceral fat in adults and elderly. PLoS One 2014, 9(7):e103499.
61. Kahn HS, Cheng YJ. Longitudinal changes in BMI and in an index estimating excess lipids among white and black adults in the United States. Int J Obes. 2008;32:136–43.
62. Bredella MA. Sex differences in body composition. Adv Exp Med Biol. 2017;1043:9–27.
63. Hokanson JE, Austin MA. Plasma triglyceride level is a risk factor for cardiovascular disease independent of high-density lipoprotein cholesterol level: a meta-analysis of population-based prospective studies. J Cardiovasc Risk. 1996;3:213–9.
64. Elffers TW, de Mutsert R, Lamb HJ, de Roos A, Willems van Dijk K, Rosendaal FR, et al. Body fat distribution, in particular visceral fat, is associated with cardiometabolic risk factors in obese women. PLoS One. 2017;12(9):e0185403.
65. de Mutsert R, Gast K, Widya R, de Koning E, Jazet I, Lamb H, et al. Associations of abdominal subcutaneous and visceral fat with insulin resistance and secretion differ between men and women: the Netherlands epidemiology of obesity study. Metab Syndr Relat Disord. 2018;16(1):54–63.
66. Wakabayashi I. Influence of age and gender on lipid accumulation product and its relation to diabetes mellitus in Japanese. Clin Chim Acta. 2014;431:221–6.
67. Li R, Li Q, Cui M, Ying Z, Li L, Zhong T, et al. Visceral adiposity index, lipid accumulation product and intracranial atherosclerotic stenosis in middle-aged and elderly Chinese. Sci Rep. 2017;7(1):7951.
68. Dai D, Chang Y, Chen Y, Chen S, Yu S, Guo X, et al. Visceral Adiposity Index and Lipid Accumulation Product Index: Two Alternate Body Indices to Identify Chronic Kidney Disease among the Rural Population in Northeast China. Int J Environ Res Public Health. 2016;13:12.
69. Dai H, Wang W, Chen R, Chen Z, Lu Y, Yuan H. Lipid accumulation product is a powerful tool to predict non-alcoholic fatty liver disease in Chinese adults. Nutr Metab (Lond). 2017;14:49.
70. Bozorgmanesh M, Hadaegh F, Azizi F. Diabetes prediction, lipid accumulation product, and adiposity measures; 6-year follow-up: Tehran lipid and glucose study. Lipids Health Dis. 2010;9:45.
71. Han TS, McNeill G, Seidell JC, Lean ME. Predicting intra-abdominal fatness from anthropometric measures: the influence of stature. Int J Obes Relat Metab Disord. 1997;21:587–93.
72. Simoes GM, Campagnaro BP, Tonini CL, Meyrelles SS, Kuniyoshi FH, Vasquez EC. Hemodynamic reactivity to laboratory stressors in healthy subjects: influence of gender and family history of cardiovascular diseases. Int J Med Sci. 2013;10(7):848–56.
73. Talukder MAH, Johnson WM, Varadharaj S, Lian J, Kearns PN, El-Mahdy MA, et al. Chronic cigarette smoking causes hypertension, increased oxidative stress, impaired NO bioavailability, endothelial dysfunction, and cardiac remodeling in mice. Am J Physiol Heart Circ Physiol. 2011;300(1):388–96.
74. Leng J, Wang P, Shao P, Zhang C, Li W, Li N, et al. Passive smoking increased risk of gestational diabetes mellitus independently and synergistically with prepregnancy obesity in Tianjin, China. Diabetes Metab Res Rev. 2017;33:3.
75. Nazare JA, Smith JD, Borel AL, et al. Ethnic influences on the relations between abdominal subcutaneous and visceral adiposity, liver fat, and cardiometabolic risk profile: the international study of prediction of intra abdominal adiposity and its relationship with Cardiometabolic risk/ IntraAbdominal adiposity. Am J Clin Nutr. 2012;96:714–26.

Resource use and clinical outcomes in patients with atrial fibrillation with ablation versus antiarrhythmic drug treatment

Julian W. E. Jarman[1], Wajid Hussain[1], Tom Wong[1], Vias Markides[1], Jamie March[2], Laura Goldstein[2], Ray Liao[3], Iftekhar Kalsekar[4], Abhishek Chitnis[4] and Rahul Khanna[4*]

Abstract

Background: The objective of our study was to compare resource use and clinical outcomes among atrial fibrillation (AF) patients who underwent catheter ablation versus antiarrhythmic drug (AAD) treatment.

Methods: A retrospective cohort design using the Clinical Practice Research Data-Hospital Episode Statistics linkage data from England (2008–2013) was used. Patients undergoing catheter ablation treatment for AF were indexed to the date of first procedure. AAD patients with at least two different AAD drugs were indexed to the first fill of the second AAD. Patients were matched using 1:1 propensity matching. Primary endpoints including inpatient and outpatient visits were compared between ablation and AAD cohorts in the 4 months-1 year period after index. Secondary endpoints including heart failure, stroke, cardioversion, mortality, and a composite outcome were compared for the 4 months-3 years post-index period in the two groups. Cox-proportional hazards models were estimated for clinical outcomes comparison.

Results: A total of 558 patients were matched in the two groups for resource utilization comparison. The average number of cardiovascular (CV)-related outpatient visits in the 4–12 months post-index period were significantly lower in the ablation group versus the AAD group (1.76 vs 3.57, $p < .0001$). There was no significant difference in all-cause and CV-related inpatient visits and all-cause outpatient visits among the two groups. For secondary endpoints comparison, 615 matched patients in each group emerged. Ablation patients had 38% lower risk of heart failure (hazard ratio [HR] 0.62, $p = 0.0318$), 50% lower risk of mortality (HR 0.50, $p = 0.0082$), and 43% lower risk of experiencing a composite outcome (HR 0.57, $p = 0.0009$) as compared to AAD treatment cohort.

Conclusion: AF ablation was associated with significantly lower CV-related outpatient visits, and lower risk of heart failure and mortality versus AAD therapy.

Keywords: Atrial fibrillation, Catheter ablation, Anti-arrhythmic drugs

Background

Atrial fibrillation (AF) affects approximately 2% of the population and is a significant risk factor for stroke and heart failure [1–3]. Recent estimates suggest that AF prevalence is increasingly on a yearly basis in the United Kingdom (UK), and the number of patients with AF is expected to increase from 700,000 in 2010 to as high as 1.8 million by 2060 [4]. Besides causing significant morbidity, AF is associated with considerable healthcare utilization and economic burden. In the UK, the direct costs are estimated to be as high as £244 million (2004) of which hospitalizations and prescription drugs account for 70% of the expenditure [5]. In Europe, AF has a substantial economic burden, ranging from €660 million to €3286 million; direct costs comprise up to 80% of costs [6, 7].

Treatments for AF include both pharmaceutical and non-pharmaceutical options; however, a large proportion of patients are left untreated [3, 8, 9]. Undertreatment is the result of multiple factors, including improper assessment, over-estimation of the risk of bleeding and

* Correspondence: rkhann14@its.jnj.com
[4]Medical Device Epidemiology, Johnson and Johnson, 410 George Street, New Brunswick, NJ 08901, USA
Full list of author information is available at the end of the article

underestimation of the risk of stroke. Clinical trials demonstrate that AF ablation supports sinus rhythm more effectively than antiarrhythmic drugs (AAD) in patients with symptomatic, paroxysmal AF [10, 11]. Ablation treatment has been shown to be cost-effective as compared to AAD treatment for AF [12], and is associated with improvement in patient-reported health-related quality of life [13]. In addition, retrospective cohort studies using large databases have found significantly lower rate of stroke and other adverse outcomes associated with AF ablation as compared to other treatment alternatives including AAD drugs [14, 17]. In one such study, Jarman et al. (2017) found significantly lower rates of stroke among AF patients undergoing ablation procedure as compared to AF patients who did not have an ablation or had cardioversion [15].

The current study builds on earlier clinical and observational research on understanding the difference between ablation and AAD treatment for AF. The primary objective of the study was to compare health care resource use over a 1-year period among patients with AF who underwent catheter ablation as compared to AAD treatment. Secondary objectives included comparison of stroke/transient ischemic attack (TIA), heart failure, direct current cardioversion (DCCV), death, and a composite of these outcomes among AF patients with ablation versus AAD treatment.

Methods

Data source(s)

The UK Clinical Practice Research Datalink (CPRD), a longitudinal database of more than 11 million patients representing 7% of the total UK population [18], was used for the current study. CPRD data has been utilized in over 1800 publications including drug safety, practice guidelines and clinical guidelines (www.cprd.com). Along with CPRD, linkage with Hospital Episode Statistics (HES) was performed to identify the patients with and without ablation for AF. HES data contains detailed information on the fields from the admitted patient, outpatient, accident and emergency (A&E) and adult critical care.

Study design

This retrospective longitudinal cohort design studied patients ≥18 years of age diagnosed with AF and treated with either ablation or AADs (specified as amiodarone, disopyramide, dronedarone, flecainide, propafenone, and sotalol) during an evaluation period from 2008 to 2013. For the ablation cohort, the earliest date of the ablation procedure was defined as the index date. Since catheter ablation is recommended only for patients that have failed to show improvement on prior AAD therapy, patients in the AAD cohort were required to have prescriptions for at least two different AAD drugs during the study period, to ensure comparisons between the two cohorts were conducted between like populations (e.g., all patients had failed or lacked sufficient improvement on first AAD). For the AAD cohort, the date of the second AAD was defined as the index date. All patients were required to have 12 months of complete medical record data prior to index date (referred to as the baseline or pre-index period), as well as 12 months of post-index data. Consistent with past approaches and treatment guidelines [11, 19], we implemented a 3-month blanking period for outcomes assessed across both groups.

Patients were excluded if any of the following criteria were met: ablation procedures performed during the 12-month pre-index period (ablation cohort) or ablation procedures performed during 12-months pre- and post-index period (AAD medication cohort); procedural code for implantation of a pacemaker or implantable cardioversion defibrillator in the 12-month pre-index period; surgical ablation performed in the 12-month pre-index period including those ablation procedures that are performed concomitantly with open heart surgery for valvular, ischemic, or congenital heart disease; valvular procedures performed in the 12-month pre-index period; and left atrial appendage occlusion procedure in the 12-month pre-index period.

Study measures

Patient age and gender were recorded on the index date. Patient comorbidities were recorded during the baseline (pre-index) period based on the presence of specific ICD codes and included ischemic heart disease with and without myocardial infarction, heart failure, cardiomyopathy, hypertensive heart disease without heart failure, valvular heart disease, conduction system disease, Wolff-Parkinson-White syndrome, other arrhythmias, hypertension, diabetes, obstructive sleep apnea, chronic obstructive pulmonary disease (COPD), acute renal failure, stroke/TIA, DCCV, and hyperthyroidism. The Charlson comorbidity index (CCI), which is an aggregate measure of comorbidity created by using select diagnoses associated with chronic disease (e.g., heart disease, cancer), was also assessed. The CCI includes 17 medical conditions and weights these conditions from + 1 to + 6 [20, 21]. Patients' stroke risk was measured using the $CHADS_2$-VASc index with a maximum score of 9; it was calculated using the presence of congestive heart failure, hypertension, Type II Diabetes Mellitus (T2DM), stroke, age, prior MI disease. Cardiovascular-related inpatient and outpatient visits in the 12-month pre-index period were assessed. Lastly, rate-control and anticoagulant medications used in the 12-month pre-index period were also assessed.

Outcome measures

Primary outcome measures, assessed during the post-blanking 4-month to 12-month period, were defined as the average number of all-cause and cardiovascular-related inpatient admissions and outpatient visits. Secondary outcome measures included inpatient readmissions with any recorded diagnosis of heart failure, stroke/transient ischemic attack (TIA), DCCV, death, and a composite measure of these outcomes occurring during the post-blanking 4-month to 3-year period. Patients were followed from the index date until record of event, death, or end of follow-up, whichever came first.

Data analysis

The ablation and AAD cohorts were first matched using the propensity score matching technique, implementing a multivariate logistic regression between patients who underwent ablation and those receiving AADs to assess factors predicting the use of ablation procedure among AF patients. Factors included in matching were age and gender (recorded at index date), comorbidities at baseline, drug utilization, and baseline resource use. After propensity score matching, the average number of inpatient admissions and outpatient visits (primary outcome measures) were compared between cohorts. Comparisons between groups were performed using 2-sample t-test. As part of the secondary outcomes assessment, a separate propensity score matching was conducted, as the pre-match ablation and AAD sample involved was different than the pre-match sample for the primary objective assessment. For secondary objectives, the ablation and AAD sample were followed for a period of three years and were therefore not required to have 12-month post-index continuous enrollment (unlike primary objective assessment, where this criterion was applied). Secondary outcomes were studied in the propensity-matched sample using log-rank test. Further, regression analysis using Cox Proportional Hazards modeling was conducted to examine the relationship between treatment status and secondary outcome adjusting for any significant standardized differences emerging post-matching. All analyses were conducted using SAS for Windows and statistical significance was set a-priori at $p < 0.05$ (two-sided).

Results

A total of 1508 patients in the ablation cohort and 920 patients in the AAD cohort were included (Fig. 1). After applying propensity score matching, a total of 558 patients were included in each cohort. The post-match sample balanced well on study variables as indicated by standardized difference scores (which were less than 0.10 for all variables except index year and Wolff-Parkinson White syndrome) between the two groups (Table 1).

No significant differences in the ablation and AAD cohort emerged in terms of the average number of all-cause hospitalizations (0.70 vs 0.75, $p = 0.086$), cardiovascular-related hospitalizations (0.55 vs.0.58, $p = 0.355$), and all-cause outpatient visits (7.95 vs.8.79, $p = 0.203$). However, the average number of cardiovascular-related outpatient visits were significantly lower for the ablation cohort as compared to the AAD cohort (1.76 vs.3.57, $p <$ 0.0001, Table 2).

For the secondary outcomes assessment, where patients were followed for a period of three years, a total of 1528 patients in the ablation cohort and 927 patients in the AAD cohort emerged as part of the pre-match sample. Significant standardized differences in the pre-match study cohorts were observed. After propensity matching, a total of 615 matched patients were included in each cohort, and were analyzed with respect to the secondary outcomes. The two cohorts matched well in terms of standardized differences (Table 3), with only index year emerging as significant post-matching, which was adjusted in a Cox regression model.

Figure 2 (a-e) depicts the survival curves for the ablation and AAD cohort for secondary outcomes. Results from comparing survival curves for heart failure were significant, with the ablation cohort having lower likelihood of heart failure over the three-year period as compared to the AAD cohort ($p = 0.0342$ for the log-rank test; Fig. 2a). No significant differences in survival curves for stroke/TIA ($p = 0.579$ for log-rank test; Fig. 2b) or DCCV ($p = 0.2018$ for log-rank test; Fig. 2c) emerged between the two cohorts. The ablation cohort was found to have a significantly lower rate of death ($p = 0.0112$ for log-rank test; Fig. 2d) and of the composite outcome ($p = 0.0012$ for log-rank test; Fig. 2e) as compared to AAD cohort.

Results from the regression analysis revealed that patients in the ablation cohort had a 38% lower rate of heart failure (Hazard Ratio [HR]: 0.624; $p = 0.0318$) as compared to the AAD cohort. Patients in the ablation cohort had ~ 50% lower mortality rate as compared to the AAD cohort (HR: 0.507, $p = 0.008$). The ablation cohort was ~ 43% less likely to incur any defined events (composite outcome) during the three-year follow-up as compared to the AAD cohort (HR: 0.578; $p = 0.001$). No significant difference in likelihood of stroke/TIA (HR: 0.82; $p = 0.623$) and DCCV (HR:0.793; $p = 0.169$) were observed between the ablation and AAD cohort.

Discussion

Current guidelines for AF management recommend AADs as the first-line therapy [11, 19, 22–25]. The 12-month AF recurrence rate for patients treated with AADs ranges from 24 to 63% [11, 22, 25]. Among drug refractory AF patients, catheter ablation is the recommended treatment option [19]. A meta-analysis of nine studies found significantly better success rate for AF treatment with catheter ablation both in the short-term (< 1 year) [OR, 10.84; 95% CI, 5.83–20.16; $P < 0.001$] and long-term (> 1 year) [OR,

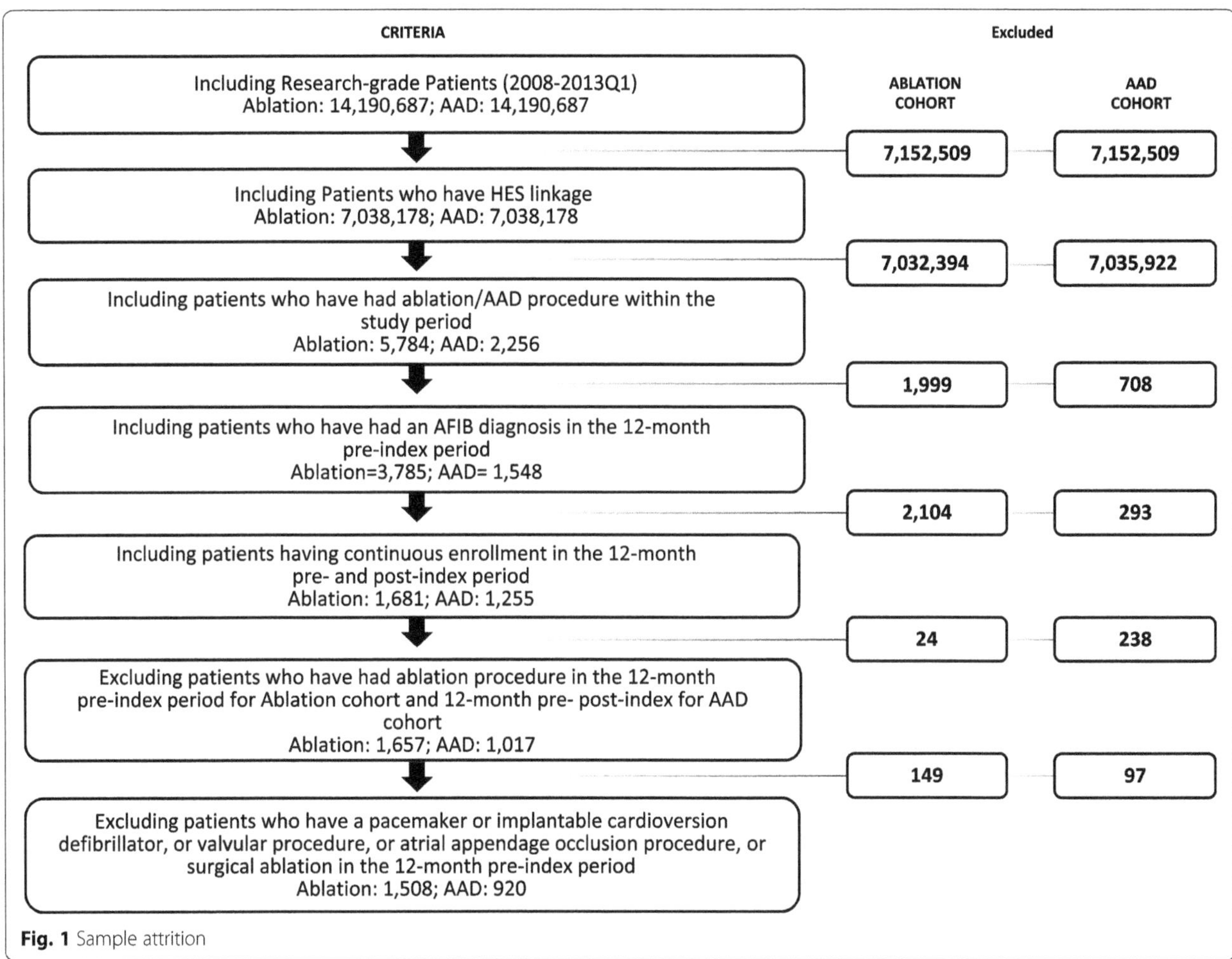

Fig. 1 Sample attrition

7.65; 95% CI, 1.97–29.73; $P = 0.03$] as compared to AADs [26]. While existing randomized controlled trial (RCT) experience demonstrates superior efficacy in terms of reduction of AF recurrence and symptoms with ablation over AADs [11, 22, 23, 25], it is important to explore the outcome variation in other parameters such as resource utilization and clinical events/hospitalizations among the two treatments in a real-world environment.

Using one of the largest nationally representative databases in the UK, our study provided insights into a short- and long-term outcomes comparison between ablation and AAD treatment among patients with AF. When assessing the cost-effectiveness of ablation treatment as compared to AAD treatment among AF patients, Rizzo et al. (2012) found an incremental cost-effectiveness ratio of £12,500 to £15,300 per quality-adjusted life-year for the ablation cohort as compared to the AAD cohort (QALY) [12]. Further, the authors reported the quality-adjusted life expectancy to be between 11.75 to 12.20 years for catheter ablation and 11.00 to 11.35 years for AAD cohort [12]. We conducted propensity score matching to minimize heterogeneity between the groups and normalize key influential factors including demographics, and underlying comorbidity status. Our study adds to the existing evidence highlighting the clinical outcome and resource utilization benefit associated with ablation as compared to AADs among AF patients.

Consistent with past studies, our study indicates lower resource use and better outcomes associated with ablation treatment as compared to AAD treatment among patients with AF. In the 12-month period post-index treatment, AF patients treated with AADs had more than twice the average number of cardiovascular-related outpatient visits as compared to those treated with ablation (3.57 [SD: 5.09] vs. 1.76 [SD: 3.83], $p < 0.0001$). When assessing outcomes over a longer term (3-year period), AF patients treated with ablation procedure were found to have ~ 38% lower likelihood of heart failure, ~ 50% lower likelihood of death, and ~ 43% lower likelihood of a composite outcome (including heart failure, stroke/TIA, DCCV, death) as compared to those treated with AADs. These results are consistent with earlier observational evidence supporting ablation procedure. In a recent observational study, Mansour et al. (2018) found 41% greater likelihood of thromboembolic event and 13%

Table 1 Pre-match and post-match sample characteristics for primary outcome assessment

Variable	Before Propensity Score Matching			After Propensity Score Matching		
	AAD cohort (*n* = 920)	Ablation cohort (*n* = 1508)	Standardized difference	AAD cohort (*n* = 558)	Ablation cohort (*n* = 558)	Standardized difference
Age	68	62	−0.5075	65	65	−0.0535
CCI score	0.7	0.72	0.0445	0.7	0.7	0.0027
CHA_2DS_2-VASc score	2.11	1.63	−0.322	1.9	1.9	0.0168
Cardiovascular-related outpatient visits (pre-index)	2.99	2.98	−0.3613	1.2	1.28	0.06
Cardiovascular-related inpatient visits (pre-index)	1.38	2.12	0.5151	1.75	1.83	0.0593
Female	45.65%	28.58%	0.359	34.41%	35.30%	−0.0188
Year of index date						
2008	20.11%	13.26%		19.53%	15.05%	
2009	19.24%	15.72%		19.89%	15.41%	
2010	19.24%	19.76%		18.46%	18.10%	
2011	17.72%	17.71%		17.20%	15.05%	
2012	13.80%	18.04%		12.72%	19.18%	
2013	9.89%	15.52%	0.2698	12.19%	17.20%	0.2653[a]
DCCV	19.78%	25.73%	0.1422	24.37%	23.84%	−0.0126
Ischemic heart disease	17.07%	14.46%	−0.0716	18.28%	19.53%	0.032
Heart failure	8.37%	9.81%	0.0503	9.68%	8.60%	−0.0373
Cardiomyopathy	2.39%	4.97%	0.1374	3.58%	3.23%	−0.0198
Valvular disease	6.63%	10.81%	0.1485	8.42%	7.89%	−0.0196
Wolff Parkinson	0.11%	2.19%	0.1961	0.18%	1.08%	0.1137[a]
Other arrhythmia	10.33%	22.35%	0.3296	14.16%	15.95%	0.0501
Hypertension	36.09%	39.66%	0.0736	41.22%	42.29%	0.0218
Diabetes	9.57%	12.00%	0.0786	11.65%	11.47%	−0.0056
Obstructive sleep apnea	0.54%	2.19%	0.1421	0.90%	1.25%	0.0348
COPD	5.54%	6.76%	0.0508	6.45%	6.63%	0.0072
Renal failure	1.20%	1.06%	−0.0127	0.54%	0.72%	0.0227
Stroke/TIA	3.59%	1.92%	−0.1018	2.69%	2.15%	−0.035
Conduction system disease	14.67%	30.97%	0.3958	19.53%	20.97%	0.0357
Hyperthyroidism	0.98%	0.20%	−0.102	0.18%	0.36%	0.0346
Rate control meds	89.57%	75.13%	−0.3855	84.77%	85.84%	0.0304
Anticoagulants	60.98%	76.46%	0.3386	72.94%	68.64%	−0.0947

[a]is significant

Table 2 Average number of visits during the post-blanking 4-month to 12-month follow-up

		AAD Cohort *N* = 558	Ablation Cohort *N* = 558	*p*-value
All-cause inpatient visits	Mean	0.75	0.70	0.0859
	Std	1.80	1.25	
Cardiovascular-related inpatient visits	Mean	0.58	0.55	0.3547
	Std	1.38	0.99	
All-cause outpatient visits	Mean	8.79	7.95	0.2029
	Std	7.41	6.45	
Cardiovascular-related outpatient visits	Mean	3.57	1.76	<.0001
	Std	5.09	3.83	

Table 3 Pre-match and post-match sample characteristics for secondary outcome assessment

Variable	Before Propensity Score Matching			After Propensity Score Matching		
	AAD cohort ($n = 927$)	Ablation cohort ($n = 1528$)	Standardized difference	AAD cohort ($n = 615$)	Ablation cohort ($n = 615$)	Standardized difference
Age	68	62	−0.5428	65	66	0.0613
CCI score	0.7	0.71	0.0255	0.74	0.75	0.0205
CHA_2DS_2-VASc score	2.11	1.63	−0.3626	1.24	1.23	0.0517
Cardiovascular-related outpatient visits (pre-index)	1.46	0.96	−0.3568	1.23	1.17	−0.0449
Cardiovascular-related inpatient visits (pre-index)	1.38	2.13	0.4898	1.76	1.80	0.0349
Female	45.63%	28.86%	0.3747	34.15%	36.26%	−0.0443
Year of index date						
2008	20.28%	13.29%		18.05%	13.98%	
2009	18.99%	15.58%		19.02%	16.26%	
2010	19.20%	19.90%		19.35%	19.19%	
2011	17.80%	17.67%		16.59%	15.45%	
2012	13.81%	18.06%		14.47%	18.05%	
2013	9.92%	15.51%	0.2612	12.52%	17.07%	0.1942[a]
DCCV	19.31%	25.59%	0.1473	25.37%	26.18%	0.0186
Ischemic heart disease	17.04%	14.53%	−0.0852	16.42%	17.56%	0.0303
Heart failure	8.41%	9.75%	0.0363	9.59%	9.92%	0.011
Cardiomyopathy	2.37%	4.91%	0.1332	3.25%	2.93%	−0.0188
Valvular disease	6.69%	10.73%	0.138	8.94%	9.11%	0.0057
Wolff Parkinson	0.11%	2.23%	0.1951	0.16%	0.65%	0.0767
Other arryhthmias	10.46%	22.58%	0.3094	14.80%	16.26%	0.0404
Hypertension	36.14%	39.66%	0.0308	41.30%	39.67%	−0.0331
Diabetes	9.39%	11.98%	0.0611	11.54%	11.71%	0.0051
Obstructive sleep apnea	0.54%	2.23%	0.1268	1.14%	1.46%	0.0287
COPD	5.50%	6.68%	0.0572	6.99%	6.34%	−0.0261
Renal failure	1.19%	1.05%	−0.0397	0.81%	0.65%	−0.0191
Stroke/TIA	3.56%	1.90%	−0.103	2.93%	1.95%	−0.0633
Conduction system disease	14.89%	31.02%	0.3682	21.14%	22.28%	0.0276
Hyperthyroidism	1.08%	0.20%	−0.0968	0.16%	0.16%	0
Rate control meds	89.64%	75.13%	−0.3948	84.88%	84.72%	−0.0045
Anticoagulants	60.95%	76.46%	0.3266	72.68%	70.57%	−0.0469

[a]is significant

greater likelihood of cardiovascular hospitalization among AF patients undergoing AAD therapy as compared to ablation treatment [16]. Besides resource use and clinical outcome benefit, the significant reduction in mortality observed among AF patients treated with ablation in our study highlights the potential health benefit accrual associated with ablation as compared to AAD therapy. Similar to our study, Jarman et al. (2017) observed lower likelihood of morality among AF patients undergoing ablation procedure as compared to AF patients who did not had ablation or had cardioversion [14]. As healthcare resources become scarce, treatment approaches including ablation for AF could offer payers significant economic benefits as compared to conventional drug treatment.

Study limitations

As with all observational studies, our study also has some limitations. Considering that we used a secondary healthcare database for this study, coding errors and misclassifications could have influenced results. Under-reported or missing diagnoses, based on patient's choice (not to seek care) or access challenges may also exist, though the extent of such occurrences may be minimal. The study did not assess patient quality of life differences between the two cohorts associated with long term use of AADs or ablation

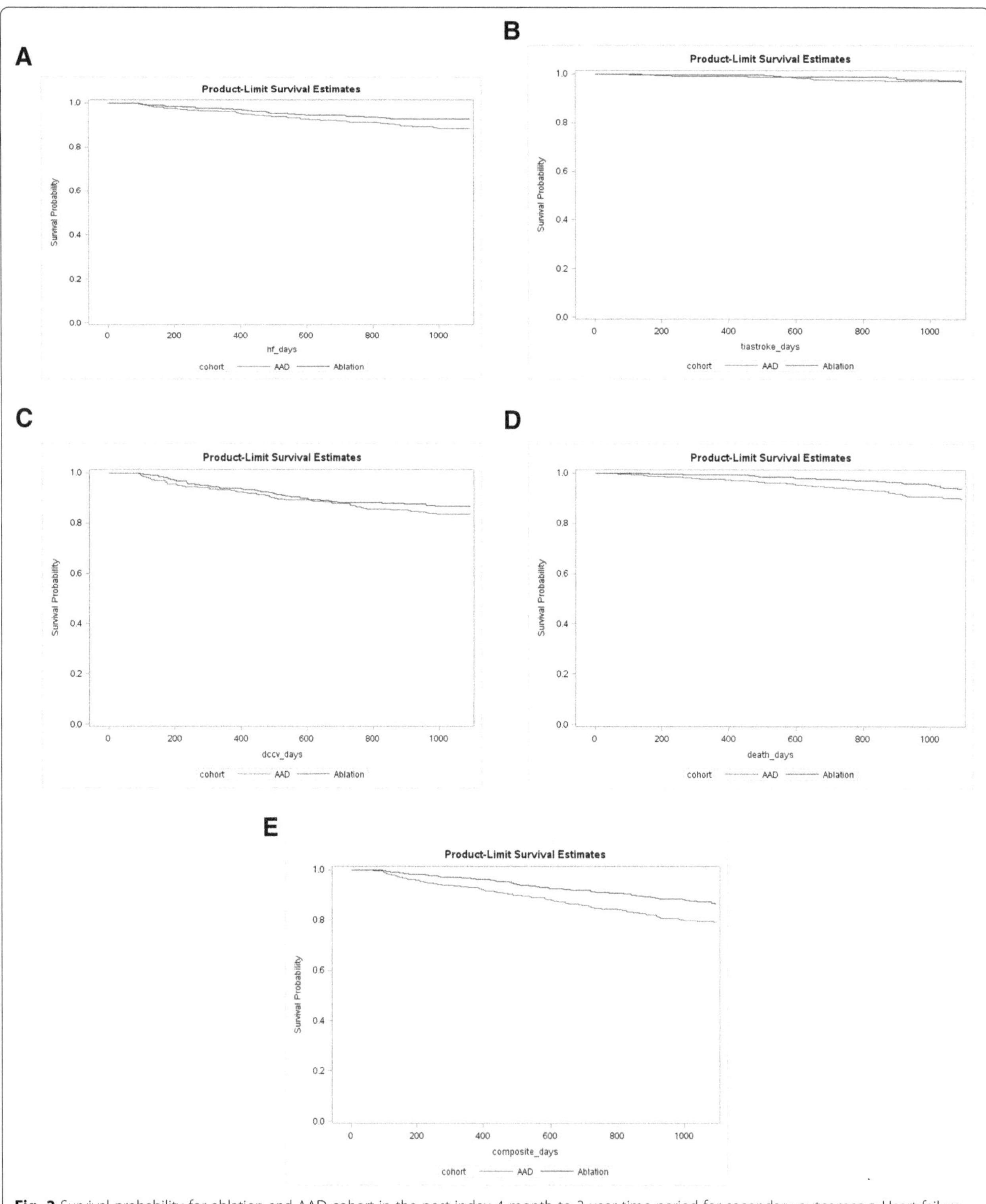

Fig. 2 Survival probability for ablation and AAD cohort in the post-index 4-month to 3-year time-period for secondary outcomes **a** Heart failure. **b** Stroke/TIA. **c** DCCV. **d** Death. **e** Composite outcome (including heart failure, stroke/TIA, DCCV, death)

because these measures are not routinely captured in healthcare databases. The database used in the study did not have any procedure-related details. For example, we were unable to examine the catheter technology, procedure time, and fluoroscopy time. As ablation catheter technology has evolved, there are likely to be variation in success rate within ablation catheters, with newer catheters having improved outcomes as compared to earlier generations. For instance, the contact force-sensing radiofrequency ablation catheters are shown to lead to 37% decrease in AF recurrence over a 12-month follow-up period when compared to radiofrequency catheters without contact force-sensing technology [27]. Future studies that have technology information available could examine the variation in outcomes between AADs and newer ablation catheters. Lastly, one of the main limitations of observational studies like ours is the lack of randomization. Unlike clinical trials, where randomization could be used to alleviate selection bias, observational studies like ours must rely on other techniques to reduce such bias. Though we achieved good balance among the two groups for primary and secondary outcome comparison using the propensity score matching technique, unmeasured confounders could have existed and influenced the results.

Conclusions

This study builds on existing literature highlighting the significant reduction in resource utilization as well as improvement in morbidity and mortality outcomes associated with ablation as compared to AAD treatment for AF. For patients, payers, and providers, the incremental benefits indicate ablation to be a valuable treatment approach for AF as compared to drug therapy. For patients, the morbidity and mortality benefit associated with ablation are likely to translate to clinical benefits over AAD therapy. For providers, ablation offers a useful approach to treat AF with improved clinical outcomes, and for payers, ablation is likely to lead to sustained economic savings as compared to AAD therapy.

Abbreviations

AAD: Antiarrhythmic drugs; AF: Atrial fibrillation; CPRD: Clinical Practice Research Datalink; DCCV: Direct Current Cardioversion; HES: Hospital Episode Statistics; TIA: Transient Ischemic Attack; UK: United Kingdom (UK)

Acknowledgements

Authors would like acknowledge Siva Arul (Mu Sigma) for his assistance in data analysis, and Zenobia Dotiwala (eMAX Health) for her assistance in manuscript writing.

Funding

This study was sponsored by Johnson & Johnson.

Authors' contributions

JJ, JM, RL, IK, AC, and RK contributed in design of the study, data interpretation, and manuscript editing. LG, WH, TW, and VM contributed in data interpretation and critical revisions of the manuscript. All authors read and approved the final manuscript.

Competing interests

JM, LG, RL, IK, AC, and RK are employees of Johnson and Johnson. JJ, WH, and TW do not have any conflict of interest to declare. VM has a consulting agreement and has received honoraria from Biosense Webster.

Author details

[1]Heart Rhythm Centre, NIHR Cardiovascular Research Unit, The Royal Brompton Hospital, and National Heart and Lung Institute, Imperial College, London, UK. [2]Franchise Health Economics and Market Access, Johnson & Johnson, Irvine, CA, USA. [3]Janssen R&D US, Raritan, NJ, USA. [4]Medical Device Epidemiology, Johnson and Johnson, 410 George Street, New Brunswick, NJ 08901, USA.

References

1. Wolf P, Abbott R, Kannel W. Atrial fibrillation as an independent risk factor for stroke: the Framingham Study. Stroke. 1991;22:983–8 originally published August 1, 1991.
2. Stewart S, Hart C, Hole D, McMurray J. A population-based study of the long-term risks associated with atrial fibrillation: 20-year follow-up of the Renfrew/Paisley study. Am J Med. 2002;113(5):359–64.
3. European Heart Rhythm A, European Association for Cardio-Thoracic S, Camm AJ, et al. Guidelines for the management of atrial fibrillation: the task force for the management of atrial fibrillation of the European Society of Cardiology (ESC). Eur Heart J. 2010;31(19):2369–429.
4. Lane DA, Skjøth F, Lip GY, Larsen TB, Kotecha D. Temporal trends in incidence, prevalence, and mortality of atrial fibrillation in primary care. J Am Heart Assoc. 2017;6(5):e005155.
5. Stewart S, Murphy N, Walker A, et al. Cost of an emerging epidemic: an economic analysis of atrial fibrillation in the UK. Heart. 2004 Mar;90(3):286–92.
6. Wolowacz SE, Samuel M, Brennan VK, Jasso-Mosqueda JG, Van Gelder IC. The cost of illness of atrial fibrillation: a systematic review of the recent literature. Europace. 2011;13(10):1375–85.
7. Ball J, Carrington MJ, McMurray JJ, Stewart S. Atrial fibrillation: profile and burden of an evolving epidemic in the 21st century. Int J Cardiol. 2013;167(5):1807–24.
8. Verdino RJ. Untreated atrial fibrillation in the United States of America: understanding the barriers and treatment options. J Saudi Heart Assoc. 2015;27(1):44–9.
9. Casciano J, Dotiwala Z, Martin BC, Kwong J. The costs of warfarin underuse and nonadherence in patients with atrial fibrillation: a commercial insurer perspective. J Manag Care Pharm. 2013;19(4):302–16.
10. Wazni OM, Marrouche NF, Martin DO, et al. Radiofrequency ablation vs antiarrhythmic drugs as first-line treatment of symptomatic atrial fibrillation: a randomized trial. JAMA. 2005;293(21):2634–40.
11. Wilber DJ, Pappone C, Neuzil P, et al. Comparison of antiarrhythmic drug therapy and radiofrequency catheter ablation in patients with paroxysmal atrial fibrillation: a randomized controlled trial. JAMA. 2010;303(4):333–40.
12. Rizzo JA, Mallow P, Cirrincione A. PMD69 Cost-Effectiveness of Catheter Ablation Versus Antiarrhythmic Drug Therapy for the Treatment of Atrial Fibrillation in the UK. Value in Health. 2012;15(7):A357.
13. Reynolds MR, Walczak J, White SA, et al. Improvements in symptoms and quality of life in patients with paroxysmal atrial fibrillation treated with radiofrequency catheter ablation versus antiarrhythmic drugs. Circ Cardiovasc Qual Outcomes. 2010;3(6):615–23.
14. Jarman JW, Hunter TD, Hussain W, et al. Mortality, stroke, and heart failure in atrial fibrillation cohorts after ablation versus propensity-matched cohorts. Pragmat obs res. 2017;8:99.
15. Jarman JW, Hunter TD, Hussain W, et al. Stroke rates before and after ablation of atrial fibrillation and in propensity-matched controls in the UK. Pragmat obs res. 2017;8:107.
16. Mansour M, Heist EK, Agarwal R, et al. Stroke and cardiovascular events after ablation or antiarrhythmic drugs for treatment of patients with atrial fibrillation. Am J Cardiol. 2018;121(10):1192–9.
17. Reynolds MR, Gunnarsson CL, Hunter TD, et al. Health outcomes with catheter ablation or antiarrhythmic drug therapy in atrial fibrillation: results of a propensity-matched analysis. Circ Cardiovasc Qual Outcomes. 2012;5(2):171–81.
18. Herrett E, Gallagher A, Bhaskaran K, et al. Data Resource Profile: Clinical Practice Research Datalink (CPRD). Int J Epidemiol. 2015;44(3):827–36.
19. January CT, Wann LS, Alpert JS, et al. 2014 AHA/ACC/HRS guideline for the management of patients with atrial fibrillation: a report of the American College of Cardiology/American Heart Association task force on practice guidelines and the Heart Rhythm Society. J Am Coll Cardiol. 2014;64(21):e1–76.
20. Deyo RA, Cherkin DC, Ciol MA. Adapting a clinical comorbidity index for use with ICD-9-CM administrative databases. J Clin Epidemiol. 1992;45(6):613–9.

21. Quan H, Li B, Couris CM, et al. Updating and validating the Charlson comorbidity index and score for risk adjustment in hospital discharge abstracts using data from 6 countries. Am J Epidemiol. 2011;173(6):676–82. https://doi.org/10.1093/aje/kwq433 Epub 2011 Feb 17.
22. Santangeli P, Biase L, Natale A, et al. Ablation versus drugs: what is the best first-line therapy for paroxysmal atrial fibrillation? Circ Arrhythm Electrophysiol. 2014;7:739–46.
23. Dagres N, Lewalter T, Lip G, et al. Current practice of antiarrhythmic drug therapy for prevention of atrial fibrillation in Europe: The European Heart Rhythm Association survey. EP Europace. 2013;15(4):478–81.
24. Calkins H, Hindricks G, Cappato R, et al. HRS/EHRA/ECAS/APHRS/SOLAECE expert consensus statement on catheter and surgical ablation of atrial fibrillation. Heart Rhythm. 2017;14(10):e275–444.
25. 25. Komatsu T. Current strategies of antiarrhythmic drug therapy for paroxysmal atrial fibrillation. J Arrhythmia. 2012;28(3):162–9.
26. Cheng X, Li X, He Y, et al. Catheter ablation versus anti-arrhythmic drug therapy for the management of atrial fibrillation: a meta-analysis. J Interv Card Electrophysiol. 2014;41(3):267–72.
27. Afzal MR, Chatta J, Samanta A, et al. Use of contact force sensing technology during radiofrequency ablation reduces recurrence of atrial fibrillation: a systematic review and meta-analysis. Heart Rhythm. 2015;12(9):1990–6.

Association of sodium intake and major cardiovascular outcomes: a dose-response meta-analysis of prospective cohort studies

Yaobin Zhu[1†], Jing Zhang[2†], Zhiqiang Li[1*], Yang Liu[2], Xing Fan[2], Yaping Zhang[3] and Yanbo Zhang[4*]

Abstract

Background: The association of sodium intake with the risk of cardiovascular morbidity and mortality is inconsistent. Thus, the present meta-analysis was conducted to summarize the strength of association between sodium intake and cardiovascular morbidity and mortality.

Methods: PubMed, Embase, and the Cochrane Library were searched systematically to identify the relevant studies up to October 2017. The effect estimates for 100 mmol/day increase in sodium intake were calculated using 95% confidence intervals (CIs) of cardiac death, total mortality, stroke, or stroke mortality for low (< 3 g/d), moderate (3–5 g/d), or heavy (> 5 g/d) sodium intake, and minimal sodium intake comparison.

Results: A total of 16 prospective cohort studies reported data on 205,575 individuals. The results suggested that an increase in sodium intake by 100 mmol/d demonstrated little or no effect on the risk of cardiac death ($P = 0.718$) and total mortality ($P = 0.720$). However, the risk of stroke incidence ($P = 0.029$) and stroke mortality ($P = 0.007$) was increased significantly by 100 mmol/day increment of sodium intake. Furthermore, low sodium intake was associated with an increased risk of cardiac death ($P = 0.003$), while moderate ($P < 0.001$) or heavy ($P = 0.001$) sodium intake was associated with an increased risk of stroke mortality.

Conclusions: These findings suggested that sodium intake by 100 mmol/d increment was associated with an increased risk of stroke incidence and stroke mortality. Furthermore, low sodium intake was related to an increased cardiac death risk, while moderate or heavy sodium intake was related to an increased risk of stroke mortality.

Keywords: Sodium intake, Cardiovascular outcomes, Dose-response, Meta-analysis, Prospective cohort studies

Background

Cardiovascular diseases (CVD) are the major causes of mortality and morbidity in the general population, accounting for approximately 17.5 million deaths worldwide. The World Health Organization (WHO) estimated over 30% of all the deaths worldwide annually due to CVDs [1]. Several studies have recommended several lifestyle factors such as intake of yogurt [2], dietary magnesium [3], nuts [4], whole grains [5], dietary fibers [6], milk [7], and saturated and trans unsaturated fatty acids [8] that prevent the progression of CVD. However, the relatively high residual risk for CVD should be addressed, and it is necessary to understand the association of individual dietary components with CVD at the population level to alter the dietary habits and improve the health conditions.

Dietary sodium intake has been documented as a modifiable risk factor for blood pressure, which in turn, is associated with the progression of CVD [9–12]. Currently, WHO recommends a sodium intake of < 2 g/d, which is largely based on the small and short-term clinical trials that evaluated the effect of modest salt reduction on blood pressure in general population [13]. However, the effect of dietary

* Correspondence: cardiacsurgeon@yeah.net; yanbozhang@126.com
†Yaobin Zhu and Jing Zhang contributed equally to this work.
[1]Cardiovascular Surgery II, Beijing Children's Hospital, Capital Medical University, National Center for Children's Health, Beijing 100045, China
[4]National Clinical Research Center of Cardiovascular Diseases, State Key Laboratory of Cardiovascular Disease, Fuwai Hospital, Chinese Academy of Medical Sciences and Peking Union Medical College, Beijing 100037, China
Full list of author information is available at the end of the article

sodium intake on subsequent cardiovascular morbidity and mortality is limited and inconclusive.

Several prospective studies have indicated that long-term interventions aiming at sodium reduction may reduce the risk of CVD [14, 15]. Moreover, the results of another prospective study did not show any correlation between sodium intake and CVD [16]. Furthermore, several studies suggested that high sodium intake may decrease the risk of cardiac death [17, 18]. Hence, clarifying the optimal daily intake of sodium is essential in the general population as it has not yet been determined. Herein, we attempted to investigate the available prospective cohort studies on a large-scale to determine the association of sodium intake and cardiovascular morbidity and mortality.

Methods

Data sources, search strategy, and selection criteria

This study was conducted and reported according to the Preferred Reporting Items for Systematic Reviews and Meta-Analysis (PRISMA) guidelines [19]. Studies with a prospective cohort design evaluating the impact of sodium intake and the risk of major cardiovascular outcomes, without any language bias (English or another language), were included in this meta-analysis. Electronic databases, such as PubMed, Embase, and Cochrane Library were searched for literature published up to October 2017. The core search terms used were "dietary salt" OR "sodium" AND ("cardiovascular disease" OR "stroke" OR "cardiac death" OR "mortality" OR "death" OR "CVD" OR "myocardial infarction" OR "coronary events") AND "clinical trials" AND "human". The reference lists from potentially relevant studies were searched to select the additional eligible studies. Parameters such as the study topic, design, participants' status, exposure, and reported outcomes were employed to identify the relevant studies.

The literature search and study selection was conducted by two authors independently, and any inconsistencies were settled by group discussion until a consensus was reached. The inclusion criteria for the studies were as follows: (1) prospective cohort design; (2) evaluation of the impact of sodium intake and the risk of major cardiovascular outcomes; (3) reported at least 1 of the following outcomes:

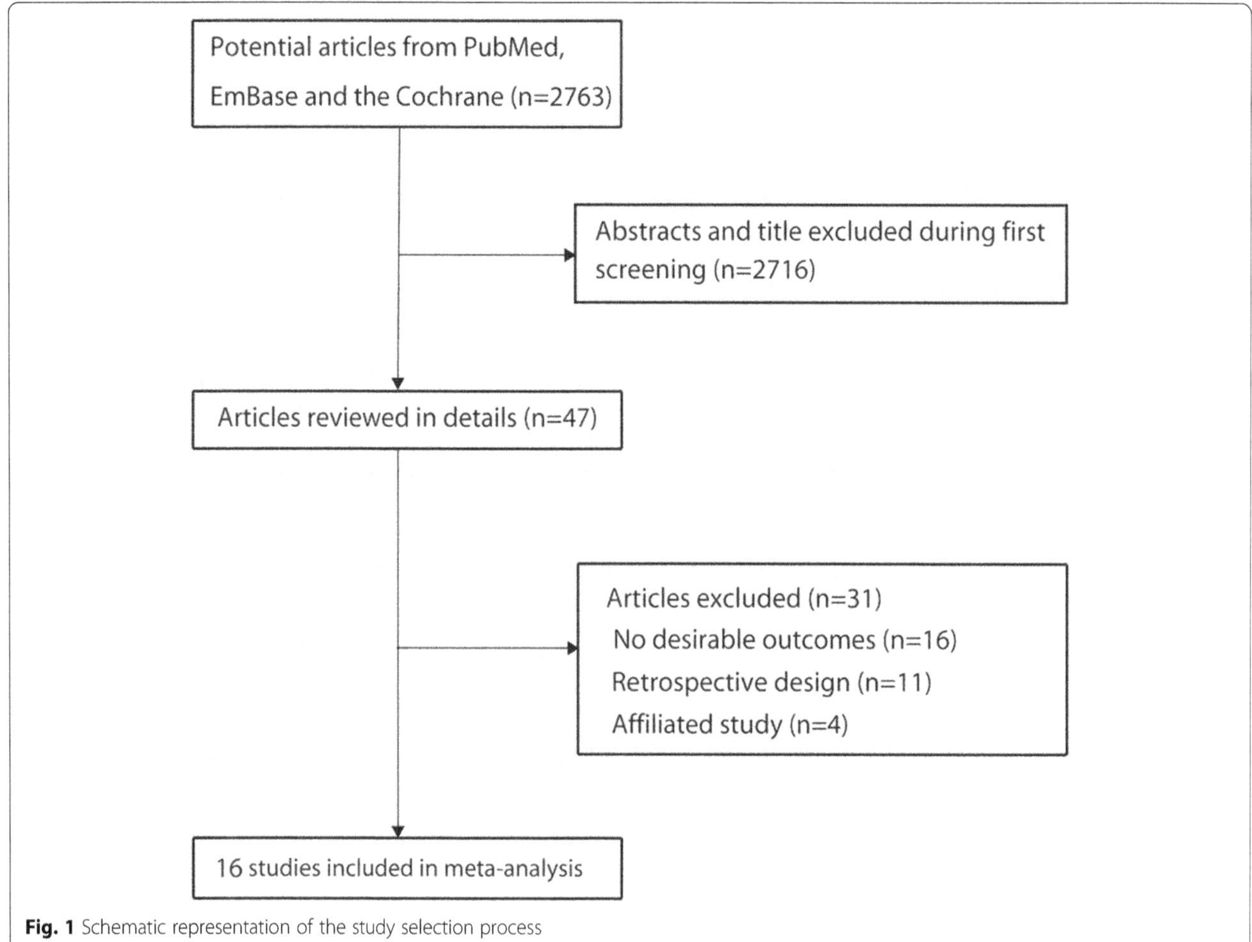

Fig. 1 Schematic representation of the study selection process

Table 1 Baseline characteristic of studies included in this meta-analysis

Study	Publication year	Country	Sample size	Age at baseline	Percentage male (%)	Assessment of exposure	Reference category of sodium intake	Reported outcomes	Follow-up (year)	Adjusted factors	NOS score
Alderman [31]	1995	US	2937	53.0	64.7	24 h urine collection	Quartile I	Stroke	3.5	Age, and race	7
Tunstall-Pedoe [32]	1997	Scotland	11,629	40.0–59.0	49.5	24 h urine collection	129.6 mmol/day	Cardiac death, total mortality	7.6	Age	8
He [33]	1999	US	9485	25.0–74.0	38.9	24 h urine collection	Quartile I	Cardiac death, stroke, stroke mortality, total mortality	19.0	Age, sex, race, SBP, SC, BMI, DM, diuretic use, PA, education, alcohol, smoking, EI	9
Tuomilehto [34]	2001	Finland	2436	25.0–64.0	48.2	24 h urine collection	< 159 mmol/day	Cardiac death, stroke, total mortality	8.0	Age, study year, smoking, HDL, SBP, and BMI	9
Nagata [35]	2004	Japan	29,079	> 35.0	49.6	FFQ		Stroke mortality	7.0	Age, EI, marital status, education, BMI, smoking, alcohol, PA, hypertension, DM, and intake of protein, potassium, and vitamin E	9
Cohen [36]	2008	US	8699	> 30.0	44.9	FFQ		Cardiac death, total mortality	8.7	Age, sex, race, education, added table salt, PA, alcohol, smoking, DM, history of cancer, SBP, TC, dietary potassium, weight, antihypertensive drug	9
Larsson [37]	2008	Finland	26,556	50.0–69.0	100	FFQ		Stroke	13.6	Age, supplementation group, smoking, BMI, SBP and DBP, SC, serum HDL, DM and CVD, PA, alcohol and EI	8
Umesawa [14]	2008	Japan	58,730	40.0–79.0	39.4	FFQ		Cardiac death, stroke mortality	12.7	BMI, smoking, alcohol, history of hypertension, DM, menopause, HRT, PA, educational, perceived mental stress, calcium, and potassium intake	9
Ekinci [38]	2011	Australia	638	64.0	56.0	24 h urine collection		Cardiac death, total mortality	9.9	Age, sex, previous CVD, eGFR, atrial fibrillation, SBP, DM duration	6
Stolarz-Skrzypek [18]	2011	Belgium	3595	40.9	47.3	24 h urine collection		Cardiac death, stroke, total mortality	7.9	Study population, sex, age, BMI, SBP, potassium excretion, antihypertensive drug, smoking, alcohol, DM, TC, and educational	9
Yang [16]	2011	US	12,267	> 20.0	48.1	FFQ		Cardiac death, total mortality	14.8	Sex, race/ethnicity, educational, BMI, smoking, alcohol, TC, HDL, PA, family history of CVD, and EI	9
O'Donnell [39]	2011	Canada	28,880	> 55.0	70.6	24 h urine collection		Cardiac death, stroke, total mortality	4.8	Age, sex, race/ethnicity, history of stroke or MI, creatinine, BMI, comorbid vascular risk factors, treatment allocation, fruit and vegetable, PA, SBP, and urinary potassium	7
Gardener [40]	2012	US	2657	69.0	36.0	FFQ		Stroke	10.0	Age, sex, race/ethnicity, education, alcohol, smoking, PA, EI, total fat, saturated fat, carbohydrates, protein, DM, hypercholesterolemia, hypertension, previous CVD, BMI	9
Mills [41]	2016	US	3757	57.8	55.6	FFQ		Stroke	6.8	Age, sex, race, clinic site, education; waist circumference, BMI, smoking; alcohol, PA, LDL, glucose; history of CVD; use of antidiabetic, lipid-lowering, and BP- lowering medications, urinary creatinine excretion, baseline estimated GFR	9

Table 1 Baseline characteristic of studies included in this meta-analysis *(Continued)*

Study	Publication year	Country	Sample size	Age at baseline	Percentage male (%)	Assessment of exposure	Reference category of sodium intake	Reported outcomes	Follow-up (year)	Adjusted factors	NOS score
Kalogeropoulos [42]	2015	US	2642	74.6	48.8	FFQ		Total mortality	10.0	Age, sex, race, BMI, smoking, PA, previous CVD, pulmonary disease, DM, depression, BP, heart rate, electrocardiogram abnormalities, and serum glucose, albumin, creatinine, and SC	9
Horikawa [43]	2014	Japan	1588	58.7	52.5	FFQ		Total mortality	7.0	Age, sex, BMI, HbA1c, DM duration, LDL, HDL, log-transformed triglycerides, insulin, lipid-lowering agents, smoking, alcohol, EI, and PA	7

**BMI* body mass index, *BP* blood pressure, *CHD* coronary heart disease, *CVD* cardiovascular disease, *DBP* diastolic blood pressure, *DM* diabetes mellitus, *EI* energy intake, *FFQ* food frequency questionnaire, *eGFR* estimated glomerular filtration rate, *GFR* glomerular filtration rate, *HbA1c* glycated hemoglobin, *HDL* high density lipoprotein, *HRT* hormone replacement therapy, *LDL* low density lipoprotein, *MACEs* major cardiovascular events, *MI* myocardial infarction, *PA* physical activity, *SBP* systolic blood pressure, *SC* serum cholesterol, *TC* total cholesterol

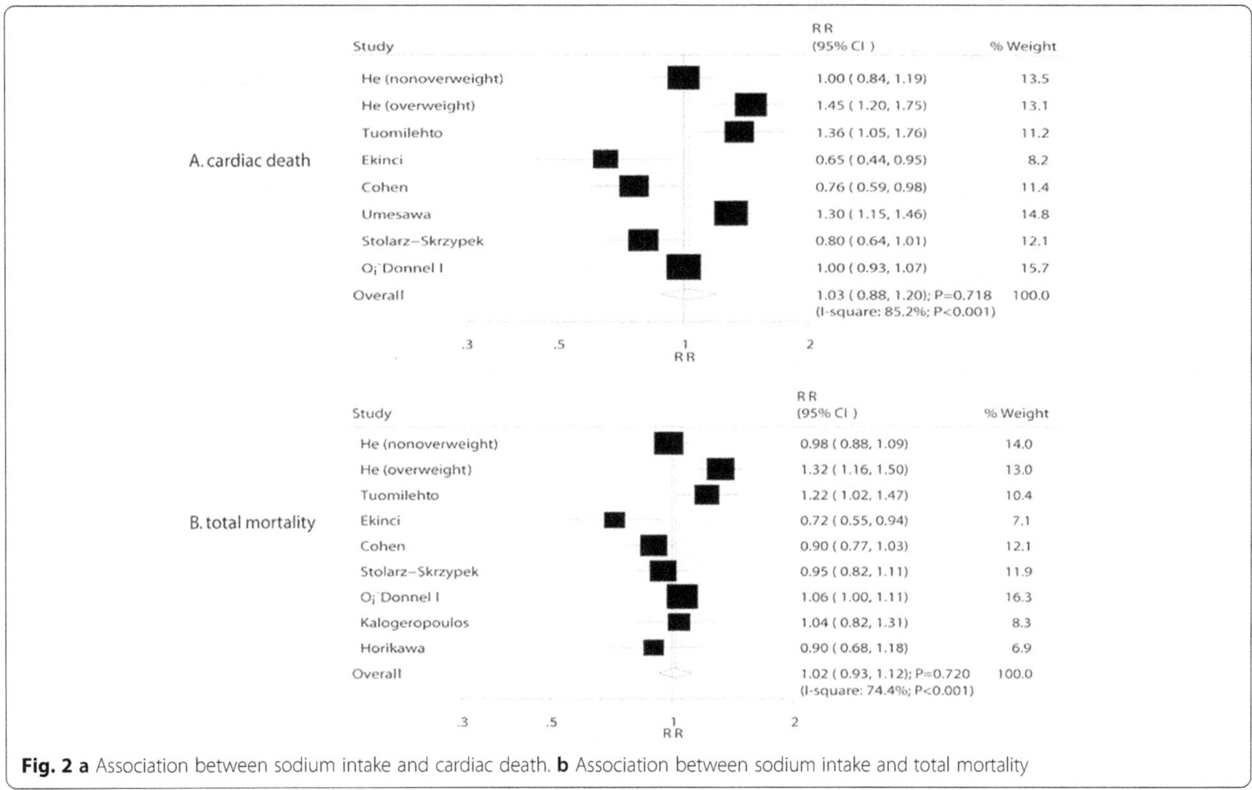

Fig. 2 a Association between sodium intake and cardiac death. **b** Association between sodium intake and total mortality

cardiac death, total mortality, stroke, or stroke mortality; (4) the data should provide the effect estimates, such as relative risk (RR), hazard ratio (HR), or odds ratio (OR,) and 95% confidence intervals (CIs) or crude data that compared the different categories of sodium intake vs. the minimal sodium intake with respect to 100 mmol/day increments and the risk of major cardiovascular outcomes. All the retrospective observational studies were excluded as various confounding factors could bias the results.

Data collection and quality assessment

The data collected from the eligible studies included the first author's name, publication year, country, sample size, age at baseline, percentage male, assessment of exposure, reference category of sodium intake, reported outcomes, follow-up duration, and covariates in the fully adjusted model. Also, the crude data on the number of cases/persons or person-years, effect of different exposure categories, and the 95% CIs were collected. In addition, the effect estimates that were maximally adjusted for potential confounders, if the study provided several adjusted effect estimates, were selected.

The comprehensive Newcastle–Ottawa Scale (NOS) has been partially validated for evaluating the quality of the observational studies in the meta-analysis, and hence, was used to evaluate the quality of the study method [20]. The NOS evaluated the quality of the observational studies based on selection (4 items), comparability (1 item), and outcome (3 items). The maximum score was 9, and the minimum score was 0 (Additional file : Table S1). The data were extracted and quality assessed by 2 authors independently, and any inconsistencies were referred to the original studies by an additional author.

Statistical analysis

To evaluate the impact of sodium intake and the risk of major cardiovascular outcomes, we collected the effect estimates (RR, HR, or OR) and the 95% CIs or the relevant crude data from each study. The summary RRs and 95%

Table 2 Summary results for different categories of sodium and subsequent major cardiovascular outcomes

Outcomes	Low sodium	*P* value	Moderate sodium	*P* value	Heavy sodium	*P* value
Cardiac death	1.19 (1.06–1.33)	0.003	0.91 (0.71–1.15)	0.421	1.02 (0.92–1.13)	0.762
Total mortality	1.02 (0.89–1.18)	0.779	0.98 (0.85–1.14)	0.806	1.09 (0.94–1.27)	0.257
Stroke	1.25 (0.85–1.85)	0.260	1.11 (1.00–1.24)	0.058	1.02 (0.93–1.11)	0.720
Stroke mortality	1.20 (0.96–1.50)	0.117	1.50 (1.20–1.88)	< 0.001	1.81 (1.29–2.55)	0.001

Table 3 Subgroup analyses for cardiac death

Factor	Subgroup	RR and 95% CI	*P* value	Heterogeneity (%)	*P* value for heterogeneity	*P* value between subgroups
Publication year	Before 2010	1.15 (0.94–1.41)	0.170	82.7	< 0.001	< 0.001
	2010 or after	0.85 (0.67–1.08)	0.174	73.8	0.022	
Sample size	≥ 10,000	1.13 (0.88–1.47)	0.334	92.8	< 0.001	0.513
	< 10,000	0.98 (0.76–1.25)	0.846	84.8	< 0.001	
Percentage male (%)	≥ 60.0	1.00 (0.93–1.07)	1.000	–	–	0.023
	< 60.0	1.03 (0.83–1.26)	0.812	85.7	< 0.001	
Assessment of exposure	FFQ	1.01 (0.59–1.70)	0.982	92.9	< 0.001	0.025
	24 h urine collection	1.03 (0.86–1.23)	0.746	82.2	< 0.001	
Follow-up duration (years)	≥ 10.0	1.24 (1.02–1.50)	0.034	78.0	0.011	< 0.001
	< 10.0	0.91 (0.74–1.11)	0.329	77.4	0.001	
Adjusted BMI	Yes	1.13 (0.96–1.32)	0.146	85.2	< 0.001	< 0.001
	No	0.72 (0.59–0.90)	0.003	0.0	0.506	
Adjusted smoking	Yes	1.09 (0.88–1.33)	0.433	85.3	< 0.001	0.003
	No	0.84 (0.56–1.27)	0.415	78.5	0.031	
Adjusted alcohol	Yes	1.04 (0.83–1.31)	0.735	87.5	< 0.001	0.028
	No	0.99 (0.74–1.34)	0.959	80.4	0.006	
Adjusted Previous CVD	Yes	0.84 (0.56–1.27)	0.415	78.5	0.031	0.003
	No	1.09 (0.88–1.33)	0.433	85.3	< 0.001	
Adjusted DM	Yes	0.98 (0.78–1.23)	0.855	87.4	< 0.001	0.125
	No	1.14 (0.84–1.53)	0.400	80.3	0.024	
Adjusted PA	Yes	1.09 (0.91–1.30)	0.355	87.2	< 0.001	0.113
	No	0.90 (0.59–1.38)	0.636	85.0	0.001	
Adjusted potassium	Yes	0.97 (0.78–1.19)	0.744	88.2	< 0.001	0.070
	No	1.10 (0.82–1.46)	0.533	83.6	< 0.001	

**BMI* body mass index, *CI* confidence interval, *CVD* cardiovascular disease, *DM* diabetes mellitus, *FFQ* food frequency questionnaire, *PA* physical activity, *RR* relative risk

CIs for the low (< 3 g/d), moderate (3–5 g/d), or heavy (> 5 g/d) sodium intake vs. and the minimized intake of sodium and the risk of major cardiovascular outcomes were calculated using the random-effects model [21, 22]. Next, we evaluated the estimates of the RR associated with every 100 mmol/day increase in sodium by the generalized least-squares method for trend estimation [23], assuming the presence of a linear relationship between the natural logarithm of the RR and increasing sodium intake. The mid-point for closed categories and median for open categories putatively determined each sodium intake category, presuming a normal distribution for sodium intake. The summary RRs for 100 mmol/day increase in sodium intake was calculated using random-effects meta-analysis [22, 24].

The heterogeneity among the included studies was assessed using the I^2 and Q statistic, and a *P*-value < 0.10 was considered as significant heterogeneity [25, 26]. Subgroup analyses were conducted for cardiac death, total mortality, and stroke according to publication year, sample size, percentage male, assessment of exposure, following-up duration, and with or without adjusted body mass index (BMI), smoking, alcohol, previous CVD, diabetes mellitus (DM), physical activity (PA), and level of potassium. The *P*-value between subgroups was evaluated by chi-square test and meta-regression [27]. A sensitivity analysis was evaluated the impact of individual studies by removing individual study from the meta-analysis [28]. Funnel plot and Egger [29] and Begg [30] tests investigated the outcomes that were also used to evaluate any potential publication bias. All the reported *P*-values are 2-sided, and $P < 0.05$ was considered statistically significant. The statistical analyses were conducted using STATA software (version 10.0; Stata Corporation, College Station, TX, USA).

Results

Literature search

The results of the study selection process were presented in Fig. 1. A total of 2763 articles were identified in the initial electronic search. Of these, 2716 were excluded as they were duplicates and irrelevant studies. Thus, a total of 47

Table 4 Subgroup analyses for total mortality

Factor	Subgroup	RR and 95% CI	*P* value	Heterogeneity (%)	*P* value for heterogeneity	*P* value between subgroups
Publication year	Before 2010	1.09 (0.91–1.30)	0.351	85.2	< 0.001	0.328
	2010 or after	0.96 (0.85–1.08)	0.493	60.2	0.040	
Sample size	≥ 10,000	1.06 (1.01–1.12)	0.029	–	–	0.428
	< 10,000	1.00 (0.89–1.14)	0.958	77.1	< 0.001	
Percentage male (%)	≥ 60.0	1.06 (1.01–1.12)	0.029	–	–	0.428
	< 60.0	1.00 (0.89–1.14)	0.958	77.1	< 0.001	
Assessment of exposure	FFQ	0.93 (0.83–1.04)	0.212	0.0	0.570	0.032
	24 h urine collection	1.05 (0.93–1.17)	0.441	80.4	< 0.001	
Follow-up duration (years)	≥ 10.0	1.11 (0.90–1.37)	0.343	83.9	0.002	0.139
	< 10.0	0.97 (0.87–1.09)	0.616	69.6	0.005	
Adjusted BMI	Yes	1.07 (0.98–1.17)	0.146	68.2	0.004	0.001
	No	0.83 (0.67–1.02)	0.082	51.4	0.151	
Adjusted smoking	Yes	1.04 (0.92–1.17)	0.522	74.5	0.001	0.991
	No	0.89 (0.61–1.30)	0.560	87.0	0.005	
Adjusted alcohol	Yes	1.01 (0.87–1.17)	0.908	80.4	< 0.001	0.471
	No	1.02 (0.87–1.19)	0.804	70.8	0.016	
Adjusted Previous CVD	Yes	0.95 (0.77–1.17)	0.649	74.1	0.021	0.999
	No	1.04 (0.91–1.19)	0.573	78.8	< 0.001	
Adjusted DM	Yes	0.98 (0.85–1.12)	0.716	77.7	< 0.001	0.132
	No	1.11 (0.97–1.25)	0.119	52.4	0.147	
Adjusted PA	Yes	1.04 (0.94–1.15)	0.475	74.2	0.002	0.291
	No	0.96 (0.74–1.24)	0.735	81.4	0.005	
Adjusted potassium	Yes	0.99 (0.88–1.10)	0.790	64.0	0.062	0.341
	No	1.03 (0.88–1.21)	0.712	79.8	< 0.001	

**BMI* body mass index, *CI* confidence interval, *CVD* cardiovascular disease, *DM* diabetes mellitus, *FFQ* food frequency questionnaire, *PA* physical activity, *RR* relative risk

potentially eligible studies were selected. After a detailed evaluation, 16 prospective cohort studies were selected for the final meta-analysis [14, 16, 18, 31–43]. A manual search of the reference lists of these studies did not yield any new eligible studies. The general characteristics of the included studies were presented in Table 1.

Study characteristics

A total of 16 prospective cohort studies with 205,575 individuals were eligible for this study. The follow-up period of the participants ranged from 3.5–19.0 years and 638–58,730 individuals were included in each study. A total of 7 studies were conducted in the USA [16, 31, 33, 36, 40–42], 4 in Europe [18, 32, 34, 37], 3 in Japan [14, 35, 43], 1 in Australia [38], and 1 in Canada [39]. Seven studies used 24-h urine collection [18, 31–34, 38, 39], and the remaining 9 studies used food frequency questionnaires (FFQ) to assess the dietary sodium exposure [14, 16, 35–37, 40–43]. The study quality was assessed using the NOS (Table 1). A score of ≥7 was considered as high quality for the study. Overall, 10 studies had a score of 9 [14, 16, 18, 33–36, 40–42], 2 had a score of 8 [32, 37], 3 had a score of 7 [32, 39, 43], and the remaining 1 study had a score of 6 [38].

Cardiac death

A total of 7 studies reported an association between sodium intake and cardiac death. The summary RR showed that a 100 mmol increment per day in sodium intake was not associated with cardiac death (RR, 1.03; 95% CI, 0.88–1.20; $P = 0.718$; Fig. 2a); however, accumulating evidence suggested significant heterogeneity ($I^2 = 85.2\%$, $P < 0.001$). Sensitivity analysis indicated that the conclusion was unaffected after sequential exclusion of each study from the pooled analysis. Furthermore, the low sodium intake was found to be associated with an increased risk of cardiac death (RR: 1.19; 95% CI: 1.06–1.33; $P = 0.003$), while moderate (RR: 0.91; 95% CI: 0.71–1.15; $P = 0.421$) and heavy (RR: 1.02; 95%CI: 0.92–1.13; $P = 0.762$) sodium intake did not demonstrate a significant effect (Table 2). Subgroup analysis indicated that an increment of 100 mmol/day in sodium intake exerted detrimental effects on cardiac death if the duration of follow-up was ≥10 years (RR: 1.24; 95% CI: 1.02–1.50; $P = 0.034$; Table 3). Conversely,

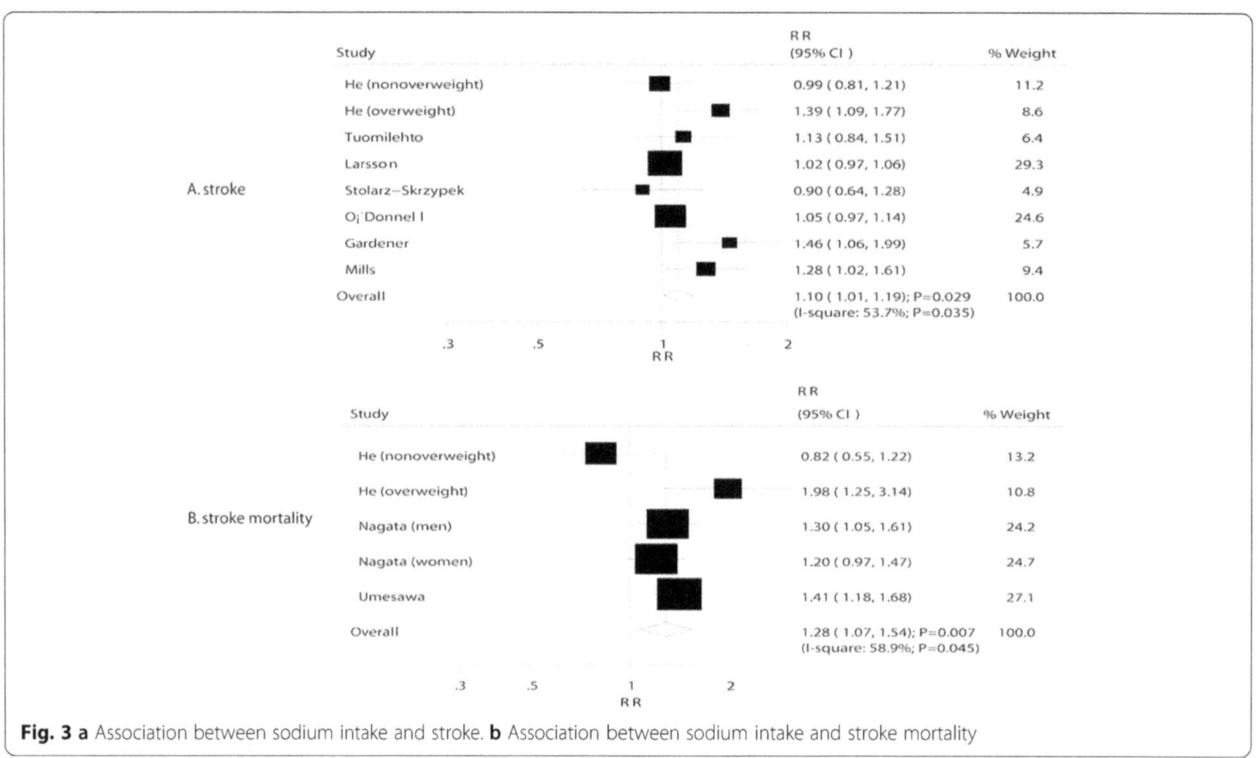

Fig. 3 a Association between sodium intake and stroke. **b** Association between sodium intake and stroke mortality

increased sodium intake was associated with the reduced risk of cardiac death if the study was not adjusted for BMI (RR: 0.72; 95% CI: 0.59–0.90; $P = 0.003$; Table 3).

Total mortality

A total of 8 studies reported a correlation between sodium intake and total mortality. However, the results did not reveal any significant association of 100 mmol increments per day in sodium intake with the total mortality risk (RR: 1.02; 95% CI: 0.93–1.12; $P = 0.720$; Fig. 2b). Although substantial heterogeneity was observed in the magnitude of the effect across the studies ($I^2 = 74.4\%$, $P < 0.001$), after sequential exclusion of each study from pooled analyses, the conclusion was not affected by the exclusion of any specific study. Furthermore, the low (RR: 1.02; 95% CI: 0.89–1.18; $P = 0.779$), moderate (RR: 0.98; 95% CI: 0.85–1.14; $P = 0.806$), and heavy (RR: 1.09; 95% CI: 0.94–1.27; $P = 0.257$) sodium intake was not associated with the risk of total mortality (Table 2). Subgroup analysis indicated that an increment of 100 mmol/day in the sodium intake was associated with an increased risk of total mortality if the sample size was ≥10,000 (RR: 1.06; 95% CI: 1.01–1.12; $P = 0.029$; Table 4), and the percentage male was ≥60.0%.

Stroke and stroke mortality

A total of 7 studies reported an association between sodium intake and stroke, and 3 studies reported the association of sodium intake and stroke mortality. Pooled analysis of stroke and stroke mortality indicated that a 100 mmol increment per day in sodium intake exerted a harmful effect (stroke: RR, 1.10; 95% CI, 1.01–1.19; $P = 0.029$, Fig. 3a; stroke mortality: RR, 1.28; 95% CI, 1.07–1.54; $P = 0.007$, Fig. 3b). Heterogeneity was observed in the magnitude of the effect across the studies ($I^2 = 53.7\%$, $P = 0.035$ for stroke; $I^2 = 58.9\%$, $P = 0.045$ for stroke mortality). However, the conclusion was not affected by excluding any specific study after sequential exclusion of each study from all the pooled analyses. Furthermore, low (RR: 1.25; 95% CI: 0.85–1.85; $P = 0.260$), moderate (RR: 1.11; 95% CI: 1.00–1.24; $P = 0.058$), and heavy (RR: 1.02; 95% CI: 0.93–1.11; $P = 0.720$) sodium intake did demonstrate any effect on the subsequent stroke risk (Table 2). In addition, low sodium intake did not affect the stroke mortality (RR: 1.20; 95% CI: 0.96–1.50; $P = 0.117$), while moderate (RR: 1.50; 95% CI: 1.20–1.88; $P < 0.001$) and heavy (RR: 1.81; 95% CI: 1.29–2.55; $P = 0.001$) sodium intake was associated with a high risk of stroke mortality (Table 2). In addition, subgroup analysis suggested that a 100 mmol per day increment in sodium intake was associated with an increased risk of stroke if the sample size was < 10,000 (RR: 1.18; 95% CI: 1.02–1.36; $P = 0.029$), the proportion of males was < 60.0% (RR: 1.18; 95% CI: 1.02–1.36; $P = 0.029$), the study adjusted for BMI (RR: 1.10; 95% CI: 1.01–1.19; $P = 0.029$), smoking status (RR: 1.13; 95% CI: 1.00–1.28; $P = 0.048$), and PA(RR: 1.11; 95% CI: 1.01–1.22; $P = 0.026$), and the study not adjusted for the level of potassium (RR: 1.16; 95% CI: 1.02–1.33; P = 0.029) (Table 5). The subgroup analysis for stroke mortality was not conducted due to the small number of studies included

Table 5 Subgroup analyses for stroke

Factor	Subgroup	RR and 95% CI	*P* value	Heterogeneity (%)	*P* value for heterogeneity	*P* value between subgroups
Publication year	Before 2010	1.09 (0.95–1.24)	0.211	54.5	0.086	0.248
	2010 or after	1.14 (0.96–1.35)	0.127	58.2	0.067	
Sample size	≥ 10,000	1.03 (0.99–1.07)	0.181	0.0	0.537	0.020
	< 10,000	1.18 (1.02–1.36)	0.029	46.5	0.096	
Percentage male (%)	≥ 60.0	1.03 (0.99–1.07)	0.181	0.0	0.537	0.020
	< 60.0	1.18 (1.02–1.36)	0.029	46.5	0.096	
Assessment of exposure	FFQ	1.19 (0.95–1.50)	0.125	76.0	0.016	0.503
	24 h urine collection	1.08 (0.96–1.21)	0.190	36.8	0.176	
Follow-up duration (years)	≥ 10.0	1.15 (0.97–1.37)	0.116	72.4	0.012	0.453
	< 10.0	1.08 (0.98–1.20)	0.136	18.2	0.300	
Adjusted BMI	Yes	1.10 (1.01–1.19)	0.029	53.7	0.035	–
	No	–	–	–	–	
Adjusted smoking	Yes	1.13 (1.00–1.28)	0.048	60.2	0.020	0.865
	No	1.05 (0.97–1.14)	0.236	–	–	
Adjusted alcohol	Yes	1.14 (0.99–1.31)	0.072	66.2	0.011	0.744
	No	1.06 (0.98–1.14)	0.174	0.0	0.636	
Adjusted Previous CVD	Yes	1.09 (0.99–1.20)	0.074	64.4	0.038	0.395
	No	1.10 (0.91–1.32)	0.317	49.7	0.114	
Adjusted DM	Yes	1.14 (0.99–1.31)	0.072	66.2	0.011	0.744
	No	1.06 (0.98–1.14)	0.174	0.0	0.636	
Adjusted PA	Yes	1.11 (1.01–1.22)	0.026	64.6	0.015	0.892
	No	1.03 (0.82–1.29)	0.811	0.0	0.326	
Adjusted potassium	Yes	1.04 (0.96–1.13)	0.309	0.0	0.396	0.963
	No	1.16 (1.02–1.33)	0.029	65.2	0.013	

**BMI* body mass index, *CI* confidence interval, *CVD* cardiovascular disease, *DM* diabetes mellitus, *FFQ* food frequency questionnaire, *PA* physical activity, *RR* relative risk

in this investigation on the association of sodium intake and stroke mortality.

Publication bias

The review of the funnel plots did not exclude the potential for publication bias for cardiac death, total mortality, stroke, and stroke mortality (Fig. 4). The Egger and Begg test's results did not show any evidence of publication bias for cardiac death (*P*-value for Egger: 0.794; *P*-value for Begg: 0.266), total mortality (*P*-value for Egger: 458; *P*-value for Begg: 0.466), stroke (P-value for Egger: 0.105; *P*-value for Begg: 0.386), and stroke mortality (*P*-value for Egger: 0.858; *P*-value for Begg: 1.000).

Discussion

The current study included the prospective cohort studies and explored the possible correlations between sodium intake and the outcomes of cardiac death, total mortality, stroke, and stroke mortality. This quantitative meta-analysis included a total of 205,575 individuals from 16 prospective cohort studies with a broad range of populations. The meta-analysis findings suggested that an increment of 100 mmol/day in sodium intake did not affect the incidence of cardiac death and total mortality. However, a 100 mmol per day increment in sodium intake significantly increased the risk of stroke and stroke mortality. Furthermore, parameters such as sample size, the proportion of males, assessment of exposure, follow-up duration, and several other adjusted factors were found to be associated with the correlation between sodium intake and major cardiovascular outcomes.

A previous meta-analysis suggested that high sodium intake was associated with a significantly increased risk of stroke and total cardiovascular diseases [44]. However, other 2 meta-analysis studies based on randomized controlled trials suggested that the reduced dietary salt did not affect the cardiovascular morbidity or mortality [45, 46]. The inherent limitation of this study included shorter duration of follow-up period than that required to show a clinical benefit, especially when the rate of events was lower than expected, which

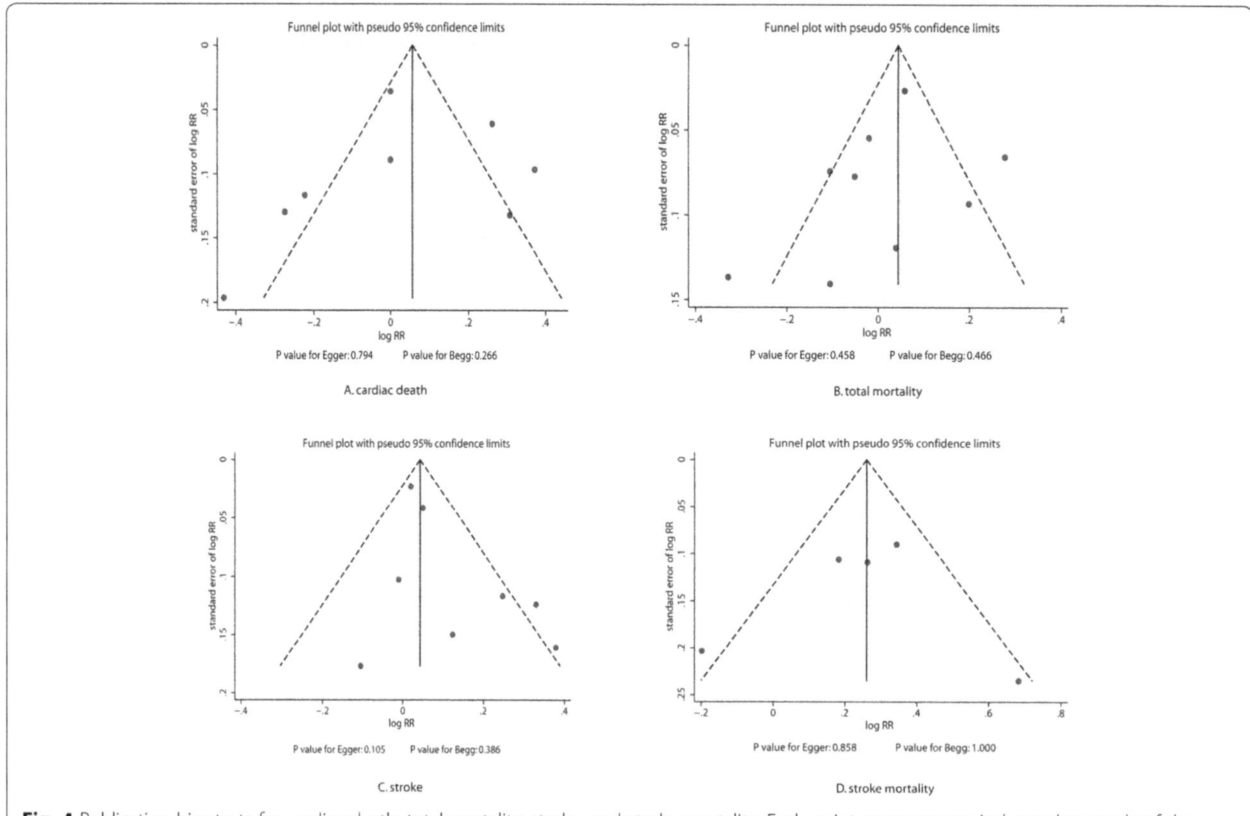

Fig. 4 Publication bias tests for cardiac death, total mortality, stroke, and stroke mortality. Each point represents an independent study of the indicated association

without any statistically significant difference. Furthermore, reduced dietary sodium intake seems to be associated with the degree of control achieved. Finally, the range of sodium intake and the cut-off values for the three categories differed among various studies. Therefore, we conducted a dose-response meta-analysis of these prospective studies for evaluating the optimal dose of sodium intake.

The current findings were in agreement with a recently published large cohort study conducted in Manhattan [40]. Our meta-analysis study included 2657 individuals and found that the participants who consumed > 4000 mg/d sodium demonstrated a 159% increased risk of stroke. Also, the risk percentage of stroke was increased by 17% for each increase in 500 mg/d. He et al. suggested that high sodium intake was strongly and independently associated with an increased risk of stroke mortality in overweight individuals, thereby significantly increasing the risk of total mortality [33]. Also, the current study indicated that increased sodium intake significantly elevated the risk of stroke and stroke mortality, while no effect on cardiac death and total mortality was demonstrated, which might be attributed to the increased blood pressure and hypertension due to high sodium levels by stiffening the endothelial cells, thickening and narrowing of resistance arteries, and blocking of nitric oxide synthesis [47].

The current study did not demonstrate a significant difference between 100 mmol increments of sodium intake per day and the risk of cardiac death. However, inconsistent results were reported by individual studies. O'Donnell et al. indicated that sodium excretion > 7 g/d was associated with an increased risk of cardiac death and coronary heart disease (CHD) as compared to sodium excretion of 4–5.99 g/d [39]. Furthermore, TunstallPedoe et al. suggested that high sodium intake significantly increased the cardiac death and CHD by 36% and 34%, respectively [32]. This phenomenon might be attributed to the inclusion of other prospective studies encompassing general individuals; however, these 2 studies specifically included individuals with high risk of cardiovascular disease, rendering them susceptible to extreme sodium intake.

Subgroup analysis suggested that a 100 mmol increment of sodium intake per day was associated with cardiac death reduction if the study was not adjusted for BMI; also, the risk of cardiac death was increased significantly if the follow-up duration was ≥10 years. In addition, the risk of total mortality was increased if the sample size was ≥10,000 and percentage male was ≥60.0%. Finally, and increased sodium intake by 100 mmol per day was associated with an elevated risk of stroke if the sample size was < 10,000, the percentage of males was < 60.0%, the study adjusted for BMI, smoking status, PA, and the study not adjusted for potassium level. However, these conclusions might be unreliable due to the inclusion of small cohorts in each subset. Therefore, this study provided a relative result as well as a synthetic and comprehensive review.

The three strengths of our study should be highlighted. Firstly, only prospective cohort studies were included, which eliminated the selection as well as recall bias and could be a concern for retrospective case-control studies. Secondly, a large sample size allowed us to quantitatively assess the association of sodium intake with the risk of cardiovascular morbidity and mortality, which in turn, demonstrated that our findings are potentially more robust than any individual studies. Thirdly, the pooled analysis included a wide range of sodium intake levels, which subsequently allowed an accurate assessment of the relation of sodium intake and major cardiovascular risk outcomes.

Nevertheless, the present study had some limitations as follows: (1) the adjusted models used in the included studies are different, and these factors might play a critical role in the development of CVDs; (2) the minimal intake of sodium in individual study varied, which might introduce uncontrolled biases and potential heterogeneity; (3) heterogeneity across included studies was high, and hence, the results of publication bias test were not reliable; (4) high heterogeneity was not investigated by subgroup analysis due to the minimal intake of sodium and cutoff value, and the adjusted factors were not consistent among included studies; (5) the meta-analysis used pooled data due to the unavailability of individual data, which restricted a detailed and relevant analysis in order to obtain comprehensive results.

Conclusions

In conclusion, the results of this study suggested that increased sodium intake might play a major role in the risk of stroke morbidity and mortality. However, the increased sodium intake did not have a significant effect on cardiac death and total mortality. Nevertheless, future studies focusing on specific populations for analyzing the secondary prevention of major cardiovascular outcomes are warranted.

Abbreviations

BMI: Body mass index; CHD: Coronary heart disease; CIs: Confidence intervals; CVD: Cardiovascular diseases; HR: Hazard ratio; NOS: Newcastle–Ottawa Scale; OR: Odds ratio; RR: Relative risk

Funding

This study was supported by the Beijing Natural Science Foundation (No. 7184204, No. 7182042), Beijing Municipal Health Bureau High-Level Talent Cultivation (Nos. 2014-3-043, 2015-3-048, and 2015-3-051), and Beijing Municipal Administration of Hospital Incubating Program (PX20166046).

Authors' contributions

YBZ1 (YZ) and JZ conducted the studies, participated in data collection, and drafted the manuscript. ZQL and YL performed the statistical analysis and participated in the experimental design. XF, YPZ, and YBZ2 (YZ) helped in drafting the manuscript. All authors read and approved the final manuscript.

Competing interests

The authors declare that they have no competing interests.

Author details

[1]Cardiovascular Surgery II, Beijing Children's Hospital, Capital Medical University, National Center for Children's Health, Beijing 100045, China. [2]Pediatric Heart Center, Beijing Anzhen Hospital, Capital Medical University, Beijing 100029, China. [3]The Heart Center, Beijing Friendship Hospital, Capital Medical University, Beijing 100050, China. [4]National Clinical Research Center of Cardiovascular Diseases, State Key Laboratory of Cardiovascular Disease, Fuwai Hospital, Chinese Academy of Medical Sciences and Peking Union Medical College, Beijing 100037, China.

References

1. Collaborators GMaCoD. Global, regional, and national age-sex specific all-cause and cause-specific mortality for 240 causes of death, 1990-2013: a systematic analysis for the global burden of disease study 2013. Lancet. 2015;385:117–71.
2. Wu L, Sun D. Consumption of yogurt and the incident risk of cardiovascular disease: a meta-analysis of nine cohort studies. Nutrients. 2017;9:3.
3. Fang X, Wang K, Han D, He X, Wei J, Zhao L, et al. Dietary magnesium intake and the risk of cardiovascular disease, type 2 diabetes, and all-cause mortality: a dose-response meta-analysis of prospective cohort studies. BMC Med. 2016;14:210.
4. Aune D, Keum N, Giovannucci E, Fadnes LT, Boffetta P, Greenwood DC, et al. Nut consumption and risk of cardiovascular disease, total cancer, all-cause and cause-specific mortality: a systematic review and dose-response meta-analysis of prospective studies. BMC Med. 2016;14:207.
5. Li B, Zhang G, Tan M, Zhao L, Jin L, Tang X, et al. Consumption of whole grains in relation to mortality from all causes, cardiovascular disease, and diabetes: dose-response meta-analysis of prospective cohort studies. Medicine (Baltimore). 2016;95:e4229.
6. Kim Y, Je Y. Dietary fibre intake and mortality from cardiovascular disease and all cancers: a meta-analysis of prospective cohort studies. Arch Cardiovasc Dis. 2016;109:39–54.
7. Larsson SC, Crippa A, Orsini N, Wolk A, Michaelsson K. Milk consumption and mortality from all causes, cardiovascular disease, and Cancer: a systematic review and meta-analysis. Nutrients. 2015;7:7749–63.
8. de Souza RJ, Mente A, Maroleanu A, Cozma AI, Ha V, Kishibe T, et al. Intake of saturated and trans unsaturated fatty acids and risk of all cause mortality, cardiovascular disease, and type 2 diabetes: systematic review and meta-analysis of observational studies. BMJ. 2015;351:h3978.
9. Group ICR. Intersalt: an international study of electrolyte excretion and blood pressure. Results for 24 hour urinary sodium and potassium excretion. Intersalt cooperative research group. BMJ. 1988;297:319–28.
10. Iso H, Stampfer MJ, Manson JE, Rexrode K, Hennekens CH, Colditz GA, et al. Prospective study of calcium, potassium, and magnesium intake and risk of stroke in women. Stroke. 1999;30:1772–9.
11. Whelton PK, Appel LJ, Espeland MA, Applegate WB, Ettinger WH Jr, Kostis JB, et al. Sodium reduction and weight loss in the treatment of hypertension in older persons: a randomized controlled trial of

nonpharmacologic interventions in the elderly (TONE). TONE collaborative research group. JAMA. 1998;279:839–46.

12. Group ToHPCR. Effects of weight loss and sodium reduction intervention on blood pressure and hypertension incidence in overweight people with high-normal blood pressure. The trials of hypertension prevention, phase II. The trials of hypertension prevention collaborative research group. Arch Intern Med. 1997;157:657–67.
13. He FJ, MacGregor GA. Effect of modest salt reduction on blood pressure: a meta-analysis of randomized trials. Implications for public health. J Hum Hypertens. 2002;16:761–70.
14. Umesawa M, Iso H, Date C, Yamamoto A, Toyoshima H, Watanabe Y, et al. Relations between dietary sodium and potassium intakes and mortality from cardiovascular disease: the Japan collaborative cohort study for evaluation of Cancer risks. Am J Clin Nutr. 2008;88:195–202.
15. Cook NR, Cutler JA, Obarzanek E, Buring JE, Rexrode KM, Kumanyika SK, et al. Long term effects of dietary sodium reduction on cardiovascular disease outcomes: observational follow-up of the trials of hypertension prevention (TOHP). BMJ. 2007;334:885–8.
16. Yang Q, Liu T, Kuklina EV, Flanders WD, Hong Y, Gillespie C, et al. Sodium and potassium intake and mortality among US adults: prospective data from the third National Health and nutrition examination survey. Arch Intern Med. 2011;171:1183–91.
17. Cohen HW, Hailpern SM, Fang J, Alderman MH. Sodium intake and mortality in the NHANES II follow-up study. Am J Med. 2006;119:275.e7–14.
18. Stolarz-Skrzypek K, Kuznetsova T, Thijs L, Tikhonoff V, Seidlerova J, Richart T, et al. Fatal and nonfatal outcomes, incidence of hypertension, and blood pressure changes in relation to urinary sodium excretion. JAMA. 2011;305:1777–85.
19. Moher D, Liberati A, Tetzlaff J, Altman DG, PRISMA group. Preferred Reporting Items for Systematic Reviews and Meta-Analyses: The PRISMA Statement. Plos Med. 2009;6:e1000097.
20. Wells GA, Shea B, O'Connell D. The Newcastle-Ottawa scale (NOS) for assessing the quality of nonrandomised studies in meta-analyses. Ottawa (ON): Ottawa hospital research institute; 2009. http://www.ohri.ca/programs/clinical_epidemiology/oxford.htm
21. DerSimonian R, Laird N. Meta-analysis in clinical trials. Control Clin Trials. 1986;7:177–88.
22. Ades AE, Lu G, Higgins JP. The interpretation of random-effects meta-analysis in decision models. Med Decis Mak. 2005;25:646–54.
23. Orsini N, Bellocco R. Generalized least squares for trend estimation of summarized dose-response data. Stata J. 2006;6:40–57.
24. Greenland S, Longnecker MP. Methods for trend estimation from summarized dose-response data, with applications to meta-analysis. Am J Epidemiol. 1992;135:1301–9.
25. Deeks JJ, Higgins JPT, Altman DG. Analyzing data and undertaking meta-analyses. In: Higgins J, Green S, editors. Cochrane Handbook for Systematic Reviews of Interventions 5.0.1., edn. Oxford: The Cochrane Collaboration; 2008.
26. Higgins JP, Thompson SG, Deeks JJ, Altman DG. Measuring inconsistency in meta-analyses. BMJ. 2003;327:557–60.
27. Deeks JJ, Altman DG, Bradburn MJ. Statistical methods for examining heterogeneity and combining results from several studies in meta-analysis. In: Egger M, Davey Smith G, Altman DG, editors. Systematic reviews in health care: Metaanalysis in context. 2nd ed. London: BMJ Books; 2001. p. 285–312.
28. Tobias A. Assessing the influence of a single study in meta-analysis. Stata Tech Bull. 1999;47:15–7.
29. Egger M, Davey Smith G, Schneider M, Minder C. Bias in meta-analysis detected by a simple, graphical test. BMJ. 1997;315:629–34.
30. Begg CB, Mazumdar M. Operating characteristics of a rank correlation test for publication bias. Biometrics. 1994;50:1088–101.
31. Alderman MH, Madhavan S, Cohen H, Sealey JE, Laragh JH. Low urinary sodium is associated with greater risk of myocardial infarction among treated hypertensive men. Hypertension. 1995;25:1144–52.
32. Tunstall-Pedoe H, Woodward M, Tavendale R, A'Brook R, McCluskey MK. Comparison of the prediction by 27 different factors of coronary heart disease and death in men and women of the Scottish heart health study: cohort study. BMJ. 1997;315:722–9.
33. He J, Ogden LG, Vupputuri S, Bazzano LA, Loria C, Whelton PK. Dietary sodium intake and subsequent risk of cardiovascular disease in overweight adults. JAMA. 1999;282:2027–34.
34. Tuomilehto J, Jousilahti P, Rastenyte D, Moltchanov V, Tanskanen A, Pietinen P, et al. Urinary sodium excretion and cardiovascular mortality in Finland: a prospective study. Lancet. 2001;357:848–51.
35. Nagata C, Takatsuka N, Shimizu N, Shimizu H. Sodium intake and risk of death from stroke in Japanese men and women. Stroke. 2004;35:1543–7.
36. Cohen HW, Hailpern SM, Alderman MH. Sodium intake and mortality follow-up in the third National Health and nutrition examination survey (NHANES III). J Gen Intern Med. 2008;23:1297–302.
37. Larsson SC, Virtanen MJ, Mars M, Mannisto S, Pietinen P, Albanes D, et al. Magnesium, calcium, potassium, and sodium intakes and risk of stroke in male smokers. Arch Intern Med. 2008;168:459–65.
38. Ekinci EI, Clarke S, Thomas MC, Moran JL, Cheong K, MacIsaac RJ, et al. Dietary salt intake and mortality in patients with type 2 diabetes. Diabetes Care. 2011;34:703–9.
39. O'Donnell MJ, Yusuf S, Mente A, Gao P, Mann JF, Teo K, et al. Urinary sodium and potassium excretion and risk of cardiovascular events. JAMA. 2011;306:2229–38.
40. Gardener H, Rundek T, Wright CB, Elkind MS, Sacco RL. Dietary sodium and risk of stroke in the northern Manhattan study. Stroke. 2012;43:1200–5.
41. Mills KT, Chen J, Yang W, Appel LJ, Kusek JW, Alper A, et al. Sodium excretion and the risk of cardiovascular disease in patients with chronic kidney disease. JAMA. 2016;315:2200–10.
42. Kalogeropoulos AP, Georgiopoulou VV, Murphy RA, Newman AB, Bauer DC, Harris TB, et al. Dietary sodium content, mortality, and risk for cardiovascular events in older adults: the health, aging, and body composition (health ABC) study. JAMA Intern Med. 2015;175:410–9.
43. Horikawa C, Yoshimura Y, Kamada C, Tanaka S, Tanaka S, Hanyu O, et al. Dietary sodium intake and incidence of diabetes complications in Japanese patients with type 2 diabetes: analysis of the Japan diabetes complications study (JDCS). J Clin Endocrinol Metab. 2014;99:3635–43.
44. Strazzullo P, D' Elia L, Kandala N. Salt intake, stroke, and cardiovascular disease: metaanalysis of prospective studies. BMJ. 2009;339:b4567.
45. Taylor RS, Ashton KE, Moxham T, Hooper L, Ebrahim S. Reduced dietary salt for the prevention of cardiovascular disease: a meta-analysis of randomized controlled trials (Cochrane review). Am J Hypertens. 2011;24:843–53.
46. Taylor RS, Ashton KE, Moxham T, Hooper L, Ebrahim S. Reduced dietary salt for the prevention of cardiovascular disease. Cochrane Database Syst Rev. 2011;12:Cd009217.
47. Bussemaker E, Hillebrand U, Hausberg M, Pavenstadt H, Oberleithner H. Pathogenesis of hypertension: interactions among sodium, potassium, and aldosterone. Am J Kidney Dis. 2010;55:1111–20.

Permissions

All chapters in this book were first published in CD, by BioMed Central; hereby published with permission under the Creative Commons Attribution License or equivalent. Every chapter published in this book has been scrutinized by our experts. Their significance has been extensively debated. The topics covered herein carry significant findings which will fuel the growth of the discipline. They may even be implemented as practical applications or may be referred to as a beginning point for another development.

The contributors of this book come from diverse backgrounds, making this book a truly international effort. This book will bring forth new frontiers with its revolutionizing research information and detailed analysis of the nascent developments around the world.

We would like to thank all the contributing authors for lending their expertise to make the book truly unique. They have played a crucial role in the development of this book. Without their invaluable contributions this book wouldn't have been possible. They have made vital efforts to compile up to date information on the varied aspects of this subject to make this book a valuable addition to the collection of many professionals and students.

This book was conceptualized with the vision of imparting up-to-date information and advanced data in this field. To ensure the same, a matchless editorial board was set up. Every individual on the board went through rigorous rounds of assessment to prove their worth. After which they invested a large part of their time researching and compiling the most relevant data for our readers.

The editorial board has been involved in producing this book since its inception. They have spent rigorous hours researching and exploring the diverse topics which have resulted in the successful publishing of this book. They have passed on their knowledge of decades through this book. To expedite this challenging task, the publisher supported the team at every step. A small team of assistant editors was also appointed to further simplify the editing procedure and attain best results for the readers.

Apart from the editorial board, the designing team has also invested a significant amount of their time in understanding the subject and creating the most relevant covers. They scrutinized every image to scout for the most suitable representation of the subject and create an appropriate cover for the book.

The publishing team has been an ardent support to the editorial, designing and production team. Their endless efforts to recruit the best for this project, has resulted in the accomplishment of this book. They are a veteran in the field of academics and their pool of knowledge is as vast as their experience in printing. Their expertise and guidance has proved useful at every step. Their uncompromising quality standards have made this book an exceptional effort. Their encouragement from time to time has been an inspiration for everyone.

The publisher and the editorial board hope that this book will prove to be a valuable piece of knowledge for researchers, students, practitioners and scholars across the globe.

List of Contributors

Stephen Jan
The George Institute for Global Health, Sydney Medical School, University of Sydney, King George V Building, 83–117 Missenden Rd, Camperdown, NSW 2050, Australia

Stephen W-L. Lee
Queen Mary Hospital, Hong Kong, SAR, China

Jitendra P. S. Sawhney
Sir Ganga Ram Hospital, New Delhi, India

Tiong K. Ong
Sarawak General Hospital, Kuching, Malaysia

Chee Tang Chin
National Heart Centre Singapore, Singapore, Singapore

Hyo-Soo Kim
Seoul National University Hospital, Seoul, South Korea

Rungroj Krittayaphong
Siriraj Hospital, Bangkok, Thailand

Vo T. Nhan
Cho Ray Hospital, Ho Chi Minh City, Vietnam

Stuart J. Pocock
London School of Hygiene and Tropical Medicine, London, UK

Ana M. Vega
Observational Research Centre, Global Medical Affairs, AstraZeneca, Madrid, Spain

Nobuya Hayashi
AstraZeneca, Osaka, Japan

Yong Huo
Peking University First Hospital, Beijing, China

Ping Zhu, Xin Zhou, Chenliang Zhang, Huakang Li, Zhihui Zhang and Zhiyuan Song
Department of Cardiology, Southwest Hospital, Third Military Medical University (Army Medical University), Chongqing, China

Shuo Yang, Li Sheng Zhao, Chuan Cai, Quan Shi, Ning Wen and Juan Xu
Department of Stomatology, Chinese People's Liberation Army General Hospital, 28 Fuxing Road, Beijing 100853, China

Nkengla Menka Adidja
Faculty of Health Sciences, University of Buea, Buea, Cameroon
Djeleng Sub-divisional Hospital, Bafoussam, Cameroon

Valirie Ndip Agbor
Ibal Sub-divisional Hospital, Oku, Cameroon
Faculty of Medicine and Biomedical Sciences, University of Yaoundé 1, Yaoundé, Cameroon

Jeannine A. Aminde
Faculty of Health Sciences, University of Buea, Buea, Cameroon
Etoug-Ebe Baptist Hospital, Yaoundé, Cameroon

Calypse A. Ngwasiri
Bamendjou District Hospital, Bamendjou, Cameroon
Clinical Research Education, Networking and Consultancy (CRENC), Douala, Cameroon

Leopold Ndemnge Aminde
Faculty of Medicine, School of Public Health, The University of Queensland, Brisbane, Australia

Kathleen Blackett Ngu
Faculty of Medicine and Biomedical Sciences, University of Yaoundé 1, Yaoundé, Cameroon

John Munkhaugen
Department of Medicine, Drammen Hospital, Vestre Viken Health Trust, Dronninggata 41, 3004 Drammen, Norway
Department of Behavioural Sciences in Medicine and Faculty of Medicine, University of Oslo, Oslo, Norway

Jøran Hjelmesæth
Morbid Obesity Centre, Vestfold Hospital Trust, Tønsberg, Norway

Department of Endocrinology, Morbid Obesity and Preventive Medicine, Institute of Clinical Medicine, University of Oslo, Oslo, Norway

Jan Erik Otterstad
Department of Medicine, Vestfold Hospital Trust, Tønsberg, Norway

Ragnhild Helseth
Centre for Clinical Heart Research, Department of Cardiology, Oslo University Hospital Ullevål, Oslo, Norway
Faculty of Medicine, University of Oslo, Oslo, Norway

Stina Therese Sollid, Erik Gjertsen and Einar Husebye
Department of Medicine, Drammen Hospital Trust, Drammen, Norway

Lars Gullestad
Department of Cardiology, Oslo University Hospital Rikshospitalet, Oslo, Norway
Faculty of Medicine, University of Oslo, Oslo, Norway

Joep Perk
Linneus University, Kalmar, Sweden

Torbjørn Moum and Toril Dammen
Department of Behavioural Sciences in Medicine and Faculty of Medicine, University of Oslo, Oslo, Norway

Ehsan Razmara
1Department of Medical Genetics, Faculty of Medical Sciences, Tarbiat Modares University, Tehran, Iran

Masoud Garshasbi
Department of Medical Genetics, Faculty of Medical Sciences, Tarbiat Modares University, Tehran, Iran
Department of Medical Genetics, DeNA laboratory, Tehran, Iran

Yintao Chen, Xiaofan Guo, Guozhe Sun, Zhao Li and Yingxian Sun
Department of Cardiology, The First Hospital of China Medical University, Shenyang 110001, People's Republic of China

Liqiang Zheng
Department of Clinical Epidemiology, Library, Shengjing Hospital of China Medical University, Shenyang, Liaoning, China

Fan Wang, Mengyun Zhu, Xiaoyu Wang, Wei Zhang, Yang Su, Yuyan Lu, Xin Pan, Di Gao, Xianling Zhang, Wei Chen, Yawei Xu, Yuxi Sun and Dachun Xu
Department of Cardiology, Shanghai Tenth People's Hospital, Tongji University School of Medicine, NO. 301 Middle Yanchang Road, Shanghai 200072, China

Halldora Ögmundsdottir Michelsen, Ingela Sjölin, Alexandru Schiopu and Margret Leosdottir
Department of Coronary Disease, Skåne University Hospital, Inga Marie Nilsson gata 47, Malmö, Sweden
Department of Clinical Sciences Malmö, Faculty of Medicine, Lund University, Box 117, SE-221 00 Lund, Sweden

Marie Nilsson and Fredrik Scherstén
Department of Coronary Disease, Skåne University Hospital, Inga Marie Nilsson gata 47, Malmö, Sweden

I. Wozniak-Skowerska, A. Hoffmann, S. Nowak, A. M. Wnuk-Wojnar and K. Mizia-Stec
First Department of Cardiology, School of Medicine in Katowice, Medical University of Silesia, Katowice, Poland

M. Skowerski and T. Skowerski
Department of Cardiology, School of Health Sciences, Medical University of Silesia, Katowice, Poland

M. Sosnowski
Unit of Noninvasive Cardiovascular Diagnostics, Medical University of Silesia, Katowice, Poland

Claudius Hansen
Herz- und Gefäßzentrum am Krankenhaus Neu-Bethlehem, Humboldtallee 6, 37073 Göttingen, Germany

Christian Loges
SLK-Kliniken Heilbronn Klinikum am Plattenwald, Bad Friedrichshall, Germany

Karlheinz Seidl
Klinikum Ingolstadt, Ingolstadt, Germany

Frank Eberhardt
Evangelisches Krankenhaus Kalk, Köln, Germany

Herbert Tröster
Marienhospital Stuttgart, Stuttgart, Germany

Krum Petrov
Kreiskliniken Böblingen Standort Sindelfingen, Sindelfingen, Germany

Gerian Grönefeld
Asklepios Klinik Barmbek, Hamburg, Germany

Peter Bramlage
Institut für Pharmakologie und Präventive Medizin, Cloppenburg, Germany

Frank Birkenhauer
Abbott - St. Jude Medical GmbH, Eschborn, Germany

Christian Weiss
Städtisches Klinikum Lüneburg gGmbH, Lüneburg, Germany

Christine K. Kissel
Department of Cardiac Sciences and Libin Cardiovascular Institute of Alberta, Cumming School of Medicine, University of Calgary, Calgary, AB, Canada
Department of Cardiology, University Heart Center, University Hospital Zurich, Rämistrasse 100, CH-8091 Zürich, Switzerland

P. Diane Galbraith and Todd J. Anderson
Department of Cardiac Sciences and Libin Cardiovascular Institute of Alberta, Cumming School of Medicine, University of Calgary, Calgary, AB, Canada

Guanmin Chen and Danielle A. Southern
O'Brien Institute of Public Health, Cumming School of Medicine, University of Calgary, Calgary, AB, Canada
Department of Community Health Sciences, Cumming School of Medicine, University of Calgary, Calgary, Canada

Boonsub Sakboonyarat and Ram Rangsin
Department of Military and Community Medicine, Phramongkutklao College of Medicine, Bangkok 10400, Thailand

Jing Li, Ying Zhou and Jingang Zheng
Department of Cardiology, China-Japan Friendship Hospital, No. 2, Yinghua Road, Beijing 100029, China

Yaowen Zhang
Medieco Group Co. Ltd, B901 Building No.20 Hepingxiyuan, Beijing 100029, China

Christian Fastner, Michael Behnes, Siegfried Lang, Martin Borggrefe and Ibrahim Akin
First Department of Medicine, University Medical Centre Mannheim (UMM), Faculty of Medicine Mannheim, University of Heidelberg, European Centre for AngioScience (ECAS), and DZHK (German Centre for Cardiovascular Research) partner site Heidelberg/Mannheim, Theodor-Kutzer-Ufer 1-3, 68167 Mannheim, Germany

Lea Hoffmann and Mohamed Aboukoura
Department of Cardiology, University Hospital Rostock, Rostock, Germany

Christoph A. Nienaber
Royal Brompton Hospital, London, United Kingdom and National Heart and Lung Institute, Imperial College London, London, UK

Wanyu Wang, Yonghong Shi, Yihua Lin and Wen Luo
Pneumology Department of the First Affiliated Hospital of XiaMen University, The first clinical medical college of Fujian Medical University Teaching hospital of Fujian Medical University, Xiamen, China

Ailing Song
Pneumology Department of Wuxi Branch of Rijin Hospital affiliated to Shanghai jiaotong university medical college, Wuxi, China

Yiming Zeng, Xiaoyang Chen and Yixiang Zhang
Department of Pulmonary and Critical Care Medicine of the Second Affiliated Hospital of Fujian Medical University, Sleep and Breathing Disorders Research Institute of Fujian Medical University, No.34 Zhongshan North Road, Licheng District, Quanzhou 362000, Fujian, China

Tongtong Yu, Chunyang Tian, Jia Song, Dongxu He, Jiake Wu, Zongyu Wen, Zhijun Sun and Zhaoqing Sun
Department of Cardiology, Shengjing Hospital of China Medical University, Shenyang, Liaoning, People's Republic of China

Zhi-jie Zheng
School of Public Health, Shanghai Jiaotong University School of Medicine, South Chongqing Road No, Shanghai 227, China

Oumin Shi
School of Public Health, Shanghai Jiaotong University School of Medicine, South Chongqing Road No, Shanghai 227, China
Institute for Clinical Evaluative Sciences, G1 06, 2075 Bayview Avenue, Toronto, ON, Canada

Anam M. Khan and Mohammad R. Rezai
Institute for Clinical Evaluative Sciences, G1 06, 2075 Bayview Avenue, Toronto, ON, Canada

Cynthia A. Jackevicius
Institute for Clinical Evaluative Sciences, G1 06, 2075 Bayview Avenue, Toronto, ON, Canada
Western University of Health Sciences, 309 E 2nd St, Pomona, California, USA
University of Toronto, 27 King's College Circle, Toronto, ON, Canada

Madhu K. Natarajan
Department of Medicine, Hamilton Health Sciences, McMaster University, 1200 Main St W, Hamilton, ON, Canada

Clare L. Atzema
Institute for Clinical Evaluative Sciences, G1 06, 2075 Bayview Avenue, Toronto, ON, Canada
Sunnybrook Health Sciences Centre, 2075 Bayview Avenue, Toronto, ON, Canada

Jafna Cox
Dalhousie University, 6299 South St, Halifax, NS, Canada

Laurie J. Lambert
Cardiology Evaluation Unit, Institut national d'excellence en santé et en services sociaux (INESSS), 2021, Avenue Union, Bureau 10.083, Montréal,Québec, Canada

Dennis T. Ko and Jack V. Tu
Institute for Clinical Evaluative Sciences, G1 06, 2075 Bayview Avenue, Toronto, ON, Canada
Schulich Heart Centre, Sunnybrook Health Sciences Centre, 2075 Bayview Avenue, Toronto, ON, Canada
University of Toronto, 27 King's College Circle, Toronto, ON, Canada

Thérèse A. Stukel
Institute for Clinical Evaluative Sciences, G1 06, 2075 Bayview Avenue, Toronto, ON, Canada
University of Toronto, 27 King's College Circle, Toronto, ON, Canada

Zhonghai Wei, Jian Bai, Qing Dai, Han Wu, Shuaihua Qiao, Biao Xu and Lian Wang
Department of Cardiology, Drum Tower Hospital, Medical School of Nanjing University, 321 Zhongshan Road, Nanjing 210008, Jiangsu Province, China

Tan Li, Hai-yang Sun and Jun Yang
Department of Cardiovascular Ultrasound, the First Hospital of China Medical University, No.155 Nanjing Bei Street, Heping District, Shenyang 110001, China

Bo Jiang, Xuan Li and Xin-tong Li
Department of Vascular and Thyroid Surgery, the First Hospital of China Medical University, Shenyang 110001, China

Jing-jing Jing
Tumor Etiology and Screening Department of Cancer Institute and General Surgery, the First Hospital of China Medical University, Shenyang 110001, China

Alina S. Kerimkulova, Olga S. Lunegova, Saamay S. Abilova, Malik P. Nabiev, Ksenia V. Neronova, Erkaiym E. Bektasheva, Ulan M. Toktomamatov and Jyldyz E. Esenbekova
Kyrgyz State Medical Academy named after I.K. Akhunbaev, T.Moldo street 3, Bishkek 720040, Kyrgyz Republic

Aibek E. Mirrakhimov
Kyrgyz Society of Cardiology, Bishkek, Kyrgyz Republic

Erkin M. Mirrakhimov
Kyrgyz State Medical Academy named after I.K. Akhunbaev, T.Moldo street 3, Bishkek 720040, Kyrgyz Republic
National Center of Cardiology and Internal Medicine named after academician M.M. Mirrakhimov, Bishkek, Kyrgyz Republic

Irena Kasacka and Żaneta Piotrowska
Department of Histology and Cytophysiology, Medical University of Bialystok, Mickiewicza 2C street, 15-222 Białystok, Poland

Anna Filipek
Nencki Institute of Experimental Biology, Laboratory of Calcium Binding Proteins, Ludwika Pasteura 3 street, 02-093 Warszawa, Poland

Wojciech Lebkowski
Department of Neurosurgery, Medical University of Bialystok, Marii Skłodowskiej-Curie 24A street, 15-276 Białystok, Poland

Nele Laleman, Geert Goderis and Gijs Van Pottelbergh
Department of Public Health and Primary Care, Universiteit Leuven (KU Leuven), Kapucijnenvoer 33, Blok J, 3000 Leuven, Belgium

Séverine Henrard and Bert Vaes
Department of Public Health and Primary Care, Universiteit Leuven (KU Leuven), Kapucijnenvoer 33, Blok J, 3000 Leuven, Belgium
Institute of Health and Society, Université catholique de Louvain (UCL), Brussels, Belgium

Marjan van den Akker and Frank Buntinx
Department of Public Health and Primary Care, Universiteit Leuven (KU Leuven), Kapucijnenvoer 33, Blok J, 3000 Leuven, Belgium
Department of Family Medicine, Maastricht University, Maastricht, The Netherlands

Anne Jokilammi
Institute of Biomedicine, University of Turku, Kiinamyllynkatu 10, FIN-20520 Turku, Finland

Deepankar Chakroborty
Institute of Biomedicine, University of Turku, Kiinamyllynkatu 10, FIN-20520 Turku, Finland
Turku Doctoral Programme of Molecular Medicine, University of Turku, Turku, Finland

Juho Heliste
Institute of Biomedicine, University of Turku, Kiinamyllynkatu 10, FIN-20520 Turku, Finland
Turku Doctoral Programme of Molecular Medicine, University of Turku, Turku, Finland
Institute for Molecular Medicine Finland, University of Helsinki, Helsinki, Finland

Ilkka Paatero
Institute of Biomedicine, University of Turku, Kiinamyllynkatu 10, FIN-20520 Turku, Finland
Turku Centre for Biotechnology, University of Turku and Åbo Akademi University, Turku, Finland

Christoffer Stark and Timo Savunen
Research Center of Applied and Preventive Cardiovascular Medicine, University of Turku, Turku, Finland

Maria Laaksonen
Medisapiens Ltd., Helsinki, Finland

Klaus Elenius
Institute of Biomedicine, University of Turku, Kiinamyllynkatu 10, FIN-20520 Turku, Finland
Medicity Research Laboratories, University of Turku, Turku, Finland
Department of Oncology, Turku University Hospital, Turku, Finland

José González-Costello, Josep Comín-Colet, Lara Fuentes and Nicolás Manito
Area de Enfermedades del Corazón, Hospital Universitari de Bellvitge, IDIBELL, Universitat de Barcelona, L'Hospitalet de Llobregat, Feixa Llarga SN, 08907 Barcelona, Spain

Cristina Enjuanes, Pedro Moliner-Borja and Nuria Farré
Servicio de Cardiología, Hospital del Mar, IMIM, Universitat Autònoma de Barcelona, Barcelona, Spain.

Josep Lupón, Marta de Antonio, Antoni Bayés-Genis and Elisabet Zamora
Unidad de Insuficiencia Cardíaca, Hospital Universitari Germans Trias i Pujol, Universitat Autònoma de Barcelona, Badalona, Barcelona, Spain

Ramón Pujol
Servicio de Medicina Interna, Hospital Universitari de Bellvitge, IDIBELL, University of Barcelona, L'Hospitalet de Llobregat, Barcelona, Spain

Wenzhi Zhao, Jian Zhang, Ai Zhao, Meichen Wang, Wei Wu, Shengjie Tan, Mofan Guo and Yumei Zhang
Department of Nutrition and Food Hygiene, School of Public Health, Peking University Health Science Center, Xueyuan Road 38, Haidian District, 100191 Beijing, China

Jian Song, Xue Chen, Jing Mi, Xuesen Wu and Huaiquan Gao
School of public health, Bengbu medical college, 2600 Donghai Road, Bengbu 233000, Anhui Province, China

Yingying Zhao
Bengbu health board, 568 Nanhu Road, Bengbu 233000, Anhui Province, China

Julian W. E. Jarman, Wajid Hussain, Tom Wong and Vias Markides
Heart Rhythm Centre, NIHR Cardiovascular Research Unit, The Royal Brompton Hospital, and National Heart and Lung Institute, Imperial College, London, UK

Jamie March and Laura Goldstein
Franchise Health Economics and Market Access, Johnson and Johnson, Irvine, CA, USA.

Ray Liao
Janssen R&D US, Raritan, NJ, USA

Iftekhar Kalsekar, Abhishek Chitnis and Rahul Khanna
Medical Device Epidemiology, Johnson and Johnson, 410 George Street, New Brunswick, NJ 08901, USA

Yaobin Zhu and Zhiqiang Li
Cardiovascular Surgery II, Beijing Children's Hospital, Capital Medical University, National Center for Children's Health, Beijing 100045, China

Jing Zhang, Yang Liu and Xing Fan
Pediatric Heart Center, Beijing Anzhen Hospital, Capital Medical University, Beijing 100029, China

Yaping Zhang
The Heart Center, Beijing Friendship Hospital, Capital Medical University, Beijing 100050, China

Yanbo Zhang
National Clinical Research Center of Cardiovascular Diseases, State Key Laboratory of Cardiovascular Disease, Fuwai Hospital, Chinese Academy of Medical Sciences and Peking Union Medical College, Beijing 100037, China

Index